Delmar's Dental Assisting

A COMPREHENSIVE APPROACH

Donna J. Phinney, CDA, BA, MEd
Spokane Community College

Judy H. Halstead, CDA, BA
Spokane Community College

Africa • Australia • Canada • Denmark • Japan • Mexico • New Zealand • Philippines
Puerto Rico • Singapore • Spain • United Kingdom • United States

NOTICE TO THE READER

Delmar Staff:
Business Unit Director: William Brottmiller
Executive Editor: Cathy L. Esperti
Acquisitions Editor: Marlene McHugh Pratt
Developmental Editor: Melissa Riveglia
Editorial Assistant: Maria Perretta
Executive Marketing Manager: Dawn Gerrain
Project Editor: Bill Trudell
Production Coordinator: Linda Helfrich
Art/Design Coordinator: Richard Killar
Cover Design: Charles Cummings Advertising/Art Inc.

COPYRIGHT © 2000
Delmar is a division of Thomson Learning. The Thomson Learning logo is a registered trademark used herein under license.

Printed in the United States of America
5 6 7 8 9 10 XXX 04 03 02 01

For more information, contact Delmar, 3 Columbia Circle, PO Box 15015, Albany, NY 12212-0515; or find us on the World Wide Web at http://www.delmar.com

Library of Congress Cataloging-in-Publication Data

Phinney, Donna.

Delmar's introduction to dental assisting / by Donna Phinney and Judy Halstead.
p. cm.
Includes bibliographical references and index.
ISBN 0-8273-9073-4
1. Dental assistants. 2. Dentistry. I. Halstead, Judy. II. Title.
III. Title: Introduction to dental assisting
RK60.5 .P48 1999
617.6'0233—dc21   98-55682
                                    CIP

CONTENTS

PREFACE

INTRODUCTION

The world of health care has changed rapidly over the past few years. As we enter the 21st century, health care professionals will encounter more challenges than ever before. But with challenge comes opportunity. Job prospects for dental assistants have never been better. The Bureau of Labor Statistics expects employment to grow much faster than average for all occupations through the year 2006. Population growth and greater retention of natural teeth will fuel demands for dental services. As the health care industry requires more work to be done by dentists, the dental assistant will be more valuable and needed than ever before.

As dental assistants, you'll be expected to take on an increasing number of clinical and administrative responsibilities to stay competitive. Now is the time to equip yourselves with the range of skills and competencies you'll need to excel in the field. Now is the time to maximize your potential, to expand your base of knowledge, and to dedicate yourself to becoming the multifaceted dental assistant required in the 21st century.

As a dental assisting student, Delmar's new text and complete learning system, *Delmar's Dental Assisting: A Comprehensive Approach,* will guide you on this journey. The result of years of research, writing, and testing, this system is designed to prepare the dental assisting student for Dental Assisting National Board (DANB) certification. It presents information in a unique manner, using a variety of formats that account for the many ways in which today's students learn.

To receive the full value of *Delmar's Dental Assisting: A Comprehensive Approach,* it's important to understand the structure of the text, chapters, and supplements, and how they're all integrated into a complete learning system. Together, these materials will make your dental assisting education comprehensive and meaningful, providing you with the skills, knowledge, principles, values, and understanding to excel in your chosen profession into the 21st century!

THE LEARNING SYSTEM

The components of the learning system were developed with today's learner in mind. The authors and Delmar Publishers recognize that students learn in different ways—they read, write, listen, watch, interact, and practice. For this reason, we've created a variety of products learners can use to fully comprehend and retain what they're taught. An instructor's manual ties the components together, making classroom integration easy and fun.

- **The Text (Donna J. Phinney, CDA, BA, MEd and Judy H. Halstead, CDA, BA)**
  Comprehensive coverage, supported by more than 1,500 full-color illustrations and photographs, and 141 step-by-step procedures, of dental assisting theory and practice, in 8 sections. Section I—*Introduction*—introduces learners to the profession and its history. Section II—*Basic Dental Sciences*—covers the basics of dental anatomy, embryology, histology, tooth morphology, charting, and microbiology, creating a foundation on which learners can move forward to skills training. Section III—*Preclinical Dental Skills*—prepares students in the areas of infection control, hazardous materials management, patient care, pharmacology, and emergency management, critical elements to the profession. Section IV—*Clinical Dental Procedures*—covers chairside assisting, instruments, management of pain and anxiety, and dental radiography. Section V—*Dental Specialties*—introduces learners to the specialized areas of endodontics, oral maxillofacial surgery, oral pathology, orthodontics, pediatric dentistry, periodontics, fixed prosthodontics, and removable prosthodontics. Section VI—*Restorative and Laboratory Materials and Techniques*—covers chairside restorative materials and techniques, and laboratory and impression materials and techniques. Section VII—*Expanded Functions*—introduces advanced techniques, such as dental dam placement, coronal polish, and retraction cord placement, that can be performed in various states' practices. Section VIII—*Dental Practice Management*—contains chapters on dental office management, dental computer software, dental insurance, employment portfolios, and legal and ethical considerations, important components for managing a dental practice properly.

  Each textbook comes with **free practice software,** bound in the back. The disk contains over 1,500 exercises, utilizing a variety of formats—multiple choice, short answer, true/false, matching, and concentration—to further reinforce content.

HANDWASHING

GLOVES

**MASK AND
PROTECTIVE EYEWEAR**

BASIC SETUP

EF

**EXPANDED
FUNCTIONS**

LEGAL

SAFETY

SAFETY

TECH

TECHNOLOGY

**GLOBAL/CULTURAL
ISSUES**

CDA

**DANB EXAM
COMPONENT**

"How to Use the Text" and "How to Use the Software" sections guide instructors and students through the text and software program, enabling teaching and learning in the best way possible. Appendices and a comprehensive glossary and index are also included.

Chapters include the following pedagogical features:

- chapter outline
- objectives
- key terms with page references (key terms also appear in color in the text)
- pronounciation of difficult terms the first time they appear in the text
- introduction
- step-by-step procedures with icons indicating handwashing, gloves, mask and protective eyewear, basic set-up, and expanded functions
- in-text icons identifying legal, safety, technology, global/cultural issues, and DANB exam components
- boxed information containing tips and summaries
- summary
- case studies
- review questions, including critical thinking

- ## Student Workbook (Karen Waide, CDA, EFDA, AAS)
  The workbook, which corresponds to the text, contains chapter objectives, summaries, key terms, exercises in a variety of formats, skill sheets to test competencies, and critical thinking scenarios/case studies.

- ## Exam Review (Melissa Thibodeaux, CDA, RDA, BS)
  The exam review provides a review and practice for the DANB exam. 500 questions, rationale, and a practice test prepare students for certification.

- ## Dental Drug Reference (Elena Bablenis Haveles, PharmD)
  Over 300 drugs are reviewed in detail, including their dental concerns. Also introduced are sections on drug classification, drug interactions of specific concern to dental health professionals, client/family teaching, antibiotic prophylaxis for bacterial endocarditis, and elements of a prescription and prescription writing.

- ## Dental Terminology (Charline Dofka)
  This book of common dental terms utilizes "sounds like" pronounciations for over 1,300 terms used in the dental practice. Terms are grouped by specialty, and are supported by review exercises, illustrations, and an appendix on word elements. A 60-minute audiotape provides actual pronounciations to help learners master the vocabulary.

- ## Dental Office Management (Ellen Dietz, CDA, AAS, BS)
  This comprehensive book takes readers through the various tasks associated with front-office dental procedures, preparing them for the office of the 21st century. Five sections—*the business of dentistry, practice communications, clinical records management, business and financial records management,* and *employment opportunities*—are supported by learning objectives, key terms, and key concepts. Skill-building for Success Student Activities (role-plays and problem-solving activities) and Skills Mastery Assessments Post-tests are provided at the end of the chapter.

- ## Instructor's Manual
  The Instructor's Manual ties the learning system together, providing the traditional components of course objectives, lesson plans, answers to text/workbook questions, and transition guides. In addition, a "How To" section explains the learning system and its rationale, and provides cross references to components, integrating them into the appropriate text chapters to ensure that students get maximum benefits from using the system.

- ## Computerized Test Bank (Deborah McGrath, CDA, BS)
  A 1,500 question text bank provides instructors with questions geared to text chapters and the DANB exam.

- **Transparencies**

  50 four-color transparencies support text concepts.

- **Image Library**

  Over 1,500 illustrations from the text are contained on a single CD, which can be used to provide visual support in the classroom via the computer or as transparencies. It can also be modified with your own teaching materials, customized to your course needs.

- **Dental Assisting Video Series**

  A series containing 5 individual tapes: 1) *Introduction to Chairside Assisting;* 2) *Dental Radiography;* 3) *Infection Control Techniques;* 4) *Restorative Dental Materials;* and 5) *Laboratory Impressions, Materials & Techniques.*

When you use all these components together, you'll discover an innovative, comprehensive system of teaching and learning that prepares students for success in the 21st century.

ABOUT THE AUTHORS

Donna J. Phinney is the chair for Spokane Community College's Allied Health department and the Program Director for the Dental Assisting Program. She has spent more than 20 years in the dental field as a dental assistant, dental office consultant, office manager, and educator. Donna holds a bachelor of arts from Eastern Washington University, a masters in education from Whitworth College, and an Associate of Science and certificate in dental assisting from Spokane Community College. A Certified Dental Assistant, she is active in the Washington State Dental Assisting Association, where she served as president from 1992–1993.

Judy H. Halstead is a dental assisting instructor at Spokane Community College. She has more than 20 years' experience teaching, and more than 10 years' experience as a dental assistant. She was a Program Director for dental assisting in a private college and for a high school skills center. Judy holds a bachelor of arts from Eastern Washington University, is a Certified Dental Assistant, and has an Expanded Functions Certificate. She has been a member of local, state, and national Dental Assistants Associations for the past 25 years. She served as president of the Washington State Dental Assisting Association from 1994–1995.

ACKNOWLEDGMENTS

The authors would like to thank Delmar Publishers and staff whose assistance and encouragement in this pursuit are greatly appreciated, especially Melissa Riveglia, Developmental Editor, whose weekly and sometimes daily phone calls encouraged and aided us in completing this text. We would also like to thank Rich Killar, Art and Design Coordinator; Marlene Pratt, Acquisitions Editor; William Trudell, Project Editor; Stratford Publishing Services; and the many others who worked so diligently to bring this text to reality.

We would also like to thank the many dentists that we have had the opportunity to work with and who made dental assisting a career to be proud of.

We would like to thank our peers across the nation and especially the Allied Health Department and staff and friends at Spokane Community College who continued to encourage us throughout this endeavor. The students, who in the end make everything worthwhile, are to be thanked for their desire to learn and the ongoing challenge they present to their instructors.

Last but never least, we would like to thank our husbands, Dwayne and Chuck, and our families who gave us ongoing support and encouragement throughout this project. Their understanding, patience, and love allowed us to stay on track and complete the task at hand. Thank you!

We also want to thank the following individuals and facilities for providing valuable assistance in the development and production of this project:

- Pat Norman, CDA, who continues to give so much; we appreciate all her help in obtaining the figures for the text and the many other areas where she picked up the slack for us.
- Julie Davitt, CDA, who supported and encouraged us throughout this project.

- Peg Jacobs Bloy, CDA, RDH, MS and Middlesex Community College for the coordination and assistance while allowing us to photograph in their facility.
- Rita Johnson, CDA, COA, RDH, MA and Dr. Vincent DeAngelis, who provided assistance, and many pictures for the text.
- Dr. Clifton Caldwell, who continues to help us with our endeavors both in student education and now publishing.
- Dr. Dale Ruemping, Dr. Steven Crump, Dr. Ola England, Dr. George Velis, Dr. Gary Shellerud, Dr. Dwight Damond, Dr. Earl Ness, Drs. Rodney Braun and Chris Chaffin, and Dr. Steven Gregg, who continue to help us with student education and provided prictures for the text.
- The reviewers who spent their time and energy to make this a better text.
- Anderson's dental laboratory, for continuing to help us with student education and providing pictures and models for the text.
- Dr. Joseph Konzelman, who provided many pictures for the text.
- Mark Rea, our photographer, for his artistic touches and easy-to-get-along-with attitude over long days of shooting, to produce the high-quality photographs used in this textbook.

REVIEWERS

Peg Jacobs Bloy, CDA, RDH, MS
Middlesex Community College
Lowell, Massachusetts

Lori Burch, RDA
Corinthian College
Reseda, California

Robin Caplan, CDA, EFDA, DRT
Medix School
Owings Mills, Maryland

Sheila Cooper, CDA
Mission Trails Regional Occupations
Salinas, California

Ellen Dietz, CDA, AAS, BS
Mesa, Arizona

Ellen DiGiacomo, CDA, MEd
Dynamic Dental Seminars
& Consulting Services
Concord, Massachusetts

Tammy Erickson, CDA, RDA
Lakeland Academy
Minneapolis, Minnesota

Thomas French, PhD
University of Health Sciences Center
Denver, Colorado

Linda Kay Hughes, RDA, NRDA
Excelle Medical and Dental College
San Diego, California

Darlene Hunziker, CDA, RDA
Eton Technical Institute
Everett, Washington

Jill Jaroski-Graf, RDH, MS, DABFE
Mount Senario College
Ladysmith, Wisconsin

Rita Johnson, CDA, COA, RDH, MA
Dynamic Dental Seminars
& Consulting Services
Concord, Massachusetts

Sharon LeMaster, PhD
Gwinett Technical Institute
Lawrenceville, Georgia

Stella Lovato, CDA, MA, MSHP
San Antonio College
San Antonio, Texas

Deborah McGrath, CDA, BS
Fayetteville Technical Community
College
Fayetteville, North Carolina

Debbie Reynon, CDA, RDA, AA, AS
Monterey Peninsula College
Monterey, California

Fred Rich
Gwinett School of Dental Assisting
Lilburn, Georgia

Betty Scott, CDA, CDPMA, AAS
East Central College
Union, Missouri

Melissa Thibodeaux, CDA, RDA, BS
San Joaquin Valley College
Bakersfield, California

Mea Weinberg, DMD, MSD, RPh
New York University College of
Dentistry
New York, New York

HOW TO USE THIS TEXT

Dental Assisting is an ever-evolving profession full of opportunity and challenge. *Delmar's Dental Assisting: A Comprehensive Approach* is designed to help you acquire the knowledge, skills, and values necessary to become a successful dental assistant. The text is organized into eight main sections which reflect the broad areas of dental assisting responsibility. The sections are then divided into a total of 31 chapters of related information. The text has many unique features which will make it easier for you to learn and integrate theory and practice, including:

CHAPTER OUTLINE

At the beginning of each chapter is an outline listing the main headings covered within the chapter. Review these headings of topic areas before you study the chapter. They'll be a roadmap to the material in the chapter.

OBJECTIVES

Learning objectives identify the key information to be gained from the chapter. Use these objectives, together with the review questions, to test your understanding of the chapter's content.

KEY TERMS

All key terms are listed at the beginning of each chapter with a page number reference. Turn to the page to understand the term used in context; turn to the glossary for the term definition. Within the text, the term is always blue boldface at its first occurrence for easy identification.

ICONS

Graphic icons pinpoint information that relates to legal, safety, technology, global or cultural issues, and certified dental assisting (CDA) competencies.

PROCEDURES

Step-by-step procedures give detailed information on dental assisting competencies. Icons at the beginning of procedures indicate which function, instruments, and protective equipment are required for the procedure.

COLOR ILLUSTRATIONS, PHOTOS, AND TABLES

Full-color illustrations and photos with detailed captions reinforce chapter material. Tables summarize important facts or concepts presented in the text.

CHAPTER SUMMARY

The chapter summary emphasizes key concepts from the chapter to help you focus your study.

CASE STUDIES

The case studies and review questions present real-life scenarios requiring a problem/solution approach. Use the case studies to put your knowledge into practice and to arrive at a deeper understanding of the dental assisting profession.

REVIEW QUESTIONS

Test your comprehension of the chapter with structured multiple choice questions and open-ended critical thinking questions that require you to combine an understanding of chapter material with your personal insight and judgement.

HOW TO USE THE PRACTICE SOFTWARE

The Student Practice Software has been designed to accompany *Delmar's Dental Assisting: A Comprehensive Approach*. By using these exercises and games, you'll challenge yourself and other students, making your study of medical assisting more effective and fun!

Getting started is easy. Follow the simple directions on the disk label to install the program on your computer. Then take advantage of the following features:

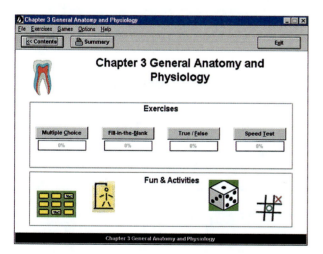

MAIN MENU

The main menu follows the chapter organization of the text exactly—which makes it easy for you to find your way around. Just click on the button for the chapter you want, and you'll arrive at the chapter opening screen.

TOOLBAR

The button at the top left of every screen allows you to retrace your steps, while the Exit button gets you out of the program quickly and easily. As you navigate through the software, check the toolbar for other features that help you use individual exercises or games.

ON-LINE HELP

If you get stuck, just press F1 or click on the *Help* menu for assistance. The on-line help includes instructions for all parts of the Student Practice Software.

THE CHAPTER SCREEN

Here you have the opportunity to choose how you want to learn the material. Select one of the exercises for additional practice, review, or self-testing. Or click on a game to practice the content for that chapter in a fun format.

Minimum System Requirements:
Operating System: Windows 3.1 or higher
Computer: 386 or higher
Memory: 4 MB
Graphics; 16 bit color VGA
Hard Drive Space: 2 MB

EXERCISES

The Student Practice Software acts as your own private tutor. For each exercise, it chooses from a bank of over 1,500 questions covering all 31 chapters. Putting these exercises to work for you is simple:

- Choose an exercise from those displayed, e.g., multiple choice, true or false, fill-in-the-blank, matching, or labeling exercise.
- You'll encounter a series of 8-10 questions for each exercise format; each question gives you two chances to answer correctly.
- Instant feedback tells you whether you're right or wrong—and helps you learn more quickly by explaining why an answer was correct or incorrect.
- The Practice Software displays the percentage of correct answers on the chapter screen. An on-screen score sheet (which you can print) lets you track correct and incorrect answers.
- Review your previous questions and answers in an exercise for more in-depth understanding. Or start an exercise over with a new, random set of questions that gives you a realistic study environment.
- When you're ready for an additional challenge, try the timed Speed Test. Once you've finished, it displays your score and the time you took to complete the test, so you can see how much you've learned.

FUN & GAMES

To have fun while reinforcing your knowledge, enjoy each of the four simple games on the software. You can play alone, with a partner, or on teams.

- **Concentration:** match terms to their corresponding definitions under the cards as the timer runs.
- **Hangman:** review your spelling and vocabulary by choosing the correct letters to spell dental words appropriate to the chapter before you're "hanged."
- **Board Game:** challenge your classmates and increase your knowledge by playing this question-and-answer game.
- **Tic-Tac-Toe:** you or your team must correctly answer a dental question before playing an ✕ or an ○.

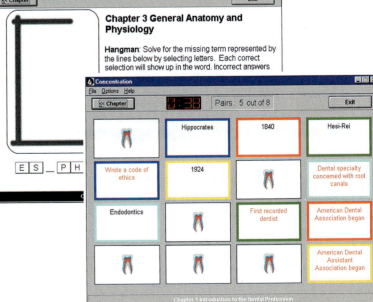

Introduction

1 Introduction to the Dental Profession

Introduction to the Dental Profession

OBJECTIVES

The student should strive to meet the following objectives and demonstrate an understanding of the facts and principles presented in this chapter:

1. Identify oral disease indications from the beginning of time.

2. List the names of individuals who had a great impact on the profession of dentistry.

3. Identify the people who promoted education and organized dentistry.

4. Explain what DDS and DMD stand for.

5. Identify the eight specialties of dentistry.

6. Describe generally what career skills are performed by dental hygienists, dental assistants, and dental laboratory technicians.

7. List the education required for and the professional organizations that represent each profession.

KEY TERMS

American Dental Assistants Association (ADAA) (p. 10)

American Dental Association (ADA) (p. 8)

American Dental Hygienists' Association (ADHA) (p. 9)

American Dental Laboratory Technician Association (ADLTA) (p. 11)

certified dental assistant (CDA) (p. 10)

Dental Assisting National Board, Inc. (DANB) (pp. 9–10)

dental public health (p. 8)

Dr. C. Edmund Kells (p. 9)

Dr. Greene Vardiman Black (p. 7)

endodontics (p. 6)

forensic dentistry (p. 9)

Juliette Southard (p. 10)

oral and maxillofacial surgery (p. 8)

oral pathology (p. 8)

orthodontics (p. 6)

pediatric dentistry (p. 8)

periodontics (p. 8)

Pierre Fauchard (p. 5)

prosthodontics (p. 9)

Wilhelm Conrad Roentgen (p. 5)

INTRODUCTION AND HISTORY

Humans, from the very beginning of time, have been plagued with dental problems. Over the years, a number of different "dental treatments" were tried and perfected. Tools of all different types were developed and used to repair and clean teeth.

It is important to be familiar with the historic struggles in and contributions to dentistry that took place in order to advance the profession into what it is today (Figure 1-1).

Early Times

Beginning in the very earliest of times, dental work was done by physicians. Often, each physician specialized in only one area of care for one part of the body. In fact, during the fifth century B.C., a Greek historian named **Herodotus** wrote from his observations that medicine had become so separate that each physician was a specialist in a disease. "All the country is full of physicians, some of the eyes, some of the teeth, some of what pertains to the belly and some of the hidden diseases." One Egyptian doctor of teeth, named **Hesi-Re** (the first dentist whose name was recorded), practiced in 3000 B.C.

Much of the dentistry practice of the time was the removal of teeth if pain occurred. Some evidence of drilling holes near the roots to allow infection to drain so that pressure in an abscessed tooth could be relieved is noted on human skulls that have been found. Other dental problems that humans from early times had was from their food preparation techniques. Grains were ground in stone bowls with stone pestles. During this process, particles of stone mixed with the grain. This grit in the food caused severe wear of the biting (occlusal) surfaces of the teeth and possible pulp exposure.

The father of medicine, **Hippocrates** (460–377 B.C.), attempted to explain health and disease. He suggested that four main fluids in the body, namely blood, black bile, yellow bile, and phlegm, along with heat, cold, dry air, and wet air, must remain in balance. Disruption of these four fluids and four elements would result in dis-

Beginning of time	Tooth decay is noted
3000 B.C.	First dentist whose name is recorded (Hesi-Re)
460–377 B.C.	Oath of Hippocrates (Hippocrates)
384–322 B.C.	Attention to oral hygiene (Aristotle)
1300–1368	Hygienic rules (Guy de Chauliac)
1452–1519	Tooth morphology (Leonardo da Vinci)
1678–1761	Founder of modern dentistry (Pierre Fauchard)
1895	X-rays discovered (Wilhelm Conrad Roentgen)
1760–1819	John Greenwood, George Washington's dentist Josiah Flagg, developed the dental chair
1840	Horace Hayden and Chapin Harris established the Baltimore College of Dental Surgery
1836–1915	G.V. Black, the "grand old man of dentistry" and inventor and dean of dental school
1840	American Society of Dental Surgeons began
1859	American Dental Association (ADA) began
1885	"Lady in Attendance," Dr. C. Edmund Kells
1913	Fones School of Dental Hygiene began
1923	American Dental Hygiene Association (ADHA) began
1924	American Dental Assistants Association (ADAA) began, first president is Juliette Southard
1947	Dental Assisting National Board, Inc. (DANB) began

FIGURE 1-1 Time line of dental progress.

ease. Among Hippocrates' numerous writings is a book titled *On Affections.* In this book he wrote, "Teeth are eroded and become decayed partly by the mucus, and partly by food, when they are by nature weak and badly fixed in the mouth." Even though much of what Hippocrates thought about health and teeth is untrue, his writings gave much-needed information for the progression of medicine. Even today, the **Oath of Hippocrates** is used as a basis for the code of ethics utilized by the medical and dental professions in regard to the solemn obligation these professionals undertake when caring for patients.

During **Aristotle**'s time (384–322 B.C.), some attention was given to oral hygiene. An Athenian physician, Diocles of Carystus, stated that oral hygiene should get proper attention, and he even gave instructions to this end. During the next couple of centuries, more importance was placed on good oral hygiene. A number of cleaning powders were made from crushed bones, oyster, and egg shells. At times, these substances were mixed with honey to make a paste to clean with. Guests in the homes of the wealthy who were invited to dinner were given silver- and even gold-decorated toothpicks with which to clean their teeth after the meal. At the time, picking one's teeth was proper etiquette.

Later Progress

In France, a surgeon named **Guy de Chauliac** (1300–1368) became one of the most influential authors of the fourteenth century on surgery. He also wrote hygienic rules for oral hygiene.

Hygienic Rules for Oral Hygiene, Written by Guy de Chauliac

1. Avoid food that putrifies readily.
2. Avoid food or drink that is either too hot or too cold, and especially avoid swallowing extremely cold food after extremely hot food, and vice versa.
3. Do not bite into things that are too hard.
4. Avoid foods that stick to the teeth, such as figs and confections made with honey.
5. Avoid certain foods known to be bad for the teeth [his example was leeks].
6. Clean the teeth gently with a mixture of honey and burnt salt to which some vinegar has been added.

It is now known that the information given by de Chauliac was not entirely true. However, because it was based on sound logic, much of it is used today. For example, it is well known that sticky, sweet foods increase dental decay. In his writings, de Chauliac noted that surgery on the teeth should be performed under the supervision of doctors but could be done by "barbers or dentators." This notation was the first to refer to "dentatores," the specific group of practitioners caring for the oral cavity and the teeth.

During the fifteenth and sixteenth centuries, artists became more interested in the human anatomy in order to enhance the accuracy of their artwork. **Leonardo da Vinci** (1452–1519) painstakingly dissected the human skull and then drew his discoveries. He was the first to make a distinction between premolars and molars. His written documents further define the morphology of teeth.

Pierre Fauchard (1678–1761) organized all known information about dentistry in a book that was clearly written and had step-by-step pictures that depicted easy-to-follow procedures. He rejected the idea that a toothworm caused decay and noted that caries (his term for decay) were a result of a "hormonal imbalance." Fauchard wrote of his perceived causes of decay and prevention techniques and was an early advocate of treatment of diseased gingival tissue. Fauchard perfected a number of dental treatments that are still used in part today, almost three centuries later. Many refer to Pierre Fauchard as the founder of modern dentistry.

Wilhelm Conrad Roentgen (1845–1923), a German physicist, discovered x-rays in 1895. This discovery allowed dentists to further their knowledge of the diseases and the structures of the mouth (see Chapter 17, Dental Radiography).

Progress of Dentistry in the United States

One of the first dentists to arrive in the United States from England was **Robert Woofendale**. Woofendale placed an advertisement in the *New York Mercury* on November 17, 1766, that stated that he "performs all operations upon the teeth, sockets, gums, and palate, likewise fixes artificial teeth, so as to escape discernment." Soon after Robert Woofendale arrived, **John Baker** came and started advertising in the Boston area. He spoke and wrote about fillings and artificial teeth. John Baker was well known and was one the dentists who treated George Washington. It was **John Greenwood** (1760–1819) who was said to be the first president's favorite dentist. John Greenwood had very little formal education but was a proficient practitioner in the eighteenth century. He thought children should care for their teeth and offered parents reduced rates for children's dental care. He also thought that tartar came from bad breath and was adamant about the regular removal of it for good oral health.

George Washington, at one time or another, was probably treated by every notable dentist of the time. A number of references in his diary note continual pain and discomfort from his teeth. At the time the picture that is currently on the one-dollar bill was taken, the president had only one tooth left, a lower left bicuspid (premolar). In fact, the artist had to pad out the cheeks and lips with cotton to give the president's sunken face a more normal appearance. Washington's last set of dentures, made by John Greenwood, were made of ivory and gold and had two springs holding them together (Figure 1-2). A number of different dentures were made for the president, but, contrary to popular belief, they were not made of wood.

Paul Revere (1735–1818), a silversmith, was involved in dentistry for several years, but his greatest contribution was making artificial teeth and surgical instruments. He may have had a part in training a notable dentist of the late 1700s, **Josiah Flagg**. Flagg's father was a partner of Paul Revere. Flagg was a skilled surgeon, accomplishing corrective procedures on cleft lips, orthodontics, endodontics, and operative dentistry. However, one of his major contributions to future dentistry was the construction of a dental chair. It had an extension on the arm to hold dental instruments and an adjustable head rest.

In the early 1800s, dentistry took a giant leap forward in America. The establishment of a popular democracy, with the chance of personal financial gain, free public-school education, and the growth in population, prompted some of the most notable dentists in the world to relocate to America. The literature and knowledge expanded a great deal during this time. Most of the large cities now had resident dentists rather than the traveling barbers who extracted teeth and sold tooth powders. The dentists of the time were better educated and involved in the communities they served. The profession was progressing far beyond massive tooth removals and occasional cleanings. Additionally, dental materials improved and developed as techniques did.

EDUCATION AND ORGANIZED DENTISTRY

Horace H. Hayden (1769–1844) sought out dental care from John Greenwood (the dentist who cared for George Washington) (Figure 1-3). Hayden was inspired and encouraged to take up dentistry as a vocation. He became very active in the profession of dentistry, writing for journals and lecturing on medical and dental topics.

One of the students who studied with Hayden was **Chapin A. Harris** (1806–1860) (Figure 1-4). Harris believed in education and built up an extensive library of dental literature, including his publication, *The Dental*

FIGURE 1-3 One of the founders of professional dentistry in America, Horace Hayden. *(Courtesy of the National Museum of Dentistry, Baltimore, MD)*

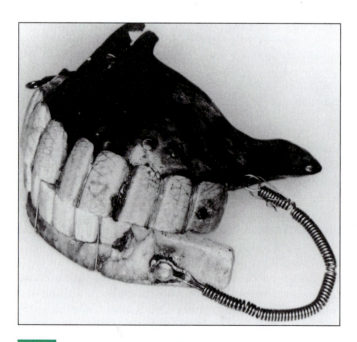

FIGURE 1-2 The last dental prosthesis worn by George Washington was made for him by John Greenwood. It is made of gold and ivory and is held together with springs. *(Courtesy of the National Museum of Dentistry, Baltimore, MD)*

FIGURE 1-4 One of the founders of professional dentistry in America, Chapin Harris. He also helped establish the first periodontal and first national association. *(Courtesy of the National Museum of Dentistry, Baltimore, MD)*

FIGURE 1-5 The "grand old man of dentistry," G.V. Black. *(Courtesy of the National Museum of Dentistry, Baltimore, MD)*

Art: A Practical Treatise on Dental Surgery. Due to the efforts of Hayden and Harris, the first dental college in the world, Baltimore College of Dental Surgery, was founded on March 6, 1840. It is now called the School of Dentistry at the University of Maryland.

Dr. Greene Vardiman Black (1836–1915), known as G.V. Black, taught in dental schools such as the University of Iowa and the Northwestern University Dental School in Chicago (Figure 1-5). As the dean, he increased the library holdings and authored more than 500 articles and several books. He invented numerous machines for testing alloys and instruments to refine the cavity prep. Dr. Black later enlarged these instruments for demonstration to students in the classroom. Many refer to him as the "grand old man of dentistry." His son, **Arthur D. Black**, followed in his footsteps, becoming the dean of the Northwestern University Dental School in Chicago. He developed the *Index to Dental Periodical Literature in the English Language* in 1921. This allowed not only researchers to access the literature, but general practicing dentists

who wanted to improve their knowledge and skills could also access it.

Lucy Beaman Hobbs was the first woman to graduate from the Ohio College of Dental Surgery in 1866. In 1869, Robert Tanner Freeman was the first African American to graduate from Harvard School of Dental Medicine.

American Dental Association

At a time when education and literature were developing, it was thought that organizing the dentists together would promote sharing of information concerned with excellence in dentistry. Horace Hayden and Chapin Harris collaborated on endeavors such as forming the first nationwide association of dentists. In 1840, the **American Society of Dental Surgeons** was formed and was later dissolved in 1856. Harris had long believed in the need for an informative dental periodical and was instrumental in founding it in 1839. This journal was called the **American Journal of Dental Science** (*AJDS*). Later, in 1859, twenty-five delegates gathered in Niagara Falls, New York, and organized the American Dental Association (ADA) (Figure 1-6). The association was small at first, but, after grouping all local associations according to states and then all states having representation to the national organization, the membership began to increase. Each state now has its own organization with bylaws approved by the American Dental Association, and each local (regional) organization has ADA-approved bylaws that are sent to each state organization. For instance, Texas is represented by the Texas State Dental Association to the ADA and the Texas State Dental Association comprises individual local dental associations. The official publication of the ADA is the *Journal of American Dental Association* (*JADA*). The ADA also has a Web site, ADAONLINE (http://www.ada.org), which provides a link to the ADA for dental professionals and dental consumers.

THE DENTAL TEAM

Dentists

Once dentistry was established as a profession, the need for formal education became apparent. Only half of the dentists practicing at this time had formal educations. The requirements finally set forth for a dental education include an undergraduate education and graduation from a dental school approved by the ADA, Commission on Dental Accreditation. Currently, three to four years of undergraduate work and four years of dental school (five at Harvard) are required to achieve a dental

FIGURE 1-6 Logo for dentistry.

degree. Depending on the program emphasis, a Doctor of Dental Surgery (DDS) or a Doctor of Medical Dentistry (DMD) degree is granted. Specialist training includes two or more additional years of postgraduate education in an approved, specialized training area. All dentists must take and pass both written and clinical examinations in the states in which they practice. All dental team members are responsible for following the regulations set up in their states. These regulations are defined in each state's dental practice act. The dental practice acts are defined to protect the public. The act specifies what legally can be performed by the dental professionals in that specific state. The dentist supervises the dental team members in his or her office.

Dental Specialists. A dentist who practices all phases of dentistry is called a general dentist. The general dentist may have cases in which additional treatment that goes beyond the scope of his or her training is required. The general dentist would refer these cases to a dental specialist. The ADA recognizes the following eight specialties:

1. **Dental public health** is the specialty concerned with the prevention of dental disease. The public health dentist works with the community to promote dental health.

2. **Endodontics** is concerned with the pathology and morphology of the dental pulp and surrounding tissues due to injury and disease. If a patient is referred for a root canal, he or she would see an endodontist.

3. **Oral pathology** is the specialty concerned with the diagnosis and nature of the diseases that affect the oral cavity. A patient who has a lesion unknown to the general dentist may be referred to the oral pathologist for further treatment and diagnosis.

4. **Oral and maxillofacial surgery** is concerned with the diagnosis and surgical treatment of the oral and maxillofacial region due to injury, disease, or defects. A patient having third molars (wisdom teeth) removed may be referred to an oral and maxillofacial surgeon.

5. **Orthodontics** is concerned with diagnosis, supervision, guidance, and correction of the malocclusion in the dentofacial structures. Braces for straightening teeth are placed by the orthodontist.

6. **Pediatric dentistry** is concerned with prevention of oral disease and the diagnosis and treatment of oral care in children, from birth through adolescence. Other patients requiring special care due to emotional, mental, or physical problems are referred to the pediatric dentist.

7. **Periodontics** is the specialty concerned with the diagnosis and treatment of the diseases of the supporting and surrounding tissues of the tooth. The periodontist is also concerned with the prevention

of disease in this area. If a patient has plaque and calculus buildup and has lost some of the bone around the tooth due to periodontal disease, he or she would be referred to the periodontist for further evaluation and treatment.

8. **Prosthodontics** is concerned with the diagnosis, restoration, and maintenance of oral functions. This specialty is also concerned with the replacement of missing teeth through artificial means.

Another area that requires additional training but is not regarded as a specialty of dentistry is **forensic dentistry**. This is a relatively new area that deals with a wide range of services, such as identification of bite marks on the body and/or identification of an individual through tooth restorations and morphology utilizing dental records.

The specialist works with the general dentist to provide the optimum oral health and patient care. During and once the specialty treatment is completed, the patient continues regular visits with his or her general dentist.

FIGURE 1-7 Logo for American Dental Hygienists' Association.

Dental Hygienists

Early in the 1900s in Bridgeport, Connecticut, several dentists, along with a leader named **Dr. Alfred Civilon Fones**, stated, that they would not be able to be surgeons and to give preventive treatments. It was suggested that women be trained to clean teeth because "they have smaller and more gentle hands." At that time, it was uncommon for women to be working outside the home. A dental assistant, Irene Morgan, was the first to be trained by Dr. Fones in dental hygiene. Dr. Fones developed a school in 1913, and it survives today as the Fones School of Dental Hygiene, University of Bridgeport. Graduates of either two- or four-year dental hygiene schools receive the title registered dental hygienist (RDH) after passing both written and clinical tests in the states in which they practice, and they are granted licenses. Dental hygienists specialize in providing dental prophylaxis, including the removal of plaque, stains, and calculus from the teeth, along with patient education. Many state practice acts allow licensed hygienists to apply tooth sealants; to expose, process, and mount dental radiographs; and to chart the conditions in the oral cavity. Some of the states allow hygienists to place restorative materials and to administer local anesthetics.

American Dental Hygienists' Association. The **American Dental Hygienists' Association (ADHA)** was formed in 1923 in Cleveland in conjunction with the ADA annual meeting (Figure 1-7). In 1927, the *Journal of the American Dental Hygienists' Association* was founded and continues to be the official publication of the organization. This organization, like the ADA, has the leadership of national, state, and local societies working together to promote oral health.

Dental Assistants

Prior to the early twentieth century, dentists hired men and boys to assist them in their dental practices. **Dr. C. Edmund Kells**, who practiced in New Orleans, hired a female to replace a male assistant in 1885. He wanted this "lady assistant" to be "quick, quiet, gentle, and attentive." A number of dentists were unsure about a female in the dental office, but the public accepted it quickly. It now allowed a woman to go to a dental office without being accompanied by her husband or maiden aunt. Due to the popularity of "Ladies in Attendance," dentists advertised the fact that they had hired female dental assistants by displaying signs in their windows.

Today, the educationally qualified dental assistant normally graduates from an institution accredited by the American Dental Association Commission on Dental Accreditation. Training is approximately one academic year in length and includes didactic, laboratory, and clinical content. Each state has a dental practice act that governs which duties dental assistants can perform. This varies from performing invasive procedures, such as placing retraction cord and dental dams, to noninvasive procedures, such as patient education. Dental assistants enable dentists to care for many more patients and to produce much more dentistry than they could alone. Almost all dental offices employ one or more dental assistants. In the office, the person working directly with the dentist during patient procedures is the dental assistant.

Certified Dental Assistants. A 104-hour course was developed in 1947, along with a certifying board, to give credentials to assistants who passed the written and clinical examination. The **Dental Assisting National**

Board, Inc. (DANB), provides a means for competent, qualified dental assistants to obtain credentials. By passing a comprehensive written examination from DANB, the dental assistant can use the title of **certified dental assistant (CDA)**. Other specialized certification can be obtained in areas such as Certified Dental Practice Management Assistant (CDPMA), Certified Orthodontic Assistant (COA), and Certified Oral and Maxillofacial Surgery Assistant (COMSA). Some state dental practice acts allow assistants to obtain the credential of registered dental assistant (RDA). Others may require registration in expanded functions (functions and skills considered to be above the normal scope of dental assisting, such as performing a coronal polish and placing a dental dam), therefore earning the title of registered dental assistant in expanded functions (EDAEF) (see Chapter 30, Employment Strategies).

Dental Receptionists/Dental Practice Management Assistants. The **dental receptionist** position is becoming a more specialized area of dental assisting with the use of computers and computerized insurance claims. The dental receptionist or practice management assistant attends seminars to upgrade skills in front office, computer technology, marketing, and accounting.

American Dental Assistants Association. The **American Dental Assistants Association (ADAA)** was founded in 1924 by **Juliette Southard**, its first president (Figures 1-8 and 1-9). It was founded on four principles: education, efficiency, service, and loyalty. Membership offers a voice in national affairs regarding the career of dental assisting, opportunities in continuing education, professional liability insurance, and the interaction with

FIGURE 1-9 Juliette Southard, founder and first president of the American Dental Assistants Association. *(Courtesy of the American Dental Assistants Association, Chicago, IL)*

other professionals in the field. Members of the ADAA can remain current with their knowledge through the ADAA publication *The Dental Assistant, Journal of the American Dental Assistants Association* or by accessing the ADAA Web site (http://members.aol.com/adaa1/index.html).

Dental Laboratory Technicians

The dental laboratory technician may not work in the dental office with the other members of the team but is an essential member of the team. Some dental laboratory technicians are employed by the dentist; others work in privately owned dental laboratories.

Originally, dentists performed their own laboratory procedures; however, they eventually became too busy

FIGURE 1-8 Logo for American Dental Assistants Association.

to complete the laboratory work and hired trained technicians to perform these skills. Dental laboratory technicians were established. The first commercial dental laboratory was opened in Boston in 1883 by **Dr. William H. Stowe**, a dentist, and **Frank F. Eddy**, a toolmaker. By the turn of the century, dental laboratories were going strong and were firmly established. Today, whether the technicians are in the dental office or outside in a commercial dental laboratory, they provide such extra oral services as fabricating gold and porcelain restorations and partial and full dentures.

In most states, a dental laboratory technician is not required to have formal training and may be trained on the job. A large number of technicians have graduated from two-year ADA-accredited dental laboratory technician programs. These programs require extensive knowledge in dental anatomy and dental materials and the development of detailed mechanical skills. Individuals seeking credentials must pass an examination to become certified dental technicians (CDTs). Membership in the **American Dental Laboratory Technician Association (ADLTA)** is also offered to dental technicians.

Chapter Summary

It is important to know the historic struggles in and contributions to dentistry that advanced the profession into what it is today. Organized dentistry was formed with the intent to promote the sharing of information concerned with excellence in dentistry. To provide excellence in dentistry, additional dental team members would become recognized and add contributing roles. Therefore, the dental assistant will need to be able to identify and define those who contribute to the dental profession.

Case Study

Lori Ann Smith was eighteen years old in 1880 and was seeking a position in a dental office. The opinion of the dentists was to not allow women access to the profession. Lori's career dreams were denied. Over 100 years later, her great-great-granddaughter, Traci Lynd, was seeking a position in a dental office and found a very different environment. What changes and advancements took place for dental assistants during that time frame to allow Traci to reach her goal?

Case Study Review

1. When were gender barriers eliminated for dental assistants?

2. What career changes for dental assistants took place over four generations?

3. With the current education advancements in the profession, what credentials are available to dental assistants today?

 To complete your study of this chapter, work the review activities that follow. Also, refer to the software that accompanies this text.

Review Questions

Multiple Choice

1. The father of medicine, who gave us the basic code of ethics utilized by the medical and dental professions, is
   a. Aristotle.
   b. Leonardo da Vinci.
   c. Pierre Fauchard.
   d. Hipprocrates.

2. Who is the teacher and inventor recognized as the "grand old man of dentistry"?
   a. Chapin A. Harris.
   b. G.V. Black.
   c. John Greenwood.
   d. Josiah Flagg.

3. Which of the following is *not* a dental specialty?
   a. Endodontics.
   b. Oral pathology.
   c. Forensic dentistry.
   d. Pediatric dentistry.

4. Which of the following dental team members specializes in the fabrication of partials and dentures?
   a. Dental assistants.
   b. Dental hygienists.
   c. Dental laboratory technicians.
   d. Dentists.

5. The first president of the American Dental Assistants Association was
   a. Juliette Southard.
   b. Lucy Hobbs.
   c. Dr. C. Edmund Kells.
   d. Dr. Alfred Fonds.

Critical Thinking

1. If a patient fell and fractured his anterior tooth midway down the crown and it seemed to have pulpal involvement and the lip was cut badly, what specialists could the general dentist refer the patient to?

2. Who would you contact for information about dental assisting organizations?

3. Which dental team member (nationally), besides the dentist, requires a license?

Basic Dental Sciences

Oral Health and Nutrition

OBJECTIVES

The student should strive to meet the following objectives and demonstrate an understanding of the facts and principles presented in this chapter:

1. Describe how plaque forms and affects the tooth.

2. Identify motivation tips for oral hygiene for each age group.

3. Identify the oral hygiene aids available to all patients, including manual and automatic.

4. Demonstrate the five toothbrushing techniques.

5. Identify types of dental floss and demonstrate flossing technique.

6. Describe fluoride and its use in dentistry.

7. Define fluoridation and describe its effectiveness on tooth development and the post eruption stage.

8. List and explain the forms of fluoride. Describe how to prepare a patient and demonstrate fluoride application.

9. Describe how an understanding of nutrition is used in the profession of dental assisting.

10. Define nutrients found in foods, including carbohydrates, fiber, fats, proteins, and amino acids. Explain how they affect oral hygiene.

11. Define a calorie and basal metabolic rate.

12. Identify and explain the function of vitamins, major minerals, and water.

KEY TERMS

Calories (p. 36)

caries (p. 16)

demineralization (p. 16)

dentifrice (p. 20)

diet (p. 35)

diuretics (p. 40)

enamel hypo-calcification (p. 32)

enamel hypoplasia (p. 32)

essential amino acids (p. 36)

fluoropatite crystal (p. 31)

fluoridation (p. 30)

fluorosis (p. 31)

halitosis (p. 20)

hydroxyl ion (p. 31)

malnutrition (p. 35)

metabolism (p. 35)

mottled enamel (p. 30)

nutrients (p. 35)

plaque (p. 16)

undernourished (p. 35)

xerostomia (p. 30)

INTRODUCTION

An important role for dental assistants in the dental office is in preventive dentistry. Dentistry is about preventing oral disease, such as dental decay, and caring for periodontal disease. It is important to educate the public on how to prevent disease. The dental assistant must be knowledgeable about the many products available to aid patients in maintaining their teeth and gums. The dental assistant must be a good listener and be able to evaluate the needs of the patients. Dental assistants must also know how to motivate patients to be effective in their oral hygiene care. Fluoride has been proven to be effective in reducing dental caries. The dental assistant will need to have background knowledge of fluoride in order to educate patients in its usage and benefits. A final area of oral health and prevention is nutrition. Many patients will not be knowledgeable about the kinds of foods that will aid them in cleansing their teeth or which foods perpetuate the problem of decay. The dental assistant, after discussions with the patient, can identify nutritional concerns and further assist the patient in choosing foods that will benefit his or her oral health.

PREVENTIVE DENTISTRY

The goal of preventive dentistry is that each individual maintain optimal oral health. Preventive concepts are woven throughout each modern dental practice. To be effective in preventive dentistry, the dental assistant must first care for his or her teeth properly and practice good nutrition.

▶ Brush and floss daily to remove plaque and bacteria.

▶ Disclose periodically to evaluate the effectiveness of brushing and flossing.

▶ Follow a fluoride program while the teeth are developing to allow them to be strong and decay resistant. The fluoride program includes office applications and home treatments.

▶ Follow a good nutrition and exercise program to maintain overall health. Good nutrition over a lifetime allows strong teeth and bones to develop and be maintained.

▶ Schedule regular dental visits for a thorough examination, cleaning, and any necessary dental treatment.

Plaque Formation

Dental **plaque** is a sticky mass that contains bacteria and grows in colonies on the teeth (Figure 2-1). Most people have missed areas while brushing their teeth and noted that a soft, white, sticky mass forms. This is plaque and other soft deposits. The bacteria in plaque is fed by the sugar in foods we eat. The bacteria-rich plaque converts the sugar into acid. After a period of time, the acid attacks the tooth and eventually causes **demineralization**, where the minerals, calcium, and phosphate are lost from the enamel surface (Figure 2-2). People who have had orthodontic appliances may have demineralization on the tooth surface where the brackets were located. When the brackets are removed, demineralization appears as a whitish area on the tooth. It developed because plaque was not removed routinely around the brackets. If plaque continues to attack the tooth, it will cause decay, or **caries**. Once dental decay has begun, the area should be restored by a dentist.

Dental decay (caries) equation.

Sugar + Plaque = Acid + Tooth = Decay

FIGURE 2-1 Plaque on the gingival surface of the teeth shown as a soft, white, sticky mass.

FIGURE 2-2 Demineralization of the enamel of the tooth appears as a white, chalky area. (*Courtesy of Dwight H. Damon, DDS, MSD*)

Patient Motivation

Preventing dental disease is ultimately the responsibility of the patients, but dental auxiliaries spend a great deal of time educating and motivating patients to care for their teeth and oral cavities. The first aspect of patient motivation is for the dental assistant to assess oral hygiene and listen to the patient. Listening to the patient will give insight into the patient's attitude toward oral hygiene and will allow the assistant to get a better idea how to motivate and communicate with the patient. It will be best to work with the patients to help them recognize their dental problems, problem solve together to develop solutions, and then provide motivation and aid them in setting oral hygiene goals.

Each patient should be treated as an individual, taking into consideration the patient's age, oral hygiene knowledge, skills, attitude, and any special considerations. Different age groups have characteristics that are normally identifiable; however, these characteristics are not absolute. The following are a few general characteristics pertaining to each age group.

Infants. An infant's oral hygiene must be accomplished by the parents or caregiver. The dental assistant can show parents how to lay the child back in their arms and use a washcloth or an infant toothbrush to remove any plaque in the area. It should be stressed that this initial contact with oral hygiene should be positive. The idea of making this a fun activity will set the stage as the infant develops (Figure 2-3).

Preschool Children. Preschool children have an active interest in visual aids, such as amusing toothbrushes or puppets. They do not have highly developed motor skills, normally are unable to read, and their attention span is less than five minutes. The child's first appointment with the dentist takes place around age three and should be a very positive contact. The dentist may not accomplish as much as desired during this appointment, but it is most important that it is a pleasant experience. The dental assistant can use a puppet to show oral hygiene instructions. Mr. "Air," the three-way syringe, can be used to

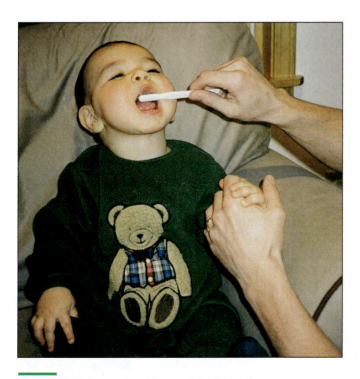

FIGURE 2-3 Parent brushing an infant's teeth.

blow "wind" on the tooth after Mr. "Water" gives the child a drink from the same syringe. Counting the "upstairs" and "downstairs" teeth for the child is another fun activity to get the child to open his or her mouth. The child can be shown how to put the toothbrush in his or her mouth and tickle the teeth and gum tissue. Even if a child chews on the brush, some plaque is being removed.

At home, parents can instruct the child to sit down and watch television or listen to a story while brushing his or her teeth. If this happens on and off throughout the day, the teeth will have some care. Parents can also brush their teeth in front of the television without toothpaste to role play what the child is to do. Children of this age love to imitate their parents. Keep in mind that the child likes active, short procedures that give positive reinforcement. Parents must ensure that at least once (at bedtime) the child's teeth get a thorough, monitored brushing. Twice a day (morning and night) is best, especially if the parent can floss between the child's molars once daily.

Ages Five through Eight. Ages five through eight are when many changes take place in a child's life and his or her attention span increases to ten to fifteen minutes. Children at this age are learning to read and their vocabulary is growing. They like to please adults and enjoy learning. They love facts and require constant guidance as they strive for immediate goals with positive reinforcement. A dental assistant could teach a child of this age to improve his or her brushing techniques and floss because the child's dexterity is getting better. Videos lasting under ten minutes with cartoons describing brushing and flossing could be used for this age group. Pictures to color, find an item in a picture, or match a picture are also popular activities for this age group. The dental assistant can design hygiene pictures or purchase commercial ones. The American Dental Association has videos and other aids that are available for hygiene instruction.

Ages Nine through Twelve. Nine- through twelve-year-olds are very concerned with fitting into a group and doing what others in that group are doing. They can brush and floss proficiently and have great curiosity to learn. They only like realistic visual aids at this age and their attention span is normally around thirty minutes. They have a mixed dentition of primary and permanent teeth that may require special directions to achieve proper hygiene in some areas. The dental assistant may provide hygiene instructions in a group of this age or may give rewards for good hygiene. One technique is to take pictures of the patients in this age group that have had success with oral hygiene. These pictures can then be posted on a bulletin board in the office. The patients love to find their friends and may strive to have their pictures among the others on the wall.

Ages Thirteen through Fifteen. Patients in the thirteen- through fifteen-year-old group are extremely motivated by peer pressure and personal appearance. The rapid growth of individuals in this age group makes coordination a problem. Some may have to work hard at flossing and it is crucial that they do not feel silly in front of others. Another problem with adolescents in this age group is that their nutrition is poor. Snacking is routine and, along with sporadic dental hygiene, the rate of decay rises. Motivation for this group will be individual and may change from office visit to office visit. Listen carefully to what is said at each visit and adapt the instruction to meet the current needs of the patient. Sincere positive reinforcement will be necessary to motivate this group of adolescents.

Ages Sixteen through Nineteen. Sixteen- through nineteen-year-olds are still very aware of peer pressure, along with an increase in health and personal appearance. This group seems to question authority, so approach them as a friend, allowing them to accept responsibility for their own oral hygiene. The nutritional habits still are in decline at this age and time management is a problem. Suggestions by the dental assistant as to when oral hygiene can fit into the patient's schedule may be helpful. One area that will aid in motivating individuals of this age group is the desire to avoid having bad breath. Talk to the individuals in this age group about the disadvantages of using a breath aid that has sugar in it. The dental assistant can give education about the process of plaque formation and tooth decay. Also, show them how to brush and floss in order to maintain good hygiene and fresh breath. Their growth has leveled off and their coordination should be improved. Share with the patients of this age group how a good smile will aid them in future employment.

Ages Nineteen through Sixty. Patients in the nineteen through sixty age group will have specific needs and concerns that originate from their own diverse backgrounds. One of the main concerns with this age group for the dental assistant is to help patients to unlearn the habits that are not beneficial to their dental care. Help these individuals identify the problem and solve it. The patient must be involved and motivated in the action plan or no change will be made.

Patients Sixty Plus. Sixty-plus years allow patients to think about the necessity of keeping their teeth for a lifetime. Patients of this age should be made aware that tooth loss is not a part of aging. They would like to keep their teeth and be able to chew their food properly. Their dental restorations and appliances may have been placed many years prior and may need to be repaired or replaced. Routine dental appointments will assist in identifying concerns. Talk with the patients in this age group to help problem solve the life changes affecting their oral health. For example, arthritis may hamper adequate toothbrushing and flossing. The dental assistant may suggest to a patient with arthritis a larger, more pliable, handled toothbrush and a floss holder to ensure that a proper grasp can be accomplished.

Many of the patients in this group may be taking medications and need to understand what happens to their oral health when taking medications. The drug may cause the mouth to be dry and saliva is an aid in fighting the acidity of plaque. Patients may choose to suck on hard candy to overcome the dryness in the mouth. The patient may not think of the effect on the teeth, and decay may develop rapidly between check-ups.

Home Care

The patient has the ultimate responsibility of caring for his or her oral health at home. The dental assistant can suggest ideas that will make this task simpler to accomplish while still meeting the goal of having every section of every tooth cleaned every day. The dental assistant's goals should closely resemble the ideas that stimulated the patient's desire to meet these goals. These ideas, of course, will be different for each patient. If what the patient has been doing is working and he or she is not developing periodontal disease or dental decay, then acknowledge that he or she is doing a good job and encourage him or her to keep it up.

Patients should be made aware that the gingival tissue may be sore and may bleed when they first start a vigorous oral hygiene program. This means that the tissues are not healthy but will improve over time. It is much like the rest of the body. If a body is out of shape and an exercise program is started including sit ups, the abdominal area will be sore for a week or so until the area is in shape. The same is true for the gingival tissue. In about a week, the tissue will firm up and become more healthy if the patient maintains the program. The patient should be told to expect the soreness and bleeding for the first few days and not to stop because of it. He or she should be encouraged to continue the daily routine in order to maintain healthy gingival tissues and prevent decay.

Oral Hygiene Aids

A number of oral hygiene aids are on the market today for patient use. It is important to keep in mind that the more simple the task, the more chance of getting it accomplished. Adding a large number of steps will make it more difficult to accomplish the task daily. There are some aids that may help some patients. Suggestions for the proper aid will come from the dental team members. The dental assistant should stay abreast of the aids on the market and know how they can help specific patients.

Disclosing Agents. Most individuals are visual in their approach to life. Being able to see plaque makes it easier for the dental assistant to show what it is and how and when it should be removed. Disclosing agents have been around for a number of years and are used as a motivating factor in oral hygiene. The agent is a temporary coloration (normally red) that makes plaque visible. The disclosing agent comes in a tablet that can be chewed, a solution that the dental assistant can paint on the teeth, or a drop that can be placed on the tongue (Figure 2-4). The color will adhere to the plaque. Disclosing agents

PROCEDURE

2-1 Applying Disclosing Agent for Plaque Identification

The procedure is performed by the dental assistant or dental hygienist. During the hygiene appointment, disclosing would be done to identify plaque and its location for the patient and operator. In some offices, a record of plaque location is charted and referred to during future appointments. Means of removing the plaque then are discussed and demonstrated.

EQUIPMENT AND SUPPLIES

▶ Basic setup: mouth mirror, explorer, and cotton pliers

▶ Saliva ejector, evacuator tip (HVE), and air/water syringe tip

▶ Cotton rolls, cotton tip applicator, and gauze sponges

▶ Petroleum jelly (lubricant)

▶ Disclosing agent (liquid or tablet) and dappen dish

▶ Plaque chart and red pencil

PROCEDURE STEPS

1. The operator examines the oral cavity and reviews the health history.

2. The operator applies the petroleum jelly (lubricant) to the patient's lips (some dentists may want the petroleum jelly on any tooth-colored restorations to prevent staining).

3. The operator applies the liquid using the dappen dish and a cotton tip applicator. Each attainable surface of the teeth should be covered with the disclosing solution.

4. If using the tablet, the patient chews and swishes around for fifteen seconds.

5. The remaining solution is rinsed and evacuated from the area.

6. The patient uses a hand mirror to see the plaque and the operator uses a mouth mirror and an air/water syringe to identify and chart the plaque (Figure 2-5).

7. Demonstrate methods of brushing and flossing for plaque removal to the patient.

FIGURE 2-4 Examples of disclosing solutions (tablets and liquids).

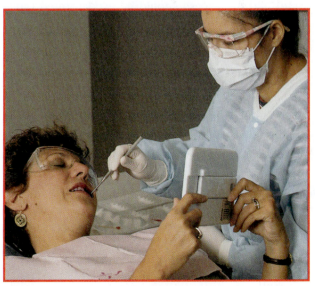

FIGURE 2-5 Dental assistant working with a patient to identify dental plaque. Disclosing agent on a patient's teeth identifying plaque.

can be used either in the dental office or at home to identify patients' plaque. The patient should be warned that the oral cavity will change color due to the use of the disclosing agent. Prior to use, it is advisable to place petroleum jelly on the lips to prevent the color from sticking to the tissue. The color will go away within thirty minutes, but the patient may not want it noticeable when he or she leaves the office.

Dentifrice. Dentifrice (**DEN**-ti-fris) is the toothpaste used along with brushing and flossing for patient oral hygiene self-care. As with all products used in the care of oral hygiene, use those that have been tested and approved by the American Dental Association. The ADA Seal of Acceptance will be located on the packaging if the American Dental Association, Council on Dental Therapeutics, has examined the product and classified it as such. The ADA can find products to be accepted, provisionally accepted, or unaccepted. The accepted classification is awarded to products that the ADA has found to be safe and effective for self-care. The provisionally accepted classification would be for products that the ADA has found to be safe but do not present clear evidence of dental usefulness. The unaccepted classification is for products that present questionable safety and no evidence of dental usefulness. These classifications are noted for three years.

Toothpaste is a product used by most individuals for dental care. It should be chosen carefully according to the abrasives, as well as caries control. The dentifrice (toothpaste) most often recommended is one that contains fluoride, especially for children and adults who are prone to caries. A small, pea-sized amount should be expelled onto the toothbrush for use. Toothpaste should not be ingested (because of the possibility of surplus fluoride) and the excess should be expectorated (spit) into the sink. A toothpaste with low abrasives is also recommended, due to the fact that extremely high abrasives can cause permanent damage to the patient's teeth with repeated use (they actually abrade the tooth structure). If a patient is prone to calculus (hard deposits mineralized on the teeth), there are toothpastes on the market that have ingredients in them that inhibit the growth of supragingival calculus. Other specialized toothpaste products whiten teeth or reduce gingival sensitivity if used routinely.

Mouth Rinses. Mouth rinses are used for cosmetic or therapeutic reasons. The advertisements may lead patients to believe that mouthwashes do more than is possible. Vigorous rinsing with mouthwashes may loosen debris and give the patient a pleasant taste, feel, and temporarily eliminate halitosis (bad breath). They can also reduce the total number of microorganisms in the mouth, but mouth rinses should not be used to replace brushing and flossing. The ADA has given approval to oral rinses that contain fluoride, which aid in reducing dental decay and supragingival plaque. Individuals using these rinses must follow manufacturer's directions. They are often not

recommended for use by small children due to the fact that, if swallowed, the fluids can cause harm.

Chewing Gum. Chewing gum designed specifically for oral hygiene purposes is a fairly new aid on the market. It is recommended for use after the intake of carbohydrates. The chewing of gum stimulates saliva that buffers the plaque acid and is said to have carious inhibition properties. The chewing action also helps dislodge particles from the teeth.

 Interdental Aids. Interdental aids are used to aid in cleaning the area between the teeth and to stimulate the gingival tissue in that area. In ancient oriental cultures, women would put spices between the teeth to have good breath. These women did not develop periodontal disease at the same rate as other individuals and it was found that the spices being placed and removed routinely cleaned the plaque in that area, therefore eliminating periodontal disease. In other early cultures, it was said that a "chew stick" was used to clean the interproximal areas of the teeth. It resembled the toothpick and, after the end was chewed, the small fibers spread out slightly. As it was inserted into the area between the teeth, it cleaned the opposing surfaces. Some individuals today use the toothpick in this manner and it is quite effective at removing plaque between the teeth. A number of other products are on the market for use today.

The interproximal brush is a hand-held, small brush with soft nylon bristles twisted in wire and adapted into a handle (Figure 2-6). It comes in different shapes and sizes and can be disposable. The brush is placed in the interproximal area and rotated back and forth using light pressure. Patients who have open contact areas or have a substantial amount of bone loss due to periodontal disease would benefit from the interproximal brush. This brush is also useful to individuals who have open bifurcation or trifurcation areas (where the roots of the teeth come together). It is also handy to use around orthodontic brackets to clean the difficult-to-access areas.

Rubber and wooden dental stimulators are placed into the interproximal area, angling them toward the occlusal (biting) surface and rotating them in a circular pattern. This action stimulates the soft tissues and removes plaque in this area. Many toothbrushes have a rubber stimulator at one end that can be used for this purpose (Figure 2-7). Wooden stimulators often come in

FIGURE 2-6 Interproximal brush.

FIGURE 2-7 Rubber tip stimulator.

FIGURE 2-8 Floss holder. *(Courtesy of Floss Aid Corporation)*

a pack much like a book of matches. These elongated, soft-wood wedges are first moistened before use. The wood, normally balsam, has a little give as it stimulates the tissue. Another type of wooden dental stimulator has a plastic handle device that holds a moistened toothpick tip to be utilized in the same manner as the rubber and wooden stimulators.

The floss holder is a Y-shaped device with a handle used by some individuals to hold the floss tightly as it is placed into the interproximal area of the teeth and then around the posterior of the last tooth in each quadrant (Figure 2-8). The floss holder makes flossing easier for individuals who have arthritis, poor manual dexterity, or hands that seem too large to allow access to the posterior teeth. The patient starts in one area and cleans the side of each tooth while rotating the floss holder around the arch and then in the same manner on the opposing arch. The floss holder is placed into each area and moved up and down on the sides of the tooth and into the sulcus area (space between the tooth and the gingival tissue) to remove plaque and clean the area.

The floss threader is used to remove the plaque and debris from under fixed bridges, orthodontic wires, and retainers (Figure 2-9). The floss threader comes in a variety of shapes and is made from stiff plastic and is designed like a needle with a large eye. The floss is threaded through the eye of the threader and the needle (stiff end) portion is then threaded through the intended area by the patient. Upon the floss reaching the opposite side, the floss threader can be removed, leaving the floss to clean this difficult-to-reach area. This allows the patient to direct the floss under the appliance and clean away the plaque and debris. After the entire area is cleaned, the floss can be removed. The area should be flossed daily using the threader to maintain proper oral hygiene.

A water irrigation device is used to clean away debris from orthodontic brackets and other prosthetic devices. It does not remove plaque and should not replace brushing and flossing. The pulsating water flow allows food debris to be removed easily and some patients place mouthwash in the fluid-holding container to gain fresh breath in the process. The patients should be instructed to use the water irrigation device carefully, because it can cause tissue damage if turned on high and directed toward the gingival sulcus (it could force debris into the tissue and damage the periodontium). It should be used at a lower speed and in a direction that forces debris to be pushed away from the gingival area.

Toothbrushing

Most patients use toothbrushes; however, many have never been shown proper techniques and the methods recommended today. The patients should be shown that the toothbrush only cleans three of the five surfaces of the tooth. The proximal (between the teeth) tooth surfaces normally are not accessible with a toothbrush. Patients have a variety of toothbrushes to select from today. Dental assistants need to stay informed of the current choices available so that they can answer the patients' questions appropriately. There are miscellaneous styles and designs of both manual and automatic toothbrushes on the market today. **Manual**

(A)

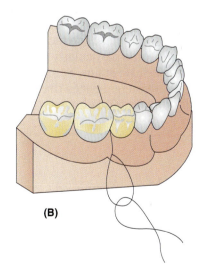

(B)

FIGURE 2-9 (A) Floss threader. (B) Floss threader threaded under the pontic area of a 3-unit bridge.

toothbrushes are powered by the human hand. **Automatic** toothbrushes are powered by electricity or batteries—The toothbrush itself does the moving while merely held by the individual. Automatic toothbrushes normally come with recharging units.

Correct toothbrush design is sized and shaped to allow for efficient cleaning and easy management. The toothbrush should be durable, inexpensive, and have bristles that are flexible and soft (normally polished on the end), allowing for repeated use. The handle must be firm and strong as well as lightweight. The choosing of a toothbrush is individual according to needs. Some adult patients will use a child's toothbrush to gain access to the teeth in the most posterior position in their mouths.

Manual Toothbrushes.
The parts of a manual toothbrush are the head, shank, and the handle (Figure 2-10). The bristles are placed on the head of the brush and can be multi-tufted or spaced and in a number of patterns. Normally, the handle, shank, and head are in a relatively straight plane. Nylon bristles are recommended because they maintain their form longer than natural bristles and they dry out quickly. The ends of the nylon bristles are often run over a flame to cause rounded ends that will not abrade the tooth. Soft bristles are recommended over medium and hard because they will not abrade the tooth or the gingival surface.

Automatic Toothbrushes.
Many patients use automatic toothbrushes (Figure 2-11). Like the manual toothbrushes, there are many available models on the market today. They have larger handles and chargers (the handles have to be larger to hold the rechargeable battery and circuit board). The heads of the automatic toothbrush can move in several different motions. Dental assistants need to be familiar with each kind of motion to be able to recommend the appropriate toothbrushing method for use with each motion. The motions can be reciprocating, orbital, vibratory, arcuate, elliptical, or a combination of two or more of these motions (Figure 2-12). The newer models also incorporate the sonic action that seems to be particularly effective in removing plaque and extrinsic stains. Some of the automatic units have built-in timing devices that allow thirty seconds for each of the four quadrants and stop when the

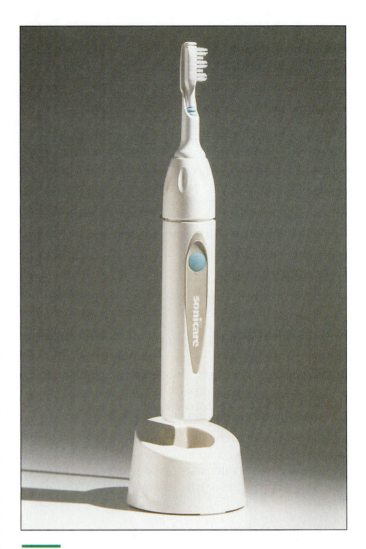

FIGURE 2-11 Automatic toothbrush. *(Courtesy of Sonicare)*

two minutes are completed. An automatic toothbrush can be used in place of a manual toothbrush. Care should be taken to apply light pressure and let the action of the bristles clean the teeth and gums.

Brushing Techniques for the Manual Toothbrush

There are several toothbrushing techniques that can be used to obtain proper oral hygiene. Any technique should allow for all the surfaces of all the teeth to be cleaned. Brushing will not clean the interproximal areas. Some patients will be successful in noting the amount of time spent on brushing by using a timer. Normally, two to three minutes is recommended to clean the facial, lingual, occlusal, and incisal surfaces of all the teeth. A pattern should be developed by the patient to ensure that no area is missed. Some patients like the counting system where five to ten strokes are made in each area. Starting at the same point each time when brushing is a good idea. The area could be the maxillary

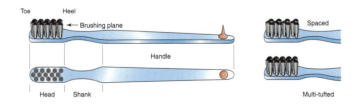

FIGURE 2-10 Manual toothbrush parts identified.

MOTION	ILLUSTRATION
Reciprocating motion– moves back and forth in a line	
Orbital motion– moves in a circle	
Vibratory motion– vibrates quickly back and forth	
Accurate motion– moves in an arc	
Elliptical motion– moves in an oval	

FIGURE 2-12 The motions of automatic toothbrushes.

(upper) right facial surface (cheek and lip side), then continue around the entire surface to the maxillary left. From that position, the lingual side (tongue side) of the arch can be cleaned from the left to the right. The mandibular (lower) teeth can be cleaned in the same manner starting from the right, continuing to the left, and then cleaning the lingual side from the left to the right. It does not matter what the pattern is; it only matters that no teeth are left uncleaned. The heel or the toe of the toothbrush can be used effectively on the more narrow anterior areas. There are five commonly used brushing techniques: Bass or modified Bass, Charters, Modified Stillman, Rolling Stroke, and the Modified Scrub. The Bass or modified Bass is the most popular in the dental community.

Bass or Modified Bass Brushing Technique. The Bass technique is named for Dr. C. Bass, a dentist who was an early advocate of preventive dentistry. The Bass brushing technique is used to remove plaque next to and directly beneath the gingival margin (Procedure 2-2).

Charters Brushing Technique. Charters brushing technique is used to loosen plaque and debris and to stimulate the gingiva, both the marginal and interdental (Procedure 2-3). The primary difference from the Bass technique is the angle of the toothbrush placement.

Modified Stillman Brushing Technique. The modified Stillman technique is designed to do a good overall cleaning, remove plaque, and stimulate and massage the gingiva (Procedure 2-4). Again, the bristles are placed in a different manner than either the Bass or the Charters technique. They are positioned so that the bristles point apically (toward the root of the tooth), with the toothbrush handle level with the biting surface of the tooth.

Rolling Stroke Brushing Technique. The rolling stroke is a method used to remove food debris and plaque from teeth and to stimulate the gingival tissue (Procedure 2-5). The brush is placed parallel to the tooth with the bristles pointed apically.

Modified Scrub. The modified scrub brushing technique uses a scrubbing motion to remove plaque and to stimulate the gingival tissue (Procedure 2-6).

Tongue Brushing

For centuries, individuals have known that it is important to clean the surface of the tongue. Bacteria can collect in the irregular dorsal (top) surface of the tongue. The daily ritual of oral hygiene historically included the scraping of the tongue with a tongue scraper (Figure 2-20). There are several different tongue cleaners on the market today. A conventional toothbrush is most often used to ensure cleaning of the tongue surface. The size of the toothbrush head may limit access to the posterior area of the tongue because it may initiate gagging. To clean the tongue, the toothbrush should be placed as far back as is comfortable and then drawn forward to the tip, allowing the bristles to clean the debris that has accumulated. Repeat this process until the entire tongue has been cleaned.

2-2 Bass or Modified Bass Brushing Technique

This procedure is explained to an individual in order to teach a toothbrushing technique.

EQUIPMENT AND SUPPLIES

▶ Toothbrush

PROCEDURE STEPS

Bass

1. Grasp the brush and place it so that the bristles are at a 45-degree angle, with the tips of the bristles directed straight into the gingival sulcus (Figure 2-13).

2. Using the tips of the bristles, vibrate back and forth with short, light strokes for a count of 10, allowing the tips of the bristle to enter the sulcus and cover the gingival margin.

3. Lift the brush and continue into the next area or group of teeth until all areas have been cleaned.

4. The toe bristles of the brush can be used to clean the lingual (tongue) anterior area in the arch.

Modified Bass

1. Follow all the steps of the Bass technique.

2. After the vibratory motion has been completed in each area, sweep the bristles over the crown of the tooth, toward the biting surface of the tooth.

FIGURE 2-13 The initial position of the toothbrush when using the Bass technique.

2-3 Charters Brushing Technique

This procedure is explained to an individual in order to teach a toothbrushing technique.

EQUIPMENT AND SUPPLIES

▶ Toothbrush

PROCEDURE STEPS

1. Grasp the brush and place it so that the back of the head is directed apically (toward the end of the root), with the bristles placed downward on the maxillary and upward on the mandibular (Figure 2-14).

2. The bristles should be placed over the gingival, where the tooth and gingiva meet.

3. Press the bristles into the space between the teeth.

4. Vibrate gently back and forth while maintaining the position. Count to 10.

5. Reposition and repeat the technique for each subsequent area.

6. For the anterior areas, hold the brush parallel to the teeth and use the sides of the toe bristles to clean the area. Count to 10.

Maxillary

FIGURE 2-14 The initial position of the toothbrush when using the Charters technique.

2-4 Modified Stillman Brushing Technique

This procedure is explained to an individual in order to teach a toothbrushing technique.

EQUIPMENT AND SUPPLIES

▶ Toothbrush

PROCEDURE STEPS

1. Place the toothbrush so that the bristles are pointing apically and the handle of the brush is level with the biting surface of the tooth (Figure 2-15).
2. Rotate the bristles downward and vibrate back and forth until the brush has rotated over the entire surface of the tooth (Figure 2-16). Do this motion slowly and count to 10.
3. Repeat this motion over the same area at least five times.
4. Continue until each area and every tooth have been cleaned in this manner.

Maxillary

FIGURE 2-15 The initial position of the toothbrush when using the Modified Stillman technique.

FIGURE 2-16 The brush stroke used with the Modified Stillman technique.

2-5 Rolling Stroke Brushing Technique

This procedure is explained to an individual in order to teach a toothbrushing technique.

EQUIPMENT AND SUPPLIES

▶ Toothbrush

PROCEDURE STEPS

1. Grasp the brush and place it parallel to the tooth so that the bristles are pointing apically, upward for the maxillary arch and downward for the mandibular arch, as was done in the modified Stillman method (Figure 2-17).
2. Firmly but gently press the bristles against the gingiva and roll them slowly over the tissue and the teeth, toward the biting surface (Figure 2-18).
3. Repeat this rolling stroke over the same surface a total of five times.
4. Move the brush to the next area and repeat the five rolling strokes.
5. Use the heel or the toe of the toothbrush to clean the lingual surfaces of the anterior teeth. The bristles

will still need to be pressed gently into the area and rolled toward the biting surface.

Maxillary

FIGURE 2-17 The initial position of the toothbrush when using the Rolling Stroke technique.

FIGURE 2-18 The brush stroke used with the Rolling Stroke technique.

2-6 Modified Scrub Brushing Technique

This procedure is explained to an individual in order to teach a toothbrushing technique.

EQUIPMENT AND SUPPLIES

▶ Toothbrush

PROCEDURE STEPS

1. Grasp the brush and place the bristles at a right angle to the tooth surface (Figure 2-19).

2. Use gentle but firm pressure and place the bristles over the area where the tooth and gingiva come together.

3. Activate the brush with back and forth scrubbing strokes.

4. Repeat this action throughout the mouth until all areas have been cleaned.

Maxillary

FIGURE 2-19 The initial position of the toothbrush when using the Modified Scrub technique.

FIGURE 2-20 Automatic tongue scraper. *(Courtesy of Oralgiene USA, Inc.)*

Flossing

Dental flossing is the second essential element of a good oral hygiene program and should be done daily. Dental floss has been shown to be the most effective way to remove bacterial plaque and other debris from otherwise inaccessible areas, the proximal surfaces of the teeth.

Types of Floss. Dental floss is available in several forms. The correct choice of floss should be determined according to the patients' manual skills, dental restorations, and preferences. Following the office philosophy, the dental assistant can make suggestions to the patient that will meet the patient's dental needs. Historically, patients have been advised to use unwaxed dental floss with small, individual filaments that aid in plaque removal as the floss is moved over the surface of each tooth. Some patients become frustrated while using unwaxed floss because it is thinner and more likely to shred or catch on old dental restorations, making it difficult to remove from the interproximal areas. These patients should be encouraged to use waxed, lightly waxed, or non-shredding dental floss. Waxed floss will slide over the surface with greater ease for patients who have tight contacts and roughened surfaces.

Dental floss also can be purchased in extra fine, larger flat tape, or even in a tufted texture that when tightened will change sizes. Some patients will be attracted to the different colors and flavors available on the market today. The colored and flavored floss does not perform better than the plain floss, but it may serve to motivate the patients to routinely use it. Daily flossing is more important than the type of floss that is used.

Hygienic Care of Prosthetic Devices

An individual may have prosthetic devices that require special oral hygiene care to obtain the desired plaque-free result each day. Professional knowledge and guidance will aid patients in the care of their prosthetic

P R O C E D U R E

2-7 Dental Flossing Technique

This procedure is explained to an individual in order to teach a dental flossing technique.

EQUIPMENT AND SUPPLIES

▶ Dental floss

PROCEDURE STEPS

1. Obtain the appropriate dental floss and dispense 18 inches in length.
2. Wrap the ends of the floss around the middle or ring finger as anchors (Figure 2-21).

FIGURE 2-21 Adapting floss to the fingers for use.

3. Grasp the floss between the thumb and index finger of each hand, allowing ½ to 1 inch to remain between the two hands (Figure 2-22).

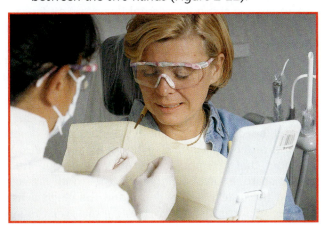

FIGURE 2-22 Floss adapted between fingers, prepared for use.

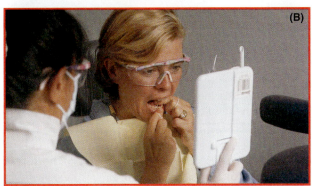

FIGURE 2-23 (A) Finger position on the floss for the maxillary arch. (B) Finger and thumb positions on the floss for the mandibular arch.

4. For the maxillary teeth, pass the floss over the two thumbs or a thumb and finger, and direct the floss upward (Figure 2-23A). For the mandibular teeth, pass the floss over the two index fingers and guide it downward (Figure 2-23B).
5. Direct the floss to pass gently between the teeth, using a sawing motion. Try not to snap the floss through the contacts because it may damage the interdental papilla (gingival point between teeth).
6. Curve the floss in a C-shape to wrap it around the tooth and allow access into the sulcus area (Figure 2-24). When a resistance is felt, it indicates that the bottom of the gingival sulcus has been reached.
7. Move the floss gently up and down the surface of the tooth to remove the plaque.
8. Lift slightly and wrap the floss in the opposite direction in a C-shape over the adjacent tooth.

(continued)

P R O C E D U R E   2 - 7   *continued*

9. Move the floss gently up and down the surface of this tooth prior to removing it from the area.

10. Rotate the floss on the fingers to allow for a fresh section to be used each time, and continue to clean between every tooth. It does not matter where an individual begins with floss, but it is best to proceed in a systematic method to ensure that no area is missed.

11. Use the dental floss around the distal surface of the most posterior tooth by wrapping it in a tight C-shape and moving it gently up and down with a firm pressure (Figure 2-25). Do the most posterior teeth in all four quadrants in the same manner.

FIGURE 2-24 Placing the dental floss around the tooth, wrapped into the sulcus.

FIGURE 2-25 Patient placing the dental floss around the last molar.

devices, such as fixed bridges, implants, orthodontic brackets, and full and partial dentures.

Fixed Bridge. A fixed bridge that is anchored on both sides with a pontic in the middle will not allow for normal flossing to be accomplished. The patient will need special instructions on how to use a floss threader (see information on floss threader) to remove the plaque and debris from under the bridge. The patient may also need special brushing instructions in order to clean the gingival area more carefully.

Implants. More and more patients have dental implants to replace their missing teeth. The implants are a great advancement in dental care. The long-term success of implants will be determined partially by the patients and how well they maintain the areas. Patients can use yarn in place of floss or a disposable elastomeric cleaning appliance and interproximal brushes to clean around the implants (Figure 2-26). A plastic scaler is used in the dental office to thoroughly clean and remove any calculus.

Full and Partial Dentures. All removable dentures and appliances should be carefully cleaned daily and rinsed following a meal or as needed. A denture brush is used to brush the appliance (Figure 2-27). It is a larger brush that can be utilized with toothpaste or a mild soap. A soft brush should be used on the tissue underneath the appliance to clean and to stimulate circulation in that area.

Commercial cleaning agents can be used for a denture on a daily basis. These chemical agents are used to remove stain and to help freshen breath. The dentures normally are immersed in solutions according to the manufacturer's directions and rinsed after the specified time has elapsed. The soaking solutions can be made at home with the following ingredients:

▶ Warm water (1 cup)

▶ Bleach (1 tsp.) (NOTE: The bleach should not be used with a partial denture as it may corrode the metal.)

▶ An anticorrosive agent (2 tsp.)

If calculus is heavy, a solution of 1 cup warm water with a teaspoon of vinegar can be used. These home solutions should be used only once a week.

Orthodontic Appliances. As stated earlier in the chapter, special oral hygiene techniques must be practiced in order to maintain orthodontic appliances. It is essential that the appliances be kept plaque free. If proper care is not maintained, the tooth structure around the brackets may decay and the gingival tissue will become irritated and virtually grow over the appliances. There are special orthodontic toothbrushes and aids that can be used (Figure 2-28A). The bristles of the brush are designed to allow contact with the orthodontic appliance while still achieving contact with the surface of the tooth. In special cases, an interproximal brush can be

FIGURE 2-26 Aids for dental hygiene around implant. (A) Proxi-Floss. (B) Proxi-Pic. *(Courtesy AIT Dental, Inc.)*

used to gain access to difficult areas. In addition to removing food and debris with a toothbrush and flossing, a water irrigation device also can be used for overall cleaning.

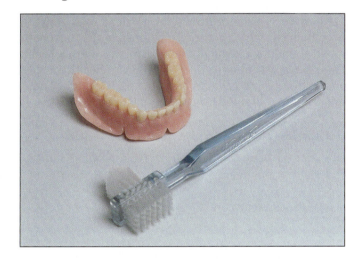

FIGURE 2-27 Denture and denture toothbrush.

FIGURE 2-28 (A) Orthodontic oral hygiene aids. (B) Brushing and flossing aids for patients who have difficulty.

Oral Hygiene for Patients with Special Needs

Dental assistants may be called upon to become creative to meet the oral hygiene needs of patients with special needs (Figure 2-28B). Patients who are mentally or physically compromised are often fed soft foods that lack the cleaning effects of normal foods. Devices can be developed to clean these patients' teeth. The dental assistants may need to show the caregiver how to clean the patient's teeth routinely. For example, putty can be wrapped over the handle of a toothbrush to allow the patient to grasp it more easily, or the handle may be extended with a tongue depressor or ruler so that the patient can reach his or her oral cavity. Keep the focus on the desired outcome and establish methods to meet these goals. A moist washcloth can be used to wipe the surfaces of the teeth, if necessary. Be creative in meeting the needs of the patients.

Pregnant Patients. Pregnant patients may require special dental hygiene techniques, due to the nausea that often accompanies pregnancy. Regurgitation will bring the acid from the stomach repeatedly over the surface of the teeth (this will also be a concern for patients with bulimia). Patients should be educated as to the possible destruction of the teeth from this repeated acid contacting the teeth. In addition, placing a toothbrush into the mouth may cause the patient to gag. Problem solve with the patient and find a way to meet the goal of proper oral hygiene. Normally, eliminating toothpaste and identifying specific times of the day when the pregnant patient is less nauseated allows toothbrushing and flossing to be made more comfortable during pregnancy. The dental assistant should tell the obstetrical patient that increased gingival bleeding is normal and that routine prophylaxis (cleaning) is recommended during pregnancy. Any dental treatment should be approved by the patient's physician.

Patients with Cancer. Patients with cancer may have a number of oral manifestations due to the cancer and the therapy. Loss of muscle function, gingival bleeding, rampant caries, and xerostomia (**zee**-roh-**STOH**-me-ah) may compromise skills of good oral hygiene. **Xerostomia** is abnormal dryness of the mouth and may be due to radiation or chemotherapy treatments. The patient may have a number of problems to overcome such as root caries. Home topical fluoride treatments are often suggested to help eliminate these problems. Listen and problem solve together with the patient. It will be important that infection does not perpetuate in the oral cavity and compound the patient's condition. The dental assistant may suggest that an extra-soft toothbrush or a moistened foam toothbrush be used on the tender tissues with a non-abrasive fluoride toothpaste. Maintaining the teeth and tissues will allow the patient to eat properly and regain a healthier state. Use empathy, encouragement, and sincerity to motivate the patient.

Patients with Heart Disease. Patients with heart disease may express a number of the same problems that cancer patients have due to medication usage. Many have xerostomia, gingival bleeding, and rampant caries. Patients with congestive heart disease will be uncomfortable in the chair if the chair is reclined (this brings increased fluid around the heart and the patient feels as if he or she is suffocating). Be aware of the patient's health status, address the problems that are identified, and aid the patient through education and understanding to seek a method to accomplish good oral hygiene.

Older Patients. Many older patients have arthritis and holding floss and a toothbrush is difficult. There are toothbrushes that have larger, soft handles that will help these patients. A floss holder can be used to secure the floss tightly as it is placed between the teeth. Listen to these patients and keep in mind that they want to save their teeth to be able to eat properly. Many are afraid of having dentures. The wonderful thing about older patients is that often they have the time available to listen carefully to oral hygiene directions and to ask questions to clarify what is required of them to meet their oral hygiene goals.

Additional Preventive Procedures Performed in the Dental Office

Other procedures that are performed in the dental office to aid patients in good oral hygiene are topical fluoride treatments and pit and fissure sealants (See Chapter 28, Advanced Chairside Functions, for further information).

▌FLUORIDE

Introduction to Fluoride

The use of fluoride in dentistry is based on the knowledge that when the fluoride content of the teeth is increased to the "optimum level," there is significant reduction in dental caries. Once, fluoride was thought to be beneficial only during tooth development years, but through further research fluoride has been proven to have additional benefits.

Fluoride is a natural mineral nutrient. It is derived from fluorine, which comes from fluospar, the thirteenth most abundant chemical element in the earth's crust. Fluoride is essential to the formation of healthy bones and teeth, just as calcium and phosphorous are. These minerals are obtained from water and certain foods.

Fluoride content in the bones and teeth.

▶ Normal bone contains 0.01 to 0.3 percent fluoride.
▶ Dental enamel contains 0.01 to 0.02 percent fluoride.
▶ Carious teeth contain as little as 0.0069 percent fluoride.

History of Fluoride in Dentistry

Early in the 1900s, Dr. G.V. Black and Dr. F. McKay of Colorado first revealed the fact that people with **mottled enamel** (discolorations) did not have as much dental decay. In the 1930s, a chemist found a definite relationship between fluoride and mottled enamel. Eventually, an "optimum" level of fluoride was found. This level prevents dental caries without mottling the teeth. The **optimum level** was found to be **1 part per million (1 ppm)**. In some climates, this level may be adjusted slightly. For example, in hot climates where people are likely to drink more water, the level may be reduced.

Fluoridation

Fluoridation is the process of adding fluoride to the water supply. The first city to test the benefits of fluoride through fluoridation was Grand Rapids, Michigan. In 1945, 1 ppm fluoride was added to the water supply. Several other cities also fluoridated their water supplies when it was proven that dental caries in Michigan were reduced by approximately 60 percent. Since then, numerous cities have added fluoride to their water supplies.

Adding fluoride to community water supplies is a very controversial issue in many areas. It has been proven that adjusting the amount of fluoride to the optimum level does reduce dental caries, but there are some people who oppose fluoridation. Much has been written about the fluoride controversy and dental assistants need to stay up-to-date on what is going on in their communities. Knowing whether the water is fluoridated, the benefits of fluoridation, and the effects of too much fluoride will better prepare the assistant to answer patients' questions.

Effects of Fluoride

Fluoride is a natural substance needed for the development of healthy teeth and bones. It is absorbed almost entirely through the blood stream from the gastrointestinal tract. Fluorides also are absorbed through the lungs, as in industrial settings where people have occupational exposure to fluorine.

Once fluoride is absorbed by the body and deposited in the bones and teeth, the remaining fluoride is excreted. The developing child requires more fluoride than a forty-year-old person and so the body adjusts the amount and excretes the excess fluoride.

Tooth Development

When the fluoride reaches the tooth, it replaces part of the tooth structure called the **hydroxyl ion**. The hydroxyl ion is on the surface of the apatite crystal in the enamel. The new tooth structure that is formed is called a **fluoropatite crystal**.

Fluoride affects the tooth both before and after the tooth has erupted into the oral cavity. During the **pre-eruption stage**, the fluoride ion replaces the hydroxyl

ion when the teeth are calcifying. Fluoride is supplied from drinking water, some foods, and fluoride tablets or drops. It is during this stage that excessive amounts of fluoride may disturb the normal pattern of development. This condition is known as **fluorosis**, or mottled enamel (Figure 2-29).

Children who are given prescribed doses of fluoride at birth and continue receiving fluoride during the development of both the deciduous and permanent teeth benefit the most in reducing the number of dental caries.

During the **post-eruption stage**, the absorption rate of fluoride is the highest just after the tooth has erupted; then, it tapers off as the enamel matures. The absorption is also affected by the amount of fluoride exposure. Once the teeth have erupted, they receive fluoride through the blood stream and also through exposure in the oral cavity to fluoride in toothpastes, tablets, gels, and rinses.

Fluoride in Dental Plaque

Fluoride in dental plaque has been found to have a favorable effect. The amount of fluoride in the plaque is relative to the amount of fluoride exposure. Fluoride in the plaque is bound within bacteria. This condition causes an **antibacterial effect** that inhibits the production of acids responsible for dental decay.

Fluoride Toxicity

Fluoride, like many other substances, can be toxic when absorbed in excessive amounts. Today, fluorides are regulated carefully by occupational health legislation and governmental agencies. Over the years, it has been found that toxicity of fluoride depends on the duration and the dosage of ingestion. Fluoride used in dentistry presents little or no risk for acute toxicity. However, the dental assistant should be aware of the possibilities of fluoride poisoning and when and where it has occurred, because patients may have questions.

(A)

(B)

FIGURE 2-29 (A) Dental fluorosis and shade guide. (B) Post op completed veneers. *(Courtesy of Dr. Ola J. Englund, DDS, PS, Spokane, WA.)*

Dangers Associated with Fluoride Ingestion.
Acute fluoride poisoning is extremely rare. Large amounts of fluoride are ingested, inhaled, or absorbed into the body at one time. The lethal dose varies from *2.5 to 10 grams in adults* to as low as *0.25 grams in infants*. A medical doctor should be contacted any time excessive amounts of fluoride are ingested at one time.

Chronic fluoride poisoning is ingestion of high fluoride levels in the water or combinations of several fluoride sources over a period of time. Two effects of chronic fluoride overdose are crippling fluorosis (skeletal hypermineralization of ligaments) and mottled enamel. With today's health and safety controls in industry, crippling fluorosis can be avoided. Mottled enamel is caused by excess exposure of fluoride during the time of tooth development. When the fluoride level is from 1.8 ppm to 2.0 ppm, the enamel shows varying degrees of white areas, brown lines, or **enamel hypoplasia**. Because high levels of fluoride occur naturally in some areas, mottled enamel would be more common unless the amount of fluoride is adjusted to the optimum level.

Mottled enamel is pitted because of a deficiency in the number of ameloblasts (enamel-forming cells) and chalky because of a lack of mineral deposits. See Table 2-1 for the appearance of teeth with varying degrees of mottled enamel.

Benefits of Fluoride

The dental health benefits of fluoride have been shown in numerous studies. The benefits are in proportion to the length of time an individual received fluoride and the amount of fluoride given. The primary benefit is the reduction of dental caries in both primary and permanent dentition, but there are also long-term effects with the reduction of need for extensive dental care and the time and cost of such care. Through the use of fluoride, primary teeth are not lost prematurely to decay. This results in less malocclusion in permanent dentition; therefore, the need for orthodontic treatment is reduced. There is also less permanent tooth loss at early ages.

Thus, adults require fewer bridges, partials, or dentures. Improved bone density can affect bone resorption and resistances to local factors. With stronger alveolar bone and less decay, the periodontal tissues stay healthier.

Forms of Fluorides Used in Dentistry

Fluorides are available for dental health care needs in two forms: **systemic fluoride** and **topical fluoride**. The fluoride compounds used in dentistry are **sodium fluoride**, **stannous fluoride**, and **acidulated phosphate fluoride**.

Systemic Fluoride. Systemic fluoride is ingested and then circulated through the body to the developing teeth. Sources of systemic fluoride include fluoridated water, foods with fluoride, fluoride tablets, and drops.

▶ Fluoridation—Fluoride may be added to the community or school water supply. The level of natural fluoride is evaluated in order to adjust water supplies to the optimum level prescribed for dental health.

▶ Foods such as meat, vegetables, cereals, and citrus fruits naturally contain small amounts of fluoride. Tea and fish have slightly higher amounts of fluoride.

▶ Tablets and drops—Require a prescription from a dentist or physician. They are prescribed from birth until the second permanent molar erupts. Vitamins with fluoride are also available.

▶ The ADA's Council on Dental Therapeutics recommends specific amounts of fluoride be prescribed according to the age and weight of the child.

▶ Studies have shown a 50 to 65 percent reduction in caries for patients who have received the optimum prescribed amount of fluoride during tooth development.

▶ Not all bottled water contains fluoride. Be sure to check the label if you want fluoride benefits and you rely on bottled water for your water supply.

The amount of natural fluoride in a water supply can be determined by tests done by laboratories and state and county agencies. In rural areas and cities without

TABLE 2-1 APPEARANCE OF TEETH WITH EXPOSURE TO FLUORIDE

Amount of Fluoride Exposure	Appearance of the Teeth
Exposure between 0.7 and 1.2 ppm—the optimum level depending on the temperature of the area	Teeth are white, opaque, and shiny without blemishes.
Exposure up to 1.8 ppm	The structure of the enamel is not affected, but chalky bands or flecks can be seen on the surface.
Exposure over 1.8 ppm	Chalky bands or flecks appear on the surface and the enamel structure is affected; this is known as **enamel hypocalcification**. The chalky bands and flecks discolor with time. With increased exposure to fluoride, the enamel may become cracked and pitted.

fluoridated water, children should receive topical fluoride. The dentist will assist the parents in determining the best methods and the amount of fluoride the child should receive for maximum benefit. It is important that the fluoride supplement be taken continuously during tooth development to be most effective.

Topical Fluoride

Topical fluoride is another method to make the tooth more resistant to demineralization and also to assist in the remineralization of decalcified areas. Because topical fluoride only penetrates the outer layer of the enamel, it is most effective if the tooth is cleaned prior to application. The cleaning can be accomplished by toothbrushing or a rubber-cup polish.

Topical fluoride is available for direct application in a variety of forms, such as gels, rinses, foams, and liquids. Polishing paste and dentifrice that are applied to the teeth also contain fluoride.

> **Dual benefit of chewing fluoride tablets.**
>
> If fluoride tablets are chewed before being swallowed, the teeth benefit both from topical and systemic fluoride applications.

Topical Fluoride Application in the Dental Office

For a child to achieve the most benefit when the drinking water supply is not fluoridated, topical fluoride is applied to clean teeth once or twice a year in the dental office. Using this method, caries can be reduced by 40 to 50 percent.

In the dental office, fluoride gels, foams, and rinses are commonly applied (Procedure 2-8). The gels and foam solutions are convenient to use and stay in the fluoride tray better. Fluorides come in many flavors and usually the dental office will have several for the patients to choose from. The dental assistant should read and follow the directions for the type of fluoride being applied to determine the length of application and helpful hints. The most common agents used are **2 percent sodium fluoride**, **8 percent stannous fluoride**, and **1.23 percent acidulated phosphofluoride**.

Advantages and Disadvantages of Fluoride Preparations

Neutral—2 Percent Sodium Fluoride Sodium fluoride solutions are relatively stable, have an agreeable taste, are non-irritating to soft tissue, and do not discolor the teeth or restorative materials. The disadvantage is that they must be used at one-week intervals for four weeks. Sodium fluoride solutions are applied after an initial prophylaxis of the crowns. The teeth are isolated and air dried and fluoride is applied for three minutes. The complete series is performed at ages three, seven, eleven, and thirteen.

8 Percent Stannous Fluoride The aqueous solution of 8 percent stannous fluoride is not stable and must be made up immediately before application. The 8 percent solution has a disagreeable taste, is astringent, causes gingival blanching, and causes discoloration of the teeth. This discoloration is due to the tin and not the fluoride.

1.23 Percent Acidulated Phosphate Fluoride (APF) APF solutions and gels are commonly preferred because of patient acceptability and greater uptake of the fluoride by the surface enamel of the tooth. They are not irritating to soft tissue, do not discolor teeth or restorative material, and are slightly astringent. They are stored in plastic containers because they become more acidic when stored in glass. The application procedure involves prophylaxis, isolation, and drying of teeth, then application of solution or gel for one or four minutes (both are available). The single application is repeated at either six- or twelve-month intervals. The choice of solution or gel is up to the individual practitioner, but gels appear to be more popular at this time.

The trays used with fluoride gels and foams come in a variety of materials and sizes (Figure 2-30). It is important to select a tray that covers all the erupted teeth and does not extend beyond the most posterior tooth. Some trays come with the maxillary and mandibular arches connected so they are placed at the same time. Others are individual for each arch, with the maxillary arch being slightly larger. Often, the trays are color coded for different sizes.

Fluoride Rinses

Fluoride rinses are available as a means of fluoride treatment. The fluoride comes in a liquid that is a higher concentration and, because it is easy to swallow, the patient must be reminded *not to swallow after rinsing.*

After the patient's teeth have been cleaned with a toothbrush or a rubber-cup polish, apply the fluoride

FIGURE 2-30 Variety of fluoride trays.

PROCEDURE

2-8 Fluoride Application

This procedure is performed by the dental assistant after the rubber-cup polish has been completed. In some states, the application of fluoride may be an expanded function.

EQUIPMENT AND SUPPLIES

▶ Basic setup: mouth mirror, explorer, and cotton pliers

▶ Saliva ejector, evacuator tip (HVE), air-water syringe tip

▶ Cotton rolls, gauze sponges

▶ Fluoride solution

▶ Appropriately sized trays

▶ Timer (for one or four minutes)

PROCEDURE STEPS (Follow aseptic procedures)

1. Seat the patient in an upright position, review health history, and confirm that he or she has not had allergic reactions to fluorides.
2. Explain the procedure to the patient. Inform the patient to try not to swallow the fluoride and show him or her how to use the saliva ejector.
3. Explain that for the fluoride to be most effective, he or she should not eat, drink, or rinse for thirty minutes after the fluoride treatment.
4. Select the trays and try them in the patient's mouth to ensure coverage of all the exposed teeth.
5. Place the fluoride gel or foam in the tray. The tray should be about one-third full.
6. Dry all the teeth with the air syringe. To keep the teeth dry while reaching for the tray, keep your finger in the patient's mouth and tell him or her to keep it open.
7. Place the tray over the dried teeth. The maxillary and mandibular arches can be done at the same time or individually (Figure 2-31).
8. Move the trays up and down to dispense the fluoride solution around the teeth.
9. Place the saliva ejector between the arches and have the patient close gently.
10. Set the timer for the designated amount of time.
11. When the timer goes off, remove the saliva ejector and the trays from the patient's mouth.
12. Quickly evacuate the mouth with the saliva ejector or the evacuator (HVE) completely to remove any excess fluoride.
13. Remind the patient not to eat, drink, or rinse for thirty minutes.
14. Make the chart entry, including the date, the fluoride solution applied, and any reactions.

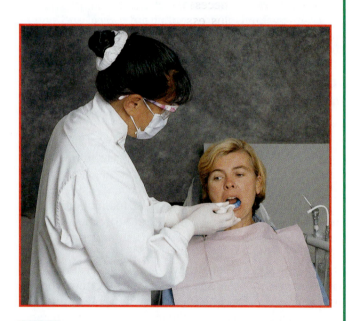

FIGURE 2-31 Dental assistant placing a loaded fluoride tray into the patient's mouth.

rinse. Follow the instructions for the individual rinse. Usually, the patient is directed to take half the dosage and then swish for a specific time (one minute). The patient then empties this amount and repeats with the second portion for the same amount of time.

Because of the taste of the fluoride, patients do not always look forward to the fluoride treatments. The dental assistant can be the motivating factor and set the stage for the patient's attitude. Children under six years of age should not use the fluoride rinses or mouthwashes because they may accidentally swallow them.

NUTRITION

To remain healthy, dental assistants must first be knowledgeable about **nutrition**, the manner in which foods are used to meet the body's needs. Dental assistants also need to be able to help patients with **diet**, the food that the individual actually eats. Many patients may have the meaning of the word diet confused with weight loss. Everything that is taken into the mouth is the diet. An **adequate diet** will meet all the individual's nutritional needs (Figure 2-32). People can eat large amounts of food and still be **undernourished**, or lacking the correct nutrients for the body. A disorder resulting from being undernourished is **malnutrition**. This is often seen in alcoholics who may experience malnutrition due to the intake of alcohol (they feel full and do not eat the food necessary for an adequate diet).

More than 50 percent of Americans are overnourished, leading to obesity and the diseases related to obesity. Americans are eating an abundance of fast foods that are high in fat content. Along with lack of exercise, the overall population gains a minimum of a half pound a year that is unnecessary.

Nutrients

Nutrients are defined as any chemical substance present in food that provides the body tissues and structures with the elements necessary for growth, maintenance, and repair. Forty-plus essential nutrients are required by the human body. These can be obtained from a diet that has foods from all the food groups. Having a variety of foods daily will help ensure that the essential nutrients are obtained and the body's **metabolism** is maintained. There are six broad classifications of nutrients: carbohydrates, fats, proteins, vitamins, minerals, and water.

Carbohydrates. Carbohydrates primarily come from fruits, grains, legumes (peas, beans, and lentils), and some vegetable roots. This group encompasses the sugars, starches, and fibers and provides quick energy to an individual. People in athletic events normally take in carbohydrates prior to the events to increase their energy levels.

The classification of carbohydrates is one that dental assistants will need to advise patients on because carbohydrates are potentially cariogenic. **Cariogenic** foods break down into simple sugars in the mouth and can be used by the bacteria to cause dental caries. Most patients will be aware that carbohydrates already broken down into simple sugars, such as candies, soft drinks, and sweet desserts, will cause decay. It will be the other carbohydrates that patients are unaware of that may cause decay, such as raisins, crackers, fruits, and a few vegetables. The intake of fruits and vegetables normally is not a problem because fruits and vegetables do not stick to the teeth and they are not converted to simple sugars until they reach the stomach.

Evaluating cariogenic foods in a patient's diet is accomplished by having the patient record his or her diet over several days. The dental assistant can review the diet and identify the cariogenic foods together with the patient. The assistant can discuss the texture of the foods and if they are retentive sugars, like caramels that remain in a concentrated sugar form on the tooth. The food could be a fruit with sugar, like an apple, which has a higher water content and provides some cleaning of the clinical portion of the tooth as it is eaten and then is washed away. Evaluation of each food in the patient's diet will provide a better understanding of which types of foods are cariogenic.

Other pertinent information the dental assistant can discuss with the patient is the number of times the cariogenic foods are being eaten, if they are eaten with other foods, and what time of day they are eaten.

One other factor in the equation of decay is that the more often the teeth are exposed to cariogenic food, the greater the probability of decay. For instance, the person who drinks a soft drink very slowly and allows the sugar to soak on the teeth over and over will have a greater chance of decay.

Eating cariogenic foods with other foods may offer some neutralization of the acid that feeds the bacteria. Eating cariogenic foods at bedtime, when the flow of saliva decreases, will increase the chance of decay. Saliva is a buffer to the acid and, if the flow rate of the saliva is inadequate, the washing away of cariogenic substances may not be accomplished.

Infants who have erupted teeth and are given bottles of milk, fruit juice, or sweet substances for long periods of time may develop **nursing bottle syndrome (NBS)**. This extensive decay of the newly formed teeth is due to the sweetened liquid frequently bathing the teeth, often at bedtime. Parents should be informed and advised of

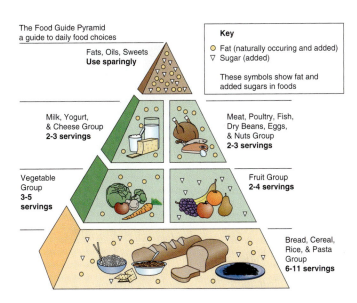

The Food Guide Pyramid
a guide to daily food choices

Key
○ Fat (naturally occuring and added)
▽ Sugar (added)

These symbols show fat and added sugars in foods

Fats, Oils, Sweets
Use sparingly

Milk, Yogurt,
& Cheese Group
2-3 servings

Meat, Poultry, Fish,
Dry Beans, Eggs,
& Nuts Group
2-3 servings

Vegetable
Group
**3-5
servings**

Fruit Group
2-4 servings

Bread, Cereal,
Rice, & Pasta
Group
6-11 servings

FIGURE 2-32 The Agriculture Department's new guide to a balanced diet takes the shape of a pyramid. *(Courtesy of U.S. Department of Agriculture)*

the possibility of NBS so that they can practice preventive measures.

Suggest to patients that they choose carbohydrates that will not remain on the teeth for great periods of time. Caution patients about medicines and mouth fresheners that have sugars in them because they dissolve in the mouth, bathing the teeth with sugar for a long period of time. These may cause a large number of caries if used over a period of time.

Fiber. Fiber is obtained from fruits, vegetables and grain food groups. It is suggested that 20 to 30 grams of fiber be eaten daily. Currently, an average of 15 grams or fewer are taken in by most Americans. Recent evidence has shown that consuming greater amounts of fiber can reduce the occurrence of colon cancer and reduce blood cholesterol levels. Increasing the levels of fiber should be done gradually to prevent unnecessary gastrointestinal problems, such as constipation.

Fats and Lipids

The classification of fats and lipids share one commonality: They are insoluble in water. The fats are derived from a solid and the lipids are the oil from a liquid. Fat provides an alternate source of energy to carbohydrates. It is often referred to as a backup source of energy. Fat also insulates the body from heat loss, protects vital organs, and aids in the transportation of fat-soluble vitamins: A, D, E, and K. There is widespread concern that Americans are consuming too much fat in their diets. The American Heart Association suggests that the diet contain 30 percent fat content but currently most Americans are consuming 40 to 45 percent fat in their diets. The excess fat has a direct correlation to cholesterol and heart disease, which is the number one cause of death of Americans over the age of forty.

Even though consumers know fat consumption is a problem, people are drawn to foods that have fat in them. Food manufacturers are aware that fat enhances the taste and smell of food. People need to read food labels and reduce the intake of fast-food products to reduce the fat in their diets.

Proteins

Found naturally in both plants and animals, protein is essential for the growth and repair of body tissue. One molecule of protein is composed of twenty different amino acids. The quality of a protein is determined by the distribution and kinds of amino acids in its structure. They are classified as "complete" if they have all ten essential amino acids and "incomplete" if they do not have all ten. Normally, animal proteins such as eggs, milk, and meat are complete and vegetable or grain proteins are incomplete. Incomplete proteins can be combined to make complete proteins if complementary foods are eaten at the same meal. For example, corn, an incomplete protein, can be eaten with beans, another incomplete protein, to make a complete protein. Macaroni with cheese, as well as cereal with milk, form complementary proteins.

Amino Acids. There are ten **essential amino acids** that the body cannot synthesize or produce in the needed amounts, so they must come from the individual's diet (Table 2-2). The non-essential amino acids can be produced or synthesized by the body.

Balancing Energy

Ideally, people should take in enough nutrition to equal the amount of energy used daily. The amount of energy that a substance is able to supply is measured in the form of **Calories**. One thousand kilo calories make up one Calorie. (When referring to a Calorie, always capitalize it or abbreviate it by using a capital C or Cal.) Carbohydrate and protein grams yield 4 Calories per gram, in contrast to 1 gram of fat that yields 9 Calories. For example:

▶ 5 grams of carbohydrates × 4 Calories = 20 Calories of carbohydrates

▶ 5 grams of proteins × 4 Calories = 20 Calories of protein

▶ 5 grams of fat × 9 Calories = 45 Calories of fat

The total of all three categories would be 85 total Calories. The fats are more energy rich than the carbohydrates or the proteins.

TABLE 2-2 ESSENTIAL AND NON-ESSENTIAL AMINO ACIDS

Essential Amino Acids	Nonessential Amino Acids
1. Arginine	Alanine
2. Histadine	Asparagine
3. Isoleucine	Aspartate
4. Leucine	Cysteine
5. Lysine	Glutamate
6. Methionine	Glutamine
7. Phenylalanine	Glycine
8. Threonine	Proline
9. Tryptophan	Serine
10. Valine	Tyrosine

The Calories are taken into the body to use as energy for everything from running to breathing. The body uses what it needs and the rest is stored as fat. The physical and chemical changes that take place in relationship to the usage of energy is called the **metabolism rate**. If the rate of metabolism is less than the consumed Calories, then the person will store fat; if the rate of metabolism is greater, the stored fat will be used.

The energy that is used when a person is at rest is called the **basal metabolic rate (BMR)**. The BMR will be higher for pregnant women, children, and leaner individuals because it takes more energy to fuel muscle than it does to store fat in the body. Optimum energy balance would include the same amount of Calories taken into the body as is used. Ideally, the majority of Calories would come from the carbohydrates. The fats and the proteins should make up less than half of the Calories taken in.

▎VITAMINS

Vitamins are a class of nutrients that do not provide the body with energy. Instead, they perform other necessary functions. *Vita* comes from the Latin word meaning life. The first vitamins were discovered by a group of scientists in 1913. They named the first vitamin A and the second vitamin B, the third C, and so on. Later, they found that Vitamin B was not one vitamin but several, so they added numbers to the letter B (e.g., Vitamin B1, B2, B3). Some of the other vitamins were given names, rather than letters or numbers. In the 1940s, a committee of scientists named the vitamins A, B, C, D, E, and K with number subscripts where applicable. All vitamins fall in one of two groups: fat soluble or water soluble.

Fat-Soluble Vitamins

The fat-soluble vitamins are vitamins A, D, E, and K. These vitamins are stored in the fatty cells, especially the liver, and they are not easily carried in the blood stream.

Vitamin A. Vitamin A has two forms: the plant form **carotene** and the animal form **retinol**. Vitamin A is essential for healthy skin and maintenance of mucous membranes and gives strength to the epithelial tissue (See Table 2-3). It aids in the continual reshaping of bone but is best known to help with the function of vision.

Vitamin D. Vitamin D can be manufactured by the body if exposed to ultraviolet rays (See Table 2-3). Dark-skinned individuals will require additional sun exposure to manufacture the same amount of Vitamin D. Individuals need Vitamin D to ensure healthy bones and good tooth development. Most milk is fortified with vitamins A and D.

Vitamin E. Vitamin E has been related to childbearing and aging. It helps nutrients by protecting them from destruction by oxidation. Scientific proof relating Vitamin E to the aging process has not been demonstrated, but many feel the vitamin is effective in conditioning the skin.

Vitamin K. The last fat-soluble vitamin is Vitamin K. It promotes the formation of **prothrombin**. Prothrombin is responsible for blood clotting and coagulation. A small amount of Vitamin K is stored in the liver.

Water-Soluble Vitamins

Vitamin C, probably the most famous of all, and the B complex vitamins fall into the group of water-soluble vitamins. The body maintains the balance of water-soluble vitamins through the function of the kidney. Any excess is excreted through the urine. Vitamin B_6 and niacin can be taken in too large of quantities and can become toxic because the kidneys cannot eliminate the surplus of these two vitamins as easily.

Vitamin C Ascorbic Acid. A large number of people take Vitamin C for everything from tooth aches to cancer (See Table 2-4). The tragic stories of individuals who developed scurvy (a disease resulting from Vitamin C deficiency) during long sea voyages, wars, and famines still carry over today. Vitamin C acts to hold cells together and is a constituent of connective tissue. Oral manifestations of Vitamin C deficiency include improper tooth development, ulcerated gums, and slow healing processes. It was discovered that citrus products prevented and treated this deficiency. Fruits and vegetables contain Vitamin C, especially citrus fruits and tomatoes.

Vitamin B Complex. Even though all the vitamins in the B classification are grouped together, they each have distinct functions (See Table 2-4). Vitamin B_1 (**thiamin**), Vitamin B_2 (**riboflavin**), and **niacin** work together in the production of energy, but they also have separate functions. For example, thiamin prevents cardiovascular changes and a disease called beri beri, riboflavin helps produce proteins and is essential in growth, and niacin prevents gastrointestinal and nervous system disturbances. Oral manifestations of Vitamin B deficiency include angular cheilosis (kee-**LOH**-sis), where lips become red and fissures develop in the corners of the mouth; glossitis (glos-**EYE**-tis), which is inflammation of the tongue and Pellagra, where mucous membranes atrophy and ulcers develop.

Vitamin B_6 is essential in the synthesis and metabolism of protein, carbohydrates, and fat. **Folic acid** and **Vitamin B_{12}** are important for the functioning of red blood cells and DNA. **Panothenic acid** and **biotin** aid in energy metabolism.

TABLE 2-3 FAT-SOLUBLE VITAMINS

Fat-Soluble Vitamins	Food Sources	Functions	Deficiency/Toxicity

Vitamin A (carotene or retinol)	Animal
	  Liver
	  Whole milk
	  Butter
	  Cream
	  Cod liver oil
	Plants
	  Dark green leafy
	    vegetables
	  Deep yellow or
	    orange fruit
	  Fortified margarine
		Dim light vision
		Maintenance of mucous
		  membranes
		Growth and develop-
		  ment of bones
		Healthy skin
			Deficiency
			  Night blindness
			  Xerophthalmia
			  Respiratory infections
			  Bone growth ceases
			Toxicity
			  Cessation of
			    menstruation
			  Joint pain
			  Stunted growth
			  Enlargement of liver

Vitamin D (cholecalciferol)	Animal
	  Eggs
	  Liver
	  Fortified milk
	Plants
	  None
		Bone growth
		Good tooth
		  development
			Deficiency
			  Rickets
			  Osteomalacia
			  Poorly developed
			    teeth
			  Muscle spasms
			Toxicity
			  Kidney stones
			  Calcification of soft
			    tissues

Vitamin E (alphatocopherol)	Animal
	  None
	Plant
	  Margarines
	  Salad dressing
		Antioxidant
		Skin conditioning
			Deficiency
			  Destruction of RBCs
			Toxicity
			  Hypertension

Vitamin K	Animal
	  Egg yolk
	  Liver
	  Milk
	Plant
	  Green leafy vegetables
	  Cabbage
		Blood clotting	Deficiency
			  Prolonged blood
			    clotting
			Toxicity
			  Hemolytic anemia
			  Jaundice

MINERALS

Major Minerals

Minerals are classified as either major or trace. A "major" classification indicates larger amounts. Minerals differ from vitamins in that they are singular elements rather than complex molecules. Some of the minerals are either positive or negatively charged and are referred to as **electrolytes**. When a person is in a healthy condition, the electrolytes are in balance.

Seven major minerals are in the body (see Table 2-5). **Calcium** (Ca) makes up the largest quantity and is found in bones and teeth. It also functions in muscle contraction, the nervous system, and the blood. **Phosphorus** (P) is found in bones and teeth and is involved in energy metabolism and maintenance of proper pH balance in the blood. **Sodium** (Na) and **potassium** (K) work together to regulate the electrolyte balance. Sodium maintains the fluid balance in the blood; potassium helps release energy and synthesize protein. **Sulfur** (S) is found in protein and is involved in energy metabolism. The last two major minerals are **magnesium** (Mg), which is involved in energy metabolism and stabilizing the components of the bones and teeth once they are formed, and **chlorine** (Cl), which maintains the correct pH balance in blood.

TABLE 2-4 WATER-SOLUBLE VITAMINS

Water-Soluble Vitamins	Food Sources	Functions	Deficiency/Toxicity

Vitamin C (ascorbic acid)	Fruits
	  All citrus
	Plants
	  Broccoli
	  Tomatoes
	  Brussel sprouts
	  Potatoes
		Prevention of scurvy
		Formation of collagen
		Healing of wounds
		Release of stress hormones
		Absorption of iron
			Deficiency
			  Scurvy
			  Muscle cramps
			  Ulcerated gums
			Toxicity
			  Raise uric acid level
			  Hemolytic anemia
			  Kidney stones
			  Rebound scurvy

Thiamin (Vitamin B_1)	Animal
	  Liver
	  Eggs
	  Fish
	  Pork
	  Beef
	Plants
	  Whole and enriched grains
	  Legumes
		Coenzyme in oxidation of glucose
		Prevention of beriberi
			Deficiency
			  Gastrointestinal tract, nervous and cardio-vascularsystem problems
			Toxicity
			  None

Riboflavin (Vitamin B_2)	Animal
	  Milk
	Plants
	  Green vegetables
	  Cereals
	  Enriched bread
		Aids release of energy from food
		Help produce proteins
		Aids in growth
			Deficiency
			  Angular cheilosis
			  Glossitis
			  Photophobia
			Toxicity
			  None

Pyridoxine (Vitamin B_6)	Animal
	  Pork
	  Milk
	  Eggs
	Plants
	  Whole-grain cereals
	  Legumes
		Synthesis of nonessential amino acids
		Conversion of tryptophan to niacin
		Antibody production
			Deficiency
			  Angular cheilosis
			  Glossitis
			Toxicity
			  Liver disease

Vitamin B_{12}	Animal
	  Seafood
	  Meat
	  Eggs
	  Milk
	Plants
	  None
		Synthesis of Red Blood Cells
		Maintenance of myelin sheaths
			Deficiency
			  Degeneration of myelin sheaths
			  Pernicious anemia
			Toxicity
			  None

Niacin (nicotinic acid)	Animal
	  Milk
	  Eggs
	  Fish
	  Poultry
		Transfers hydrogen atoms for synthesis of ATP
		Prevents gastrointestinal problems
		Prevents nervous system problems
			Deficiency
			  Pellagra
			Toxicity
			  Vasodilation of blood vessels

Folacin	Animal
	  None
	Plants
	  Spinach
	  Asparagus
	  Broccoli
	  Kidney beans
		Synthesis of Red Blood Cells	Deficiency
			  Glossitis
			  Macrocytic anemia
			Toxicity
			  None

(continued)

TABLE 2-4 *(continued)*

Water-Soluble Vitamins	Food Sources	Functions	Deficiency/Toxicity

Biotin	Animal
	    Milk
	    Liver
	Plants
	    Legumes
	    Mushrooms
		Coenzyme in carbohydrate
		    and amino acid
		    metabolism
		Niacin synthesis from
		    tryptophan
		Energy metabolism
			Deficiency
			    None
			Toxicity
			    None

Pantothenic acid	Animal
	    Eggs
	    Liver
	    Salmon
	    Yeast
	Plants
	    Mushrooms
	    Cauliflower
	    Peanuts
		Metabolism of carbo-
		    hydrates, lipids,
		    and proteins
		Synthesis of acetylcholine
		Energy metabolism
			Deficiency
			    None
			Toxicity
			    None

Trace Minerals

In smaller quantities yet as important as the major minerals are the group of trace minerals. **Copper**, **chromium**, **molybdenum**, **selenium**, and **manganese** are important to our bodies in the process of metabolism. **Iodine**, found in the thyroid gland, regulates metabolism of the body as well.

Iron primarily functions to carry the oxygen through the blood to the cells. A person who is deficient in iron becomes anemic, which reduces his or her energy level. Women tend to be more prone to this condition. **Zinc** aids in tissue growth and maintenance of the immune system. **Cobalt** helps in the functioning of red blood cells. **Fluorine** helps strengthen teeth and research also indicates that it aids in the prevention of osteoporosis (osteoporosis is a condition the elderly have in which calcium deficiency makes the bones weak and brittle).

WATER

Water, by far, is the most abundant nutrient in the body. Water makes up 60 to 70 percent of the total body weight. A turnover of 5 percent of total water each day is experienced by the average human adult. A person can go far longer without food than without water. In excessive heat, the body requires additional intake of water to prevent dehydration.

Water is used by the body in several ways, but the primary function is as a solvent for the biochemical reactions of the body to take place. For instance, a large part of the blood is composed of water and this allows for transportation and necessary reactions to occur. This solvent action also serves to remove toxic waste from the body. Water acts as a lubricant, especially in the digestive system and the joints. It also helps control the body temperature, releasing excessive heat through perspiration, and dispersing the heat evenly throughout the body.

The body does not store water and it must be replenished daily. It is lost primarily through perspiration, urination, and fecal output. Some water is obtained from foods eaten, but an additional eight glasses of water per day is recommended. It should be noted that coffee and alcohol cannot be counted as water intake; in fact, they act as **diuretics** and cause the body to lose water through increased urine output.

NUTRITION LABELS

In order for dental assistants to make good choices and be able to advise patients to do the same, it is essential that they be knowledgeable about the nutrition labels on food products (Figure 2-33). Information is provided on the label according to government standards. Manufacturers of food products know that people are attracted to words on the products like "lite" or "healthy." These titles may or may not correlate to the product inside, so it is important to read the details on the nutrition label. Information such as **preservatives** (the chemicals added to food to keep the contents fresh for a longer period of time) and artificial flavors and colors are indicated.

Listed Items on Labels. Standard information is listed on nutrition labels. The government requires that the labels be easy for the consumer to read, so nutri-

TABLE 2-5 **THE SEVEN MAJOR MINERALS AND THEIR FOOD SOURCES**

Name	Food Sources	Function	Deficiency/Toxicity

Calcium (Ca)	Milk exchanges
	  Milk, cheese
	Meat exchanges
	  Sardines
	  Salmon
	Vegetable exchanges
	  Green vegetables
		Development of bones and teeth
		Permeability of cell membranes
		Transmission of nerve impulses
		Blood clotting
		Muscle contraction
			Deficiency
			  Osteoporosis
			  Osteomalacia
			  Rickets

Phosphorus (P)	Milk exchanges
	  Milk, cheese
	Meat exchanges
	  Lean meat
		Development of bones and teeth
		Transfer of energy
		Component of phospholipids
		Maintain pH balance in the blood
			Same as calcium

Potassium (K)	Fruit exchanges
	  Oranges, bananas
	  Dried fruits
		Contraction of muscles
		Maintaining water balance
		Transmission of nerve impulses
		Carbohydrate and protein
		  metabolism
			Deficiency
			  Hypokalemia
			Toxicity
			  Hyperkalemia

Sodium (Na)	Table salt
	Meat exchanges
	  Beef, eggs
	Milk exchanges
	  Milk, cheese
		Maintaining fluid balance in blood
		Transmission of nerve impulses
		Works with potassium to regulate
		  fluid balance in the blood
			Toxicity
			  Increase in blood
			    pressure

Chlorine (Cl)	Table salt
	Meat exchanges
		Gastric acidity
		Regulation of osmotic pressure
		Activation of salivary amylase
		Energy metabolism
			Deficiency
			  Imbalance in gastric
			    acidity
			  Imbalance in blood pH

Magnesium (Mg)	Vegetable exchanges
	  Green vegetables
	Bread exchanges
	  Whole grains
		Energy metabolism
		Transmission of nerve impulses
		Activator of metabolic enzymes
		Relaxation of skeletal muscles	

Sulfur (S)	Meat exchanges
	  Eggs, poultry, fish
		Maintaining protein structure
		Formation of high-energy
		  compounds	

tional information is most often listed in a standard format. The 1990 Nutritional Labeling and Education Act was passed by Congress and enacted in 1994. This requires manufacturers to list all the ingredients in the product. Now, individuals who have special dietary needs can readily identify the ingredients and consumers can make comparisons from one product to another. The labels provide the serving size, percent of daily nutritional value, Calories, fat and cholesterol, sodium, carbohydrate, and other pertinent information on each label.

The **serving size** is listed on the label in a measurement or number of the product, for instance, ½ cup or 2 cookies for a cookie package. It will also give the total number of servings per package. The rest of the information is given on a single serving size.

The **ingredients** and the **percent of daily value** are also listed. The daily value percent is based on a diet of 2,000 calories per day for one individual. So, if the amount listed for total carbohydrate is 15 grams, this indicates that it is 5 percent of the daily value required according to the calculations for the carbohydrate group.

The total **Calories** per serving are noted along with the specific Calories derived from fat. The Calories from fat should total less than thirty percent of the total Calories. Remember that this is the Calories from one serving and not the entire package.

Fat and **cholesterol** notations are valuable to the consumer because of various health concerns, including heart disease and weight control. The listing on the sample label in Figure 2-33 breaks out the total fat as

Nutrition Facts
Serving Size: 1/2 Cup
Servings Per Container: 4

Amount Per Serving	
Calories 100 Calories from Fat 30	
	% Daily Value*
Total Fat 3g	5%
Saturated Fat 0g	0%
Cholesterol 0mg	0%
Sodium 340mg	14%
Total Carbohydrate 15g	5%
Dietary Fiber 1g	4%
Sugars 0g	
Protein 2g	

Vitamin A 0%	•	Vitamin C 0%
Calcium 0%	•	Iron 2%

*Percent Daily Values are based
on a 2,000 calorie diet. Your daily
values may be higher or lower
depending on your calorie needs:

	Calories	2,000	2,500
Total Fat	Less than	65g	80g
Sat Fat	Less than	20g	25g
Cholesterol	Less than	300mg	300mg
Sodium	Less than	2,400mg	2,400mg
Total Carbohydrate		300g	375g
Dietary Fiber		25g	30g

Calories per gram:
Fat 9 ∞ Carbohydrate 4 ∞ Protein 4

Ingredients: Flour, Water, Yeast
Vegetable Oil, Salt, Artificial
Flavor and Color.

FIGURE 2-33 Food label.

well as the saturated fat. The saturated fat primarily comes from animal sources while unsaturated fat primarily comes from vegetable sources. The total cholesterol content is also noted on the label for one serving.

Patients with heart disease or other diseases on sodium-restricted diets will want to watch the levels of **sodium** in foods. The total amount of sodium for one serving is listed on the nutritional label.

The total amount of **carbohydrates** is also listed. They may be broken down into dietary fiber (complex carbohydrates) or sugar (simple carbohydrates).

The nutritional labels will show other information, such as the protein, vitamins, and minerals included in the product.

Diet, Culture, Religion, and Group

 Dental assistants will come into contact with patients who come from a variety of cultural backgrounds. The patients may eat foods that are unfamiliar to the dental assistant. A dental assistant should be informed of patients' diet choices so that he or she can make suggestions that will aid them in better oral health (see Table 2-6).

TABLE 2-6   CULTURE, RELIGION, REGION, GROUP, DIET, AND FOOD CHOICES

Culture/Religion/ Region/Group	Diet and Food Choices
Native American	It is thought that approximately half of the edible plants commonly eaten in the United States today originated with the Native Americans. Examples are corn, potatoes, squash, cranberries, pumpkins, peppers, beans, wild rice, and cocoa beans. In addition, they used wild fruits, game, and fish. Foods were commonly prepared as soups and stews and dried. The original Native American diets were probably more nutritionally adequate than their current diets, which frequently consist of too high a proportion of sweet and salty, snack-type, empty-calorie foods. Native American diets today may be deficient in calcium, vitamins A and C, and riboflavin.
U.S. Southern	Hot breads such as corn bread and baking powder biscuits are common in the U.S. South because the wheat grown in the area does not make good quality yeast breads. Grits and rice are also popular carbohydrate foods. Favorite vegetables include sweet potatoes, squash, green beans, and lima beans. Green beans cooked with pork are commonly served. Watermelon, oranges, and peaches are popular fruits. Fried fish is served often, as are barbecued and stewed meats and poultry. There is a great deal of carbohydrate and fat in these diets and limited amounts of protein in some cases. Iron, calcium, and vitamins A and C may sometimes be deficient.
Mexican	Mexican food is a combination of Spanish and Native American foods. Beans, rice, chili peppers, tomatoes, and corn meal are favorites. Meat is often cooked

TABLE 2-6 *(continued)*

Culture/Religion/ Region/Group	Diet and Food Choices
	with the vegetable, as in chili con carne. Corn meal is used in a variety of ways to make tortillas and tamales, which serve as bread. The combination of beans and corn makes a complete protein. While tortillas filled with cheese (called enchiladas) provide some calcium, the use of milk should be encouraged. Additional green and yellow vegetables and Vitamin C-rich foods would also improve these diets.
Puerto Rican	Rice is the basic carbohydrate food in Puerto Rican diets. Vegetables commonly used include beans, plantains, tomatoes, and peppers. Bananas, pineapple, mangoes, and papayas are popular fruits. Favorite meats are chicken, beef, and pork. Milk is not used as much as would be desirable from the nutritional point of view.
Italian	Pastas with various tomato or fish sauces and cheese are popular Italian foods. Fish and highly seasoned foods are common to Southern Italian cuisine, while meat and root vegetables are common to northern Italy. The eggs, cheese, tomatoes, green vegetables, and fruits common to Italian diets provide excellent sources of many nutrients, but additional milk and meat would improve the diet.
Northern and Western European	Northern and Western European diets are similar to those of the U.S. Midwest, but with a greater use of dark breads, potatoes, and fish and fewer green vegetable salads. Beef and pork are popular, as are various cooked vegetables, breads, cakes, and dairy products.
Central European	Citizens of Central Europe obtain the greatest portion of their calories from potatoes and grain, especially rye and buckwheat. Pork is a popular meat. Cabbage cooked in many ways is a popular vegetable, as are carrots, onions, and turnips. Eggs and dairy products are used abundantly.
Middle Eastern	Grains, wheat, and rice provide energy in these diets. Chickpeas in the form of hummus are popular. Lamb and yogurt are commonly used, as are cabbage, grape leaves, eggplant, tomatoes, dates, olives, and figs. Black, very sweet (Turkish) coffee is a popular beverage.
Chinese	The Chinese diet is varied. Rice is the primary energy food and is used in place of bread. Foods are generally cut into small pieces. Vegetables are lightly cooked and the cooking water is saved for future use. Soybeans are used in many ways, and eggs and pork are commonly served. Soy sauce is extensively used, but it is very salty and could present a problem with patients on low-salt diets. Tea is a common beverage, but milk is not. This diet may be low in fat.
Japanese	Japanese diets include rice, soybean paste and curd, vegetables, fruits, and fish. Food is frequently served tempura style, which means fried. Soy sauce (shoyu) and tea are commonly used. Current Japanese diets have been greatly influenced by Western culture.
Southeast Asian	Many Indians are vegetarians who use eggs and dairy products. Rice, peas, and beans are frequently served. Spices, especially curry, are popular. Indian meals are not typically served in courses as Western meals are. They generally consist of one course with many dishes. Eating with one's fingers is considered acceptable.
Thailand, Vietnam, Laos, and Cambodia	Rice, curries, vegetables, and fruit are popular in Thailand, Vietnam, Laos, and Cambodia. Meat, chicken, and fish are used in small amounts. The wok (a deep, round fry pan) is used for sautéing many foods. A salty sauce made from fermented fish is commonly used.
Jewish	Interpretations of the Jewish dietary laws vary. Those who adhere to the Orthodox view consider tradition important and always observe the dietary laws.

TABLE 2-6   *(continued)*

Culture/Religion/Region/Group	Diet and Food Choices
	Foods prepared according to these laws are called *kosher.* Conservative Jews are inclined to observe the rules only at home. Reform Jews consider their dietary laws to be essentially ceremonial and so minimize their significance. Essentially the laws require the following: • Slaughtering must be done by a qualified person, in a prescribed manner. The meat or poultry must be drained of blood, first by severing the jugular vein and carotid artery, then by soaking in brine before cooking. • Meat or meat products may not be prepared with milk or milk products. • The dishes used in the preparation and serving of meat dishes must be kept separate from those used for dairy foods. • A specified time, six hours, must elapse between consumption of meat and milk. • The mouth must be rinsed after eating fish and before eating meat. • There are prescribed fast days—Passover Week, Yom Kippur, and Feast of Purim. • No cooking is done on the Sabbath—from sundown Friday to sundown Saturday. These laws forbid the eating of: • The flesh of animals without cloven (split) hooves or that do not chew their cuds • Hindquarters of any animal • Shellfish or fish without scales or fins • Fowl that are birds of prey • Creeping things and insects • Leavened (contains ingredients that cause it to rise) bread during the Passover Generally, the food served is rich. Fresh smoked and salted fish and chicken are popular, as are noodles, egg, and flour dishes. These diets can be deficient in fresh vegetables and milk.
Roman Catholic	Although the dietary restrictions of the Roman Catholic religion have been liberalized, meat is not allowed its adherents on Ash Wednesday and Fridays during Lent.
Eastern Orthodox	Followers of this religion include Christians from the Middle East, Russia, and Greece. Although interpretations of the dietary laws vary, meat, poultry, fish, and dairy products are restricted on Wednesdays and Fridays and during Lent and Advent.
Seventh Day Adventist	Generally, Seventh Day Adventists are ovolacto-vegetarians, which means they use milk products and eggs but no meat, fish, or poultry. They may also use nuts, legumes, and meat analogues (substitutes) made from soybeans. They consider coffee, tea, and alcohol to be harmful.
Mormon (Latter Day Saints)	The only dietary restriction observed by Mormons is the prohibition of coffee, tea, and alcoholic beverages.
Islamic	Adherents of Islam are called Muslims. Their dietary laws prohibit the use of pork and alcohol, and other meats must be slaughtered according to specific laws. During the month of Ramadan, Muslims do not eat or drink during daylight hours.
Hindu	To the Hindus, all life is sacred and small animals contain the souls of ancestors. Consequently, Hindus are usually vegetarians. They do not use eggs as they represent life.

TABLE 2-6 *(continued)*

Culture/Religion/ Region/Group	Diet and Food Choices
Vegetarian	There are several vegetarian diets. The common factor among them is that they do not include red meat. Some include eggs, some fish, some milk, and some even poultry. When carefully planned, these diets can be nutritious. They can contribute to a reduction of obesity, high blood pressure, heart disease, some cancers, and possibly diabetes. They must be carefully planned so they include all needed nutrients. Lacto-ovo vegetarians use dairy products and eggs but no meat, poultry, or fish. Lacto-vegetarians use dairy products but no meat, poultry, or eggs.
Vegan	Vegans avoid all animal foods. They use soybeans, chickpeas, and meat analogues made from soybeans. It is important that their meals be carefully planned to include appropriate combinations of the nonessential amino acids to provide the needed amino acids. For example, beans served with corn or rice, or peanuts eaten with wheat, are better in such combinations than any of them would be if eaten alone. Vegans can show deficiencies of calcium; zinc; vitamins A, D, and B_{12}; and, of course, proteins.
Zen Macrobiotic Diet	The macrobiotic diet is a system of ten diet plans developed from Zen Buddhism. Adherents progress from the lower number diet to the higher, gradually giving up foods in the following order: desserts, salads, fruits, animal foods, soups, and ultimately vegetables, until only cereals—usually brown rice—are consumed. Beverages are kept to a minimum and only organic foods are used. Foods are grouped as Yang (male) or Yin (female). A ratio of 5:1 Yang to Yin is considered important. Most macrobiotic diets are nutritionally inadequate. As the adherents give up foods according to plans, their diets become increasingly inadequate. These diets can be especially dangerous because avid adherents promise medical cures from the diets that cannot be attained, and so medical treatment may be delayed when needed.

CHAPTER SUMMARY

To be effective in preventive dentistry, the dental assistant must first care for his or her teeth properly and practice good nutrition. Becoming knowledgeable about the oral disease process will aid the dental assistant to educate the public how to prevent it. The dental assistant can then aid patients in maintaining their teeth and gums. In speaking with patients about their home care habits and nutrition, it is important to remember that the patients choose their habits for a variety of reasons including, work, student, parent, cultural, religious, or ethical beliefs. The goal of preventive dentistry is that each individual maintain optimum oral health.

CASE STUDY

Heidi Ann Jones, a seventeen-year-old, came to the dental office and was concerned with the discoloration of her teeth. After a thorough examination by the dentist, the findings showed that she had no caries, one restoration, and marginal gingivitis. What further information would be important to ask Heidi? What preventive techniques would be beneficial for Heidi?

(continued)

CASE STUDY (continued)

Case Study Review

1. Was Heidi given fluoride drops or pills during the development of the permanent teeth?

2. Was she raised in an area that had fluoridated water?

3. What oral hygiene aids and habits were used by Heidi in her daily routine?

4. Because Heidi is seeking information about her discolored teeth and not about the gingivitis, the operator first needs to make sure that Heidi also wants help with the gingivitis before proceeding with home care instruction.

5. Home care instructions should include toothbrushing and flossing appropriate for a seventeen-year-old.

 To complete your study of this chapter, work the review activities that follow. Also, refer to the software that accompanies this text.

REVIEW QUESTIONS

Multiple Choice

1. The most widely used brushing technique is the
   a. Stillman technique.
   b. Charters technique.
   c. Bass technique.
   d. Rolling Stroke technique.

2. What is the most effective way to remove bacterial plaque from the proximal surfaces of the teeth?
   a. Use of a toothbrush.
   b. Use of a tongue cleaner.
   c. Use of the interproximal brush.
   d. Use of dental floss.

3. What is the optimum level of fluoridation?
   a. 1 part per million.
   b. 5 parts per million.
   c. 10 parts per million.
   d. 25 parts per million.

4. Water-soluble vitamins are
   a. vitamins B_1, B_2, D, and niacin.
   b. vitamins D, E, K, and C.
   c. vitamins D, E, B, and K.
   d. vitamins B_1, B_2, C, and niacin.

5. The major minerals are calcium, phosphorus, potassium, sodium, chlorine, magnesium, and
   a. copper.
   b. sulfur.
   c. chromium.
   d. manganese.

Critical Thinking

1. If you have a choice of a hard candy or a candy bar, which one will be the most damaging to the teeth?
2. Can dental fluorosis occur on a permanent tooth after eruption into the mouth?
3. How can knowledge of nutrition be beneficial to the dental assistant?

General Anatomy and Physiology

OBJECTIVES

The student should strive to meet the following objectives and demonstrate an understanding of the facts and principles presented in this chapter:

1. List the body systems, body planes and directions, and cavities of the body, and describe the structure and function of the cell.

2. Explain the functions and divisions of the skeletal system, list the composition of the bone, and identify the types of joints.

3. List the functions and parts of the muscular system.

4. List the functions and the structure of the nervous system.

5. List the functions and the parts of the endocrine system.

6. Explain the dental concerns related to the reproductive system.

7. Explain the functions of the circulatory system and list and identify the parts.

8. Explain the functions and parts of the digestive system.

9. List the functions and parts of the respiratory system.

10. List the functions and parts of the lymphatic system and the immune system.

KEY TERMS

absorption process (p. 61)

alimentary canal (p. 61)

alveoli (p. 63)

articulations (p. 52)

atria (p. 59)

bronchioles (p. 63)

cancellous bone (p. 51)

cartilage (p. 52)

chyme (p. 61)

dorsal cavity (p. 50)

endocardium (p. 59)

epiglottis (p. 61)

hemostasis (p. 60)

homeostasis (p. 51)

laryngopharynx (p. 63)

myelin sheath (p. 55)

myocardium (p. 59)

nasopharynx (p. 63)

oropharynx (p. 63)

osteoblasts (p. 52)

osteoclast (p. 51)

pericardium (p. 59)

periosteum (p. 52)

ventral cavity (p. 50)

INTRODUCTION

In order to give the quality of care that each patient deserves, the dental assistant needs to be familiar with the terminology of body systems and how each system functions. **Anatomy** means the study of the body structure and **physiology** is the study of how the body functions. Both the anatomy and physiology of each body system will be briefly discussed.

Specific terms are used to establish a means for the health professional to communicate more effectively. Depending on the information and understanding needed, the human body can be studied on many different levels. The body is divided into systems, planes, cavities, and basic units. This gives common references and terms for studying and communicating information about the human body.

Body Systems

There are ten systems of the body: skeletal, muscular, nervous, endocrine, reproductive, circulatory, digestive, respiratory, lymphatic, and immune. Information about each system is presented according to its relationship with dentistry. Refer to Table 3-1 for a list of the systems and their major functions.

Refer to Table 3-2 for terms commonly used to describe areas of the body. The dental assistant will use these terms in many circumstances. For example: When discussing radiographic images, an abscess that shows on the radiograph may be mesial and superior to the root, or an abnormal lesion may be found on the dorsal surface of the tongue.

Body Planes and Directions

The body is divided into three primary planes (Figure 3-1). The **sagittal plane** divides the body into left and right halves. If the sagittal plane divided the body into equal left and right halves, it would be referred to as the **mid-sagittal plane**. The plane that divides the body into upper and lower sections is known as the **transverse plane**, sometimes called the **horizontal plane**. The **frontal plane** divides the body into front and back

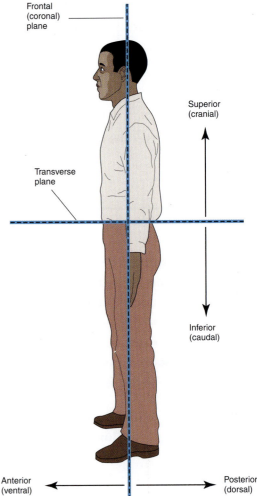

FIGURE 3-1 Body planes and directions.

TABLE 3-1 **BODY SYSTEMS**

System	Function
Skeletal	Provides the basic framework of the body; protects, shapes, and gives support to the body; source of attachment for muscles; stores minerals and manufactures blood cells.
Muscular	Muscles contract and relax to allow external body movement and production of the body's heat; internal muscles work to move food along the digestive track and keep the heart beating.
Nervous	Provides a communication system for the body; response to both internal and external stimuli.
Endocrine	Controls growth; stimulates sexual development; regulates use of calcium; aids in regulating the body's water balance; produces insulin.
Reproductive	Produces new life.
Circulatory	Carries life-sustaining substances, such as nutrients and oxygen, throughout the body; carries away waste materials; maintains a balance between intracellular and extracellular fluids.
Digestive	Takes food in, breaks it down and converts it to substances the body needs to sustain life; provides a means for the body to eliminate solid wastes.
Respiratory	Brings oxygen into the body, which is transported to all cells; the waste product, carbon dioxide, is picked up and exhaled.
Lymphatic	Provides nutrients; drains body fluids and absorbs fats.
Immune	Protects the body from disease and harmful substances.

TABLE 3-2 **TERMS TO DESCRIBE AREAS OF THE BODY**

Term	Definition	Example
Anterior	In front of; in the front of the body or body section.	The eye is anterior to the ear.
Ventral	On the front.	The belly or abdominal area of the body is on the ventral side of the body.
Posterior	In back or behind; in the back of the body or body section.	The ear is posterior to the nose.
Dorsal	On the back.	The dorsal surface is on the back of the body or organ.
Medial	Toward the middle of the body; the medial is closest to the midline.	The midline or median line divides the body into left and right halves.
Mesial	Toward the midline of the body (primarily used in dentistry).	The surface of a tooth that faces the median line is the mesial surface.
Lateral	Toward the outside or away from the midline that divides the body.	The ear is located on the lateral surface of the head.
Distal	Away from the midline of the body or body section.	The hand is the distal portion of the arm. In dentistry, the surface of a tooth that faces away from the median line is the distal surface.
Proximal	Refers to the part of the body closest to the point of attachment.	The thigh is the proximal surface of the leg.
Inferior	Below or under.	The mouth is inferior to the nose.
Superior	Above or higher.	The eyes are superior to the mouth.

sections. This vertical division divides the body into a front section, called the ventral or anterior, and a back section, referred to as the dorsal or posterior.

Body Cavities

Body cavities are spaces or areas within the body where various structures and organs are found. The body cavities are divided into two sections: the dorsal and the ventral.

The dorsal cavity is in the posterior portion of the body and contains two parts: the **spinal canal**, which contains the spinal cord, and the **cranial cavity**, which contains the brain. These two occupy one continuous space.

The ventral cavity is in the anterior portion of the body and contains three main parts: the **thoracic cavity**, **abdominal cavity**, and **pelvic cavity.** These cavities contain organs that maintain the basic life processes. The thoracic cavity or chest cavity contains the lungs, the heart, and all accessory parts needed for their functioning. The abdominal cavity is divided into upper and lower sections. The upper cavity is called the abdominal and includes most of the digestive tract and supporting organs needed for the process of digestion. The lower portion is called the pelvic cavity and contains the urinary bladder, the rectum, and the reproductive system (Figure 3-2).

Basic Structure and Functions of the Cells

The **cell** is the basic unit of all systems and the smallest functioning unit of the body (Figure 3-3). Cells differ in appearance, function, and structure according to what

FIGURE 3-3 Basic cell structures identified.

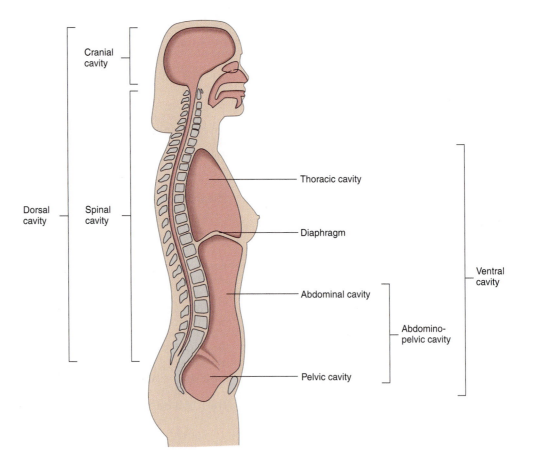

FIGURE 3-2 View of major body cavities.

they do. Specialized groups of cells form **tissues** and tissues group together to form **organs**. Tissues and organs unite to form **systems**. These cells, tissues, organs, and systems all function together to maintain harmony within the body, which is called homeostasis (**hoh**-me-o-**STAY**-sis).

SKELETAL SYSTEM

Functions of the Skeletal System

The functions of the skeletal system include support for the body's framework and overall body shape. The skeleton provides a surface for muscles to attach to and protects the delicate organs of the body. Also, the skeletal system manufactures blood cells and stores minerals for use when they are needed. An example is calcium.

Divisions of the Skeletal System

The skeleton is divided into two main divisions: the axial skeleton and the appendicular skeleton. The **axial skeleton** includes bones of the cranium, face, spinal column, ribs, and sternum. It is the framework of the head and the trunk of the body. The **appendicular skeleton** is composed of the bones from the upper and lower extremities and includes the arms, hands, legs, feet, shoulders, and hips. Together, the two divisions total 206 bones in an adult skeleton (Figure 3-4A and B).

Composition of the Bones

The bone or **osseous tissue** is composed of connective tissue. This connective tissue is rendered hard by the deposits of mineral salts. The bone tissue is 20 percent water; of the remaining 80 percent, two-thirds is minerals and inorganic matter and one-third is organic matter, including blood cells, lymphatic vessels, and nerves.

There are two types of bone tissue: cancellous or spongy bone and compact or dense bone. The cancellous bone has a sponge-like appearance and is not as strong as compact bone. Cancellous bone is found in the ends of long bones and in the middles of other bones. The **compact bone** is the strong and hard section of the bone. Compact bone is dense and forms the main shaft of long bones and the outer layer of other bones. Osteoclast cells are found in the compact bone. When bone is damaged or stressed, the osteoclasts dissolve and reabsorb the calcium salts of the bone matrix. The compact bone is covered with a layer of tough, fibrous tissue

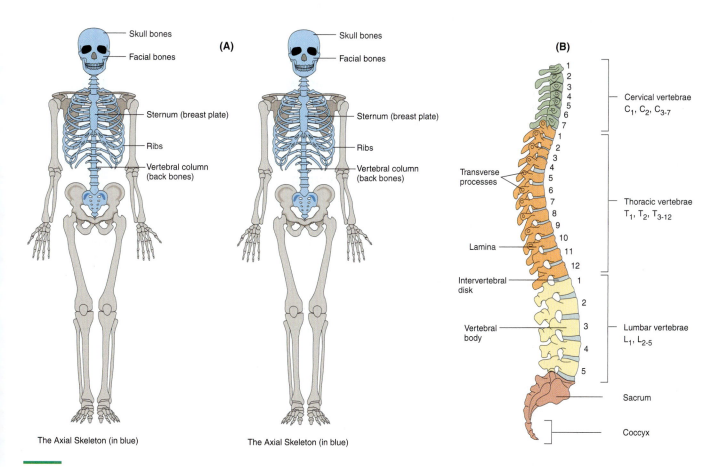

The Axial Skeleton (in blue)   The Axial Skeleton (in blue)

FIGURE 3-4 (A) Divisions of the skeletal system include the axial skeleton and the appendicular skeleton. (B) The five sections of the vertebral column.

called the periosteum. The periosteum contains blood and lymph vessels, bone-building cells called osteoblasts, and nerve tissue.

Inside the spaces of the cancellous bone is **red bone marrow**. Red marrow is filled with blood vessels and small amounts of connective tissue. Red bone marrow manufactures red and white blood cells and platelets. It is found in the ends of long bones and the middles of other bones. **Yellow bone marrow** contains mainly fat cells and is found in the center shafts of long bones. As the body ages, the active red bone marrow is slowly replaced with yellow bone marrow (Figure 3-5).

Cartilage is found where bones join together and also forms part of structures such as the nose and ears. It is a tough, non-vascular, resilient connective tissue.

Types of Joints

Joints or **articulations** are areas where two or more bones meet or form a junction. A joint is usually composed of fibrous connective tissue and cartilage. Table 3-3 illustrates the three types of joints, explains how they are divided, and gives an example of each.

Synovial joints provide movement and make up most of the joints in the body (Figure 3-6).

> The skeletal system contains the cranium and the facial bones, including the maxilla and the mandible. These bones support the teeth and surrounding tissues and are the primary focus of dentistry. Conditions of the skeletal system may alter patient treatment. The knowledge of this system aids dental assistants in correct patient positioning and movement at the dental unit, as well as sound ergonomic principles for themselves.

Diseases and Conditions of the Skeletal System

Diseases of the bone include:

▶ **Osteomyelitis** (**oss**-tee-oh-**my**-eh-**LYE**-tis)—an infection of the bone-forming tissue. There is inflammation, edema, and circulatory congestion in the bone

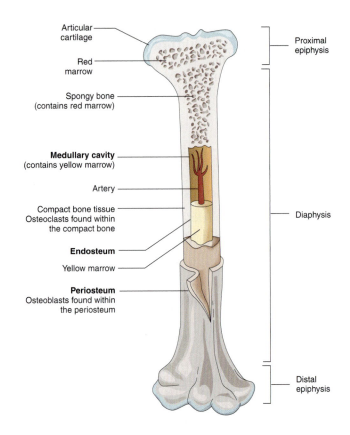

FIGURE 3-5 Anatomic features of the bone.

marrow. Pus may form and inflammatory pressure may cause small pieces of bone to fracture.

▶ **Osteoporosis**—the loss of bony material, thus leaving the bones brittle and soft.

▶ **Cleft palate**—the failure of the palate to form and join correctly.

▶ **Fractures**—breaks of the bone or cartilage.

▶ **Temporomandibular joint**—degeneration or disease of the joint where the mandible articulates with the temporal bone.

TABLE 3-3 **JOINTS**

Name of Joint	Description of Joint	Type of Movement	Example
Fibrous joint	Fibrous connective tissue	Immovable or fixed	Sutures found between the bones of the cranium.
Cartilaginous joint	Connective tissue, cartilage	Slightly movable	Joints found between bones of the vertebrae.
Synovial joint	Fluid within the joint (synovial fluid)	Considerable or free movement	There are six types of synovial joints: ball and socket, hinge, pivot, gliding, saddle, and condyloid. The temporomandibular joint is a synovial joint.

FIGURE 3-6 (A) Structures of a synovial joint and several examples of synovial joints. (B) Ball and socket joint of the hip. (C) Hinge joint of the elbow. (D) Hinge joint of the knee.

MUSCULAR SYSTEM

Functions of the Muscular System

The muscular system makes up 30 to 40 percent of the body's total weight. The muscles contract and relax to provide for all movements of the body, both internally and externally. Internal muscles move food along the digestive track and keep the heart beating. External muscles allow the body to walk, run, stand up straight, and communicate. Muscles also produce the body's heat.

Types of Muscles

There are three types of muscle tissue: striated, cardiac, and smooth. To study these muscle tissues, look at their locations, appearances, and functions (Figure 3-7).

Striated Muscles. Made up of long, thin cells that have stripes or bands across them. These muscles are in

bunches of fibers that attach to the skeleton, thus they are sometimes called skeletal muscles. This type has the largest amount of muscle tissue of the three types and its function is to provide for external body movement, from facial expression to riding a bike. The striated muscles are under voluntary control. They are the only group of muscles an individual has conscious control over and are sometimes called voluntary muscles.

Cardiac Muscles. Have the same striated or striped appearance as the striated muscles but are involuntary in action. Cardiac muscles are found only in the heart, where they receive approximately seventy-five stimuli per minute. These muscle cells are specially designed in a chain-like appearance and are able to receive an impulse and respond and relax very rapidly, thus keeping the heart beating in an even rhythm.

Smooth Muscles. Non-striated tissue. The smooth muscles are involuntary, which means they are under the autonomic nervous system and are not consciously

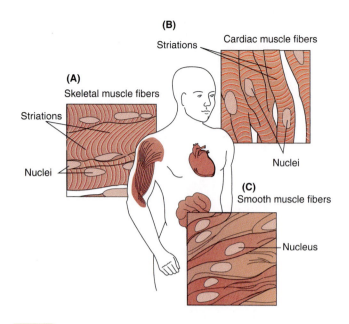

FIGURE 3-7 (A) Striated muscle. (B) Cardiac muscle. (C) Smooth muscle.

controlled. These muscles are found in internal organs (except the heart), blood vessels, skin, and ducts from glands.

Muscle Characteristics

Each muscle is made of cells in various shapes and sizes depending on its function. Groups of muscle cells are often called fibers. Each fiber is about the size of a human hair and can support 1,000 times its own weight. Humans have over a trillion fibers in over 600 muscles in their bodies. Each fiber has nerves and a supply of blood; it also has a fibrous sheet of connective tissue that covers, supports, and separates these muscle fibers. This sheet is called the **fascia**.

Muscle tissue has the capacity to respond to stimuli, called **excitability** or **irritability**. This response puts the muscle into motion or activity. **Extensibility** is the ability of the muscle to stretch or spread in order to perform tasks. **Muscle tone** is the tension of the muscular system. The brain and spinal cord continually send stimuli to the muscles on a subconscious level. The increase or decrease of the constant stimuli from the nervous system affects the muscle tone. When the muscles are used, they stay toned and ready in a healthy state, while muscles that are not used become flabby and begin to deteriorate.

Muscles work by **contracting** and **relaxing**. When muscles contract, they become shorter and thicker. When relaxed, they release and return to their normal form. There are two types of contractions: isometric and isotonic. **Isometric contraction** is when there is no change in the length of the muscle but the muscle ten-

sion is increased. Pushing against a solid object is an example of isometric contraction. Lifting weights is an example of **isotonic contractions**—the muscle tension remains the same but the muscles shorten.

Muscle Attachments

Skeletal muscles attach to the bone in a variety of ways. They may attach directly to the periosteum of the bone or they may attach through specialized connective tissue that extends beyond the muscle. When this extension is in the form of a cord, it is called a **tendon**. Tendons attach muscle to bone (Figure 3-8). Certain muscles require a broad, flattened extension called an **aponeurosis** (**ap**-oh-new-**ROH**-sis). Aponeurosis attaches muscle to bone and binds muscle to muscle. **Ligaments** are composed of bands or sheets of fibrous tissue and act to connect or support two or more bones.

The **origin** of the muscle is where the muscle attaches to the more stationary bone. The **insertion point** of the muscle is where the bone is moveable.

How Muscles Work and Function

Muscles contract and relax in order to provide movement. Most skeletal muscles function in **antagonistic pairs**. This means that while one set of muscle contracts, another corresponding set relaxes. The body moves and functions through these coordinated efforts.

It takes energy for muscles to work and function. Energy is received in the form of oxygen and glucose. Oxygen comes to the muscle through the circulating blood and glucose is stored as a substance called **glycogen**. Muscles go through chemical changes in order to provide energy for body functions. Sometimes, when the activity is too rapid, there is not enough oxygen and an incomplete breakdown of glycogen occurs, resulting in a waste product called **lactic acid**. When the activity stops, the normal metabolic process re-adjusts and sufficient oxygen is restored.

FIGURE 3-8 Muscle tissues and attachments of the arm.

Conditions and Diseases of the Muscular System

Conditions and diseases of the muscular system are numerous and varied. The following are a few examples.

▶ The muscle tissue can be **strained**, **sprained**, **cramped**, or **inflamed**.

▶ Sometimes the muscles go into **spasm**, which is a sudden, involuntary muscle contraction.

▶ If muscles are not used, they begin to deteriorate, known as **atrophy**.

▶ **Fibromyalgia** (**figh**-broh-my-**AL**-jee-ah) is chronic pain in the muscles and soft tissues surrounding the joints.

▶ **Muscular dystrophy** is a congenital disorder characterized by progressive degeneration of the skeletal muscles. It usually strikes early in childhood.

▶ **Myasthenia gravis** (my-as-**THEE**-nee-ah **GRAH**-vis) is an auto-immune disorder that leaves the muscles weak and fatigued. One of the first symptoms is a weakness in the facial or swallowing muscles.

NERVOUS SYSTEM

Functions of the Nervous System

The nervous system transmits stimuli from outside and inside the body; it is the body's communication system. It has the ability to respond and transmit stimuli to maintain the body's unity and harmony.

Structure of the Nervous System

The nervous system consists of three sections: brain, spinal cord, and nerve cells. The brain and the spinal cord make up the **central nervous system (CNS)**. All the nerves outside the central nervous system make up the **peripheral nervous system (PNS)**. There is also a specialized group of peripheral nerves that function mainly automatically; this group is called the **autonomic nervous system (ANS)**.

The basic structural unit of the nervous system is a **neuron** or **nerve cell**. The neuron structure includes a nucleus surrounded by a cell membrane with thread-like projections called nerve fibers. The nerve fibers that conduct impulses *toward* the cell body are called **dendrites**. **Axons** are nerve fibers that conduct impulses *away* from the cell body. Some dendrites and axons can be up to two feet in length. Nerve fibers move impulses from one to another through a **synapse**. This is a junction where chemicals are released from the ends of axons to allow the stimuli to jump to the next dendrite. Some nerves in the PNS are covered with layers of Schwann cells. These layers insulate and protect and are known as the myelin sheath (Figure 3-9).

Sensory neurons work together to carry messages from all over the body to the spinal cord and the brain. Neurons that carry a message away from the spinal cord and brain are **motor neurons**. Motor neurons carry messages that direct the body to act. A third type of neuron, **interneurons** or **associate neurons**, transmit impulses from sensory neurons to motor neurons within the central nervous system.

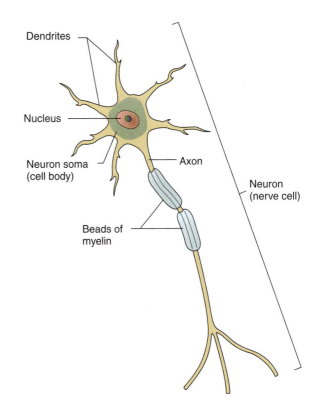

FIGURE 3-9 Structures of a neuron.

The Spinal Cord and Spinal Nerves

The spinal cord is a main part of the nervous system. The activity of the spinal cord is two-fold. First, it is a center for reflex or involuntary responses. **Reflex arc** occurs when a stimuli is sent through the sensory neurons into the spinal cord and a response is automatically processed and sent back through motor neurons for an action (Figure 3-10).

Second, the spinal cord transmits stimuli from the body to the brain, where the message is interpreted and then a response is sent back to an organ or a muscle.

There are thirty-one pairs of spinal nerves that come from the spinal cord. The nerves are named and numbered according to the closest vertebrae.

The Brain and the Cranial Nerves

The brain consists of many parts that all function together. The brain receives incoming stimuli and interprets and processes the information. Stimuli are directed to various parts of the brain, depending on what area of the body the stimuli is coming from.

There are twelve pairs of cranial nerves that mainly involve the head. They are numbered with Roman numerals beginning in the front of the brain and moving toward the back (Table 3-4).

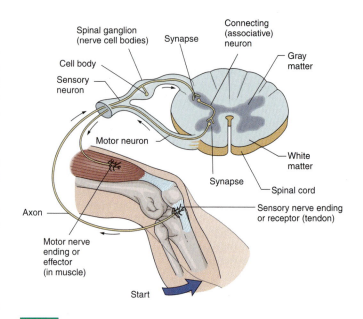

FIGURE 3-10 Simple reflex arc.

Importance to the Dental Assistant

Understanding the structure and how the nervous system works will help the dental assistant work with the dentist and the patient. Patients often fear going

TABLE 3-4 CRANIAL NERVES AND THEIR FUNCTIONS

I.	**Olfactory nerves** conduct impulses from receptors in the nose to the brain and are sensory in function.
II.	**Optic nerves** conduct impulses from receptors in the eyes to the brain and are sensory in function.
III.	**Oculomotor nerves** send motor impulses to four of the external eye muscles, as well as to certain internal eye muscles.
IV.	**Trochlear nerves** send motor impulses to one external eye muscle of each eye.
V.	**Trigeminal nerves** each divide into three branches: **Ophthalmic branches** go to the eyes and forehead. **Maxillary branches** go to the upper jaw. **Mandibular branches** go to the lower jaw.
VI.	**Abducens nerves** innervate the muscles that turn the eye to the side.
VII.	**Facial nerves** innervate the facial muscles, salivary glands, lacrimal glands, and the sensation of taste on the anterior two-thirds of the tongue.
VIII.	**Acoustic nerves** each divide into two branches. **Cochlear branches** are concerned with the sense of hearing. **Vestibular branches** are concerned with the sense of balance.
IX.	**Glossopharyngeal nerves** innervate the parotid glands, the sense of taste on the posterior third of the tongue, and part of the pharynx.
X.	**Vagus nerves** innervate part of the pharynx, larynx, and vocal cords and parts of the thoracic and abdominal viscera.
XI.	**Spinal accessory nerves** innervate the shoulder muscles. Some of the fibers of these nerves arise from the spinal cord.
XII.	**Hypoglossal nerves** primarily innervate the muscles concerned with movements of the tongue.

to the dentist because they assume that it will be a physically painful experience. Anesthesia blocks the patients' pain and makes the dental procedure possible. Dental assistants must know the nerves that are in the face and oral cavity to effectively assist the dentist during the administration of anesthetic, as well as during many types of surgical procedures. The dental team members sometimes experience physical problems themselves, especially with the sciatic nerve located in the lower back and traveling down the back of the thigh. This is due to the positions they must hold for long periods of time.

Diseases of the Nervous System

▶ **Neuritis** is the inflammation of nerves. It may be the result of a fall or blow and can affect one or more nerves within the body. The term neuritis is also used when describing degeneration of nerve tissue.

▶ **Multiple sclerosis (MS)** is a disease that usually appears in people twenty to forty years old. This disease destroys the myelin sheath of neurons in the central nervous system. When this happens, impulses are not able to transmit to their destinations.

▶ **Parkinson's disease** is a chronic nervous disease characterized by slowly spreading tremors, muscular weakness, and a peculiar gait.

▶ **Bell's Palsy** is a sudden onset of facial paralysis.

ENDOCRINE SYSTEM AND REPRODUCTIVE SYSTEM

Functions of the Endocrine System

The endocrine system, like the nervous system, is a controlling and communicating system. The nervous system acts rapidly to transmit stimuli, whereas the endocrine system is much slower and the results are longer lasting. The nervous system and the endocrine system are connected because the nervous system controls the pituitary gland and this gland controls the other glands. The endocrine system generally controls the body's growth, protects the body in stressful situations, stimulates sexual development, regulates utilization of calcium, aids in regulating the body's water balance, and produces insulin, which aids in the transport of glucose into cells (Table 3-5).

Parts of the Endocrine System

The endocrine system is made up of glands that are spread throughout the body (Figure 3-11). They are grouped together because of their structures and interrelated functions. These glands produce secretions and are ductless—There is not a tube for secretions from the glands to pass through, so the secretions empty directly into the blood stream and circulate throughout the body. These secretions are called **hormones**. Hormones are released from the endocrine glands.

Reproductive System

The reproductive system includes male and female reproduction organs. The male and female reproductive systems' main function is the creation of new life. In both sexes, primary and accessory organs must be protected in certain procedures used in dentistry. Two examples of procedures requiring protection are using a lead apron when exposing radiographs and providing adequate ventilation during nitrous oxide sedation. Safety guidelines are routinely followed in the dental office to protect the patient and the dental staff.

TABLE 3-5   MAJOR GLANDS OF THE ENDOCRINE SYSTEM

Name of Gland	Main Function(s)
Pituitary	Master gland that releases hormones that affect the workings of other glands.
Thyroid	Increases metabolic rate, which affects both mental and physical activities. Needed for normal growth.
Parathyroid	Increases the level of calcium in the blood. Regulates the calcium between bone and the blood.
Adrenal	Releases the *fight or flight* hormone, which increases heart rate and blood pressure and aids in the metabolism of carbohydrates, proteins, and fats during stress.
Pancreas (Islets of Langerhans)	Produces hormones, including insulin and glucagon.
Testes	Responsible for the development of male sexual characteristics.
Ovaries	Responsible for the development of female sexual characteristics.

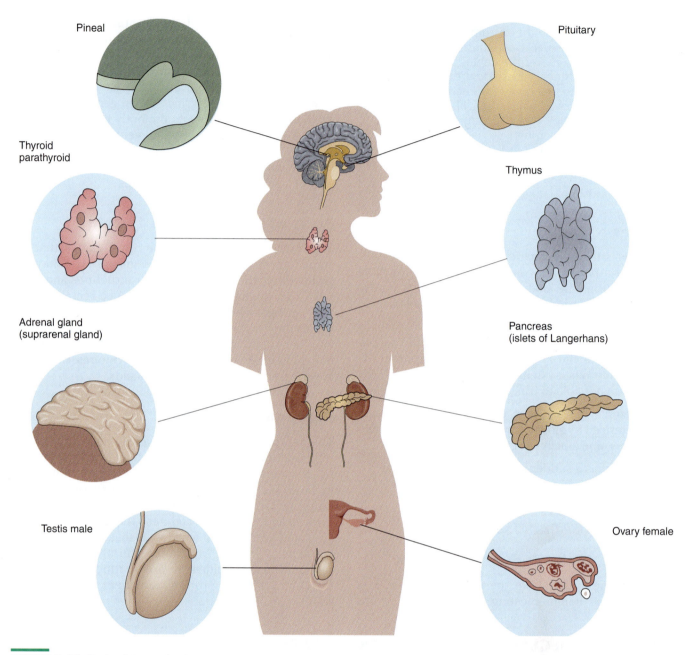

FIGURE 3-11 Parts of the endocrine system.

Importance to the Dental Assistant

There are diseases and conditions of the endocrine system, such as **diabetes**, that affect patients and how they respond to dental treatment. The dental assistant can prepare for possible emergencies and understand the patient's needs. With young patients going through puberty and older patients going through menopause, better communication and understanding will be enhanced by knowledge of this system. The dental assistant is responsible for knowing and following all precautions and standards regarding radiation and use of nitrous oxide in the dental examination room.

Diseases and Conditions of the Endocrine and Reproductive Systems

▶ **Diabetes mellitus** is a disease that occurs when the pancreas produces an insufficient amount of insulin.

▶ During **pregnancy**, dental treatments may need to be altered depending on the stage of pregnancy.

▶ **Hypothyroidism** is an underactive thyroid gland.

▶ **Hyperthyroidism** is an overactive thyroid gland with excessive secretion of hormones.

CIRCULATORY SYSTEM

Functions of the Circulatory System

The circulatory system is the body's means of transporting a continuous supply of oxygen, nutrients, hormones, and antibodies throughout the body while carbon dioxide and other cellular wastes are being removed from the body. This system maintains a balance between intracellular and extracellular fluids.

Parts of the Circulatory System

Circulation is divided into two pathways. The first pathway circulates blood through the heart to the lungs and back to the heart. This is **pulmonary circulation**. The second pathway, **systemic circulation**, carries the blood from the aorta to the smallest blood vessels and back to the heart (Figure 3-12). Main components of the circulatory system include the heart, the blood vessels (arteries, veins, and capillaries), and the blood.

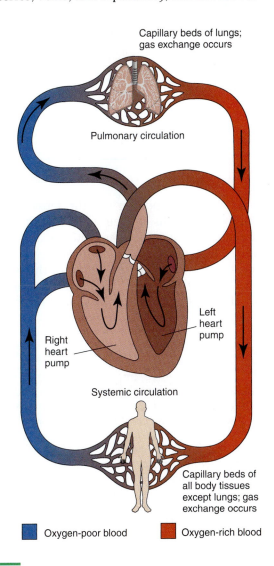

Capillary beds of lungs; gas exchange occurs

Pulmonary circulation

Right heart pump

Left heart pump

Systemic circulation

Capillary beds of all body tissues except lungs; gas exchange occurs

■ Oxygen-poor blood   ■ Oxygen-rich blood

FIGURE 3-12 Systemic and pulmonary circulation.

Heart. The **heart** is a pump that circulates the blood throughout the body. It is a triangular-shaped muscular organ that is approximately the size of a closed fist (Figure 3-13). The heart is covered with three layers: the **pericardium**, the outer layer that is composed of a double-walled sac; the **myocardium**, a tough, muscular wall; and the **endocardium**, a thin lining on the inside of the heart. A wall divides the heart into right and left halves. Each half is divided again into upper chambers called the **atria** or **auricles** and lower chambers called **ventricles**. There are four **valves** that regulate the flow of blood in one direction. The blood comes into the heart through large vessels called the **vena cava**. From the superior and inferior vena cava, the blood enters the right atrium, then is pumped through the **tricuspid valve** into the right ventricle. It then goes through the **pulmonary valve** into the pulmonary artery, which carries the blood to the lungs to get rid of waste and gases, and picks up fresh oxygen. From the lungs, the blood is carried by the pulmonary vein to the left atrium, then through the **mitral (bicuspid) valve** into the left ventricle and then through the **aortic valve** into the aorta to be distributed to all parts of the body (Figure 3-13).

Blood Vessels, Arteries, Veins, and Capillaries. The **arteries** carry oxygenated blood *from the heart to the capillaries* of the tissues. The walls of the arteries are tough and composed of three layers to withstand the pressure. The largest artery is the **aorta**, which receives blood directly from the heart; the **arterioles** are the smallest arteries.

The **veins** carry blood that has drained *from the capillaries back to the heart*. The walls of the veins are composed of three layers like the arteries, but they are much thinner and less muscular. Within the inner layer are folds that form valves that keep the blood flowing toward the heart.

The **capillaries** are the connection between the arteries and the veins. It is in the capillaries that the exchange is made between the blood and body cells. Here, oxygen and nutrients are delivered to the cells and carbon dioxide and wastes are removed. The walls of the capillaries are one thin layer, which is the extension of the lining of the arteries and veins. There are thousands of miles of connecting capillaries in the body.

Blood. The **blood** has three main functions: *transportation* of nutrients, gases, waste products, and hormones; *regulation* of the amount of body fluids, the pH balance, and the body temperature; and *protection* against pathogens and blood loss after injury through the clotting mechanism. Blood is a thick fluid that varies in color from bright red to a darker brownish red. The average adult has four to six quarts of blood. The liquid portion of the blood, **plasma**, is 91 percent water and carries nutrients, hormones, and wastes. The cells or solid portion of the blood are called **corpuscles**. There are three types of corpuscles: erythrocytes, leukocytes, and platelets.

FIGURE 3-13 Structures of the heart.

▶ **Erythrocytes** or *red blood cells* contain the protein **hemoglobin**, which gives the erythrocytes the ability to carry oxygen.

▶ **Leukocytes** or *white blood cells* protect the body from infection and disease. There are five types of leukocytes, all with specific tasks to defend the body against viruses, bacteria, or other foreign substances.

▶ **Thrombocytes** or *platelets* are fragments or pieces of cells that are necessary for the blood to clot (coagulate). The process by which the body controls bleeding is called **hemostasis**.

Blood Groups. There are five main classifications of blood type: A, AB, B, O, and ABO system. The ABO system is primarily used for blood transfusions. Refer to Table 3-6 for blood types, donors, and recipients. If a patient were to receive blood that was not compatible with his or her own blood type, the result could be fatal. Additionally, the **Rh factor** should be considered when treating patients who may require blood transfusions from a donor. Serious transfusion reactions could occur if the Rh factor is not matched. The Rh factor is also an important consideration during pregnancy; if the child is Rh positive and the mother is Rh negative, incom-

patibility between the mother and the fetus may result. People with the Rh antigen are Rh positive and those without are Rh negative. The mother may become sensitized by the blood of the Rh positive fetus. To prevent problems in future pregnancies, if the fetus is Rh positive, during the second trimester of the first pregnancy the mother is given Rhogam. Rhogam is an immunoglobulin.

Importance to the Dental Assistant

The circulatory system is important to the dental assistant as our population is aging and geriatric dentistry is growing. Understanding heart disease and the medications frequently prescribed will help the assistant to be alert for possible complications. Another consideration is to be prepared for an emergency—Dental treatment can present a stressful situation to an already compromised patient.

Diseases and Conditions of the Circulatory System

▶ **Bacterial endocarditis** is an inflammation of the lining of the heart. Patients who have histories of rheumatic

TABLE 3-6 BLOOD TYPES, DONORS, AND RECIPIENTS

Blood Group/ Type	Percent of Population	Antigen/ Agglutinogen on Red Blood Cells	Antibody/ Agglutinin in Plasma	Can Receive	Can Donate to
A	41	A	Anti-B	A or O only	A or AB only
B	12	B	Anti-A	B or O only	B or AB only
AB	3	A and B	None	A, B, AB, O Universal recipient	AB only
O	44	None	Anti-A and Anti-B	O only	A, B, AB, O Universal donor

fever, congenital heart disease, open-heart surgery, joint replacement, or dental implants should always be treated with antibiotics before dental treatment.

▶ A disorder called **hemophilia** is the failure of the blood to clot.

▶ **Leukemia** is a malignant, progressive disease of the blood-forming organs that is marked by unrestrained growth of abnormal leukocytes. Leukemia cells infiltrate the bone marrow and lymph tissue. These cells then advance to the blood stream and various body organs.

DIGESTIVE SYSTEM

Functions of the Digestive System

The digestive system provides a means for consumed food to be prepared for use by the body, circulated to all cells, and then the wastes eliminated. This is done by **digestion**, breaking down the food into small nutrient molecules that the cells can use. After food has gone through digestion, it is transferred into the blood stream; this is the **absorption process**. Here, the small nutrient molecules are circulated by the blood stream to all cells of the body. Another function of the digestive system is the process of **elimination**, which provides a means for the body to eliminate solid wastes.

Parts of the Digestive System

The digestive system is divided into two groups: the **alimentary canal** and **accessory organs**. The alimentary canal forms a canal or tube from the mouth to the anus. The canal includes the mouth (oral cavity), pharynx, esophagus, stomach, small intestine, and large intestine. The accessory organs aid in the process of digestion. Included are the teeth, tongue, salivary glands and ducts, liver, gallbladder, and pancreas (Figure 3-14).

Alimentary Canal

The **mouth (oral cavity)** receives food and begins the process of breaking the food down. The teeth, tongue, lips, cheeks, and salivary glands all work together to mechanically break food into small pieces and then move the food to the throat area.

The **pharynx** provides a connection from the oral cavity to the esophagus. It is where the food is swallowed. The pharynx also functions as part of the respiratory system. Therefore, sometimes during the process of swallowing, food may go into the larynx instead of the esophagus. To prevent this from occurring, the **epiglottis** (a small, leaf-shaped cartilage) covers the larynx. Swallowing is a complex, multi-stepped process that is controlled by the medulla part of the brain.

The **esophagus** extends from the pharynx to the stomach. Muscles help to keep food moving toward the stomach, even when the body is reclined. The lower esophageal sphincter (**SFINK**-ter) muscle, at the end of the esophagus, relaxes to allow food into the stomach and then contracts to prevent it from flowing backward.

The **stomach** is an organ that extends from the esophagus to the small intestine. It is located in the upper left area of the abdominal cavity and can expand to hold a half gallon of food. The stomach acts as a storage area and a churn to mix the food with gastric juices. Two components of gastric juices are hydrochloric acid and pepsin. These gastric juices are secreted by glands in the lining of the stomach. Then, the muscular movement of the walls mix food with gastric juices and break it down to a mixture called **chyme**. After about three hours, chyme leaves the stomach in spurts and enters the small intestine.

The **small intestine** connects the stomach to the large intestine. It is approximately twenty feet in length and one inch in diameter. The first section of the small intestine is called the **duodenum**. Here, other digestive juices enter and the breakdown process continues. In the walls of the small intestine are finger-like projections called

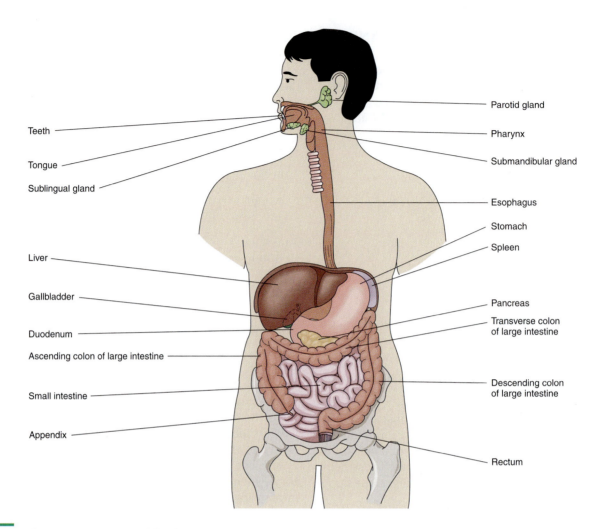

FIGURE 3-14 Major structures of the digestive system.

villi. Here, the digested food is absorbed into the blood stream.

The **large intestine** extends from the small intestine to the rectum. The large intestine is shorter in length, approximately five feet long, and one-half to two and one-half inches in diameter. The large intestine stores and excretes the waste products of digestion.

The Accessory Organs

The accessory organs each have specific functions, but each organ relies on the functions of the others in order to complete the digestive process.

▶ The **teeth** begin the digestive process by biting, tearing, and grinding the food.

▶ The **tongue** moves food from the anterior teeth to the posterior teeth and gathers the food before it is swallowed.

▶ The **salivary glands** produce saliva to dissolve food, facilitate the process of chewing (mastication), and coat food for ease in swallowing. There are three salivary glands that surround the mouth. More informa-

tion on the salivary glands is found in Chapter 4, Head and Neck Anatomy.

▶ The **liver** is the largest of the glandular organs and is located on the right side of the body, just below the diaphragm. The liver has many functions that aid in the digestive process, but the main function is the production of **bile**. Bile contains salts that emulsify fats.

▶ The **gallbladder** is a muscular sac that stores bile from the liver. It is located on the right side on the inferior surface of the liver.

▶ The **pancreas** produces pancreatic juices that are emptied into the duodenum to aid digestion and produce insulin.

Importance to the Dental Assistant

The digestive system begins with the oral cavity, which is the focus in dentistry. Knowing the components of this system and how each contributes to the processing of food will enable the dental assistant to detect disease and communicate with the patient.

Diseases and Conditions of the Digestive System

There are many diseases and conditions of the digestive system that directly relate to dentistry.

▶ **Tooth decay** is destruction of the tooth surface.

▶ **Periodontal disease** is inflammation and deterioration of the periodontal tissues.

▶ **Bulimia** is a disease in which individuals "purge" or vomit after eating large quantities of food. With time, the hydrochloric acid from the stomach, left in the oral cavity after vomiting, can cause serious dental problems for bulimic patients. The acid eventually dissolves tooth structure.

▶ **Hepatitis** is inflammation of the liver that is caused by several viruses. There are three main hepatitis viruses: Hepatitis A, Hepatitis B, and Hepatitis C. Hepatitis B is contracted by exposure to body fluids of infected individuals and is of the most concern because of the serious prognosis of the disease. More information is found in Chapter 8, Microbiology.

RESPIRATORY SYSTEM

Functions of the Respiratory System

Breathing is the main function of the respiratory system. Air is inhaled through the nose into the lungs, where it is absorbed into the blood system and carried to all cells of the body. Once the oxygen reaches the cells, it is exchanged for the waste product carbon dioxide. Carbon dioxide is then transported by the blood back to the lungs and exhaled.

Parts of the Respiratory System

The respiratory system consists of the nose, pharynx, larynx, trachea, bronchi, and lungs (Figure 3-15).

The **nose** is the passage for outside air to enter the body. The nose contains two **nasal cavities**, which are divided by the **nasal septum**. The inner surface of the nose is lined with **nasal mucosa**, which warms and humidifies the air as it passes through. The nose also contains the **olfactory receptors**, which facilitate the sense of smell.

The **pharynx**, or throat, serves as a passage for two systems: the respiratory and the digestive systems. Air and food pass through the pharynx as they move downward. This tube is about five inches long and is divided into three sections. The first is the nasopharynx, the upper section behind the nasal cavity. The **eustachian** (you-STAY-shun) (auditory) **tubes** open into the pharynx. The oropharynx (o-ro-FAIR-inks), the middle section, is the portion behind the mouth. It is lined with the same mucosa as found in the oral cavity. The lower section, the laryngopharynx (lah-ring-goh-FARE-inks), divides and has an opening in the front to the larynx and in the back to the esophagus.

The **larynx**, or voice box, connects the pharynx and the trachea. The larynx is made up of cartilage and is supported by muscles. At the upper end of the larynx is the leaf-shaped **epiglottis**. Its function is to close off the larynx during swallowing to prevent food from entering. The thyroid cartilage, or Adam's Apple, is a large cartilage that lies anterior to the larynx. In the interior of the larynx, the **vocal cords** stretch across the width of the larynx to produce sound.

The **trachea**, or windpipe, the next section of passage for air, is four to five inches long and extends to the lungs. The trachea consists of C-shaped cartilage, which allows for expansion of the esophagus during the process of swallowing. The trachea can become blocked by the inhalation of an object or from swelling.

The **bronchi** are the two branches that form at the end of the trachea and enter the lungs. The bronchi branches divide into smaller tubes called bronchioles. At the end of the bronchioles are **alveolar sacs**, which resemble clusters of grapes. These alveolar sacs consist of individual alveoli. It is here in the alveoli where the gaseous exchange takes place. The thin walls of the alveoli make for easy passage of air entering and leaving the blood capillaries.

The **lungs** are two cone-shaped organs located inside the rib cage. Each lung consists of a spongy mass that is pink at birth and then darkens to a blue-gray or black, depending on the air quality and personal habits. Each lung is surrounded by a sac called the **pleura**.

Respiration is the process of breathing and exchanging gases (oxygen and carbon dioxide) between the body and its environment. There are two phases to this process: inhalation and exhalation. During **inhalation**, muscles contract, the chest enlarges, and air flows into the lungs. **Exhalation** occurs when the muscles relax and the air is moved out of the lungs.

Importance to the Dental Assistant

The dental assistant should watch the patient for signs of discomfort or problems with breathing. Allergic reactions can and do occur in the dental office. A patient could choke on materials that fall to the back of the throat and respiratory diseases or conditions can make treatment difficult. Understanding the respiratory system could save a patient's life.

Diseases of the Respiratory System

▶ **Asthma** is the muscular spasm of the walls of the bronchi. The air passages are constricted so the person cannot exhale easily.

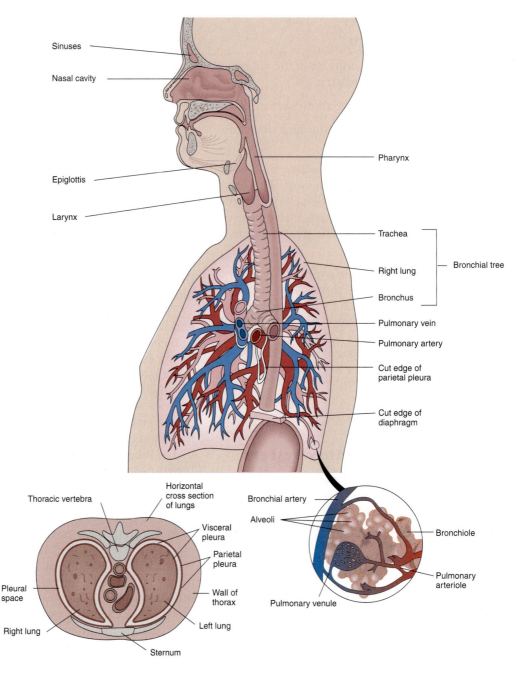

FIGURE 3-15 Structures of the respiratory system.

▶ **Tuberculosis** is a highly contagious disease of the respiratory system. Tuberculosis is transmitted by an individual breathing or swallowing droplets contaminated by the TB bacillus.

▶ **Lung cancer** is a malignancy of the lung tissue. It is a very common form of cancer and is often perpetuated by cigarette smoking.

▶ Other conditions include the common cold, pneumonia, and bronchitis, which affect the respiratory system. Following Standard Precautions will protect the office staff and the patient when treatment is required during times of infection.

LYMPHATIC SYSTEM AND IMMUNE SYSTEM

Functions of the Lymphatic System

The lymphatic system is a network of vessels that drains and filters the tissue fluid that surrounds cells.

Parts of the Lymphatic System

The parts of the lymphatic system include the lymph, the lymph vessels, the lymph nodes, the spleen, and the thymus gland (Figure 3-16).

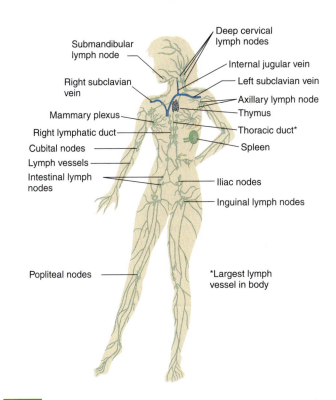

FIGURE 3-16 Parts of the lymphatic system.

Lymph, also called **tissue fluid**, is a clear liquid formed in tissue spaces. The lymph enters the lymphatic capillary system and drains away excess fluid and carries proteins back to the blood stream.

Lymph is transported through a specialized network of vessels called **lymphatic capillaries**. These capillaries are very thin walled and only allow lymph to travel in one direction on the way back to the general circulation system.

Lymph nodes are found in groups along the lymphatic vessels. They are small, round masses that vary in size and location. The lymph nodes most commonly known are the ones located in the armpit, neck, and groin. The purpose of the lymph nodes is to filter the lymph as it journeys back to the blood stream and to manufacture antibodies and other active materials of the immunity process.

The **spleen**, located behind the stomach, is protected by the rib cage. It is the largest lymphoid organ in the body and contains a very rich blood supply. If the spleen is damaged, it may have to be removed in order to stop the blood loss. As the blood moves through the spleen, it removes bacteria and other foreign materials, filters out old red blood cells, produces red blood cells before birth, and acts as a storage for blood in case of hemorrhage. Humans can live without the spleen because other lymphoid tissues take over its functions. However, without the spleen, the person may be more susceptible to certain bacterial infections.

The **thymus** is located under the sternum, just below the thyroid. It is large and active from before birth

through puberty, but then shrinks and almost disappears in an adult. The thymus gland is important to the development of our immune system.

Tonsils form a protective circle around the inside of the oral cavity. They consist of masses of lymphoid tissue that guard against bacteria that may enter the body through the digestive and respiratory systems. There are three groups of tonsils: the **palatine tonsils**, located on each side of the throat; the **lingual tonsils**, on the base of the tongue; and the **pharyngeal tonsils** (adenoids), located on the posterior wall of the nasopharynx area.

Functions of the Immune System

The immune system is part of the body's defense from harmful organisms. It protects from pathogens, foreign materials, debris, and damaged cells by removing these elements. The immune system is composed of specialized cells (phagocytes and lymphocytes) and molecules (antibodies and antigens). The system is organized into defenses that are nonspecific and specific. **Nonspecific immunity** is the body's defense against any harmful agents, while **specific immunity** acts against selected agents. The immune system involves organs or vessels from several other systems (Figure 3-17).

Importance of the Lymphatic and Immune Systems to the Dental Assistant

The dental assistant is constantly exposed to disease and infection. A large responsibility of each dental team member is to maintain a safe environment. Continuing education on prevention of and protection from health risks is necessary for all dental professionals.

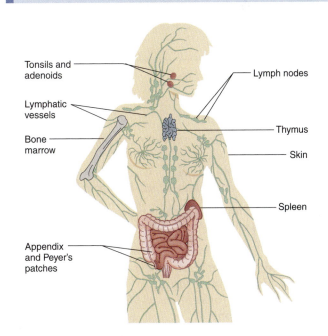

FIGURE 3-17 Organs and vessels from other body systems involved in the immune system.

Diseases and Conditions of the Lymphatic and Immune Systems

▶ **Tonsillitis** is a chronic infection of the tonsil tissue.

▶ **Hodgkin's disease** is a malignant disorder that causes enlargement of the lymph nodes.

▶ **Allergy** is a hypersensitivity to certain substances.

▶ **Cancer** is uncontrolled growth and spread of abnormal cells.

▶ **Immune Deficiency Disease** is a failure in some part of the immune system.

CHAPTER SUMMARY

Specific terms are used to establish a means for the health professional to communicate more effectively. Depending on the information and understanding needed, the human body can be studied on many different levels. The body is divided into systems, planes, cavities, and basic units. This gives common references and terms for studying and communicating information about the human body.

The dental assistant needs to be familiar with the terminology of body systems and how each system functions to give the quality of care each patient deserves. Both the anatomy and the physiology of each body system will need to be understood.

CASE STUDY

Charlie T. Smith is a twenty-three-year-old patient with a history of diabetes. The patient is in a reclined position in the dental chair. The dental assistant is placing a rubber dam clamp on a tooth when the clamp pops off and drops to the back of the patient's mouth. The patient swallows the clamp.

Case Study Review

1. List the body systems affected.

2. List the specific structures of the primary system that could become involved.

3. Would the patient's age or medical condition impact the situation?

 To complete your study of this chapter, work the review activities that follow. Also, refer to the software that accompanies this text.

REVIEW QUESTIONS

Multiple Choice

1. Which of the following divides the body into left and right halves?
   a. The horizontal plane.
   c. The sagittal plane.
   b. The transverse plane.
   d. The frontal plane.

2. The skeletal muscles are this type of muscle tissue:
   a. Striated muscle.
   c. Smooth muscle.
   b. Cardiac muscle.

3. The neurons that carry messages away from the spinal cord and brain are
   a. sensory neurons.
   c. associate neurons.
   b. motor neurons.
   d. interneurons.

4. All of the following are layers of the heart EXCEPT
   a. endocardium.
   c. pericardium.
   b. myocardium.
   d. intracardium.

5. The body system that drains and filters the tissue fluid around cells is the
   a. respiratory system.
   c. circulatory system.
   b. lymphatic system.
   d. immune system.

Critical Thinking

1. Name the synovial joint that is of significance to the dental assistant.

2. Explain why the pulmonary arteries are called arteries although they carry deoxygenated blood and the pulmonary veins are called veins although they carry oxygenated blood.

3. Why it is harder to replace lost blood in elderly patients?

Head and Neck Anatomy

OBJECTIVES

The student should strive to meet the following objectives and demonstrate an understanding of the facts and principles presented in this chapter:

1. List and identify the landmarks of the face and the oral cavity.

2. Identify the bones of the cranium and the face and identify the landmarks on the maxilla and the mandible.

3. List and identify the muscles of mastication, facial expression, the floor of the mouth, the tongue, the throat, the neck, and the shoulders. Explain their functions.

4. List and identify the nerves of the maxilla and the mandible.

5. Identify the arteries and veins of the head and the neck.

KEY TERMS

alveolar process
(p. 72)

buccal branch
(p. 80)

buccinator (p. 75)

common carotid
(p. 81)

ethmoid bone
(p. 71)

external jugular vein
(p. 83)

**external oblique
ridge** (p. 73)

**external pterygoid
muscles** (p. 74)

frena (p. 69)

**incisive nerve
branch** (p. 81)

incisive papilla
(p. 69)

**inferior alveolar
branch** (p. 80)

internal jugular vein
(p. 83)

**internal oblique
ridge** (p. 73)

**internal pterygoid
muscles** (p. 74)

labial commissures
(p. 68)

labio-mental groove
(p. 68)

lacrimal bones
(p. 72)

linea alba (p. 68)

lingual branch
(p. 80)

masseter muscles
(p. 74)

**mental nerve
branch** (p. 81)

mentalis
(p. 75)

oral vestibule
(p. 68)

papilla (p. 69)

parotid glands
(p. 70)

sphenoid bone
(p. 71)

Stensen's duct
(p. 68)

temporal muscles
(p. 74)

uvula (p. 69)

vermilion border
(p. 68)

Wharton's duct
(p. 70)

zygomatic bones
(p. 72)

INTRODUCTION

This chapter provides information on the anatomy of the head and neck. The dental assistant must be able to describe the anatomy, including the locations of the structures and their functions. Identifying the anatomy of the head, face, and neck in normal, healthy tissues will enable the dental assistant to recognize the abnormal.

LANDMARKS OF THE FACE AND ORAL CAVITY

Landmarks of the Face

The face has the following landmarks: ala of the nose, naso-labial groove, philtrum, vermilion border, vermilion zone, the tubercle of the lip, labial commissures, and the labio-mental grooves (Figure 4-1).

The **ala of the nose** is the wing of the nose or outer edge of the nostril. From the ala of the nose to the corners of the mouth is a groove called the **naso-labial groove**, or sulcus. Between the bottom of the nose and the middle of the upper lip is a shallow, V-shaped depression known as the **philtrum**. All of the above landmarks are covered with skin consistent with the skin in other parts of the face. These are areas to look at for scarring from accidents, surgeries, or physical conditions, such as cleft lip.

The lips are covered externally with skin and internally with mucous membrane. The reddish portion of the lips is called the **vermilion zone**. The vermilion zone is highly vascular and covered with a thin layer of epithelium. The **vermilion border** is where the skin meets the vermilion zone and forms a line around the lips. In the middle of the upper lip is a small projection that sometimes enlarges or thickens. It is called the **tubercle of the lip**. The corners of the mouth, where the upper lip meets the lower lip, are known as **labial com-**

missures. The commissures should be observed for cracks, color changes, and variations in form. Just below the lower lip is the **labio-mental groove,** which runs horizontally and separates the lip from the chin.

Landmarks of the Oral Cavity

Understanding the landmarks of the oral cavity will aid the dental assistant when taking radiographs, placing topical anesthetic, recognizing healthy tissue, and recording information or medical history on a patient's chart.

The landmarks of the oral cavity include the following: vestibule, vestibule fornix, labial mucosa, buccal mucosa, parotid papilla, Stensen's duct, linea alba, Fordyce's spots, alveolar mucosa, gingiva, labial frenum, and the buccal frenum.

Inside the mouth, a pocket is formed by the soft tissue of the cheeks and the gingiva. This is the **oral vestibule**. The deepest point of the vestibule is called the **vestibule fornix**. The fornix forms a U-shaped pocket that is continuous throughout the anterior and posterior areas. The tissue that lines the inner surface of the lips and cheeks is called **mucosa**. The mucosa is named according to location. The inner surface of the lips is called the **labial mucosa**, and the inner surface of the cheeks is the **buccal mucosa**. On the labial mucosa are small, yellowish glands just inside the commissures called **Fordyce's spots**, which become larger and more visible with age. On the buccal mucosa, opposite the maxillary second molar, there is a flap of tissue called the **parotid papilla**, which is where the opening of the Stensen's duct is located. On the buccal mucosa is a raised white line that runs parallel to where the teeth meet, called the linea alba (Figure 4-2). Mucosa also covers the alveolar bone that supports the teeth. It is called the **alveolar mucosa**. Alveolar mucosa is loosely attached and is highly vascular, giving the mucosa a reddish color. Moving from the alveolar mucosa toward

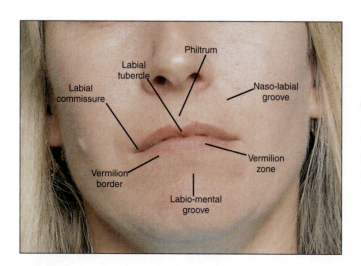

FIGURE 4-1 Landmarks of the face.

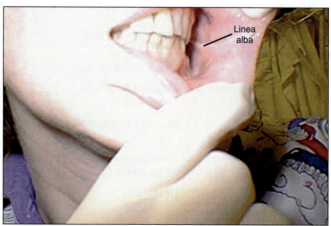

FIGURE 4-2 The oral vestibule with the linea alba on the buccal mucosa.

the teeth is the **gingiva**. The gingiva is firmly attached and usually pale pink or brownish pink, depending on pigmentation. This dense, fibrous tissue covered with mucous membrane can withstand the pressures during chewing. The portion of the gingiva that meets the tooth is called the free gingiva or marginal gingiva.

When the lips are pulled out, frena become visible. Frena (plural form of frenum) are raised lines of mucosal tissue that extend from the alveolar mucosa through the vestibule to the labial and buccal mucosa. On the labial, the main frena are between the maxillary central incisors, and the mandibular central incisors, with minor frena along the vestibule of both arches in the labial and buccal areas.

The Palate Area of the Oral Cavity

On the inside of the maxillary teeth is the **palate**, or the "roof of the mouth." The palate is divided into hard and soft sections. The hard palate, the anterior portion, is a bony plate covered with pink to brownish pink keratinized tissue. The soft palate, the posterior portion, covers muscle tissue and is darker pink or yellowish in color. On the hard palate is the incisive papilla, which is a raised area of tissue lying behind the maxillary central incisors (Figure 4-3). Extending from the back of the incisive papilla is a slightly raised line that extends down the middle of the hard palate, known as the **palatine raphe**. The ridges that run horizontally across the hard palate behind the incisive papilla are the **palatine rugae**. Occasionally, in the middle of the palate a lump or prominence of bone (exostosis) may be found. This excess bone is called a **torus** (plural is tori), or a torus palatinus, specifically.

The following landmarks are located on the soft palate and the oropharynx areas: the uvula, anterior

tonsillar pillars, posterior tonsillar pillars, palatine tonsils, and the fauces (Figure 4-3). The uvula is a projection that extends off the back of the soft palate. Extending horizontally from the uvula to the base of the tongue are folds of tissue called **anterior tonsillar pillars** or **palatoglossal arches**. Another set of arches is found farther back in the throat. This set is the **posterior tonsillar pillars** or **palatopharyngeal arches**. Between the two sets of pillars is a depressed area where the palatine tonsils are situated. The **palatine tonsils** are often marked with deep grooves and are red and inflamed due to infection. The space in the back of the oral cavity where food passes into the pharynx is called the **fauces**.

The Tongue

The **tongue** is a significant region of the oval cavity with the following landmarks: sulcus terminalis, circumvallate papilla, filiform papillae, fungiform papillae, foliate papilla, and median sulcus on the dorsal or top surface of the tongue. On the ventral or underside of the tongue are the lingual frenum, the lingual veins, and the fimbriated folds. When the tongue is extended, a shallow, V-shaped groove is apparent on the posterior portion. This is the sulcus terminalis. This groove separates the anterior two-thirds, or body of the tongue, from the base of the tongue. Anterior to the sulcus, covering the dorsal side of the tongue (Figure 4-4A), are small, raised projections called papilla, where taste buds are located. The largest papilla, mushroom shaped, are located anterior to the sulcus terminalis in a row of eight to ten and are called **circumvallate papillae**. Anterior to the circumvallate papillae and covering the dorsal side of the tongue are hair-like projections called **filiform papillae**. Papillae that give the tongue the "strawberry effect" are the **fungiform papillae**. On the lateral border of the tongue near the base are the **foliate papillae**, which are slightly raised, vertical folds of tissue. The tongue is divided in half by the **median sulcus**, which runs from the base to the tip of the tongue. The median sulcus is a groove that varies in depth from person to person.

In the middle of the ventral side of the tongue, a line of tissue extends from the tongue to the floor of the mouth, called the **lingual frenum** (Figure 4-4B). On either side of the lingual frenum are the **lingual veins**. They are bluish in color and run the length of the tongue. Lateral to the lingual veins are folds of tissue called **fimbriated folds**. Sometimes, under the tongue on the alveolar bone are excess bone formations called **torus mandibularis**.

The Floor of the Mouth

The **floor of the mouth** includes the sublingual caruncles, sublingual folds, and sublingual sulcus (Figure 4-4B). Where the lingual frenum attaches to the floor of the mouth are two small, raised folds of tissue, one on

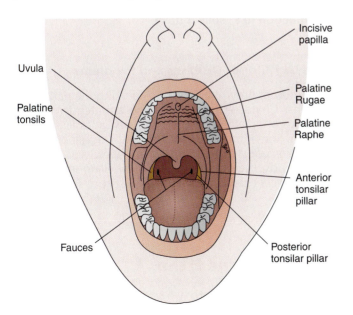

Incisive papilla

Uvula

Palatine Rugae

Palatine tonsils

Palatine Raphe

Anterior tonsilar pillar

Fauces

Posterior tonsilar pillar

FIGURE 4-3 Landmarks of the palate and oral pharynx area.

(A)

Sulcus terminalis

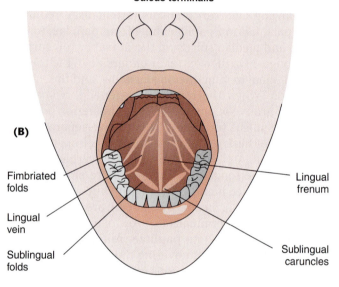

(B)

FIGURE 4-4 (A) Dorsal surfaces of the tongue. (B) Ventral surfaces of the tongue.

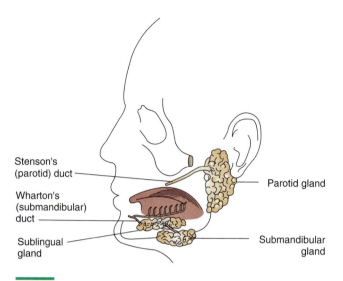

FIGURE 4-5 Salivary glands and ducts.

largest of the salivary glands are the **parotid glands**, which lie just below and in front of the ear. The parotid glands empty into the mouth through the **parotid duct** (also known as the Stensen's duct). The duct empties into the mouth through the parotid papilla, which is just opposite the maxillary second molar. The **submandibular glands** are about the size of a walnut and lie on the inside of the mandible in the posterior area. They empty the saliva into the mouth through the **Wharton's duct**, which ends in the sublingual caruncles. The third set of glands are the **sublingual**. These are the smallest of the glands and are located on the floor of the mouth. These glands either empty directly into the mouth through the **ducts of Rivinus** or through the sublingual caruncles by means of the **ducts of Bartholin**. The ducts of the sublingual glands are similar in function to a "soaker hose."

Salivary Glands Diseases and Problems

The mumps are a viral infection affecting the parotid glands. Characterized by swelling and tenderness, mumps often affect children between ages five and fifteen. Sometimes, the salivary glands develop crystallizations or stones. When these stones try to leave the glands, they block the ducts. Swelling immediately occurs and the stones must be surgically removed.

either side of the frenum. These are **sublingual caruncles**. On top of these folds of tissue lie the ducts of two salivary glands. The **sublingual folds** begin at the caruncles on either side of the frenum and run backward to the base of the tongue. To the lateral of the sublingual fold runs a horseshoe-shaped groove that follows the curve of the dental arch, called the **sublingual sulcus**. This sulcus marks the end of the alveolar ridge and the beginning of the floor of the mouth.

The Salivary Glands

There are three major pairs of **salivary glands** that supply the oral cavity: the parotid glands, submandibular glands, and sublingual glands (Figure 4-5). These glands secret saliva to assist in the process of digestion. The

BONES OF THE HEAD

The skull is divided into two sections: the **cranium** and the **face**. The cranium covers and protects the brain and is composed of eight bones. The face consists of fourteen bones, including the maxilla and the mandible.

Bones of the Cranium

The **frontal bone** forms the forehead, the main portion of the roof of the eye socket (orbit), and part of the nasal cavity. On the skull just behind the frontal bone are the two parietal bones, right and left halves joining at the midline. The **parietal bones** form most of the roof of the skull and the upper half of the sides. Below each parietal bone, forming the lower sides and the base of the skull, are the **temporal bones**. Each temporal bone contains the following landmarks: external auditory meatus, mastoid process, glenoid fossa, and the styloid process. The **external auditory meatus** is the opening for the ear. The **mastoid process** is the bony projection found on the bottom border of the temporal bone. A pit or depression found anterior to the mastoid process is the **glenoid fossa**, the location where the mandible articulates with the skull. The **styloid process** is a sharp projection on the under-surface of the temporal bone between the glenoid fossa and the mastoid process. The **occipital bone** forms the back and base of the skull. The occipital bone contains a large opening, the foramen magnum, through which the spinal cord passes. The **sphenoid bone** is a wedge-shaped bone that goes across the skull anterior to the temporal bones. It is one continuous bone, shaped like a bat with its wings spread out. The wings of the sphenoid bone are called the **pterygoid** process. The sphenoid bone forms the anterior base of the skull behind the orbit and contains the **sphenoid sinuses**. The **ethmoid bone** forms part of the nose, orbits, and the floor of the cranium. This bone is thin and spongy or honeycombed in appearance. It contains the **ethmoid sinuses** (Figure 4-6 and Table 4-1).

Bones of the Face

The **nasal bones** form the bridge of the nose. The **vomer bone** is a single bone on the inside of the nasal cavity. It forms the posterior and the bottom of the nasal septum (the nasal septum is a cartilage structure

TABLE 4-1 BONES OF THE CRANIUM

Name of Cranial Bone	Number
Frontal bone	One (1)
Parietal bones	Paired (2)
Temporal bones	Paired (2)
Occipital bone	One (1)
Sphenoid bone	One (1)
Ethmoid bone	One (1)

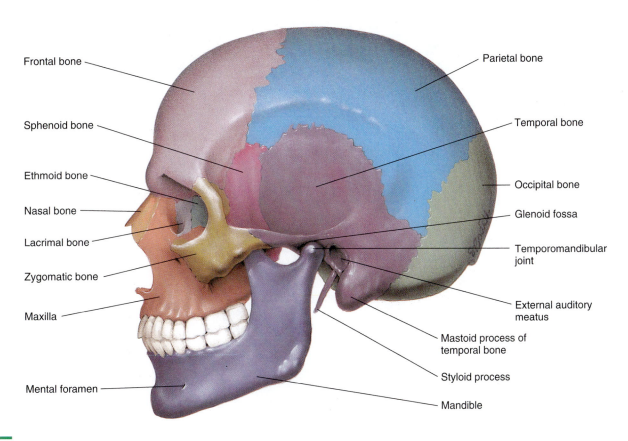

FIGURE 4-6 Lateral aspect of the cranium.

that divides the nasal cavities). On the outside of the nasal cavities are scroll-like bones called **inferior nasal conchae**. Each concha consists of thin, cancellous bone. The lacrimal bones are small and very delicate. They are anterior to the ethmoid bone, making part of the orbit (the corner of the eye). The tear ducts pass through the lacrimal bones. The zygomatic bones form the cheeks (Figures 4-6, 4-7, and Table 4-2).

Maxilla. The **maxilla** is the largest of the facial bones and is composed of two sections of bone joined at the **median suture**. The maxilla extends from the floor of each orbit and the floor and exterior walls of the nasal cavity to form the roof the mouth. The maxilla is formed by *four processes* (outgrowths of bone). The *frontal* and the *zygomatic processes* meet the frontal and the zygomatic bones. The alveolar process forms the bone that supports the maxillary teeth, and the *palatine process* is the main portion of the hard palate.

The **infraorbital foramen** (foramen means an opening) is just below the orbit on the maxillary bone and the **maxillary sinus** forms a large cavity above the roots of the maxillary molars. Just beyond the last posterior maxillary tooth is a rounded area known as the **maxillary tuberosity**.

TABLE 4-2   BONES OF THE FACE

Name of Facial Bone	Number
Nasal bone	Two (2)
Vomer bone	One (1)
Inferior nasal conchae	Two (2)
Lacrimal bones	Two (2)
Maxillae bones	Two (2)
Zygomatic bones	Two (2)
Palatine bones	Two (2)
Mandible bone	One (1)

Palatine Bones. The **palatine bones** are joined at the midline, often referred to as the median **palatine suture** (Figure 4-8). Just behind the maxillary central incisors is the incisive (nasopalatine) foramen, which is an opening for the nasopalatine nerve. In the posterior region of

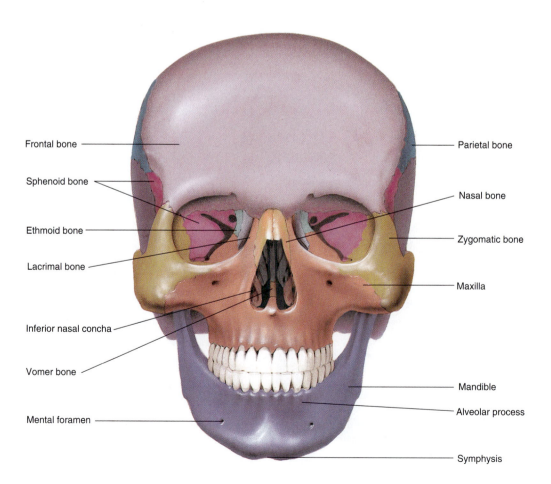

FIGURE 4-7 Bones of the face.

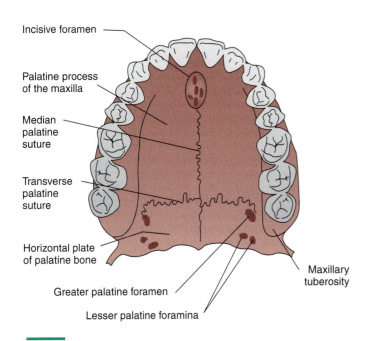

FIGURE 4-8 Landmarks of the palate.

FIGURE 4-9 (A) External surface of the mandible. (B) Internal (lingual) view of the mandible.

the hard palate there are three other openings on each side. The first of these three is the largest and is called the **greater palatine foramen**. Behind the greater foramen are two smaller or **lesser palatine foramen**.

Mandible. The **mandible** is the only movable bone of the face (Figure 4-9A). The mandible consists of a horseshoe-shaped body that is horizontal, with two vertical extensions called **rami** (plural form of ramus). At the top of the rami are two projections. The posterior projection is the **condyle** or **condyloid process**, and the anterior projection is the **coronoid process**. The condyle articulates with the temporal bone to form the **temporomandibular joint (TMJ)**. Between the two processes is a depression known as the **mandibular notch** (also referred to as the sigmoid or coronoid notch). From the top of the rami moving downward is the body of each ramus. On the inside of the body of the ramus is the **mandibular foramen**, which is the beginning of the **internal oblique ridge** (Figure 4-9B). The internal oblique ridge, also known as the **mylohyoid ridge**, follows the inside of the ramus and the body of the mandible. Where the ramus meets the body of the mandible on the outside border is the **angle of the mandible**. On the body of the mandible near the apex of the premolars is the **mental foramen**. Extending from the mental foramen, the **external oblique ridge** follows the length of the body of the mandible past the last tooth and up to the ramus. Behind the last molar is a triangular area known as the **retromolar area**. In the center of the mandible on the external surface is a concave area where two bones of the mandible are fused. This area is known as the **symphysis**. The tip of the chin is called the **mental protuberance**. On the internal surface at the center of the mandible is the **lingual fora-**

men, which is surrounded by small, bony projections called **genial tubercles**. The mandibular teeth are supported in the alveolar process.

Temporomandibular Joint (TMJ)

Once the bones of the cranium and the face have been identified, it is easy to locate the temporomandibular joint (TMJ). The joint is named for the two bones that form the union: the temporal and the mandible bones. The TMJ is composed of three parts:

1. Glenoid fossa of the temporal bone
2. Articular eminence of the temporal bone
3. Condyloid process of the mandible

These bones are covered with a thick cartilage and are surrounded by several ligaments. There are no blood vessels or nerves in this connective tissue, but a **synovial fluid** bathes these bone structures, providing nourishment and lubrication that enable the bones to glide over each other without friction. (Synovial means a thick, sticky fluid found in the joints of bones.)

The TMJ is formed by the condyle of the mandible articulating with the glenoid fossa and the articular eminence of the temporal bone (Figure 4-10). The condyle rests closer to the glenoid fossa and then moves forward to the articular eminence when the mouth opens.

Between the condyle and temporal bone is the **articular disc** (meniscus). This disc is a dense, fibrous connective tissue that is thicker at the ends. The articular disc is attached to the condyle, so when the condyle glides forward and backward, the disc moves with it.

Surrounding the articular disc is a dense, fibrous **capsule** that encloses the entire joint. The capsule is divided into upper and lower cavities by the disc, and these cavities are filled with synovial fluid.

The temporomandibular joint is supported by ligaments, and the muscles of mastication control the movements. The left and right TMJs function in unison and move in two ways: hinge (swinging) motion and gliding movement.

The hinge motion occurs in the lower joint cavity when the mouth opens. The condyles and the discs begin this hinge motion by rotating anteriorly. As this motion continues and the mouth opens wider, there is an anterior gliding movement as well. This gliding movement involves both the upper and the lower cavities. The gliding continues along the articular disc during protrusion and lateral movements of the mandible during mastication (Figure 4-11).

Some problems with the TMJ occur when the disc becomes stuck or displaced. Popping and clicking sounds may result if the disc does not stay interposed between the condyle and the temporal bone. More severe problems may occur as the condition advances.

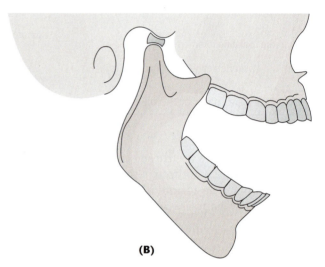

(A)

(B)

FIGURE 4-11 Movement of the TMJ. (A) Hinge joint. (B) Gliding joint movement.

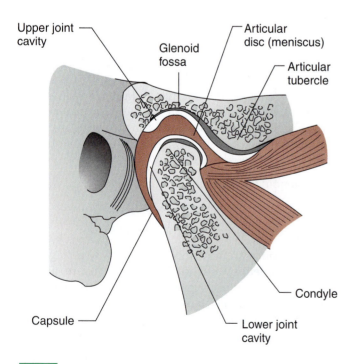

FIGURE 4-10 Temporomandibular joint (TMJ).

MUSCLES OF THE HEAD AND NECK

Muscles expand and contract to make movement possible and each muscle has an **origin** (fixed point) and **insertion** (movable point). Muscles of the head and neck include muscles of mastication, muscles of facial expression, muscles on the floor of the mouth, muscles of the tongue, muscles of the soft palate, the pharynx, and muscles of the neck.

Muscles of Mastication

There are four pairs of muscles of mastication, known as the **temporal muscles**, **masseter muscles**, **internal pterygoid muscles**, and **external pterygoid muscles**. These muscles provide movement for the mandible as they protrude, retract, elevate, and provide lateral movements (Figure 4-12). Nerves to the muscles of mastication originate from the mandibular division of the trigeminal labor. The origins, insertions, and functions (distributions of nerves) of the muscles of mastication are listed in Table 4-3.

TABLE 4-3   MUSCLES OF MASTICATION

Muscle	Origin	Insertion	Function
Temporal muscles	Fan shaped across the temporal fossa of the temporal bone.	Inserts into the coronoid process of the mandible and down the anterior border of the ramus.	Elevates the mandible—closing the jaw. Contraction of the posterior fibers retracts the mandible.
Masseter muscles	Two portions: superficial portion (strong, tendinous fibers from the zygomatic process of the maxilla and from the anterior two-thirds of the lower border of the zygomatic arch) and deep portion (muscular and smaller from the medial aspect and inferior border of the posterior one-third of the zygomatic arch).	The superficial portion inserts into the angle and lower border of the mandible; the deep portion is inserted into the upper section of the ramus and the lateral surface of the coronoid process.	Strong elevator of the jaw. This muscle is easily seen when the teeth are clenched.
Medial (internal) pterygoid muscles	Medial surface of the lateral pterygoid plate of the sphenoid bone, the lateral portion of the palatine bone, and the maxillary tuberosity.	The medial pterygoids insert into the interior surface of the angle of the mandible (opposite the insertion of the masseter muscle).	Elevates the mandible.
Lateral (external) pterygoids	Superior portion from the lateral surface of the greater wing of the sphenoid bone; inferior portion from the lateral surface of the lateral pterygoid plate.	Superior portion inserts into the articular capsule of the temporal mandibular joint; inferior portion inserts into the neck of the condyle of the mandible.	Opens jaw by depressing the mandible. If both lateral pterygoid muscles contract, the jaw protrudes; if only one contracts, the mandible shifts laterally.

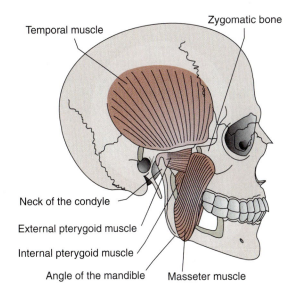

FIGURE 4-12 Muscles of mastication. Lateral view of the internal pterygoid muscle and the external pterygoid muscle. The temporal muscle and the masseter muscle.

Muscles of Facial Expression

The major muscles of facial expression include the **orbicularis oris**, **buccinator**, **mentalis**, and **zygomatic major**. These muscles allow for a wide variety of facial expressions, including smiling and whistling. The muscles of the face are innervated by the facial nerve, which is the seventh cranial nerve (Figure 4-13). The muscles of facial expression are described in Table 4-4.

Muscles of the Tongue

The muscles of the tongue are divided into intrinsic and extrinsic groups. The **intrinsic muscles** are all within the tongue and are responsible for shaping the tongue during speech, mastication, and swallowing. There are four **extrinsic muscles** to assist in the movement and functioning of the tongue: **genioglossus**, **hyoglossus**, **styloglossus**, and **palatoglossus**. (The palatoglossus is discussed with the palate) (Figure 4-14). All of the muscles of the tongue are innervated by the hypoglossal nerve except the palatoglossus muscle. See Table 4-5 for the origin, insertion, and function of each extrinsic muscle of the tongue.

TABLE 4-4 **MUSCLES OF FACIAL EXPRESSION**

Muscle	Origin	Insertion	Function
Orbicularis oris	Complex origin—There is no skeletal attachment. The origin is from muscle fibers that surround the mouth.	Insertion is into itself and the surrounding skin.	Closing the lips or protruding them.
Buccinator	Alveolar processes of the maxilla and the mandible and the pterygomandibular raphe.	Inserts into the corners of the mouth, becoming part of the muscles that surround the mouth.	Compresses the cheeks against the teeth to assist during mastication. Assists in blowing air out of the mouth.
Mentalis	Incisive fossa of the mandible.	Inserts into the skin of the chin.	Wrinkles the skin of the chin and protrudes the lower lip.
Zygomatic major	Zygomatic bone.	Insertion into the corners of the mouth.	Lifts the corners of the mouth upward and backward, as in smiling.

FIGURE 4-13 Muscles of facial expression.

TABLE 4-5   **EXTRINSIC MUSCLES OF THE TONGUE**

Muscle	Origin	Insertion	Function
Genioglossus	Genial tubercle in the center of the lingual of the mandible.	Fans out to insert in the inferior surface of the tongue and to the hyoid bone.	Most of the work of the tongue. Protrudes the tongue and retracts or depresses the tongue.
Hypoglossus	Hyoid bone.	Runs vertically to insert in the inferior sides of the tongue.	Mainly depresses the tongue.
Styloglossus	Anterior surface of the styloid process of the temporal bone.	Part of the styloglossus inserts into the sides of the tongue while the rest of the muscle continues forward to the tip of the tongue.	Retracts the tongue and raises the tip of the tongue.

Hyoid Bone.   There is also a horseshoe-shaped bone lying at the base of the tongue called the **hyoid bone**. Muscles of the tongue and the floor of the mouth attach to this bone for support (Figure 4-15).

Muscles of the Floor of the Mouth

The muscles that form the floor of the mouth are the **digastric**, **mylohyoid**, **stylohyoid**, and **geniohyoid**. These four muscles are located between the mandible and the hyoid bone. Unlike some other muscle groups, the muscles on the floor of the mouth are innervated by different nerve branches (Table 4-6 and Figure 4-15).

Muscles of the Soft Palate

There are two muscles of the soft palate, called the **palatoglossus** and **palatopharyngeal** (Table 4-7). These

muscles raise the soft palate during the swallowing process (deglutition) and are both innervated by the pharyngeal plexus (Figure 4-16).

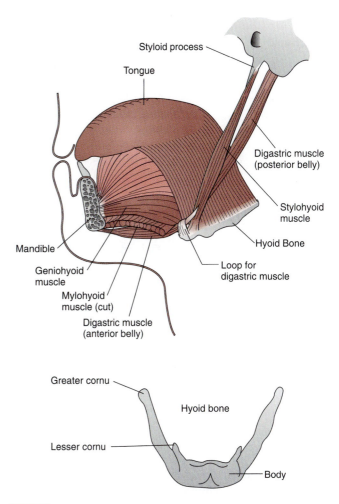

FIGURE 4-15 Muscles of the floor of the mouth and the hyoid bone.

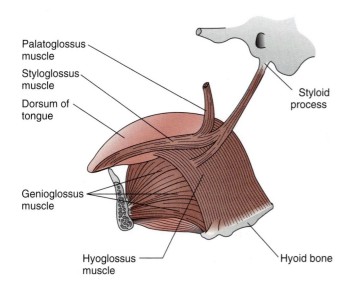

FIGURE 4-14 Extrinsic muscles of the tongue.

TABLE 4-6 **MUSCLES OF THE FLOOR OF THE MOUTH**

Muscle	Origin	Insertion	Function	Innervation
Digastric	There are two portions, called bellies. Posterior belly originates from the mastoid process of the temporal bone; anterior belly begins on the lingual surface of the mandible at the midline.	Both the posterior belly and the anterior belly insert into the intermediate tendon on the hyoid bone.	Together the digastric muscles lift the hyoid bone and assist in opening the mouth; separately, the posterior belly draws the hyoid bone posteriorly and the anterior belly pulls the hyoid bone anteriorly.	The posterior belly is innervated by the facial nerve, and the anterior belly is innervated by the mandibular branch of the trigeminal nerve.
Mylohyoid	This muscle is composed of left and right halves that join at the midline of the mandible. From the midline, each half attaches in a fan shape to the last molar area, thus following the mylohyoid line.	Inserts into the body of the hyoid bone.	Forms the floor of the mouth and assists in depressing the mandible and elevating the tongue.	The trigeminal nerve stimulates the mylohyoid muscle. The mandibular branch.
Stylohyoid	The styloid process of the temporal bone.	Inserts into the body of the hyoid bone.	Draws the hyoid bone superiorly and posteriorly and stabilizes it.	Facial nerve.
Geniohyoid	Above the mylohyoid muscle the geniohyoid originates from the genial tubercle of the mandible.	Inserts into the anterior portion of the hyoid bone.	Pulls the hyoid bone and the tongue anteriorly.	Hypoglossal nerve.

TABLE 4-7 **MUSCLES OF THE SOFT PALATE**

Muscle	Origin	Insertion	Function
Palatoglossus	This muscle forms the anterior arch on each side of the throat and arises from the soft palate.	Inserts along the posterior side of the tongue.	Elevates the posterior portion of the tongue and narrows the fauces.
Palatopharyngeal	This muscle forms the posterior arch on each side of the throat and also arises from the soft palate.	Inserts into the thyroid cartilage and the wall of the pharynx.	Constricts the nasopharyngeal passage and elevates the larynx.

Muscles of the Neck

The three muscles of the neck are the **platysma**, **trapezius**, and **sternocleidomastoid** (Figure 4-17). Knowing the muscles of the neck helps the dental assistant perform chairside functions in positions that are not tiring and will not cause injury (Table 4-8).

NERVES OF THE HEAD AND NECK

There are four cranial nerves that innervate the face and oral cavity: **trigeminal**, **facial**, **glossopharyngeal**, and **hypoglossal**. The largest cranial nerve and the most important to dental auxiliaries is the trigeminal nerve,

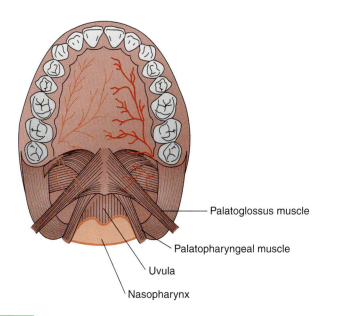

FIGURE 4-16 Muscles of the soft palate.

- Palatoglossus muscle
- Palatopharyngeal muscle
- Uvula
- Nasopharynx

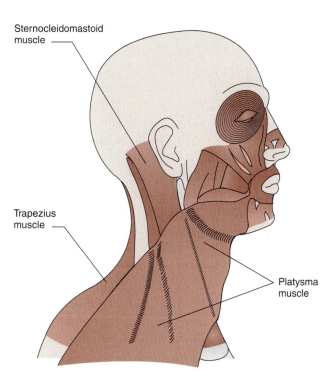

FIGURE 4-17 Muscles of the neck.

- Sternocleidomastoid muscle
- Trapezius muscle
- Platysma muscle

because this cranial nerve innervates the maxilla and the mandible. The trigeminal nerve divides at the semi-lunar (gasserian) ganglion into three branches: the ophthalmic nerve, maxillary nerve, and mandibular nerve.

The Maxillary Branch of the Trigeminal Nerve

Maxillary Nerve Branch. The **maxillary nerve branch** is a sensory nerve that innervates the nose, cheeks, palate, gingiva, maxillary teeth, maxillary sinus, tonsils, nasophynarynx, and other facial structures. The maxillary nerve branch is divided into four branches: **zygomatic**, **infraorbital**, **posterior superior alveolar**, and **pterygopalatine** (Figure 4-18).

Pterygopalatine Nerve Branch. After the maxillary nerve leaves the semi-lunar ganglion, one branch becomes the **pterygopalatine nerve branch**. This branch divides into the **greater palatine nerve**, the **lesser palatine nerve**, and the **nasopalatine nerve**. The greater palatine nerve extends downward from the pterygopalatine nerve and reaches the palate through the greater palatine foramen. This nerve serves the soft palate, hard palate, medial gingiva, and mucous membrane as far forward as the anterior teeth. The lesser palatine nerve

TABLE 4-8   MUSCLES OF THE NECK

Muscle	Origin	Insertion	Function	Innervation
Platysma	Clavicle and the shoulder.	Inserts into the inferior border of the mandible.	This sheet of muscle draws down the mandible as well as the corners of the mouth and the lower lip.	Facial nerve.
Trapezius	Protuberance on the occipital bone.	Inserts into the clavicle and shoulders.	This large muscle moves the head backward and laterally.	Spinal accessory nerve.
Sternocleido-mastoid	The top of the sternum and the clavicle.	Inserts into the mastoid process and the anterior of the occipital bone.	One on each side of the neck assists in elevating the chin.	Spinal accessory nerve.

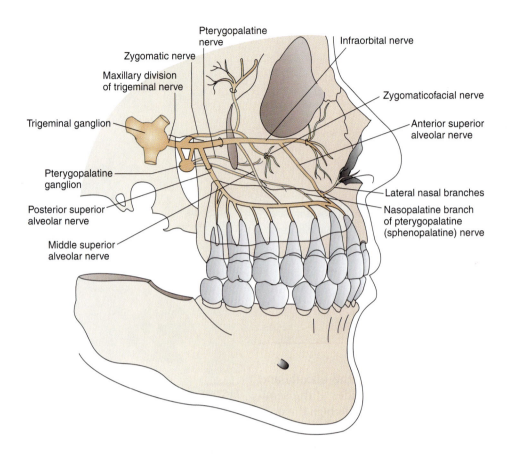

FIGURE 4-18 Nerves of the maxillary arch.

is a smaller branch that innervates the soft palate, uvula, and tonsils. The nasopalatine nerve extends anteriorly from the pterygopalatine nerve and exits through the incisive foramen. This nerve innervates the anterior hard plate, gingiva, mucous membrane, and the anterior teeth from the cuspids forward.

The Infraorbital Nerve. The **infraorbital nerve** is another branch of the maxillary nerve. There are two nerves that come from the infraorbital nerve before it exits through the infraorbital foramen. These are the **middle superior alveolar nerve** and the **anterior alveolar nerve**.

The middle superior alveolar nerve supplies the lateral wall of the maxillary sinus, gingiva, mesial buccal root of the first molar, and all the roots of the bicuspids (premolars). The anterior superior alveolar nerve is the next nerve to come from the infraorbital nerve. It innervates the anterior maxillary sinus, gingiva, cuspids, laterals, and central incisors.

Posterior Superior Alveolar Nerve. The **posterior superior alveolar nerve** branches downward from the maxillary nerve. It supplies the gingiva, maxillary sinus, cheeks, and maxillary molars with the exception of the mesial buccal root of the first molar, which is innervated by the middle superior alveolar nerve.

The Mandibular Branch of the Trigeminal Nerve

The **mandibular nerve branch** is composed of both sensory and motor neurons and is the largest division of the trigeminal nerve. There are three branches of the mandibular nerve: the **buccal branch**, **lingual branch**, and **inferior alveolar branch** (Figure 4-19).

The Buccal Nerve Branch. The buccal nerve branch passes through the buccinator muscle to the cheek, where it innervates the buccal mucosa, buccal gingiva, and the buccal of the mandibular molars.

Lingual Nerve Branch. The lingual nerve branch descends from the mandibular nerve to the underside of the tongue and extends from the posterior to the anterior of the mouth. This nerve innervates the floor of the mouth, the ventral side of the tongue, taste buds on the anterior two-thirds of the tongue, and the lingual gingiva.

Inferior Alveolar Nerve Branch. The inferior alveolar nerve branch descends from the mandibular nerve and runs parallel to the lingual nerve. The first branch is the **mylohyoid nerve branch**, which supplies the mylohyoid muscle and the anterior belly of the digastric muscle. The inferior alveolar nerve then enters through

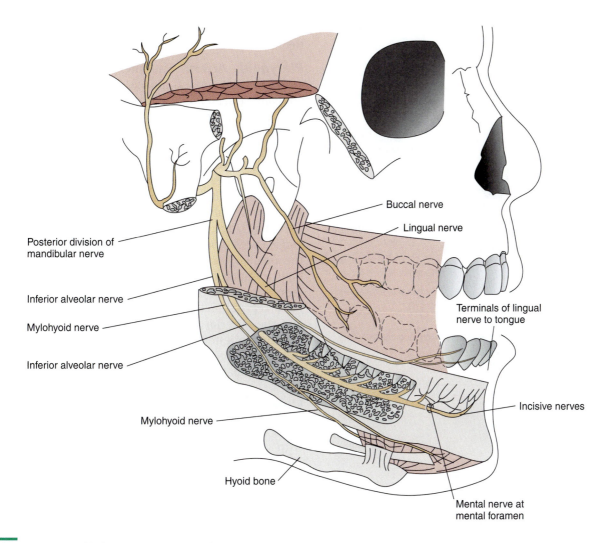

FIGURE 4-19 Mandibular nerves.

Labels in figure:
- Buccal nerve
- Lingual nerve
- Posterior division of mandibular nerve
- Inferior alveolar nerve
- Mylohyoid nerve
- Inferior alveolar nerve
- Terminals of lingual nerve to tongue
- Mylohyoid nerve
- Incisive nerves
- Hyoid bone
- Mental nerve at mental foramen

the mandibular foramen and runs through the mandibular canal. Within the canal, the inferior alveolar nerve supplies the mandibular teeth (specifically the molars and the premolars) the gingiva, and the mucosa. It then subdivides into the mental nerve branch and the incisive nerve branch. The **mental nerve branch** supplies the chin and the lower lip area, and the **incisive nerve branch** innervates the anterior teeth and labial gingiva.

CIRCULATION OF THE HEAD AND NECK

The arteries and veins of the face and oral cavity are located near each other. They supply blood and nutrients to the area and drain unoxygenated blood and waste products from the area.

Arteries of the Face and Oral Cavity

The **common carotid** supplies blood to most of the head and neck. As the common carotid ascends up the neck, it divides into the internal and external carotid arteries. The **internal carotid artery** supplies blood to the brain and eyes, while the **external carotid artery** supplies blood to the face and oral cavity and has many branches (Figure 4-20). (Information presented is limited to the arteries that supply the teeth, tongue, and surrounding tissues.)

External Carotid Artery

The external carotid artery branches go to the throat, tongue, face, and ears and to the wall of the cranium. Branches are named according to the areas they supply and are located nearer the surface (more superficial).

Lingual Artery. The lingual branch is about even with the hyoid bone and has several branches that supply the entire tongue, floor of the mouth, lingual gingiva, a portion of the soft plate, and the tonsils.

Facial Artery. The **facial artery** is above the lingual artery, near the angle of the mandible. It branches across the mandible to the corners of the mouth and

Superficial temporal artery

Posterior superior alveolar artery

Infraorbital artery

Middle superior alveolar artery

Anterior superior alveolar artery

Descending palatine artery

Maxillary artery

Facial artery

Inferior alveolar artery

Lingual artery

External carotid artery

Internal carotid artery

Thyroid cartilage

Common carotid artery

Vertebral artery

Brachiocephalic trunk

Clavicle

Subclavian artery

FIGURE 4-20 Arteries of the face and oral cavity.

then upward toward the eye. The facial artery has six branches that supply the pharynx muscles, soft palate, tonsils, the posterior of the tongue, submandibular gland, muscles of the face, nasal septum, the nose, and eyelids.

Maxillary Artery. The **maxillary artery** is the largest of the branches of the external carotid artery. It moves anteriorly across the ramus of the mandible, near the condyle, and supplies facial structures. The maxillary artery divides into three sections: mandibular, pterygoid, and pterygopalatine.

Mandibular Artery. The **mandibular artery** is behind the ramus of the mandible and branches into five arteries. The **inferior alveolar artery** descends the ramus, enters the mandibular foramen, and bifurcates around the first premolar tooth to form the incisive and the mental arteries. The mylohyoid artery and the dental arteries are additional branches. The **mylohyoid artery** branches off the inferior alveolar artery before entering the mandibular canal. It supplies the mylohyoid muscle. As the inferior alveolar artery travels through the mandibular canal, the **dental arteries** supply the roots and periodontal ligaments of the molars and premolars. The **incisive arteries** continue anteriorly to supply blood to the roots and periodontal ligaments of the anterior teeth. The **mental artery** branch of the inferior alveolar artery then exits the mandibular

canal at the mental foramen and supplies the chin and the lower lip.

Pterygoid Artery. The **pterygoid artery** supplies blood to the temporal muscle, masseter muscle, pterygoid muscles, and buccinator muscles. The pterygopalatine artery divides into branches: **posterior superior alveolar artery**, **infraorbital artery**, **middle superior alveolar artery**, **anterior superior alveolar artery**, and **greater palatine artery**. The posterior superior alveolar artery branches from the maxillary artery and descends along the maxillary tuberosity, where it enters the posterior superior alveolar foramen. This artery supplies the maxillary sinus, maxillary molar teeth, and surrounding gingiva with blood. The infraorbital artery ascends from the maxillary artery and travels anteriorly to the infraorbital foramen, where it supplies the face with blood. From the infraorbital artery, the middle superior alveolar artery branches to the maxillary premolar teeth, and the anterior superior alveolar artery branches to supply the anterior teeth. The greater palatine artery travels through the greater palatine foramen to supply the hard palate and the maxillary lingual gingiva.

Veins of the Face and Oral Cavity

Some of the veins of the face and oral cavity are located with corresponding arteries and have similar names. There are many variations of venous drainage, but ultimately the blood from the face and oral cavity drains into either the external jugular vein or internal jugular vein and then into the brachiocephalic vein, which flows into the superior vena cava. The veins are divided into the **superficial veins** and the **deep veins**. Only the primary veins of importance to the dental assistant are discussed (Figure 4-21).

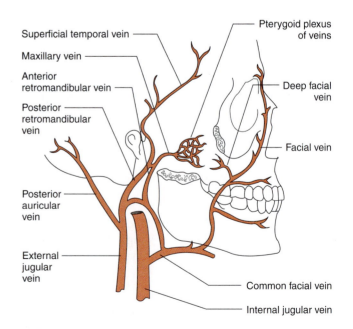

Superficial temporal vein

Maxillary vein

Anterior retromandibular vein

Posterior retromandibular vein

Posterior auricular vein

External jugular vein

Pterygoid plexus of veins

Deep facial vein

Facial vein

Common facial vein

Internal jugular vein

FIGURE 4-21 Veins of the face and oral cavity.

Superficial Veins. The **facial vein** drains the facial structures, beginning near the eye and descending toward the mandible. One of the tributaries is the **deep facial vein**, which connects the facial vein to the pterygoid plexus of veins. Near the border of the mandible, the facial vein heads posteriorily to the angle of the mandible, where it joins with the retromandibular vein. The **retromandibular vein** is frequently formed within the parotid gland. This vein drains the maxillary artery and the superficial temporal arteries. Below the facial vein is the **lingual vein**, which drains the floor of the mouth. The tongue empties into the internal jugular vein.

Deep Veins. The **maxillary vein** drains the pterygoid plexus of veins. It is a short vein that follows the maxillary artery. The **pterygoid plexus of veins** is a junction or center of veins that directly or indirectly drain a vast area, including the nasal cavity, the eye, the paranasal sinuses, the muscles of mastication, the buccinator muscle, the palate, and the teeth. The pterygoid plexus of veins is located between the temporal and pterygoid muscles.

Jugular Vein. The **external jugular vein** drains the superficial veins of the face and neck into the subclavian vein. The **internal jugular vein** receives blood from the cranium, face, and neck and drains into the brachiocephalic vein, then into the superior vena cava, which drains into the heart.

CHAPTER SUMMARY

As a vital team member, the dental assistant needs to be able to recognize factors that may influence the general physical health of the patient. The understanding of landmarks of the oral cavity, as well as being able to describe head and neck anatomy as it relates to location of structure and function, will enable the dental assistant to recognize the abnormal. For this reason, accuracy is especially important when completing the patient's dental chart. This information will provide a point of comparison for future visits.

CASE STUDY

Pat Boyer is a thirty-five-year-old patient at Dr. Olson's office. Pat has had a series of headaches and pain during mastication (chewing). She also experiences clicking and popping when opening her mouth. These symptoms have been continual for six months and seem to be worsening.

Case Study Review

1. List the components of the head and neck affected, identifying the specific anatomy.

2. Identify the possible conditions.

3. How might the dental assistant be involved in this patient's care?

To complete your study of this chapter, work the review activities that follow. Also, refer to the software that accompanies this text.

REVIEW QUESTIONS

Multiple Choice

1. What are the raised lines of mucosal tissue that extend from the alveolar mucosa to the vestibule called?
   a. Gingiva.
   b. Alveolar mucosa.
   c. Frenum.
   d. Papilla.

2. The vertical part of the mandible that articulates with the temporal bone is called the
   a. oblique ridge.
   b. ramus.
   c. maxilla.
   d. palatal.

3. Which of the following are muscles of mastication?
   a. Temporals, masseters, buccinators, and internal pterygoids.
   b. Temporal, masseters, internal pterygoids, and external pterygoids.
   c. Masseters, mentalis, buccinators, and external pterygoids.
   d. Orbicularis oris, buccinators, zygomatic major, and mentalis.

4. Which division of the common carotid artery supplies the face and the oral cavity?
   a. The external carotid artery.
   b. The internal carotid artery.
   c. The facial artery.
   d. The maxillary artery.

5. All of the following are correct statements about the veins that supply the face and the oral cavity EXCEPT
   a. the veins correspond to the arteries and often have similar names.
   b. the veins drain into the external or internal jugular vein.
   c. the veins are classified as deep or superficial veins.
   d. the lingual vein drains the muscles of mastication, the sinuses, and the palate.

Critical Thinking

1. Which maxillary nerve is involved if a patient has a toothache on tooth #4?

2. Between the bottom of the nose and middle of the upper lip is a shallow, V-shaped depression. Identify this landmark and any developmental disturbances that occur in this area.

3. Prominence of excess bone is sometimes found in the bones of the arches. What are these prominences called and where are they specially located?

Embryology and Histology

OBJECTIVES

The student should strive to meet the following objectives and demonstrate an understanding of the facts and principles presented in this chapter:

1. Identify the terms and times of the three prenatal phases of pregnancy.

2. Describe how the human face develops and changes during the zygote and embryo phases.

3. Describe the life cycle of a tooth and identify the stages.

4. Identify the four primary structures of the tooth and the location and function of each.

5. Identify the substances of enamel, dentin, cementum, and pulp and their identifying marks.

6. Identify the components of the periodontium and the considerations of the aveolar bone.

7. Describe the structures of the gingiva and the mucosa.

KEY TERMS

alveolar crest
(p. 94)

alveolar mucosa
(p. 96)

alveolar process
(p. 94)

alveolus (p. 94)

ameloblasts (p. 90)

attached gingiva
(p. 96)

attrition (p. 90)

calcification (p. 90)

cementoblasts
(p. 90)

cementum (p. 90)

cleft lip (p. 88)

cleft palate (p. 89)

cleft uvula (p. 89)

dentin (p. 90)

dentinal tubules
(p. 92)

enamel (p. 90)

epithelial
attachment
(p. 97)

fibroblasts (p. 93)

free gingiva (p. 96)

gingiva (p. 96)

gingival sulcus
(p. 97)

lamina dura (p. 94)

mucogingival
junction (p. 96)

Nasmyth's
membrane (p. 92)

odontoblasts
(p. 90)

periodontium
(p. 93)

philtrum (p. 87)

pulp (p. 90)

Sharpey's fibers
(p. 94)

stomedeum (p. 87)

zygote (p. 86)

INTRODUCTION

Dental assistants should be familiar with general embryological development of the face and the oral cavity and a background in general histology to understand the composition, formation, and eruption of the teeth. In addition to embryology and histology the chapter covers the components of the periodontium and describes the strucures of the gingiva.

EMBRYOLOGY

The study of prenatal growth and the developing process of an individual is called the science of **embryology**. Oral embryology refers to the study of the development of the oral cavity. The following information provides the dental assistant with a basic understanding of embryology.

Human pregnancy is approximately nine months (38 weeks) in duration. This time period starts immediately after conception, when the ovum is fertilized by the sperm. The following terms and times are utilized to identify the three prenatal phases of the pregnancy:

▶ Conception through the first two weeks—zygote

▶ Two weeks through the eighth week—embryo

▶ Nine weeks through birth—fetus

The **zygote** phase is when cells rapidly increase in number, or **proliferate**. During the embryonic phase, many critical changes are taking place. The cells are differentiating (developing individual characteristics) and integrating to form cell layers that develop into a human being. There are three stages of differentiation:

1. **Cytodifferentiation**—the development of different cells

2. **Histodifferentiation**—the development of different tissues

3. **Morphodifferentiation**—the development of different forms

Three primary embryonic layers are formed early in the embryo phase. The **ectoderm** layer differentiates into skin, hair, nails, the brain, the nervous system, the lining of the oral cavity, and the enamel of the teeth. The second layer, the **mesoderm**, differentiates into the lining of the abdominal cavity, the bones, the muscles, the circulatory system, the reproductive system, the internal organs, and the dentin, cementum, and pulp of the teeth. The **endoderm**, the third layer, gives rise to the epithelial linings of the respiratory system, some glandular organs, and the digestive tract. To remember the layers, recall that *derm* refers to tissue and *ecto* refers to outside, *meso* refers to middle and *endo* refers to inside (Figure 5-1). The first sign of a developing tooth is noted during the embryonic phase, in the area that will eventually become the lower mandibular anterior region (Figure 5-2).

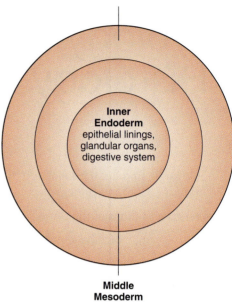

Outer
Ectoderm
skin, brain, nervous system, hair, nails, enamel of teeth, lining of the oral cavity

Inner
Endoderm
epithelial linings, glandular organs, digestive system

Middle
Mesoderm
bones, muscles, circulatory system, internal organs, reproductive system, lining of the abdominal cavity, dentin, cementum, pulp of the teeth

FIGURE 5-1 The three primary embryonic layers—ectoderm (outer), mesoderm (middle), and endoderm (inner), and associated tissues.

Primitive Facial Development

The face begins to form during the fourth week of prenatal development (Figure 5-3A). This embryonic phase involves all three embryonic layers. At this time, the

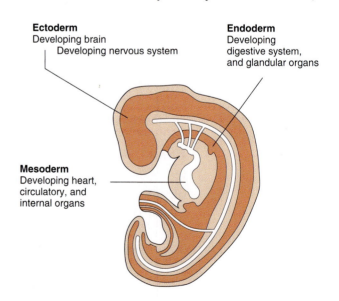

Ectoderm
Developing brain
Developing nervous system

Endoderm
Developing digestive system, and glandular organs

Mesoderm
Developing heart, circulatory, and internal organs

FIGURE 5-2 The developing embryo with primary embryonic layers identified.

future face appears to be squeezed between the bulging brain and the large heart, with the eyes and nose spread out toward the sides. The face further develops from the three embryonic layers (Figures 5-3B and C). The first area, the frontonasal process, forms the upper portion of the face, the forehead, eyes, nose, and the **philtrum** (vertical groove on the midline of the upper lip). The second area forms the middle of the face, called the maxillary (medial nasal) process. This area consists of the cheeks, sides of the upper lip, midface, secondary palate, zygomatic bones, portion of the temporal bones, and the maxilla embryonic surface. The third area, called the mandibular process, forms the two mandibular arches (first branchial arches) and makes up the lower lip, lower face, temporal area, and the mandible. The **stomedeum** (stoh-mah-DE-um), or primitive mouth, appears between the maxillary and mandibular processes. It initially appears as a shallow depression in the embryonic surface.

The face continues developing until the twelfth week, changing shape considerably during this time. The eyes move forward, the nose comes together, and the face appears much more narrow than during the first formation. The maxillary processes on each side of the face fuse at the **labial commissures**, or corners of the mouth, with the mandibular arch (Figure 5-3B). The frontonasal process fuses with the maxillary process along the line of the **nasolacrimal groove**. This groove extends from the medial corner of the eye to the nasal cavity along the maxillary process to the medial nasal process. This fusion normally is completed during the sixth week of prenatal development.

Inside the oral cavity, the **primary** (primitive) **palate** is developing. It appears as a triangular mass and contains the four maxillary incisor teeth. It serves to separate the developing oral cavities from the nasal cavities. The two palatal shelves develop and move medially toward each other, fusing to form the **secondary palate**, which will become two-thirds of the hard palate (Figure 5-4). The secondary palate contains the remaining teeth and forms the remaining two-thirds of the hard palate and the soft palate, including the uvula. During the twelfth week of prenatal development, the primary palate and the secondary palate meet and fuse together, forming the final palate. Thus, the oral cavity and the nasal cavity are completely separated.

Developmental Disturbances

Disturbances during periods of prenatal development most often occur during the embryonic period but may occur any time. Genetic and environmental factors such as drugs and infections can initiate malformations in the unborn child. Women should avoid using alcohol and drugs immediately after suspicion of pregnancy. Infants born to women who have persisted taking alcohol during pregnancy may exhibit fetal alcohol syndrome (FAS). Symptoms of FAS include, but are not limited to,

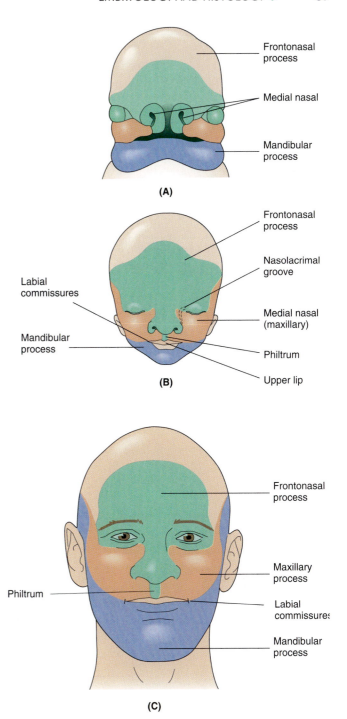

FIGURE 5-3 Embryonic facial processes shown on (A) embryo, (B) child and (C) adult.

small head circumference, low nasal bridge, indistinct philtrum, thin upper lip, and a small mandible.

Specific infections contracted by pregnant women may cause malformations and developmental disturbances in the unborn child. For example, German measles may cause heart, eye, or hearing defects in the unborn child. Syphilis, another infection, can cause paralysis, blindness, deafness, and defects in the incisors and molars.

Varying degrees of disfigurement may be caused by the failure of the tissues to fuse together. Children born

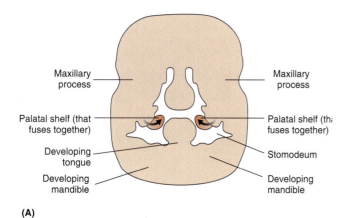

Maxillary process

Maxillary process

Palatal shelf (that fuses together)

Palatal shelf (that fuses together)

Developing tongue

Stomodeum

Developing mandible

Developing mandible

(A)

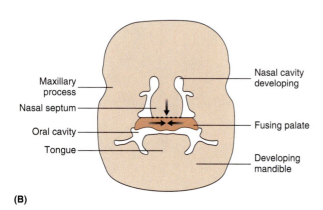

Maxillary process

Nasal cavity developing

Nasal septum

Oral cavity

Fusing palate

Tongue

Developing mandible

(B)

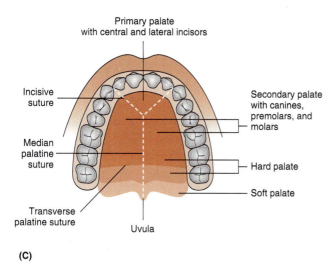

Primary palate with central and lateral incisors

Incisive suture

Secondary palate with canines, premolars, and molars

Median palatine suture

Hard palate

Soft palate

Transverse palatine suture

Uvula

(C)

FIGURE 5-4 Development of the palate. (A) Palate forming from three sections. (B) Frontal view. (C) Palatal view of the three sections and where the secondary and primary palate fuse.

with disabilities of this kind should be seen by medical and dental specialists. Initially, the infant may face problems that limit nursing and feeding. Decisions need to be made to allow proper nutritional care for the child. Developmental disturbances that deal with the failure

of tissues to fuse normally require long-term attention. If the palate has not fused, the teeth may not erupt in the proper positions, if at all. The dentist follows the case to ensure that all needed procedures are done at the proper time. Reconstructive surgery and speech and hearing therapy may be recommended.

Disturbance in the fusion may be caused by a number of factors. It is important that the pregnant mother be healthy and enjoy good nutrition. Drugs (alcohol included) taken during pregnancy may cause birth defects. Hereditary factors may play a role in birth defects also.

Cleft Lip. When the maxillary processes fail to fuse with the medial nasal process, **cleft lip** results. Cleft lip occurs in about one in 1,000 live births. These cleft lips can occur on one side or both sides of the upper lip. One side is called **unilateral** cleft lip; both sides are referred to as a **bilateral** cleft lip (Figure 5-5A). Cleft lips are more common in boys and more frequently unilateral on the left side. They are also more severe in boys than girls. Clefts can be as small as a notch in the lip to more severe cases that extend into the floor of the nostril.

FIGURE 5-5 (A) Cleft lip. (B) Cleft palate. *(Courtesy of Joseph L. Konzelman, Jr., DDS)*

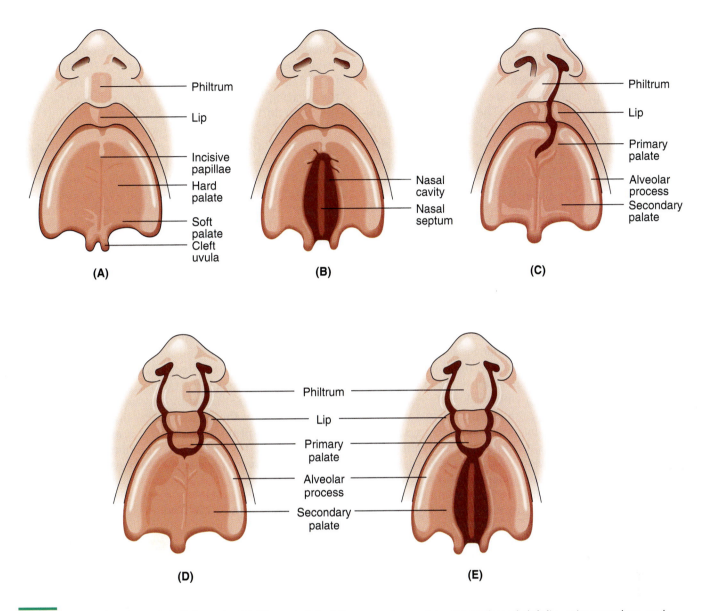

FIGURE 5-6 Cleft palates. (A) Cleft uvula. (B) Bilateral cleft of the secondary palate. (C) Unilateral cleft lip, primary palate, and alveolar process. (D) Bilateral cleft of the lip, alveolar process, and primary palate. (E) Bilateral cleft of the lip, alveolar process, and primary and secondary palate.

Cleft Palate. A **cleft palate**, the failure of the palatal shelves to fuse with the primary palate or with each other, may occur with or without a cleft lip. Cleft palate occurs in one of every 2,500 births. Cleft palate occurring alone is more common in girls than boys. A **cleft uvula** is the mildest form of a cleft palate because it does not hamper eating or speaking to the same degree that the cleft palate or the cleft lip does. With a cleft uvula, only the uvula is separated slightly (Figure 5-6A). The clefts may be bilateral in only the posterior palate or complete unilateral cleft lip and alveolar process with unilateral cleft of the primary palates (Figures 5-6B and C). The clefts may also be complete bilateral cleft lip and alveolar process with bilateral cleft of the primary palatal portions (Figure 5-6D). The most complex

is the complete bilateral cleft lip and maxillary alveolar process with bilateral cleft of the primary and secondary palates (Figure 5-6E).

▌ LIFE CYCLE OF THE TOOTH

Each tooth goes through a number of successive periods of development during its life cycle. These periods often are grouped into different stages according to the shape and development of the organ.

Bud Stage

The first stage of **odontogenesis** (origin of the tooth) is referred to as the **bud stage** (Figure 5-7A). During this stage, initiation takes place. **Initiation** is when the tooth begins formation from the **dental lamina**. The dental lamina is a growth from the oral epithelium that gives rise to the tooth buds. Therefore, on a deciduous dentition, ten growths on each arch are apparent or ten buds later become the primary teeth. The first sign of a developing tooth is noted during the embryonic phase in the area that will eventually be the lower mandibular anterior region of the child's oral cavity. The permanent teeth develop in a similar manner. Each arch has sixteen different buds developing into one tooth each. The last three molars in each quadrant develop behind the primary dentition. The six year molar begins developing at birth, the twelve-year molar starts developing when the baby is about six months old, and the third molars (wisdom teeth) start when the child is approximately five years of age.

Cap Stage

The bud of the tooth grows and changes shape during the cap stage. The organ is indented on the lower side and appears much like a cap, therefore the name **cap stage** (Figure 5-7B). The primary embryonic ectoderm layer that has developed into the oral epithelium matures into the enamel of the developing tooth. The processes of **proliferation**, when the cells multiply, and histodifferentiation, when the cells develop into different tissues, take place along with early morphodifferentiation, when the cells begin to outline the future shape of the developing organ. During this process, the primary embryonic mesoderm layer develops into connective tissue that is referred to as the **mesenchyme** tissue. This connective tissue forms an enclosed area, referred to as a **dental sac**, and further matures into the dentin, cementum, and the pulp of the tooth. A portion of the mesenchyme surrounds the outside of the enamel organ, the cementum, and the periodontal ligament of the tooth.

Bell Stage

Further specialization of the cells, or histodifferentiation, takes place in the bell stage (Figure 5-7C). The inner epithelium of the enamel organ becomes **ameloblasts**, enamel-forming cells. The peripheral cells of the dental papilla become **odontoblasts**, cells that form dentin. The **cementoblasts**, cementum-forming cells, form from the dental sac. Continued morphodifferentiation takes place, forming the organ into a shape that resembles a bell (Figure 5-7D).

Maturation Stage

The odontogenesis reaches completion in these final stages. The tissues of enamel, dentin, and cementum are formed in layers and fused together in the appropriate manner. The process of depositing calcium salts and other minerals in the formed tooth takes place during the **apposition** stage (Figure 5-7E). This process is called calcification and is the last developmental stage prior to **eruption** of the tooth (Figures 5-7F and G). The final stage of the life cycle of the tooth is attrition, or the wearing away of the incisal or occlusal surfaces of the tooth during normal function (Figures 5-7H and 5-8).

The root of the tooth does not develop fully prior to eruption. Eruption is the phase when the tooth passes through the bone and the oral mucosa and into its place in the oral cavity. An eruption schedule for the primary and permanent teeth is located in Chapter 6, Tooth Morphology. Twenty of the permanent teeth are located below and distal to the primary teeth. As the permanent teeth erupt, they apply pressure to the apices of the roots of the primary teeth. During this force, **osteoclasts**, bone resorption cells, **evanesce** (ev-a-**NES**) (dissolve) the root of the primary tooth. This resorption first takes place at the apex and continues up toward the crown of the tooth. When very little of the root structure of the primary tooth is left, the tooth loosens due to lack of support. Children often assist in the final stages of loosening the tooth by moving it back and forth until they break the attaching fibers.

The primary teeth occupy and maintain space in the dental arches for the permanent teeth and act as guides during the eruption process. If the primary teeth are removed early, the spaces may be diminished, causing crowding when the permanent teeth erupt.

▍ HISTOLOGY

The study of the microscopic structure and function of tissues is **histology**. Oral histology is the study of the tissues of the teeth and the structures of the oral cavity that surround the teeth.

▍ TOOTH STRUCTURE

Each tooth is made up of four primary structures (Figure 5-9). The enamel is the structure that covers the outside of the crown of the tooth. It is the hardest living tissue in the body. Enamel can be very brittle if not supported by dentin and a vital pulp. Dentin makes up the bulk of the tooth structure but is not normally visible. It surrounds the pulp cavity and lies under the enamel, within the anatomical crown and under the cementum within the root. The cementum is the third structure and is located around the root. It covers the dentin on the root portion of the tooth. At the center of the tooth, within the pulp cavity, is the pulp tissue. It is made up of the nerves and blood vessels that provide nutrients to the tooth. The pulp cavity is made up of a pulp chamber with pulp horns and pulp canal(s). The **pulp canal**(s) is (are) located in the root(s) of the teeth. The **pulp chamber** is a large portion of the pulp, which is located in the crown of the tooth. The **pulp horns**, pointed elonga-

(A) Initiation

Bud stage

(B) Proliferation

Cap stage (begins proliferation, histodifferentiation, and morphodifferentiation

(C) Histodifferentiation

Bell stage

(D) Morphodifferentiation

(E) Apposition

Maturation stage

(F) Calcification

(G) Eruption

(H) Attrition

FIGURE 5-7 Life cycle of the tooth.

FIGURE 5-8 Attrition of the primary dentition. *(Courtesy of Dr. Steve Gregg)*

tions of the pulp, extend toward the incisal or occlusal portion of the tooth. The pulpal portion of the tooth is often larger in primary teeth and newly formed permanent teeth. As a person ages, the pulpal portion may decrease in size. For example, adults over seventy years of age may have small pulp chambers or the pulpal portion may be totally calcified.

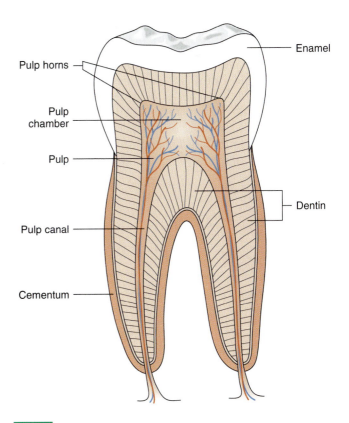

FIGURE 5-9 Tissues of the tooth.

Enamel

Enamel is thicker on the biting surfaces, occlusal cusps, and the incisal edge than in other areas. Ameloblasts aid in the developing of the enamel rods. These rods, which are not visible to the naked eye, are four micrometers in diameter, variable lengths, and shaped in the pattern of a fish (Figure 5-10). Their location in the enamel is such that the head is surrounded by the tails of two other enamel rods. The substance surrounding the inner portion, the **rod core**, of each enamel rod is the **interprismatic substance**. Of these substances, the enamel rods are hardest and the interprismatic substance is the weakest.

The enamel matrix is produced by the ameloblast cells. **Tome's process**, a secretory surface of the ameloblast, is responsible for laying down the enamel matrix. Tome's process guides the **enamel matrix** into place. As the second layer is laid down, the first becomes more mineralized and this process follows until the last layer is placed.

Enamel rods under a microscope show several developmental identification marks. The **lines of Retzius** (**RET**-zee-us) appear as incremental lines or bands around the layers, much like the growth rings on a tree. Very few lines are indicated prenatally, but one, known as the **neonatal line**, an accentuated incremental line, indicates the trauma of birth. It is found in all the primary teeth and several of the permanent teeth. Along with the lines of Retzius are the **imbrication lines**, slight ridges on the cervical third of certain teeth that extend mesiodistally, and the **perikymata** (pear-ee-**KIGH**-mah-tah), small grooves noted on some teeth.

Enamel spindles represent short, dentinal tubules that seem to have crossed over into the enamel and were trapped there during the process of enamel mineralization. Noted with bases near the dentinoenamel junction are the **enamel tufts**. They appear as small, dark brushes. Narrower and longer enamel tufts are called **enamel lamellae**. These thin structures extend from the dentinoenamel junction to the enamel surface.

Enamel rod

Head

Tail

FIGURE 5-10 Drawing representing the enamel rods.

Clinical Considerations Regarding Enamel

▶ Primary teeth may erupt with a covering over the enamel, left over from the epithelium and the ameloblasts, called the **Nasmyth's membrane**. Nasmyth's membrane may pick up stain easily. This membrane is easily removed by a thorough polishing. No lasting effects on the condition of the enamel are observed following removal of the membrane.

▶ Certain developmental disturbances can occur during the apposition stage. A loss of nutritional support may result in the surface of the teeth becoming grooved and pitted, called **enamel dysplasia**. The patient may be concerned with the appearance of the tooth, and the weakened surface is more susceptible to decay. With today's dental materials, the surface of the tooth can be restored.

▶ Fluoride can aid in strengthening the enamel to prevent demineralization. Fluoride can be ingested or applied topically.

▶ Dentists prepare the teeth for the placement of restorations in a manner in which isolated enamel rods are protected from fracture.

Dentin

Mature dentin is softer than enamel but harder than cementum and bone. If the dentin is exposed, it appears a yellowish white color. It is what gives the translucent enamel its underlying yellow hue. The cuspid is a bulky tooth with a greater amount of dentin; therefore, it appears more yellow than the teeth surrounding it. Dentin is less dense and appears rougher in surface texture than enamel. The odontoblasts form dentin, beginning at the dentinoenamel junction and continuing toward the pulp chamber. **Dentinal tubules** pass through the entire surface of the dentin. These long tubes contain the **dentinal fluid**, which is presumably tissue fluid surrounding the cell membrane of the odontoblast.

As with enamel, developmental marks are apparent in the dentin. **Imbrication lines of Von Ebner** are the stained growth rings or incremental lines in dentin. Contour lines that demonstrate a disturbance in the body metabolism are called **contour lines of Owen**. Again, the most pronounced stained contour line is the neonatal line that occurs due to the trauma of birth.

Types of Dentin. Dentin differs from area to area and is not uniform throughout. **Peritubular dentin** is the dentin that creates the wall of the dentinal tubule. Dentin found between the tubules is called **intertubular dentin**. The first predentin that is formed and matures within the tooth is called **mantle dentin**. The layer of dentin that surrounds the pulp is called **circumpulpal dentin**. Forming the bulk of the tooth is **primary dentin**, which is formed prior to the completion of the apical foramen (opening of the root's pulp canal). **Secondary dentin** forms after the completion of the apical foramen and slowly throughout the life of the tooth. Due to continued growth, the pulp chamber narrows and may become calcified later in life. **Tertiary dentin** repairs and is reactive to irritations. It forms quickly in response to localized injury. Injury may be caused by dental caries, cavity preparation, recession, attrition, or erosion. Tertiary dentin may be more irregular than primary or secondary dentin.

Clinical Considerations Regarding Dentin

▶ If the antibiotic tetracycline is taken during the formation of dentin, it binds chemically to the dentin and causes permanent yellow staining.

▶ Cavities that appear small on the outside of the tooth extend more rapidly through the dentin because it is a less dense structure than enamel.

▶ Patients may experience **dentinal hypersensitivity** if the dentin is exposed. This may be very painful for the patient. In some individuals, the enamel and cementum do not come together at the cementoenamel junction (CEJ), leaving exposed dentin; therefore, dentinal hypersensitivity exists. Using the air-water syringe in an area that is not anesthetized will cause discomfort.

Pulp

The pulp of the tooth evolves from cells similar to the dentin. Its function is to provide nourishment, support, and maintenance for the dentin. Also, when the dentin or pulp is injured, sensory nerves send the messages to the brain for interpretation. The pulp identifies the temperature and chemical changes, vibrations, and bacterial invasion of the tooth and transmits this information to the brain. It is a warning system that works as a defense system for the tooth.

The pulp is made partially from fibroblasts (cells from which connective tissue evolve), which synthesize protein fibers and **intercellular substances** (substances between the cells) to form pulp tissue. The pulp is fed continually through the opening at the apex of the root, the apical foramen.

Clinical Considerations Regarding Pulp

▶ If the pulp is damaged due to an injury, the tissue may become inflamed, causing **pulpitis**. The pressure becomes great and cannot escape. The structures of the tooth form a hard encasement and, when the tooth becomes inflamed, it causes a great deal of pressure and discomfort. The patient may need to have root canal therapy, which opens the pulp and releases the pressure.

▶ If endodontic treatment (root canal therapy) is performed on a tooth, the pulp tissue is removed and the tooth becomes non-vital.

▶ The use of water-cooled handpieces prevents overheating of the pulp during dental treatment.

▶ **Pulp stones**, calcified masses of dentin, are sometimes present in the pulp tissue. They can be attached or unattached to the pulpal wall. They are quite common and normally will cause a problem only if root canal therapy is necessary.

COMPONENTS OF THE PERIODONTIUM

The periodontium consists of portions of the tooth structure, supporting hard and soft dental tissues, and the alveolar bone. The cementum is part of the periodontium as well as the last tooth structure.

Cementum

Surrounding the root of the tooth, attaching it to the alveolar bone by anchoring the periodontal ligaments, is the **cementum** (Figure 5-11). It is a dull light yellow in color, lighter than dentin and darker than enamel. It is softer than both dentin and enamel and has a grainy feel. Cementum continues to develop throughout life, like dentin and pulp. Cementum is formed by cementoblasts and is thicker at the apex than at any other area. Cementum does not resorb and regenerate like bone, which allows orthodontic treatment to move the teeth

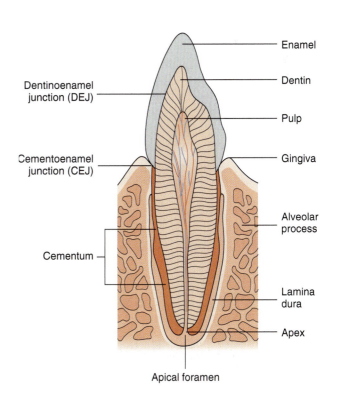

Enamel

Dentin

Dentinoenamel junction (DEJ)

Pulp

Gingiva

Cementoenamel junction (CEJ)

Alveolar process

Cementum

Lamina dura

Apex

Apical foramen

FIGURE 5-11 Tooth and surrounding tissues.

through the bone and not destroy the cementum. Within the outer part of the cementum are collagen fibers from the periodontal ligament, called **Sharpey's fibers** (Figure 5-12). They act as anchors between the alveolar bone and the tooth.

Clinical Concerns Regarding Cementum

▶ In the case of gingival recession, the cementum may become exposed. The cementum is very thin at the cementoenamel junction (CEJ) and can quickly wear away. This exposes the dentin and causes pain to the patient.

▶ **Cemental spurs** are found near the CEJ. During dental cleaning (scaling and curettage), the operator may find it difficult to differentiate cemental spurs from calculus. One difference is that the calculus is much easier to remove.

▶ If the tooth is traumatized due to force from the occlusal or incisal surface, a condition known as **hypercementosis** may take place. This causes a thickening of cementum around the apex, which may show on the x-ray as a mass at the apex.

Alveolar Bone

The bones of the mandible and maxilla are formed by **osteoblasts**, bone-forming cells. The cells that remodel and resorb bone are called **osteoclasts**. The extended areas of bone in each arch that are tooth bearing are called the **alveolar process**. The compact bone plates on the facial and lingual surfaces are called the **cortical bone**. The bone that surrounds the root of the tooth, the socket, is the **alveolus**. On a dental radiograph, the **lamina dura**, or radiopaque line, represents the thin, compact alveolus bone lining the socket. This alveolus does not actually contact the root because the periodontal ligament suspends it in place. The two cortical bone plates come together between each tooth. This is referred to as the **alveolar crest** and should be slightly below the CEJ in a healthy mouth (Figure 5-13). If the tooth has multiple roots, the bone that separates the roots is identified as **interradicular septum**. Each socket is separated by a bony projection called the **interdental septum**.

Clinical Concerns Regarding the Alveolar Bone

▶ Periodontal disease can cause the loss of bone. The bone does not regenerate and the diseased tissue must be removed.

▶ The bone is stimulated from mastication and speech. If the teeth are removed, this stimulation is lost and the bone can resorb. The bone supports the teeth and the teeth support the bone.

▶ Modern implants placed in the bone are more successful if proper dental hygiene of the area is maintained. The implant has no movement in the bone; unlike the teeth, it remains stable.

Periodontal Ligament

The **periodontal ligament**, like all connective tissue, is formed by the fibroblast cells and secures the tooth into the socket by a number of organized fiber groups. The Sharpey's fiber is attached in the cementum and to the alveolar bone. The periodontal ligament has two types

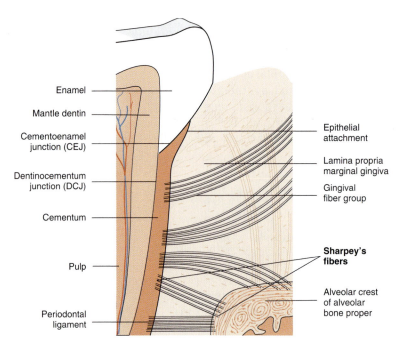

Enamel
Mantle dentin
Cementoenamel junction (CEJ)
Dentinocementum junction (DCJ)
Cementum
Pulp
Periodontal ligament

Epithelial attachment
Lamina propria marginal gingiva
Gingival fiber group
Sharpey's fibers
Alveolar crest of alveolar bone proper

FIGURE 5-12 A section of tooth identifying Sharpey's fibers and cementum.

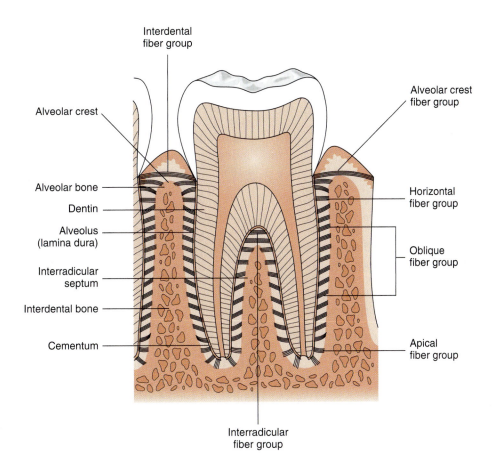

FIGURE 5-13 A section of a mandibular molar showing periodontal ligaments, group fibers of alveolar crest, horizontal, oblique, apical, interradicular, and interdental.

of nerves: one sensory and one to regulate the blood vessels. This ligament is wider at the cervix (CEJ) and at the apex and narrow between these points.

Periodontal Fiber Groups. Most of the fibers in the **periodontal fiber groups** are principle fibers, meaning they are organized into bundles or groups dependent on their functions. These fibers allow for some flexibility during mastication, speech, and other forces that would be exerted on the teeth. Six principle fiber groups consist of the five **alveolodental** (al-vee-oh-loh-**DENT**-al) **ligament** fiber groups and one interdental or transseptal ligament group (Figure 5-13).

The alveolodental dental ligaments include the following:

▶ **Alveolar crest fiber groups** function to resist rotational forces and tilting. They originate in the alveolar crest of the alveolar bone and then insert into the cervical cementum at various angles.

▶ **Horizontal fiber groups** function in much the same manner as the alveolar crest fiber group. They are, however, located in a different area. They originate in the alveolar bone, apical to the alveolar crest, and then insert into the cementum in a horizontal manner.

▶ **Oblique fiber groups** constitute the most abundant of the fiber groups. Their function is to resist intrusive forces that try to push the tooth inward. The oblique fiber group covers two-thirds of the root, attaching in the alveolar bone and extending in an oblique (diagonal) manner into the cementum.

▶ **Apical fiber groups** function to resist forces that try to pull the tooth outward, as well as rotational forces. They attach at the apex of the tooth and radiate outward to attach in the surrounding alveolar bone.

▶ **Interradicular fiber groups** are found only in multirooted teeth. Their function is to resist rotational forces and to hold the teeth in interproximal contact. They run from the cementum of one root to the cementum of the other root(s), over the interradicular septum.

▶ **Interdental (or transseptal) ligament groups** function to resist rotational forces and hold teeth in interproximal contact. They run above the crest of the alveolar bone interdentally, from the cervical cementum of one tooth to the cervical cementum of another tooth.

Clinical Considerations Regarding the Periodontal Ligaments

▶ Occlusal trauma does not cause periodontal disease but can accelerate an existing disease.

▶ Chronic periodontal disease causes the fiber groups to become disorganized and lose attachment due to resorption.

▶ The fiber group that is retained the longest during periodontal disease is the interdental ligament. As the disease progresses, this ligament reattaches itself in a more apical manner.

Gingival Fiber Groups. The **gingival fiber groups** are found in the **lamina propria**, the connective tissue of the marginal gingiva (Figure 5-14). They support the marginal gingival tissues in relationship to the tooth. They lie above the alveolar bone crest and below the epithelium.

▶ **Dentogingival fiber groups** act to maintain the gingival integrity of the marginal gingiva. They are attached to the cementum and extend into the lamina propria of the marginal gingiva.

▶ **Circular ligament fiber groups** circle and tighten the gingival margin around the neck of the tooth. This fiber group is located in the lamina propria of the marginal gingival.

▶ **Alveologingival fiber groups** aid in attaching the gingiva to the alveolar bone. They extend from the alveolar bone and diffuse into the overlying lamina propria of the marginal gingiva.

▶ **Dentoperiosteal fiber groups** are supportive fibers that anchor the tooth to the bone. They originate from the cementum, near the CEJ, and extend across the alveolar crest.

Gingiva

The **gingiva**, composed of a mucosa that surrounds the necks of the teeth and covers the alveolar processes, is commonly referred to as **gums**. It can be attached to the underlying bone or unattached (free) (Figures 5-15 and 5-16). (The plural of gingiva is gingivae.) The gingival tissue surrounds the teeth and, in a healthy state, is firm and tightly adapted to the tooth. The texture appears similar to the outside of an orange—**stippled**. The color of the gingiva may differ according to the pigmentation of the particular person.

Alveolar Mucosa. The **alveolar mucosa** appears thin and loosely attached, covering the alveolar bone. It flows into the tissue of the cheeks and lips and the inside floor of the mandible. It is found immediately apical to the mucogingival junction.

Mucogingival Junction. The **mucogingival junction** is the line of demarcation between the attached gingiva and the alveolar mucosa.

Attached Gingiva. The **attached gingiva** extends from the mucogingival junction to the gingival groove. The tissue is stippled and attached tightly to the alveolar bone.

Gingival Groove. The gingival groove, or free gingival groove, is the line of demarcation between the attached gingiva and the marginal gingiva.

Marginal Gingiva. The marginal gingiva, commonly referred to as **free gingiva**, surrounds the teeth. This tis-

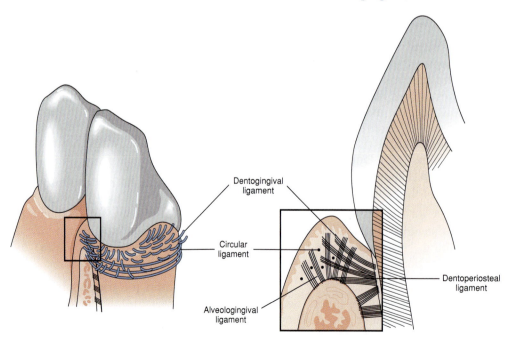

FIGURE 5-14 The gingival fiber groups: dentogingival, circular ligament, alveologingival, and dentoperiosteal.

FIGURE 5-15 The periodontium.

FIGURE 5-16 The periodontium identified on an individual.

sue, attached only at the gingival groove, appears lighter in color (if healthy) and about one millimeter in width.

Interdental Gingiva. The interdental gingiva is an extension of unattached gingiva between adjacent teeth. It is also referred to as interdental papilla.

Gingival Sulcus. The **gingival sulcus** is the space between the unattached gingiva and the tooth. In a healthy mouth, this space would not exceed two to three millimeters in depth.

Epithelial Attachment. The **epithelial attachment** is the gingiva in the floor of the gingival sulcus that attaches to the enamel surface of the teeth just above the CEJ of the teeth.

Clinical Considerations Regarding Gingival Tissue

▶ Certain drugs can affect the gingiva and cause **gingival hyperplasia**, which is an overgrowth of the tissue. An example of this would be the drug Dilantin (trade name for phenytoin sodium), taken in the treatment of epilepsy. These drugs cause the fibroblasts to increase output.

▶ The gingival tissue, rich in blood and fluid, can become inflamed to fight infection. It appears swollen and red, bleeds easily, and looses its stippled look. Correct hygiene measures can usually alleviate this condition.

CHAPTER SUMMARY

It is vital for the entire dental team to be able to communicate the structure and function of the oral cavity. Therefore, it is important for the dental assistant to understand the structure/function of tissue, the prenatal growth/development process of oral embryology, and the oral cavity that surrounds the teeth.

CASE STUDY

Joseph Tanner is a new patient at the Community Dental Clinic. He is a six-year-old with a loose primary tooth in the anterior region of the mandible. He stated that the tooth has been "wiggling" for two months. He has tried to get it out but has been unsuccessful. The dentist examines the area and documents his findings.

Case Study Review

1. Describe the process of resorption of the root of the primary tooth.

2. Identify the periodontal fibers that may remain attached around the loose tooth at this stage.

3. If the primary tooth is removed early, what are the possible complications that may occur?

To complete your study of this chapter, work the review activities that follow. Also, refer to the software that accompanies this text.

REVIEW QUESTIONS

Multiple Choice

1. The term used to identify the third prenatal phase of pregnancy from nine weeks through birth is
   a. fetus.   c. zygote.
   b. embryo.   d. ovum.

2. The embryonic layer that differentiates into enamel and the lining of the oral cavity is the
   a. ectoderm.   c. endoderm.
   b. mesoderm.   d. stomedeum.

3. Enamel-forming cells are called
   a. ameloblasts.   c. cementoblasts.
   b. odontoblasts.   d. fibroblasts.

4. An incremental line in the enamel indicating the trauma of birth, found in all primary teeth and several of the permanent teeth, is the
   a. line of Retzius.   c. Tome's process.
   b. imbrication line.   d. neonatal line.

5. The tooth structure that is the softest is the
   a. alveolar bone.   c. dentin.
   b. cementum.   d. enamel.

Critical Thinking

1. While in the hospital maternity ward, a dental assistant sees a newborn child with a severe unilateral cleft lip. Based on what he or she knows about the probability of a child having this condition, an assumption would be made that the child is what sex?

2. If a child has enamel dysplasia, a dental assistant would assume that a disturbance took place during which cycle of tooth development? Which stage?

3. If a calcified mass of dentin material is present in the pulp chamber, what procedures can it inhibit? What are such masses called?

Tooth Morphology

OBJECTIVES

The student should strive to meet the following objectives and demonstrate an understanding of the facts and principles presented in this chapter:

1. Identify the dental arches and quadrants using the correct terminology.

2. List the primary and permanent teeth by name and location.

3. Explain the eruption schedule for the primary and permanent teeth.

4. Identify the different divisions of the tooth, including clinical and anatomical divisions.

5. Identify the surfaces of each tooth and their locations.

6. List the anatomical structures and their definitions.

7. Describe each permanent tooth according to location, anatomical features, morphology, function, position, and other identifying factors.

8. Describe each deciduous (primary) tooth according to its location, anatomical features, morphology, function, position, and other identifying factors.

KEY TERMS

adjacent (p. 100)

anatomical crown (p. 104)

apical foramen (p. 105)

bifurcated (p. 105)

buccal (p. 105)

cervical line (p. 104)

cingulum (p. 105)

clinical crown (p. 104)

cusps (p. 101)

cusp of Carabelli (p. 105)

dentition (p. 100)

developmental groove (p. 106)

distal (p. 105)

facial (p. 105)

fissure (p. 106)

fossa (p. 106)

furcation (p. 106)

imbrication lines (p. 110)

incisal edge (p. 101)

lingual (p. 105)

lobes (p. 106)

mamelons (p. 106)

mandibular arch (p. 100)

marginal ridge (p. 106)

maxillary arch (p. 100)

mesial (p. 105)

midline (p. 100)

oblique ridge (p. 106)

occlusal (p. 105)

pit (p. 107)

posterior (p. 102)

ridge (p. 107)

succedaneous (p. 102)

supplemental groove (p. 107)

transverse ridge (p. 108)

triangular ridge (p. 108)

trifurcated (p. 108)

INTRODUCTION

Tooth morphology is the study of the structure and form of teeth. In this chapter, the morphology of the teeth is discussed, along with the location, eruption schedule, and function of each tooth in the primary and permanent dentition. The terms in this chapter are the building blocks for dental terminology used in the dental office.

DENTAL ARCHES

The **dentition** (natural teeth in position) are arranged in two arches. The upper arch is the **maxillary arch**, because the teeth are set in the maxilla bone. The lower teeth are located in the mandible bone, therefore located in the **mandibular arch** (Figure 6-1). The maxillary arch is fixed to the skull and the mandibular arch is movable, bringing the biting force toward the maxillary arch. Each arch has an identical number of teeth, and the teeth are designed so that proper function and positioning can be maintained. The teeth in the maxillary arch slightly over-lap the mandibular teeth when in proper alignment. The teeth in each arch touch the teeth **adjacent** (next) to them, except for the last tooth in each arch. The teeth from the maxillary arch contact the teeth from the mandibular arch each time the mouth is closed together. Each tooth supports the teeth beside it and the teeth in the opposing arch so that displacement does not occur.

DENTAL QUADRANTS

Each of the dental arches is divided in two halves by an imaginary line called the **midline** (median line), which creates two sections called **quadrants**. Thus, there are four quadrants, containing eight permanent teeth each, found in the dentition. The arrangement of the teeth is identical in each quadrant, and each quadrant is named according to its location in the dentition (Figure 6-2).

The quadrants are labeled according to the patient's right or left. Looking into the oral cavity from the front of the patient makes the directions of right and left reversed to the dental assistant.

Maxillary

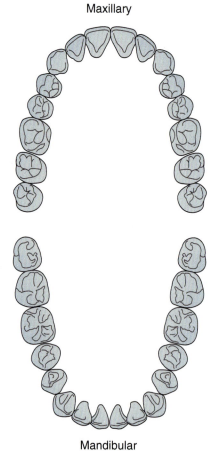

Mandibular

(A) Permanent dentition

Maxillary

Mandibular

(B) Deciduous dentition

FIGURE 6-1 (A) Maxillary and mandibular dentition of an adult (permanent dentition). (B) Maxillary and mandibular dentition of a child (deciduous dentition).

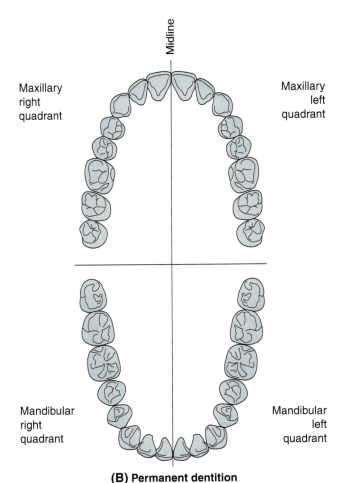

FIGURE 6-2 Dental arches of (A) primary (deciduous) dentition and (B) permanent dentition divided into quadrants with the midline identified.

TYPES OF TEETH AND THEIR FUNCTIONS

Primary Teeth

The primary (**deciduous**) teeth in each quadrant are named similar to the permanent teeth. The deciduous dentition has twenty teeth total: ten in each arch and five in each quadrant. The following teeth are found in each quadrant. Starting from the midline, the first tooth is called the **central incisor** and is used to cut or bite the food that is ingested. The second tooth from the midline, the **lateral incisor**, is also used for cutting. The third tooth from the midline is the **canine** (cuspid). This tooth is slightly more bulky in size and aids in tearing food. The next two teeth are molars and are named the first molar, which is the one closest to the midline, and the second molar. **Molars** are used to chew food.

> Both the first and the second primary teeth from the midline are incisors; to incise something is to cut it.

When compared to the permanent dentition, the deciduous dentition contains an identical number of central incisors, lateral incisors, and canines but has no premolars and one less molar per quadrant (Figure 6-3).

Permanent Teeth

Permanent teeth are arranged similar to the deciduous teeth. Adults have thirty-two permanent teeth: sixteen in each arch and eight in each quadrant. Each quadrant has the permanent central incisor, the lateral incisor, and the canine (cuspid), as did the deciduous quadrant. Directly after the canine (cuspid) in the permanent dentition are the first and second **premolars**.

The premolars are often called **bicuspids** because they usually have two (bi) **cusps** (pointed or rounded mounds on the crown of the tooth). However, two of the eight bicuspids may have three cusps; therefore, the term is not technically correct. However, it is important to be aware of the different names commonly used for the same teeth (for example, canines or cuspids and premolars or bicuspids).

The premolars are used to pulverize food. In other words, the premolars break the food down into smaller sizes to ready them for the chewing process, which is done by the molars.

After the premolars, the permanent dentition has the first, second, and third molars. The first molars are closest to the midline and the third molars, farthest from the midline, are commonly termed the "wisdom teeth."

The teeth in either arch that are toward the front of the mouth from cuspid to cuspid are the anterior teeth. The central incisors, lateral incisors, and canines (cuspids) are termed anterior teeth for both the deciduous and permanent dentition. Anterior teeth have single roots and a cutting or tearing edge called the **incisal edge**.

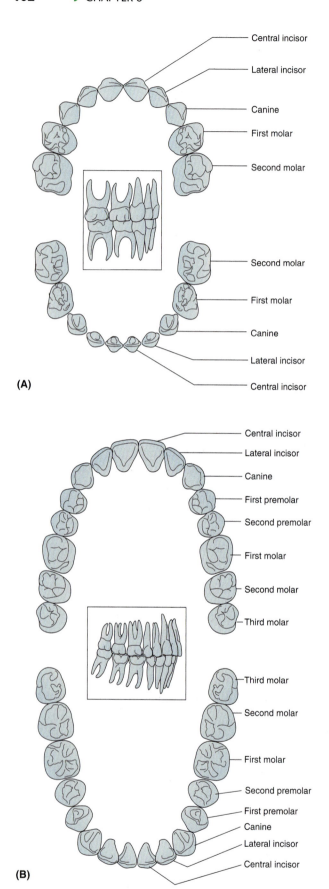

Central incisor
Lateral incisor
Canine
First molar
Second molar

Second molar
First molar
Canine
Lateral incisor
Central incisor

(A)

Central incisor
Lateral incisor
Canine
First premolar
Second premolar
First molar
Second molar
Third molar

Third molar
Second molar
First molar
Second premolar
First premolar
Canine
Lateral incisor
Central incisor

(B)

FIGURE 6-3 (A) The deciduous dentition identifying each tooth by name. (B) The permanent dentition identifying each tooth by name.

The teeth in either arch that are located in the back of the mouth are termed **posterior** teeth. The molars are posterior teeth in the deciduous dentition, and the premolars (bicuspids) and molars are posterior teeth in the permanent dentition. Posterior teeth normally have more than one root and multiple cusps for pulverizing and chewing.

ERUPTION SCHEDULE

Humans have two dentitions. The primary dentition (deciduous teeth) begins eruption (proceeds into the oral cavity) around six months of age. All twenty teeth are normally erupted by the age of three years (Table 6-1). The period when both primary teeth and permanent teeth are in the dentition is called the **mixed dentition** period (Figure 6-4). This period lasts from approximately six to twelve years of age. After the age of twelve, most of the primary teeth have **exfoliated** (shed from the oral cavity). The permanent dentition begins to erupt from about six years of age until around seventeen to twenty-one years of age (Table 6-2).

The permanent teeth that replace the primary teeth are called **succedaneous** teeth (Figure 6-5). This refers to succeeding deciduous teeth. Therefore, because there are twenty primary teeth, there are also twenty succedaneous teeth. The only permanent teeth that are not succedaneous teeth are the molars, because the premolars replace the primary molars.

DIVISIONS OF THE TOOTH

Each tooth has two basic parts: the **crown** and the **root**. The crown of the tooth is described as either

FIGURE 6-4 A mixed dentition of a seven- or eight-year-old.

TABLE 6-1 **ERUPTION AND EXFOLIATION DATES FOR PRIMARY TEETH**

Tooth	Eruption Date	Exfoliation Date	Maxillary Order
Central incisor	6–10 months	6–7 years	#1
Lateral incisor	9–12 months	7–8 years	#2
Canine	16–22 months	10–12 years	#4
First molar	12–18 months	9–11 years	#3
Second molar	24–32 months	10–12 years	#5
			Mandibular Order
Central incisor	6–10 months	6–7 years	#1
Lateral incisor	7–10 months	7–8 years	#2
Canine	16–22 months	9–12 years	#4
First molar	12–18 months	9–11 years	#3
Second molar	20–32 months	10–12 years	#5

TABLE 6-2 **ERUPTION DATES FOR PERMANENT TEETH**

Tooth	Eruption Date	Order of Eruption (Maxillary)
Central incisor	7–8 years	#2
Lateral incisor	8–9 years	#3
Canine	11–12 years	#6
First premolar	10–11 years	#4
Second premolar	11–12 years	#5
First molar	6–7 years	#1
Second molar	12–13 years	#7
Third molar	17–21 years	#8
		Order of Eruption (Mandibular)
Central incisor	6–7 years	#2
Lateral incisor	7–8 years	#3
Cuspid	9–10 years	#4
First premolar	10–11 years	#5
Second premolar	11–12 years	#6
First molar	6–7 years	#1
Second molar	11–13 years	#7
Third molar	17–21 years	#8

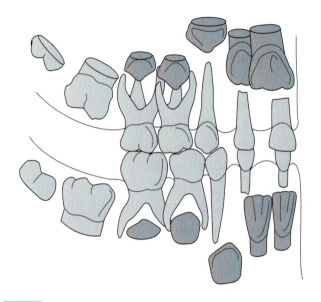

FIGURE 6-5 A dentition of a five-year-old showing the unerupted succedaneous teeth shaded.

anatomical or clinical (Figure 6-6). The **anatomical crown** is the portion of the tooth that is covered with the enamel. The **clinical crown** is the portion of the crown that is visible in the mouth. The clinical crown may be smaller than the anatomical crown if the level of the gingiva covers a portion of the crown (for example, during tooth eruption). The root of the tooth is also

divided into anatomical and clinical portions. The **anatomical root** is the portion covered with cementum, and the **clinical root** is the portion of the root seen in the oral cavity (for example, where the gingiva has receded). The **cervical line** divides the crown and the root and is where the anatomical crown and the root join together. (Cervical comes from the word *cervix,* meaning "the neck of.") The cervical line is also termed the cementoenamel junction (CEJ).

SURFACES OF THE TEETH

All teeth have five surfaces on the crown portion. Each surface, or side, has a specific name (Figure 6-7).

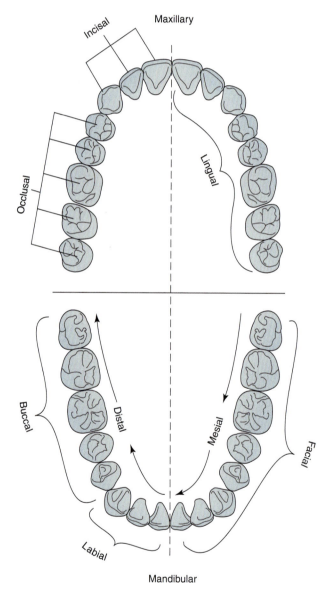

Permanent dentition

FIGURE 6-7 The surfaces of the teeth identified on the dental arches.

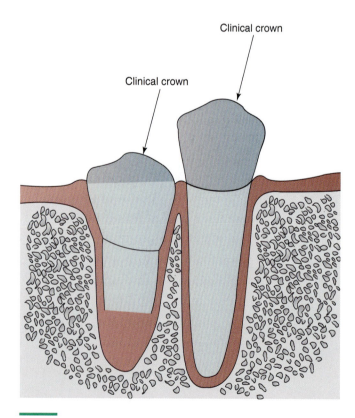

FIGURE 6-6 Clinical crown.

Anterior Teeth

▶ **Mesial**—The surface *toward* the midline.

▶ **Distal**—The surface *away* from the midline.

▶ **Labial**—The "outside" surface, which is toward the lips.

▶ **Lingual**—The "inside" surface, which is toward the tongue. On the maxillary arch, the lingual side may be referred to as the **palatal** surface.

▶ **Incisal edge**—The biting or cutting edge.

Facial Surface

The term **facial** may be used for either the labial surface of the anterior teeth or the buccal surface of the posterior teeth.

Posterior Teeth

▶ **Mesial**—The surface *toward* the midline.

▶ **Distal**—The surface *away* from the midline.

▶ **Lingual**—The "inside" surface, which is toward the tongue.

▶ **Buccal**—The "outside" surface, which is toward the cheek.

▶ **Occlusal**—The pulverizing or chewing surface.

All of the above tooth surfaces are either flat, convex, or concave (Figure 6-8). **Convex** means to bulge or curve outward, and **concave** means recessed or indented. (A clue to remember this is to think of a "cave" in concave; a cave is hollow and not bulging outward.)

ANATOMICAL STRUCTURES

It is important to be able to identify the landmarks on each individual tooth. Each area's name should be used when identifying the anatomical structures.

▶ **Apex**—At or near the end of the root (Figure 6-9).

▶ **Apical foramen**—An opening in the end of the tooth through which nerve and blood vessels enter (Figure 6-9). There may be more than one opening at the end of the root.

▶ **Bifurcated**—When there are two roots on one tooth, they are said to be bifurcated, or branched in two (bi means two and furca means fork) (Figure 6-10).

▶ **Buccal groove**—A linear depression forming a groove that extends from the middle of the buccal surface to the occlusal surface of the tooth (Figure 6-11).

▶ **Cingulum**—A convex area on the lingual surface of the anterior teeth, near the gingiva (Figure 6-12).

▶ **Cusp**—A pointed or rounded mound on the crown of the tooth (Figure 6-13).

▶ **Cusp of Carabelli**—A fifth cusp located on the mesial lingual surface of most maxillary first molars (Figure 6-14). (The name comes from the man who first described it.)

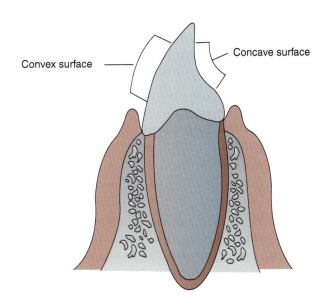

FIGURE 6-8 The concave and convex surfaces of the mandibular incisor.

FIGURE 6-9 The apex and apical foramen of a tooth.

Bifurcated roots

FIGURE 6-10 Mandibular molar showing the bifurcated roots.

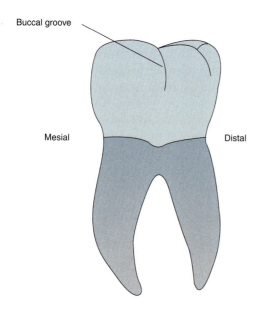

Buccal groove

Mesial

Distal

FIGURE 6-11 Mandibular molar with the buccal groove identified.

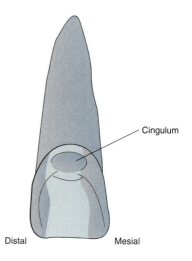

Cingulum

Distal

Mesial

FIGURE 6-12 The lingual surface of a central incisor with the cingulum shaded.

Cusps

FIGURE 6-13 A maxillary second premolar with the cusps identified.

▶ **Developmental groove**—A groove formed by the uniting of lobes during development of the crown of the tooth (Figure 6-15).

▶ **Fissure**—A developmental groove that has an imperfect union where the lobes come together (Figure 6-16). Decay often initiates in the fissure.

▶ **Fossa**—A shallow rounded or angular depression (Figure 6-17).

▶ **Furcation**—The dividing point of a multi-rooted tooth (Figure 6-18).

▶ **Lobes**—The separate divisions that come together to form a tooth (Figure 6-19). Often in the molars, the lobes become cusps.

▶ **Mamelons**—Three bulges on the incisal edge of the newly erupted central incisor (Figure 6-20). Mamelons normally disappear from normal wear.

▶ **Marginal ridges**—Elevated area of enamel that forms the mesial and distal borders of the lingual surface of the anterior teeth and the mesial and distal borders of the occlusal surface of the posterior teeth (Figure 6-21).

▶ **Oblique ridge**—Elevated area of enamel that extends obliquely across the occlusal of the tooth (Figure 6-22).

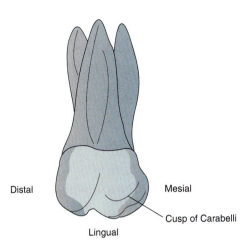

FIGURE 6-14 A maxillary first molar showing the mesial lingual side with the cusp of Carabelli identified.

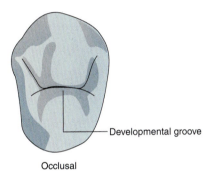

FIGURE 6-15 The developmental groove on the occlusal surface of the maxillary first premolar where the lobes were united.

FIGURE 6-16 A mandibular second premolar showing the imperfect union or fissure on the occlusal surface.

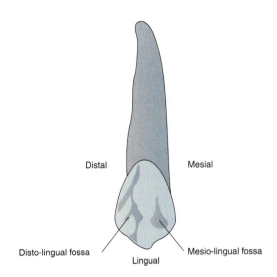

FIGURE 6-17 The lingual view of a maxillary canine with the mesio-lingual fossa and disto-lingual fossa shaded.

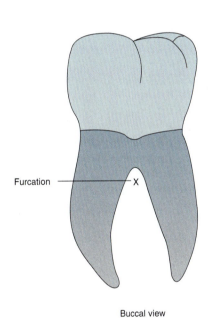

FIGURE 6-18 A mandibular first molar from the buccal side showing the furcation or dividing area where the roots fork off.

On the maxillary first molars, the oblique ridge extends from the disto-buccal cusp to the mesio-lingual cusp.

▶ **Pit**—The place where the grooves come together or the fissures cross (Figure 6-23). Decay often begins in the pit.

▶ **Ridge**—A linear elevation of enamel found on the tooth (Figure 6-24).

▶ **Supplemental groove**—Shallow, linear groove that radiates from the developmental groove (Figure 6-25). It often gives the tooth surface a wrinkled look.

Lobes

Occlusal

FIGURE 6-19 The occlusal view of the maxillary first molar showing the lobes and how they come together.

Mamelons

FIGURE 6-20 A newly erupted maxillary incisor showing the three bulges on the incisal edge, called mamelons.

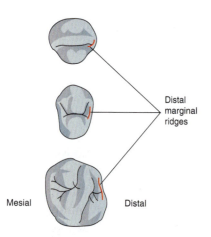

Distal marginal ridges

Mesial   Distal

FIGURE 6-21 The marginal ridges of the maxillary central, premolar, and molar.

Oblique ridge

FIGURE 6-22 A maxillary first molar with the oblique ridge identified.

Pits

FIGURE 6-23 A permanent mandibular first premolar showing the occlusal view with the pits identified.

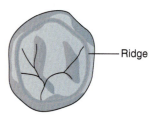

Ridge

FIGURE 6-24 The ridge identified on the occlusal surface of the mandibular second premolar.

Supplemental grooves

FIGURE 6-25 The occlusal surface of the mandibular second molar showing the shallow linear grooves called supplemental grooves.

These grooves do not denote any major divisions of the tooth.

▶ **Transverse ridge**—The union of two triangular ridges that produces a single ridge of elevation across the occlusal surface of a posterior tooth (Figure 6-26).

▶ **Triangular ridge**—A ridge or an elevation that descends from the cusp and widens as it runs down to the middle area of the occlusal surface (Figure 6-27).

▶ **Trifurcated**—Where there are three roots (tri means three) coming from the main trunk of the tooth (Figure 6-28).

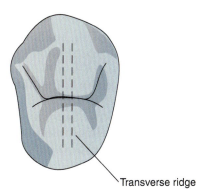

FIGURE 6-26 The maxillary right first premolar occlusal view showing the transverse ridge.

Transverse ridge

Buccal

Lingual

FIGURE 6-27 Triangular ridge identified on the occlusal surface of a maxillary second premolar.

Trifurcated roots

FIGURE 6-28 A maxillary first molar buccal showing the roots as trifurcated (three roots forked off from the main trunk).

PERMANENT TEETH DESCRIPTIONS

Maxillary Central Incisor

The maxillary central incisor is the first tooth closest to the midline (Figure 6-29). These teeth, along with the lateral incisors, play an important part in a person's appearance. Their shape, color, size, and placement directly relate to how a person looks. The position of the teeth dictates the shape of a person's profile. Normal placement will provide for correct support of the

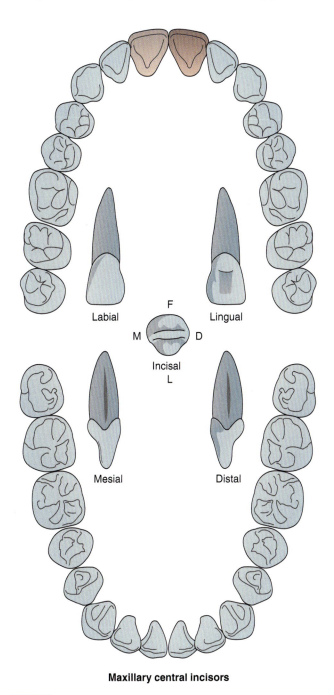

Labial

F

Lingual

M   D

Incisal

L

Mesial

Distal

Maxillary central incisors

FIGURE 6-29 The permanent dentition with the maxillary central incisors identified and the maxillary central incisor viewed from the five different surfaces.

face and lips. The incisors also play an important role in speech. To execute specific sounds, such as Ss and Ts, these teeth are necessary. The incisors also have a unique incisal edge that differs greatly from the other teeth in the mouth, which all have cusps. The ridge allows for the cutting of food into smaller particles.

The maxillary central incisor erupts with three bumps on the incisal edge, called **mamelons** (Figure 6-30). They derive from the three developing lobes coming together. The mamelons wear away from attrition (wear), and the incisal edge becomes a flattened surface. At the gingival area of the labial of the crown, small, curved lines run parallel to the CEJ. These are called **imbrication lines**. Most central incisors have imbrication lines.

The crown of the maxillary central incisor is the longest of any of the maxillary teeth. The labial surface is convex, both mesial to distal and gingival to incisal. The lingual surface is concave, except the gingival one-third where the cingulum is present. The cingulum spreads toward the mesial and distal in an arch pattern, forming the mesial and distal marginal ridges. The mesial surface is slightly longer than the distal surface. The mesial-incisal angle is rather acute, at about a ninety-degree angle, and the distal-incisal angle is more rounded. The root is about one and a half to two times the length of the crown. The root appears constricted at the CEJ and then swells in the body, tapering suddenly at the apical portion. Therefore, it ends in a rather blunt apex. The root tends to incline slightly distally.

Maxillary Lateral Incisor

The maxillary lateral incisor is the second tooth from the midline and the smallest in the maxillary arch (Figure 6-31). It initially contacts the central incisor on the mesial and the primary canine (cuspid) on the distal. It resembles the maxillary central in most ways. The difference is primarily its size, the crown being about three-tenths smaller in all directions. The root also is smaller in all directions; however, the length has been known to be similar to that of the maxillary central. The crown of the lateral incisor appears more narrow than the central, especially in females. The distal-incisal angle is more

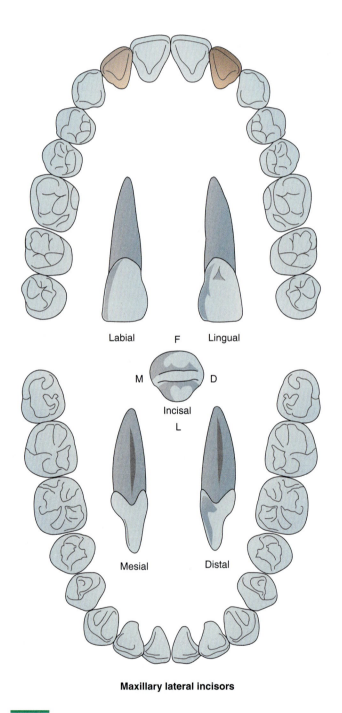

Maxillary lateral incisors

FIGURE 6-31 The permanent dentition with the maxillary lateral incisors identified and the maxillary lateral incisor viewed from the five different surfaces.

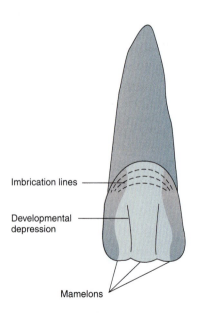

Imbrication lines

Developmental depression

Mamelons

FIGURE 6-30 The labial surface of the maxillary right central incisor with the mamelons, developmental depressions, and imbrication lines identified.

rounded than that of the central incisor, making the distal length much shorter than the mesial length.

Except for the third molars, the maxillary lateral is the tooth with the most **anomalies** (extreme variations from the norm). The most frequent is the **peg lateral**. This is a diminutive, peg-shaped crown with a smooth surface lacking contact on the mesial and distal surfaces. Maxillary laterals are sometimes congenitally missing. **Agenesis** occurs when the tooth buds do not form. Roots that are curved in unusual ways and distorted crowns may appear. Many of these deviations appear generation after generation.

Maxillary Canine (Cuspid)

The canine is often called the "cornerstone of the mouth" due to its placement, which is between the incisors and the bicuspids (Figure 6-32). It is the one tooth that turns the corner for the arch. The canine's purpose is to tear the food, which is much different from the incisors, which bite or cut the food, and the premolars and molars, which chew or grind it.

> The canine (cuspid) is one of the most important teeth for animals, because it tears the food. This term, derived from the Latin term for dog, has carried over to humans.

The canine (cuspid) is the third tooth from the midline. Because of its placement and size, it is extremely important in supporting the muscles of the face. Therefore, the canine contributes to a person's appearance.

The root is the longest in the maxillary arch and therefore the most stable. The crown of the canine is convex on the facial surface, with a ridge running vertically. The incisal edge is fairly pointed and is off center, slightly toward the mesial (the name cuspid is derived from the long cusp that ends in a point on the incisal edge). The mesial surface of the canine (cuspid) is longer than the distal surface, and as they both turn toward the incisal edge, the angle is more rounded than that of the incisors. The lingual surface has two concave fossas, one toward the mesial and the other toward the distal, with a lingual ridge dividing them in the middle. On the outer sides of the fossa is a distal marginal ridge and a mesial marginal ridge. On the lingual side of the tooth, toward the gingiva, is a cingulum. The canine appears darker than the incisors because of the bulk of the dentin.

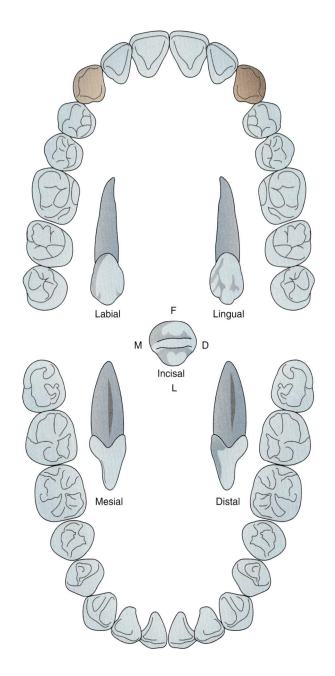

Maxillary canines (cuspids)

FIGURE 6-32 The permanent dentition with the maxillary canines (cuspids) identified and the maxillary canine viewed from the five different surfaces.

Premolar (Bicuspid)

There are eight premolars: four in each arch, two in each quadrant. They are named first and second premolars because of their positions from the midline. The first premolars, closest to the midline, line up in the fourth position. The second premolars line up in the fifth position from the midline. They are transitional teeth, placed between the cuspids and the molars. They look like the canines (cuspids) from the facial side; in fact, the buccal cusp functions much like a cuspid in tearing food, but the transitional teeth have an additional cusp on the lingual side (hence bicuspids, meaning two). The additional cusp aids in further breaking down the food or pulverizing it for the molars to chew. These posterior teeth are not as critical in personal appearance because of their placement. They do not always show when smiling or talking.

Maxillary First Premolar (Bicuspid)

The facial cusp of the maxillary first premolar is much more prominent in size than the lingual cusp (Figure 6-33). It is longer and wider across and appears much like the cuspid from the facial. The cusps come together on the occlusal surface in a central groove. This central groove extends to the mesial and distal grooves. The mesial groove is bordered by the mesial marginal ridges, and the distal groove is bordered by the distal marginal ridge. The

maxillary first premolar has a bifurcated root (two roots, one buccal and one lingual), that is slightly separated. Some first premolars have roots that are fused together; thus, one root has two canals. The roots have a depression on the mesial and distal sides running from the CEJ to the root bifurcation. The roots are shorter in length and resemble the roots of the molars in this aspect more than they do the roots of the cuspid.

This premolar is often considered for removal if the patient's teeth are overcrowded and orthodontic treatment is needed. The position allows for movement both from anterior and posterior teeth. The orthodontist closes the space and the patient's facial appearance is not changed by the removal of this tooth. Also, the depression in the root structure makes it more susceptible to periodontal disease; therefore, it is a better choice for removal than the second premolar.

Maxillary Second Premolar (Bicuspid)

The maxillary second premolar resembles the first in all but the following variations (Figure 6-34). The cusps, one on the buccal and one on the lingual, are more equal in length. The lingual cusp is slightly shorter but not as short as the cusp on the maxillary first bicuspid. The mesial buccal cusp slope is shorter than the distal buccal cusp slope. There is only one root and therefore only one root canal. There is a slight depression on the mesial root, but it is very shallow. The crowns of both the first and second bicuspids are wider bucco-lingually than mesio-distally. The second bicuspid is slightly more narrow mesial-distally than the first premolar.

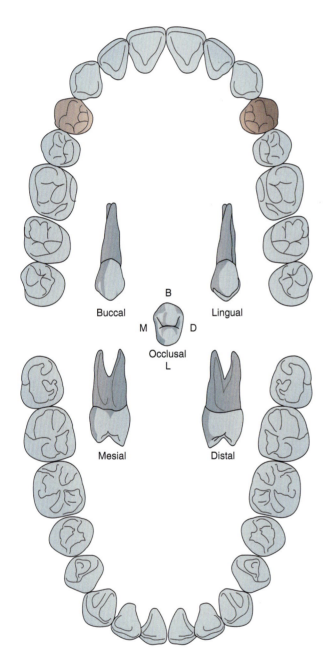

Maxillary first premolars (bicuspids)

FIGURE 6-33 The permanent dentition with the maxillary first premolars bicuspids identified and the maxillary first premolar viewed from the five different surfaces.

Maxillary Molar

The word molar is derived from the Latin word *molaris,* referring to a millstone. This seems like an appropriate term for the teeth that chew, grind, or break down the food into tiny particles for swallowing. When normal eruption occurs, the molars are the first and last permanent teeth in the mouth. There are twelve molars in the oral cavity: six in each arch and three in each quadrant. They are called the first, second, and third molars because of their placement from the midline. The first molar is the closest to the midline. The molars are the strongest teeth in the arch due to the size of their crowns and the shape and size of their roots. The first molar is the largest and the strongest; this decreases toward the posterior, leaving the third molar the weakest and smallest of the molars. Just as the cuspids are considered the cornerstones of the anterior teeth, the first molars are considered the cornerstones of the developing occlusion in the posterior teeth. The molars do not replace any primary teeth and therefore are not succedaneous teeth. They erupt posterior to the deciduous dentition.

Maxillary second premolars (bicuspids)

FIGURE 6-34 The permanent dentition with the maxillary second premolar identified and the maxillary second premolar viewed from the five different surfaces.

Maxillary first molars

FIGURE 6-35 The permanent dentition with the maxillary first molar identified and the maxillary first molar viewed from the five different surfaces.

Maxillary First Molar

The maxillary first molar is often referred to as the "six-year molar" because of its eruption time (Figure 6-35). Often, parents do not realize that this is a permanent tooth due to the age of the eruption. The crown of the maxillary first molar appears square in shape with four primary cusps present: mesio-buccal, disto-buccal, mesio-lingual, and disto-lingual. There is a fifth cusp, the **cusp of Carabelli**, located on the largest cusp, the

meso-lingual. This cusp is located about one-third the way down from the occlusal surface and appears as a "mini" cusp. The prominence of this cusp varies from tooth to tooth.

The mesio-buccal and the disto-buccal cusps are divided by a **buccal groove** that extends about half the length of the crown and ends in a depression often termed the **buccal pit**. The lingual cusps are slightly longer than the buccal cusps. The mesio-lingual cusp and the disto-lingual cusp are also divided by a lingual groove that travels about halfway down the crown on the lingual side, ending in a shallow depression called the **lingual pit**.

The root of the maxillary first molar is trifurcated. The first two roots, a meso-buccal root and a distal-buccal root, are placed on the buccal side. These buccal roots curve slightly toward each other. The third root is the largest and longest and is located on the lingual side. These three roots are spread out from each other and normally have one canal each.

On the occlusal surface of the maxillary first molars, the four primary cusps come together in a central fossa. There is an **oblique** (diagonal) **ridge** running across the occlusal surface that unites the distal cusp ridge of the mesio-lingual cusp and the lingual cusp ridge of the disto-buccal cusp. Another ridge, a **transverse ridge**, runs from the buccal cusp of the mesio-lingual cusp to the lingual cusp ridge of the mesio-buccal cusp. The occlusal surface also has a mesial ridge on the mesial of the occlusal surface and a distal ridge on the distal occlusal surface. This creates a surface with additional grooves and ridges in order to properly grind food.

Maxillary Second Molar

The second molar is called the "twelve-year molar" because of the time of eruption (Figure 6-36). It is similar to the first molar in many ways; however, it is smaller both in size of the crown and size of the root. The crown of the maxillary second molar has four cusps (no cusp of Carabelli). The cusps are located mesio-buccal, disto-buccal, mesio-lingual, and disto-lingual. The surface of the mesial of the tooth is greater across than the distal surface. The occlusal surface of the molars tapers down in size from the first molar toward the third molar.

The occlusal surface, although smaller, is much like that of the first molar. It has more supplementary grooves than the first molar, making it more wrinkled in appearance. The roots are the same in number but smaller in size and not as spread apart as the roots of the first molar. Each root has one canal, as in the maxillary first molar.

Maxillary Third Molar

The developmental variations make it impossible to describe exactly what the third molar looks like. The maxillary third molar is called the wisdom tooth because it was thought that by the time these teeth erupted into the oral cavity a person would have obtained maturity or wisdom (Figure 6-37). Many people do not develop third molars because foods are more processed and the body adapts with smaller arches. If third molars do develop, they may not erupt into the oral cavity because of lack of space in the posterior of the arches. This is the one tooth that, after careful diagnosis, that the dentist may recommend be removed.

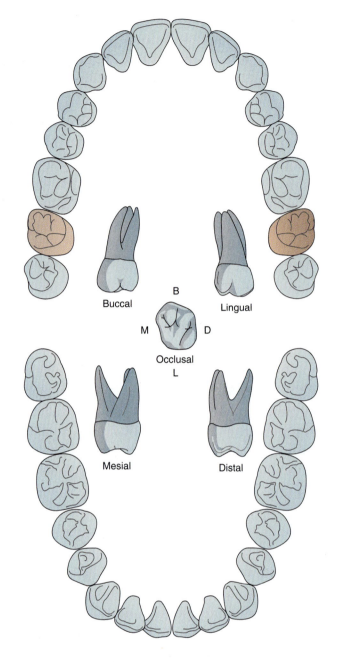

Maxillary second molars

FIGURE 6-36 The permanent dentition with the maxillary second molar identified and the maxillary second molar viewed from the five different surfaces.

When the tooth erupts normally, it resembles the second molar, only slightly smaller. It exhibits a more wrinkled appearance on the occlusal surface because many more supplemental grooves are usually present. The roots are normally fused together and vary in number.

Mandibular Central Incisor

The mandibular central incisor is the least variable tooth in the mouth (Figure 6-38). It is also the smallest tooth in the dentition. It is smaller than the mandibular lateral,

Maxillary third molars

Mandibular central incisors

FIGURE 6-37 The permanent dentition with the maxillary third molar identified and the maxillary third molar viewed from the five different surfaces.

FIGURE 6-38 The permanent dentition with the mandibular central incisors identified and the maxillary central incisor viewed from the five different surfaces.

which is not the case in the maxillary arch. The maxillary central incisor is larger than the maxillary lateral incisor.

When the mandibular central incisor erupts, it has three mamelons on the incisal edge. These wear off, leaving a fairly straight incisal edge for cutting. The crown of the mandibular incisor has a labial surface that is convex but does not appear to have the developmental depressions and imbrication lines the maxillary central has. The crown is narrow and the incisal angle makes a

sharp ninety-degree angle as it extends down the mesial and distal surfaces. The lingual is concave and has a cingulum near the gingiva. It is relatively smooth, and the structures are not as prominent as in maxillary centrals. The root is straight and ends abruptly at the apex.

This tooth is the first from the midline; therefore, the mesial surface of each central incisor contacts its counterpart. The distal surface contacts the lateral in its prospective quadrant.

Labial   F   Lingual

M   D

Incisal

L

Mesial   Distal

Mandibular lateral incisors

Labial   F   Lingual

M   D

Incisal

L

Mesial   Distal

Mandibular canines (cuspids)

FIGURE 6-39 The permanent dentition with the mandibular lateral incisors identified and the mandibular lateral incisor viewed from the five different surfaces.

FIGURE 6-40 The permanent dentition with the mandibular canines (cuspids) identified and the mandibular canine viewed from the five different surfaces.

Mandibular Lateral Incisor

The anatomy of the mandibular lateral incisor so closely resembles that of the central incisor that a detailed description is unnecessary (Figure 6-39). The mandibular incisor is slightly larger. The root is also larger and slightly longer. Concavities may be present on the mesial and distal of the root. If these occur, the mesial concavity is more shallow.

The crown of the lateral incisor is shaped the same as the central incisor except that the distal surface is

not as long. The incisal distal angle is more rounded to accommodate this change in length. This tooth does not have the developmental abnormalities that the maxillary lateral has.

Mandibular Canine (Cuspid)

The mandibular canine is the third tooth from the midline (Figure 6-40). It resembles the maxillary canine but is not as well developed. The crown of the tooth is approximately the same length as the maxillary canine, but the root is generally shorter (the root is still longer than the mandibular central and lateral roots). The cusp of the mandibular canine is not as well developed as the maxillary and not as sharp on the tip. The function, however, is the same: They both are designed to tear food.

The distal cusp slope is longer than the mesial cusp slope. The cingulum and marginal ridges are not as pronounced as on the maxillary canine, and the pronounced buccal ridge does help give shape to the face.

The canine is the longest tooth in the mandibular arch. The single root provides for stability; it is the cornerstone of the mandibular arch. The root, with one canal, has deep depressions on both the mesial and distal surfaces.

Mandibular First Premolar (Bicuspid)

The mandibular first premolar is much more of a transitional tooth than the maxillary first premolar (Figure 6-41). It does not resemble the mandibular second premolar as much as the maxillary first premolar resembles the maxillary second premolar. It looks much more like the mandibular canine: It has two cusps, one buccal and one lingual. The lingual cusp is often non-functioning; therefore, the shape is much like the canine. The buccal cusp is larger in all directions and its convex surface is more pronounced. The mesial cusp slope is shorter than the distal cusp slope.

The occlusal surface has both the mesial and distal ridges and, as the buccal and lingual cusps incline toward the occlusal groove, a transverse ridge crosses the tooth.

The single straight root of the mandibular first premolar is slightly shorter than the mandibular second premolar and a great deal shorter than the root of the mandibular canine. It sometimes bifurcates slightly at the apex.

Mandibular Second Premolar (Bicuspid)

The buccal surface of the mandibular second premolar resembles the mandibular first premolar except it is not as long and it is wider (Figure 6-42). The lingual cusps are much more developed. Instead of one lingual cusp, it has two or possibly three functioning cusps. This tooth helps with the transition from cutting and tearing to chewing. The occlusal surface of the mandibular second premolar resembles the molars, while the first mandibular premolar resembles the canine.

The cusps of the lingual surface are shorter than the buccal cusps and are divided by a lingual groove. The mesio-lingual cusp is slightly larger than the disto-lingual cusp but more equal in size than the cusps of the mandibular first bicuspid.

Three grooves divide the occlusal surface. The disto-buccal groove and the mesio-buccal groove come together with the lingual groove to form a Y shape on the occlusal surface. All the cusps slope into these

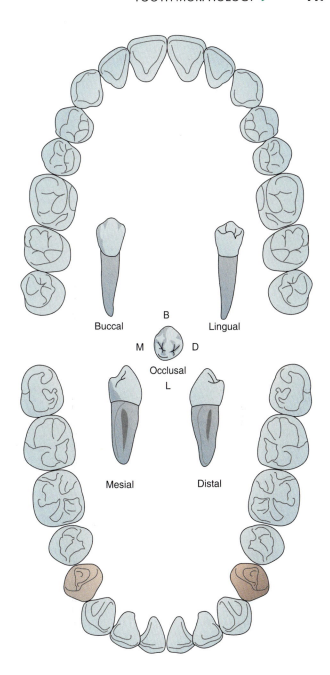

Mandibular first premolars (bicuspids)

FIGURE 6-41 The permanent dentition with the mandibular first premolars (bicuspids) identified and the mandibular first premolar viewed from the five different surfaces.

grooves in the middle of the tooth. The mesial and distal ridges outline the sides of the occlusal surface.

The root is shorter than the maxillary cuspid root but longer than the mandibular first bicuspid root. The root has a single canal and inclines slightly toward the distal.

Mandibular Molars

The mandibular molars are the largest and strongest of all the mandibular teeth.

Mandibular second premolars (bicuspids)

FIGURE 6-42 The permanent dentition with the mandibular second premolars (bicuspids) identified and the mandibular second premolar viewed from the five different surfaces.

Mandibular first molars

FIGURE 6-43 The permanent dentition with the mandibular first molars identified and the mandibular first molar viewed from the five different surfaces.

Mandibular First Molar

The mandibular first molar is referred to as the "six-year-molar" (Figure 6-43). It normally erupts slightly before the maxillary first molar and is thought to be the "keystone" of the dental arch. It has the widest crown of any tooth in the dentition and is the largest mandibular tooth.

There are normally five functioning cusps present on the occlusal surface of this tooth. The mesio-buccal cusp is the bulkiest and the longest of the three buccal

cusps; however, it is shorter than the lingual cusps. The disto-buccal cusp is a rounded cusp, found between the larger mesio-buccal cusp and the smaller distal cusp. The mesio-lingual cusp and the disto-lingual cusp are the longest and the sharpest of the five cusps. The mesio-lingual cusp may be slightly smaller than the disto-lingual cusp. All of these cusps come together on the occlusal surface in the central fossa and are divided by a groove extending between one cusp and the next. For instance, the buccal groove coming from the central fossa extends between the mesio-buccal cusp and the disto-buccal cusp and ends halfway down the buccal surface of the crown of the tooth in a buccal pit. These divisions make the occlusal surface appear as though five different lobes come together. The mesial surface of the tooth is slightly concave, and the distal side is fairly straight.

The mandibular first molar has two roots: mesial and distal. The mesial root is the wider and the stronger of the two. It normally has two different pulp canals, which is unusual because most of the teeth have one canal per root. The root is fairly flat in shape from the buccal to the lingual and tends to incline first toward the mesial of the tooth and then curve back toward the distal. The distal root is the smaller and weaker of the two. It is usually straight but occasionally will curve toward the mesial or the distal. It usually has a wider canal, and the outer surface of the root is more convex on the distal portion.

Mandibular Second Molar

The mandibular second molar is similar to the first molar but smaller (Figure 6-44). It has four cusps: mesio-buccal, disto-buccal, mesio-lingual, and disto-lingual. They are nearly the same size, but the mesio-buccal cusp is normally the largest and the disto-lingual cusp is normally the smallest. They are divided by the buccal groove on the buccal surface and the lingual groove on the lingual surface. Both of these grooves travel down the outside portion of the crown, about one-half of the surface, and end in pits or shallow depressions. The occlusal surface exhibits more supplemental grooves than the first molar.

The roots of the second molar are normally shorter than the first molar, but they do have more variations. The two bifurcated roots generally are closer together and may even be fused. They normally angle more toward the distal than the roots of the first mandibular molar. The mesial root is wider than the distal root and may have one or two canals (the distal root has one canal). They are shaped similar to the first molar, but the mesial root is flatter and the distal root is rounder.

Mandibular Third Molar

The mandibular third molar has many different variations in shape and size (Figure 6-45). If it does develop properly and erupt, this molar resembles the second molar but is smaller. The mandibular third molar has a wrinkled surface and the roots often are fused together. The roots tend to angle toward the distal in almost a horizontal position and may be four or more in number and fused together. These teeth, like the maxillary third molars, are referred to as "wisdom teeth" and may not develop or erupt at all. The dentist must determine if it is to the patient's advantage to keep these teeth. If they do erupt, they normally are difficult to keep plaque free because of their location and additional grooves.

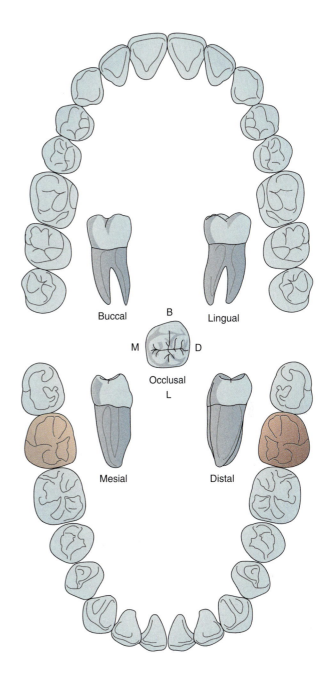

Mandibular second molars

FIGURE 6-44 The permanent dentition with the mandibular second molars identified and the mandibular second molar viewed from the five different surfaces.

DECIDUOUS (PRIMARY) TEETH DESCRIPTIONS

There are twenty deciduous teeth in the primary dentition: ten in each arch, five in each quadrant (Figure 6-46). There is a central incisor, lateral incisor, cuspid, first molar, and second molar (there are no bicuspids in the deciduous dentition). The primary teeth may be referred to as the baby teeth, milk teeth, first teeth, or primary teeth, but the correct clinical term is deciduous

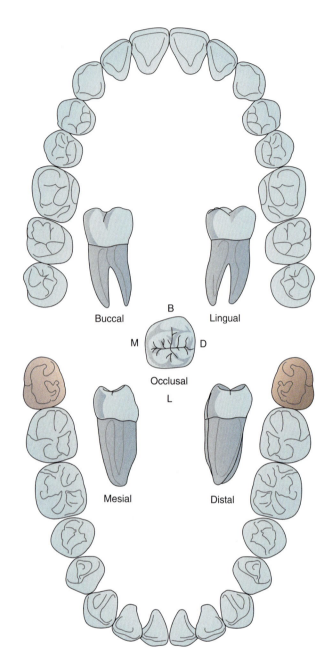

Mandibular third molars

FIGURE 6-45 The permanent dentition with the mandibular third molars identified and the mandibular third molar viewed from the five different surfaces.

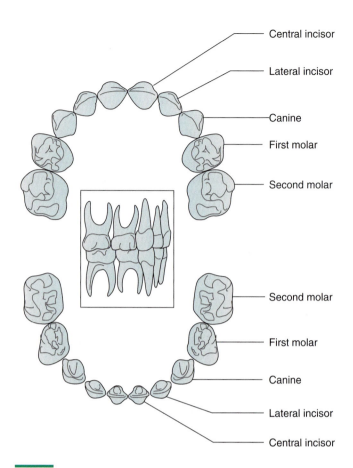

FIGURE 6-46 The deciduous dentition with tooth identification.

teeth. They begin to erupt when the child is six months of age and finish erupting when the child is approximately two to three years of age.

It seems that less importance has been placed on the deciduous teeth because they are only temporary. Some patients prefer not to restore deciduous teeth and choose to have them removed, knowing that a permanent tooth will replace them. However, the deciduous teeth play a very important role in maintaining space for the permanent teeth, and they also aid the child in

mastication and phonetics. Additionally, the appearance of the deciduous teeth play an important role in establishing a child's good self-image. Even though the deciduous teeth begin **exfoliation** by age six, they are still an important part of facial development.

The deciduous teeth are normally smaller than the permanent teeth that replace them. The crown portion is quite short in comparison to the root, and the cervical ridge is much more pronounced. The crowns of the deciduous teeth appear more white or light bluish in color, as compared to the yellow-gray color of the permanent teeth. This is because the enamel and dentin are much thinner and the pulp chamber is much larger. The deciduous molars have especially large mesial pulp horns. Knowing that the pulp is larger and closer to the surface of the deciduous tooth, a dental assistant should take great care during the coronal polish not to overheat the tooth and cause injury to the pulp.

Maxillary Deciduous Central Incisor

The maxillary deciduous central incisor resembles the permanent maxillary central in shape. It is much smaller in size than the permanent maxillary central and has a more pronounced cervical line. The crown is the only anterior tooth in either dentition to have a shorter inciso-cervical height than the mesio-distal width. This tooth erupts with no mamelons, and the labial surface is convex and smooth.

Maxillary Deciduous Lateral Incisor

The maxillary deciduous lateral incisor is similar to the central incisor except it is smaller. Another difference is that it is longer than it is wide. The incisal edge of the deciduous maxillary lateral incisor is more rounded on the mesial and distal sides than the straight incisal edge of the central incisor.

Maxillary Deciduous Canine (Cuspid)

The maxillary deciduous canine appears to be wider than it is long; however, with the pointed incisal edge, it is slightly longer than it is wide. It is more convex than the permanent maxillary canine and constricts more at the cervix of the tooth. The mesio-incisal slope has a pronounced cingulum and mesial and distal marginal ridges. The root is similar to the incisors but is longer (but nothing like the permanent canine).

Maxillary Deciduous First Molar

The maxillary deciduous first molar resembles the permanent bicuspid in many respects. It has four cusps; the mesio-buccal and the mesio-lingual are the most prominent. The mesio-lingual is the longest and the largest. The disto-lingual is the smallest or may even be absent. The tooth has transverse and oblique ridges like the permanent maxillary first molar, but they are not as prominent. The roots, like those of all deciduous molars, spread out rapidly from the crown of the tooth and are widely spaced. The maxillary deciduous first molar has three roots, like its permanent counterparts.

Maxillary Deciduous Second Molar

This tooth resembles the maxillary first permanent molar because it has four primary cusps and may even have a cusp that resembles the cusp of Carabelli. It has three roots that are widely spaced.

Mandibular Deciduous Central Incisor

This tooth more closely resembles the permanent mandibular lateral incisor than its central incisor counterpart. The crown of the tooth is slightly wider than the permanent lateral incisor. The shape and form of the incisal edge is almost exactly the same as that of the permanent lateral. The root is slender and rather long.

Mesial and distal surfaces of the root are flat, while lingual and labial surfaces are convex.

Mandibular Deciduous Lateral Incisor

The mandibular deciduous lateral resembles the mandibular deciduous central incisor except that it is slightly longer and wider. The cingulum and the mesial and distal marginal ridges are more pronounced and the fossa is not as shallow. The root curves toward the distal at the apex.

Mandibular Deciduous Canine (Cuspid)

The mandibular deciduous canine is much more delicate in form than that of the maxillary deciduous cuspid—even the root is not as large or long. The cingulum and the mesial and distal marginal ridges are less pronounced than those of the maxillary counterpart. The mesio-incisal slope is not as long as the disto-incisal slope; the maxillary incisal slopes are more nearly equal in length.

Mandibular Deciduous First Molar

This tooth resembles no other permanent or deciduous tooth. It has four cusps, with the mesio-buccal the largest and the mesio-lingual next in size. The disto-buccal and the disto-lingual are much smaller. The buccal surface is longer than that of the lingual and has a very prominent cervical ridge across the gingival area, directly above where the tooth constricts at the cervix. The tooth has two roots: a mesial root, which is much longer and wider, and a distal root. The apex of the mesial root is flattened or squared off.

Mandibular Deciduous Second Molar

The mandibular deciduous second molar closely resembles the permanent mandibular first molar. It is smaller in all dimensions and the mesio-buccal and the disto-buccal cusps are nearly equal in size, unlike in the permanent mandibular first molar. The distal root is smaller, while the mesial root is longer and wider. The permanent mandibular first molar has roots approximately the same length as this tooth.

▍ CHAPTER SUMMARY

By understanding tooth morphology, it will better prepare the assistant to record accurately for the dentist or hygienist and will make a vital contribution to those individuals to make a more accurate diagnosis. Therefore, the dental assistant will need to be able to identify each tooth form from its anatomical form.

CASE STUDY

Travis Charles, age twelve, complains of discomfort in the back of the mouth on both sides. The patient says that it feels like the skin is broken open behind his teeth.

Case Study Review

1. What probable condition is present?

2. Does the discomfort last all the time? Should Travis be concerned?

3. Is there any one thing that brings on the discomfort? Would Travis expect primary tooth loss in these areas?

 To complete your study of this chapter, work the review activities that follow. Also, refer to the software that accompanies this text.

REVIEW QUESTIONS

Multiple Choice

1. How many teeth are in the deciduous dentition?
   a. 32
   b. 16
   c. 20
   d. 24

2. The surface of the tooth that is *away* from the midline is the
   a. mesial surface.
   b. distal surface.
   c. labial surface.
   d. lingual surface.

3. Three bulges on the incisal edge of the newly erupted central incisor are
   a. marginal ridges.
   b. cingulums.
   c. mamelons.
   d. fissures.

4. Except for the third molar, the maxillary tooth that has the most anomalies is the
   a. central incisor.
   b. lateral incisor.
   c. first premolar (bicuspid).
   d. second molar.

5. The cusp on the mandibular second molar that is normally the smallest is the
   a. mesio-buccal.
   b. disto-buccal.
   c. mesio-lingual.
   d. disto-lingual.

Critical Thinking

1. If a patient has not formed a permanent mandibular first bicuspid on the left side, which deciduous tooth is retained in its place?
2. Which teeth in the maxillary arch are bifurcated?
3. Which surface of the anterior teeth is convex?

Dental Charting

OBJECTIVES

The student should strive to meet the following objectives and demonstrate an understanding of the facts and principles presented in this chapter:

1. Explain why charting is used in most dental practices.

2. Identify charts that use symbols to represent conditions present in the oral cavity.

3. List and explain the systems used for charting the permanent and deciduous dentitions.

4. Define G.V. Black's six classifications of cavity preparations.

5. List common abbreviations used to identify simple, compound, and complex cavities.

6. Describe basic terminology used in dental charting.

7. Explain color indicators and identify charting symbols.

KEY TERMS

abscess (p. 128)

bridge (p. 128)

crown (p. 128)

denture (p. 128)

drifting (p. 129)

Fédération Dentaire Internationale (FDI) system for numbering (p. 125)

gold foil (p. 129)

incipient (p. 129)

mobility (p. 129)

overhang (p. 129)

Palmer System for numbering (p. 125)

partial denture (p. 129)

periodontal pocket (p. 129)

restoration (p. 129)

root canal (p. 129)

sealant (p. 129)

Universal/National System for numbering (p. 124)

INTRODUCTION

CDA Recording the conditions present in the patient's oral cavity on a dental chart using symbols, numbers, and colors is a shorthand technique called charting. Charting is used in most dental offices. Numerous symbols and various charts are used, and the dental assistant needs to identify the doctor's preferred system in order to ensure that accurate charting is accomplished. Charting is part of the patient's legal record that is maintained in the office. As with all legal and medical records, each patient's chart should be complete and correct. The initial charting is normally accomplished during the patient's first examination. The dentist dictates his or her findings to the dental assistant, who charts them on a tooth diagram. The doctor indicates the existing conditions, the dental services that have been completed, and the dental services that need to be completed. The patient's dental record (chart) is used for billing purposes, diagnosis, and consultation. Forensic dentistry also uses the patient's dental record to provide information and to identify individuals involved in homicides, abuse, or other tragedies.

DENTAL CHARTS

There are several types of dental charts. Each chart has an area designed for dental charting and an area in which to record treatment. The most commonly used chart is one with diagrams of the teeth that may show an anatomic or a geometric representation of the teeth. Most charts show both the permanent and the primary dentition. The anatomical charts show the crown of the tooth, the crown and a small portion of the root, or the crown and the complete root. The geometric charts show the teeth as circles. Each circle represents one tooth and is sectioned into five areas indicating the corresponding surfaces of the tooth. Each dental office chooses the chart it feels best meets its needs.

NUMBERING SYSTEMS

Dental offices have several numbering systems available for their use, and the dentists indicate the preferred systems to be used in their offices. All patient records in one office are documented according to one numbering system in order to prevent confusion.

Universal/National System for Numbering

In 1968, the American Dental Association (ADA) adopted the **Universal/National System for numbering**. This numbering system is currently the most commonly used in the United States (Figure 7-1). Each permanent tooth has its own number, starting from the maxillary right

(A)   **Permanent teeth**

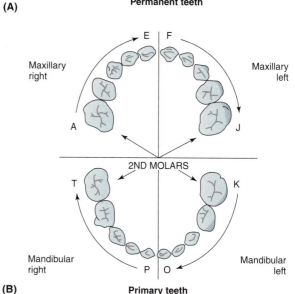

(B)   **Primary teeth**

FIGURE 7-1 (A) Permanent and (B) primary dentition showing the Universal/National numbering and lettering system.

third molar as #1 and moving in a clockwise direction to the maxillary left third molar as #16. The mandibular left third molar is #17, and the mandibular right third molar is #32. Therefore, #1 and #32 occlude together and #16 and #17 occlude together. Always remember that it is the *patient's* right side where tooth #1 and #32 are located, so that they are not reversed during charting. The primary teeth are each given a letter or a "d" with a number. The maxillary right deciduous second molar is lettered "A" or "d-1," and this continues across the maxillary arch, with the maxillary left second deciduous molar as "J" or "d-10." The mandibular left second deciduous molar is "K" or "d-11," and this continues across the mandibular arch, with the mandibular right second deciduous molar lettered as "T" or "d-20." Most standardized charts in the United States come with diagrams of the primary and permanent teeth using the Universal System for numbering .

Fédération Dentaire Internationale (FDI) System for Numbering

The International Standards Organization (ISO) TC 106 designated a system for teeth and areas of the oral cavity. It is widely used in Canada and European countries. This system is designed to provide an international system for coding teeth and the oral cavity. In 1996, the ADA adopted this system and the universal system for tooth numbering. The **Fédération Dentaire Internationale (FDI) system for numbering** can be adapted easily to the computer and is widely used in most other countries (Figure 7-2). With this system, each quadrant is assigned a number. The oral cavity is given two digits. If two 00s are noted, the whole oral cavity is designated. If 01 is used, it designates the entire maxillary arch; 02 designates the entire mandibular arch. For example, a full denture on the upper (maxillary) arch is noted as denture 01.

The permanent dentition is given 1 for the upper right quadrant, 2 for the upper left quadrant, 3 for the lower left quadrant, and 4 for the lower right quadrant. The deciduous dentition is assigned 5 though 8 for the corresponding quadrants. Each quadrant is numbered from 1 to 8, starting with the centrals and ending with the molars. The primary teeth are numbered from 1 to 5 in the same manner. When the FDI system is used, the quadrant number is recorded first. For example, the maxillary right lateral incisor is numbered 12 in the permanent dentition and the maxillary right lateral incisor in the deciduous dentition is 52.

Palmer System for Numbering

The **Palmer System for numbering** and lettering the teeth is used in some dental offices (Figure 7-3). With this system, the permanent teeth are numbered 1 through 8 in each quadrant: The centrals are 1 and the third molars are 8. With each number, a quadrant bracket is used to denote which quadrant it is referring to. For example, the maxillary right first bicuspid is charted as 4⌋. The deciduous teeth are identified in a similar manner except that the teeth are lettered "A" through "E" for each quadrant. "A" represents the central incisors and "E" represents the primary second molars. Again, the quadrant bracket is used to denote which quadrant it is referring to. For example, the deciduous mandibular right central incisor is charted as A⌉.

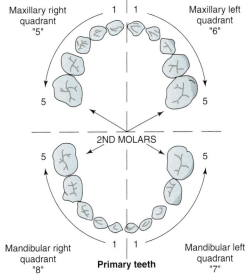

FIGURE 7-2 Permanent and primary dentition showing the International Standards Organization (ISO) TC 106 Designation System/Fédération Dentaire Internationale system.

CAVITY CLASSIFICATIONS

Five standard cavity classifications were developed by G.V. Black (the "grand old man of dentistry"), and a sixth class was added later. These classifications aid in

Permanent teeth

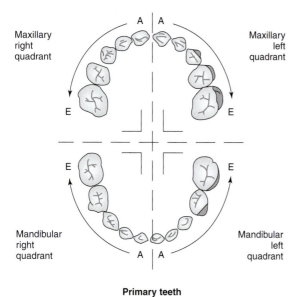

Primary teeth

FIGURE 7-3 Permanent and primary dentition with the Palmer numbering and lettering system.

recording the type of dental **caries** (cavity) on a patient's chart.

Class I

Class I caries are developmental cavities in the pit and fissures of teeth (Figure 7-4). They are located in:

▶ The occlusal surfaces of the posterior teeth (premolars and molars)

▶ The buccal or lingual pits on the molars

▶ The lingual pit near the cingulum of the maxillary incisors

Class II

Class II caries are on the proximal (mesial or distal) surfaces on the posterior teeth (premolars and molars) (Figure 7-5).

Class III

Class III caries are on the interproximal surface (mesial or distal) of anterior teeth (canines, lateral incisors, and central incisors) (Figure 7-6).

Class IV

Class IV caries are on the interproximal surface (mesial or distal) of anterior teeth and include the incisal edge (Figure 7-7).

Class V

Class V caries occur on the cervical third of the facial or lingual surface of the tooth (Figure 7-8). Often, Class V caries occur because the patient regularly sucks on sweets. Additionally, the dental assistant may see several Class V caries in one quadrant because the patient takes medications, chews gum, or drinks soft drinks over long periods of time.

Class VI

Class VI caries were not part of the original standard classification of cavities developed by G.V. Black (Figure 7-9). They were later identified in order to more clearly label cavities that involve the incisal or occlusal surface that has been worn away due to abrasion.

ABBREVIATIONS OF TOOTH SURFACES

Terms such as simple, compound, and complex are used in cavity classification. A simple cavity involves only one tooth surface, a compound cavity involves two surfaces, and a complex cavity involves more than two surfaces (See Table 7-1, on page 128).

When documenting the chart to record the surfaces of the teeth that need to be restored or that have been restored, the dental assistant abbreviates the notations. Each surface is abbreviated using the first letter of the

(A)

(B)

(C)

FIGURE 7-4 Caries shown on the (A) occlusal surfaces of the premolars and molars, (B) buccal surface on the molar, and (C) lingual surface on the maxillary incisors.

surface, capitalized. For instance, an abbreviated form of a mesial restoration on tooth #8 is #8 M. If two or more surfaces are restored, then a combined word is used. The *"al"* is normally dropped and *"o"* is substituted on the first word. For example, to identify the restoration that is on the distal and occlusal surfaces, the term is disto-occlusal restoration or DO restoration. If three surfaces are combined, the same principle is applied to the second word as well. If the tooth has a mesial-occlusal-distal restoration, the correct term is mesio-occluso-distal or MOD restoration. If a mesial surface of the tooth is restored with another surface, it is always used first. Occlusal and lingual normally fall in the last position.

Commonly Used Abbreviations

Some commonly used abbreviations for simple, compound, or complex cavities include the following:

▶ MOD   Mesio-occluso-distal

▶ DO   Disto-occlusal

(A)

MO restoration   MOD restoration

(B)

FIGURE 7-5 Caries shown on the proximal surfaces of (A) premolars and molars and (B) placed prior to an MO or MOD restoration on the surfaces of premolars and molars.

FIGURE 7-6 Caries on the proximal surfaces of incisors and cuspids.

▶ MO   Mesio-occlusal

▶ MI   Mesio-incisal

▶ DI   Disto-incisal

▶ LI   Linguo-incisal

▶ DL   Disto-lingual

▶ MODBL   Mesio-occluso-disto-bucco-lingual

▶ I   Incisal

▶ M   Mesial

▶ D   Distal

▶ B   Buccal

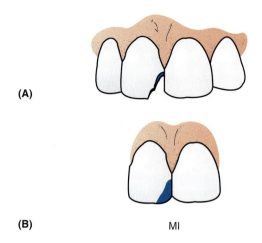

(A)

(B)   MI

FIGURE 7-7 Fractured area on (A) the proximal incisal surfaces of incisors and (B) a completed restoration on the central incisor.

FIGURE 7-8 Caries on the gingival buccal area of the teeth.

FIGURE 7-9 Caries on the occlusal surface of a mandibular incisor due to abrasion.

BASIC TERMS USED IN CHARTING

▶ **Abscess**—A localized area of infection.

▶ **Bridge**—A prosthetic device placed in the mouth where a tooth is missing, normally attached on each side and covering the space created by the missing tooth. The attaching sides are called **abutments** and the middle area is called the **pontic**. A **cantilever bridge** is attached on only one side. This kind is useful in an area that has little stress, such as a missing lateral. The abutment side could then be on the canine, which is a strong support. The **Maryland bridge** has wings on the pontic, and they are attached to the lingual sides of the adjacent (abutment) teeth.

▶ **Crown**—Often called a cap by the patient but not usually by dental professionals. Some crowns are cast in a laboratory and made to fit the patient's tooth exactly. They are made of several types or combinations of materials, such as gold, porcelain and gold, or porcelain. Crowns can be permanent or temporary or made for the anterior or posterior. Preformed (temporary) crowns are manufactured in quantities. The dentist sizes and forms the crown to fit the tooth. These crowns are usually made from stainless steel or plastic. All crowns are "fixed" or cemented into place in the patient's mouth and are not removable like partial and full dentures. Crowns cover the complete tooth, as in a full crown, or three-quarters of the tooth, as in a three-fourths crown.

▶ **Denture** (complete and partial)—A full denture replaces the complete arch of a patient's dentition. Patients sometimes refer to full dentures as their upper or lower plates. If all the natural teeth in one arch are missing, a full denture is needed. If some of the natural teeth are missing, a partial denture (artificial teeth mounted on a metal framework) can be used.

TABLE 7-1 CAVITY CLASSIFICATIONS AND TOOTH SURFACES

Classification	Identifying Terms/Tooth Surfaces
Class I	Simple—One surface
Class II	Compound—Two surfaces, or Complex—More than two surfaces
Class III	Simple—One surface
Class IV	Compound—Two surfaces
Class V	Simple—One surface
Class VI	Simple—One surface

▶ **Drifting**—All teeth are supported by each other in the dentition. If a maxillary tooth is removed, then the opposing mandibular tooth may drift, or **over-erupt**, into the space. Also, the teeth adjacent to the space created by the removed tooth can drift into the space.

▶ **Gold foil**—A restoration created when several layers of pure gold are placed in the preparation. A gold foil is a restoration not commonly used today.

▶ **Incipient**—Beginning decay that has not broken through the enamel. The doctor may choose to watch this area for further breakdown rather than immediately restoring this area. Incipient appears as a chalky area on the tooth. It is not yet decay, but the surface has begun to decalcify. Some doctors note this on the chart by placing the word "watch" on that area. Other doctors use a series of red dots, a symbol that represents an incipient area.

▶ **Mobility**—When the tooth moves in the socket, normally due to periodontal disease or trauma. A numbering system is used to indicate how many millimeters the tooth moves and is recorded in Roman numerals, or from 0–4.

▶ **Overhang**—Excessive restorative material normally found interproximally near the gingiva.

▶ **Partial denture**—A prosthetic device that replaces missing teeth. It has a metal framework and artificial teeth.

▶ **Periodontal pocket**—The space in the gingival sulcus created by periodontal disease. It is measured by a periodontal probe in millimeters. A healthy sulcus depth is 1–3 millimeters; beyond this depth it is a periodontal pocket. See Chapter 23, Periodontics.

▶ **Restoration**—An agent that is effective in replacing the missing tooth structure. Patients may refer to these as fillings. A number of different materials are used in dental restorations, including gold, amalgam, and composite.

▶ **Root canal**—When the pulp is removed and replaced with a filling material.

▶ **Sealant**—An enamel sealant is a resin material used to seal pits and fissures in order to prevent potential decay.

CHARTING COLOR INDICATIONS AND SYMBOLS

Colors and symbols are used in charting to indicate the existing condition of the patient's teeth and surrounding tissues and the restorative services required (See Table 7-2 and Figure 7-10). There are some established symbols that allow for common references when interaction takes place between dental professionals.

Red is used to represent the dentistry that needs to be done, and blue indicates that the work has been completed. Some of the symbols can be charted in either color. For instance, if a tooth is fractured but not causing any discomfort to the patient or not affecting the patient's appearance, the dentist may decide not to restore it. A notation is made on the chart that nothing is to be done at this time and it is charted in either color.

TABLE 7-2 COLOR INDICATION AND CHARTING SYMBOLS OF WORK COMPLETED

Description	Symbol
• Amalgam restoration (outlined and filled in solidly with blue, if complete, or red, if to be done)	▮ (solid blue rectangle)
• Composite restoration (outlined in red, if it is to be done, or blue, if it is complete)	▭ (outlined rectangle)
• Gold restoration (area outlined with diagonal lines drawn through it) red, if to be done, or blue if it is complete	(rectangle with diagonal lines)
• Gold foil restoration (area outlined with crosshatch lines drawn through it) red, if to be done, or blue if it is complete	(rectangle with crosshatch lines)
• Porcelain restoration (outlined with red, if it is to be done, or blue, if it is complete, and/or a P placed inside the outline)	P
• Sealant (S on occlusal surface) red, if to be done, or blue if it is complete	S
• Stainless steel (outlined with swervy lines through it or two Ss inside the outlined area) (red if to be done, or blue if it is complete).	(rectangle with swervy lines)

Missing teeth (removed or never erupted)	
Missing multiple teeth	
Teeth to be extracted	
All teeth missing	
Teeth impacted or unerupted	
Teeth that are drifting / over erupted	
Teeth that are drifting / mesial inclination	
Teeth that are drifting / distal inclination	
Teeth that need a root-canal therapy	
Tooth that has an abcess	
Tooth that has a root canal completed	
Tooth with a Class V buccal gold-foil restoration	

FIGURE 7-10 Charting symbols.

(continued on following pages)

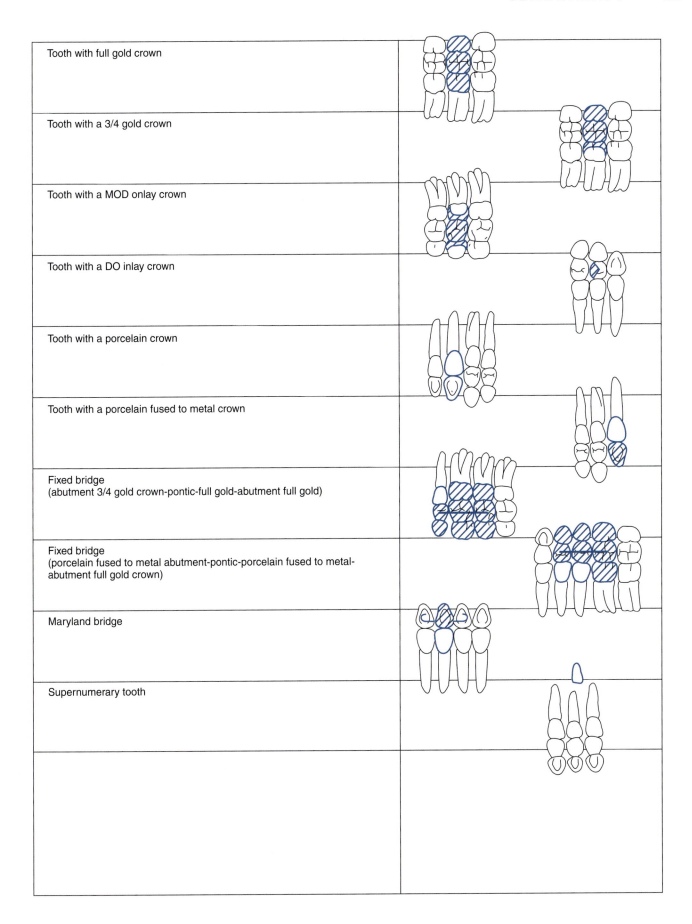

Tooth with full gold crown	
Tooth with a 3/4 gold crown	
Tooth with a MOD onlay crown	
Tooth with a DO inlay crown	
Tooth with a porcelain crown	
Tooth with a porcelain fused to metal crown	
Fixed bridge (abutment 3/4 gold crown-pontic-full gold-abutment full gold)	
Fixed bridge (porcelain fused to metal abutment-pontic-porcelain fused to metal-abutment full gold crown)	
Maryland bridge	
Supernumerary tooth	

FIGURE 7-10 *(continued)*

Periodontal pocket	
Overhang on a restoration	
Food impaction	
Open contacts	
Decalcification	
Heavy calculus	
Occlusal caries	
Occlusal amalgam restoration	
Occlusal composite restoration	
Enamel sealant	
Disto-occlusal (DO) caries	
Mesio-occluso-distal (MOD) amalgam restoration with recurrent decay	

FIGURE 7-10 *(continued)*

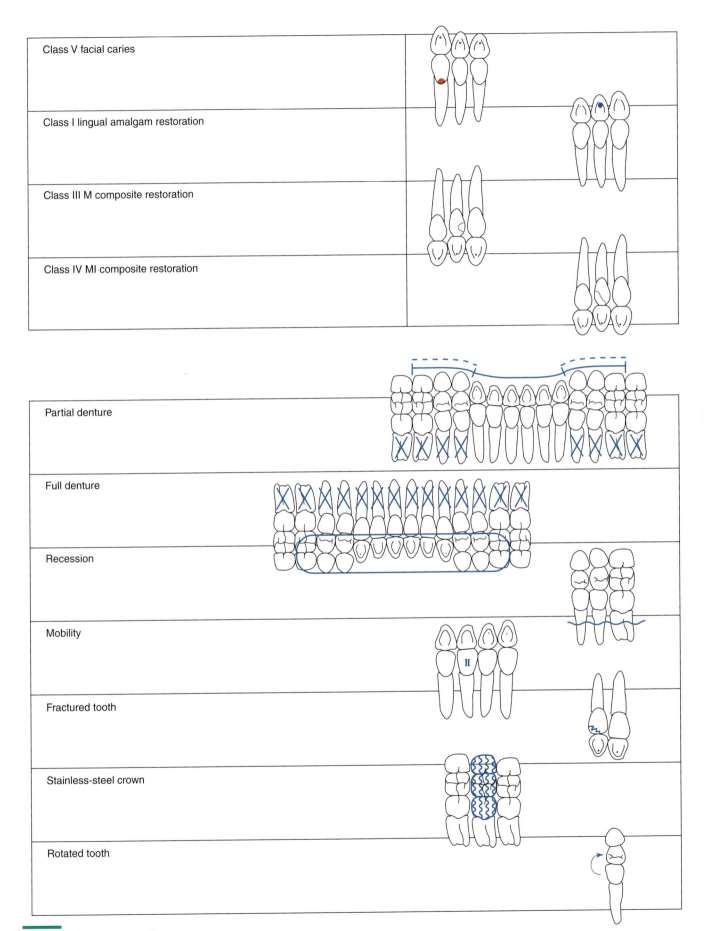

Class V facial caries	
Class I lingual amalgam restoration	
Class III M composite restoration	
Class IV MI composite restoration	
Partial denture	
Full denture	
Recession	
Mobility	
Fractured tooth	
Stainless-steel crown	
Rotated tooth	

FIGURE 7-10 *(continued)*

Diastema	
Porcelain veneer	
Dental implant	

FIGURE 7-10 *(continued)*

CHAPTER SUMMARY

Dental charting provides legal documentation of the patient's oral cavity. Utilizing the correct numbering system and charting symbols will ensure proper documentation. Therefore, accuracy in charting is critical.

CASE STUDY 1 (Charting Using the Anatomical Representation of the Teeth and the Universal System for Numbering)

Tooth	#1	impacted
	#2	Class II DO amalgam restoration present
	#4	Class II MOD amalgam restoration present
	#6	Class III M composite restoration present
	#8	Class IV MI composite restoration present
	#9	Class III M decay
	#13	Class II MOD amalgam restoration with recurrent decay
	#14	Class II MO amalgam restoration present; food impaction between 13 & 14
	#16	has been removed
	#17	partially impacted and needs to be removed
	#19	bridge present, abutment full gold crown
	#20	bridge present, pontic porcelain with gold
	#21	bridge present, abutment porcelain with gold
	#24	mobility of III, periodontal pocket on M and D of 4mm each, heavy calculus from mandibular left cuspid to mandibular right cuspid
	#25	periodontal pocket on M and D of 3mm each
	#28	needs a full gold crown with a porcelain facing
	#28	has a root canal completed
	#30	Class I O decay
	#31	Class II MO amalgam restoration present
	#32	has been removed

(continued)

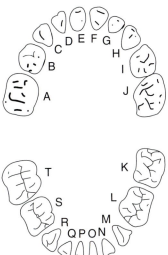

FIGURE 7-11 Charting using the anatomical teeth and the Universal numbering system.

Case Study Review

1. Which tooth has a Class III M caries?

2. How many teeth are restored?

3. Which tooth is a pontic?

CASE STUDY 2 (Charting Using the Geometric Representation of the Teeth and the International Standards Organization System for Tooth Identification)

Tooth #18   impacted

  #16   full porcelain with gold crown present

  #15   Class II MO amalgam restoration present

  #14   Class I O sealant present

  #12   Class III M composite present with recurrent decay

  #11   Class I L composite present

  #24   bridge present, abutment full porcelain with gold

  #25   bridge present, pontic full porcelain with gold

  #26   bridge present, abutment full porcelain with gold

  #28   has been removed

  #38   has been removed

  #36   has a full gold crown

  #34   has an abscess and needs a root canal

  #33   is missing and the deciduous tooth is retained

  #31   Class IV MI composite restoration present

  #42   has a fracture on the MI edge

  #45   Class II DO amalgam restoration with an overhang

  #47   has been removed

  #48   mesial inclination

Case Study Review

1. Which tooth has an enamel sealant?

2. Which primary tooth is present in the patient's mouth?

3. Which tooth needs endodontic therapy?

(continued)

CASE STUDY 2 *(continued)*

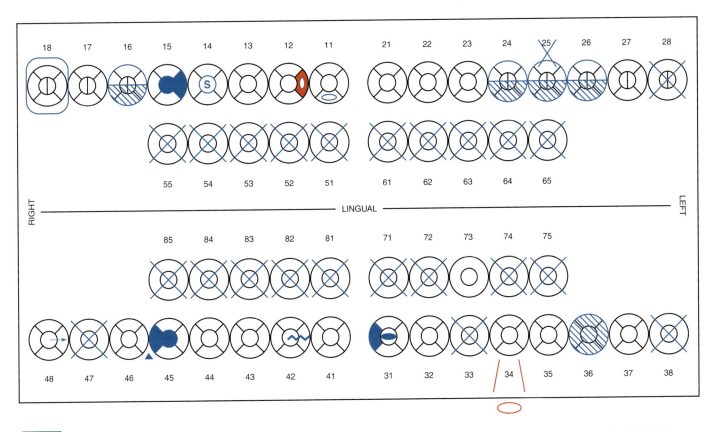

FIGURE 7-12 Charting using the geometric representation of the teeth and the International Standards Organization (ISO) TC 106 designation system for the teeth.

To complete your study of this chapter, work the review activities that follow. Also, refer to the software that accompanies this text.

REVIEW QUESTIONS

Multiple Questions

1. Which of the following charting systems utilizes brackets?
  a. Universal System for numbering.
  b. Nationale System for numbering.
  c. International Fédération Dentaire.
  d. Palmer System for numbering.

2. Cavities on the interproximal surface of the anterior teeth that do not include the incisal edge are
  a. Class I.
  b. Class II.
  c. Class III.
  d. Class IV.

3. Excess restorative material found near the gingival tissue is
  a. sealant.
  b. overhang.
  c. drifting.
  d. gold foil.

4. Restorations that need to be completed are charted in which color?
  a. Yellow.
  b. Black.
  c. Red.
  d. Blue.

5. Gold crowns are charted with which symbol?
   a. Diagonal lines.
   b. Crosshatch lines.
   c. Multiple dots.
   d. Swervy lines.

Critical Thinking

1. The five surfaces on a posterior tooth are mesial, distal, occlusal, lingual, and buccal. What are the five surfaces on an anterior tooth? Which of these surfaces are the same for both anterior and posterior?

2. A young adult broke his upper teeth at a drinking fountain, from the middle of the biting edge to the middle of each front tooth in an upside-down V pattern. Which surfaces, classifications, and teeth numbers would be involved if using the Universal System for numbering? The ISO or FDI system? The Palmer System?

3. If an anterior tooth is fractured and does not need to be restored, which color would it be charted in and why?

Microbiology

OBJECTIVES

The student should strive to meet the following objectives and demonstrate an understanding of the facts and principles presented in this chapter:

1. Identify Anton Van Leeuwenhoek, Louis Pasteur, and Robert Koch according to their contributions to microbiology.

2. Explain the groups of microorganisms and the staining procedures used to identify them.

3. Identify characteristics pertaining to the microorganism bacterium.

4. List characteristics pertaining to the microorganism protozoa.

5. Identify characteristics pertaining to the microorganism rickettsia.

6. Explain characteristics pertaining to the microorganisms yeasts and molds.

7. List characteristics pertaining to the microorganisms viruses.

8. Describe the diseases of major concern to the dental assistant and explain why they cause concern.

9. Identify how the body fights disease. Explain different immunities and routes of microorganism exposure.

KEY TERMS

**acquired
    immunodeficiency
    syndrome (AIDS)**
    (p. 146)

anaphylactic shock
    (p. 147)

antibodies (p. 147)

antigens (p. 147)

antitoxin (p. 147)

etiologic agent
    (p. 140)

**human
    immunodeficiency
    virus (HIV)**
    (p. 146)

pathogens (p. 140)

purulence (p. 147)

viral hepatitis
    (p. 146)

INTRODUCTION

The study of microorganisms is called **microbiology**. The majority of microorganisms are beneficial to humans. They are used in making vitamins, antibiotics, and some food products. However, some microorganisms are harmful to humans, such as **pathogens** (disease-producing microorganisms). In this chapter, five groups of pathogenic microorganisms are covered, along with the diseases they cause and the ways in which the body defends against them. Methods and instruments used to study microorganisms include the microscope, growing colonies in a culture medium, color or staining, and injection into an animal in order to observe the outcome.

IMPORTANT PEOPLE IN MICROBIOLOGY

Anton Van Leeuwenhoek

Born in 1632 in Holland, Anton Van Leeuwenhoek (1632–1723) ground lenses in order to magnify and view things more closely. He looked at a raindrop through these lenses and found small things that moved around, therefore seeing microorganisms for the first time. Later, he scraped his teeth and viewed the scrapings through the ground lenses and found a great number of microorganisms moving around. He was the first in his field to leave a written account of his microscopic findings and is referred to as the father of microbiology.

Louis Pasteur

Louis Pasteur (1822–1895) experimented with the process of fermentation. By isolating the causative bacteria in other diseases, some affecting man, he proved that bacteria caused disease. Pasteur found that bacteria, along with resistant spores, could be destroyed by heat. He showed that broth, when heated and kept from the microbes in the air, did not spoil and suggested that food be processed by steam under pressure in an airtight container. His work led to the food-canning process used today. The sterilizers used in dental offices are designed on his original premise that heat kills pathogens. Pasteur's name is noted in the pasteurization of milk, whereby the pathogens in milk are destroyed by heat.

Robert Koch

Robert Koch (1843–1910), a German biologist, proved that a specific type of bacteria causes a specific disease, termed the **etiologic agent** (causative agent) of the disease. He was able to determine the etiologic agent for tuberculosis. Koch is remembered for his Koch Postulates, a procedure he developed to prove that bacterium was the cause of a disease.

Koch's Postulates

1. The organism must be present in all cases of the disease.
2. The organism must be isolated in pure culture.
3. The organism must be capable of producing the disease in another person or animal.
4. The organism must be recovered again in pure culture.

GROUPS OF MICROORGANISMS

The two main groups of microorganisms that are important to dentistry are the **bacteria** and **virus** groups (Figure 8-1). When looking through a microscope, the different types of bacteria are distinguished from each other due to their characteristics, shapes, and sizes.

Often, bacteria cells are stained to further identify the groups. Dr. Christian Gram developed a staining procedure called the **Gram stain** in order to differentiate cells into two specific groups. To aid in viewing the cells, special dyes are used. The cells are placed on a slide, dried, and then stained with an alkaline solution of violet dye. The slide is rinsed with iodine and left untouched for two minutes. Then, the slide is gently rinsed with water and then rinsed with acetone alcohol. If the cell wall keeps the color, the cells are classified as **gram positive** and appear dark purple under the microscope. If they lose the color during the procedure, they are classified as **gram negative** and appear colorless under the microscope.

BACTERIA

Bacteria (back-**TEER**′-ee-uh) are tiny, simple, single-celled plants that contain no chlorophyll. If an individual

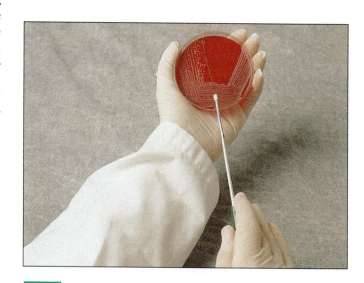

FIGURE 8-1 Microorganism being grown in a medium.

has 2,000 bacteria laying side by side together in a line, they are about the width of the period at the end of this sentence. Bacteria divide by simple fission: They elongate and divide into two separate cells and then continuously repeat this cycle. If ideal conditions (warm, dark, and moist) are present, they divide about every twenty minutes. Bacteria are often wrongly called "germs." Some bacteria are **sporulating**. One example is bacilli. These **spores** become enclosed in several protein coats that are resistant to drying, heat, and most chemicals. They also withstand boiling. Sporulating is a means of survival for bacteria, and bacteria have been known to survive for years in this state. Later, they may land on a surface that is moist and nutrient rich and then reactivate. The process is much like a seed that floats around and then lands on rich soil and begins growing. This should not be confused with reproduction; sporulating is for survival.

Bacteria's Need for Oxygen

▶ **Aerobic bacteria** must have oxygen to grow and live. Most bacteria are **aerobic**.

▶ **Anaerobic bacteria** are destroyed in the presence of oxygen and live only without oxygen.

▶ **Facultative anaerobic bacteria** grow with or without oxygen present.

The Morphology of Bacteria

The shape of bacteria (morphology) is unique to this group of microorganisms (Figure 8-2). Under a microscope, the types of microorganisms are bacilli (rod shaped), cocci (round or bead shaped), spirilla (S shaped), and vibrios (curved like a comma).

When the bacteria are grown in **colonies**, or masses, they appear differently (Figure 8-3). The prefix diplo, as in **diplococci**, identifies pairs of bacteria; **staphylococci** grow in clusters, much like grapes; and **streptococci** identifies chains of bacteria.

Disease Examples Caused by Bacteria

Tuberculosis. **Tuberculosis** is caused by mycobacterium tuberculosis and is most often found in the lungs. Several months may pass by before signs of the disease appear. A person exhibits fatigue, low-grade fever, night sweats, loss of weight, and, finally, a persistent cough. This disease is spread to others by airborne particles released while coughing, from saliva contact, and, if cross-contamination occurs, by dental treatment. Dental personnel must wear masks during dental procedures to protect from the handpiece spray that may contain infectious particles if the patient has tuberculosis. The disease can be detected by a skin test and/or chest x-ray. Treatment for this disease is normally antibiotics or other drugs.

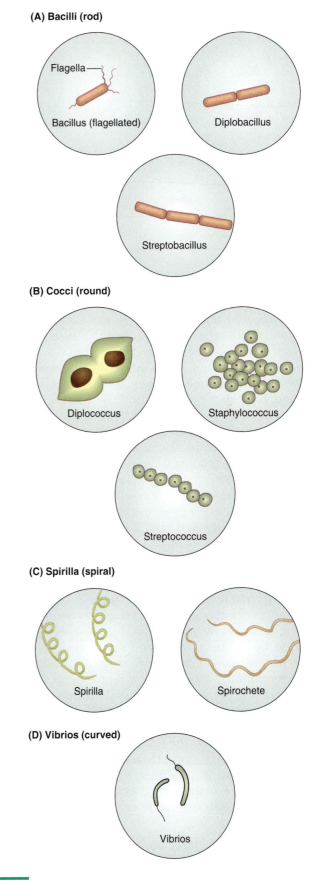

FIGURE 8-2 The unique shapes of bacteria. (A) Bacilli: rod shaped. (B) Cocci: round shaped. (C) Spirilla: S-shaped. (D) Vibrios: curved like a comma.

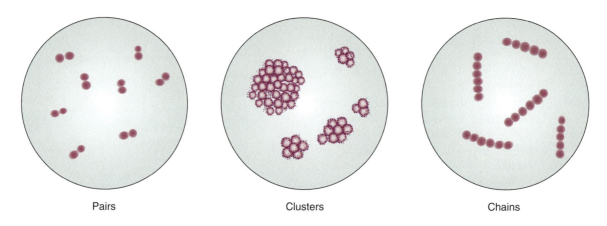

Pairs   Clusters   Chains

FIGURE 8-3 The pair, cluster, and chain shapes of bacteria colonies.

Diphtheria, Pertussis, and Tetanus. Diphtheria, pertussis, and **tetanus** are diseases caused by a bacterium microorganism. Diphtheria, caused by the microorganism bacillus corynebacterium diphtheria, appears as a severe throat infection and fever. At one time, diphtheria took the lives of thousands. Pertussis (whooping cough) is caused by the bacterium bordetella. Pertussis is a disease of the respiratory system, and it mainly affects infants and young children. Tetanus is caused by spores of bacterium clostridium tetani. The most common sign of tetanus is a stiffness of the jaw, commonly called lockjaw. All three of these diseases are prevented with a combined vaccination. The DPT immunization is given to children at two, four, and six months of age and then a booster is given at five years of age. After age five, tetanus boosters are given every ten years.

Strep Throat. Strep throat is one of the most common bacterial diseases infecting humans, caused by the streptococcus microorganism. Symptoms are sore throat, fever, and general malaise. In some cases, toxins released by the bacterium can cause a rash to develop and become a condition known as scarlet fever. **Streptococcus mutans**, a species of streptococcus, has been implicated in dental caries and endocarditis. This same group of bacteria can give rise to the diseases known as pneumonia or rheumatic fever. These infections can be prevented by the prompt use of antibiotics. The ADA recommends a prophylactic regimen be followed for any dental procedures that may cause endocarditis. It is recommended that a single dose of amoxicillin be administered one hour before the anticipated procedure.

Staphylococcal Infections. Staphylococcal infections are from the bacteria groups that grow in clusters. Some diseases in this group include the staph infection, gangrene, toxic shock syndrome, venereal diseases, and some forms of pneumonia. Antibiotics are the first line of treatment.

PROTOZOA

Protozoa (proh-tah-**ZOH**-ah) are microorganisms 100 microns in size, just below visibility of the naked eye (Figure 8-4). Often referred to as ameoba, protozoa reproduce by binary fission. (In binary fission, a transverse cell wall develops around the cell, the cell lengthens and then divides into two. The process then repeats.) They live in fluids in the blood stream, mouth, and intestinal tract and survive in polluted water in pools and ponds. Protozoa are single-celled animal life, and some are sporulating. They engulf their food as they change in shape in order to achieve mobility. Many have a long, threadlike appendage called a **flagella** projecting from them. These flagella whip around and cause additional movement for the protozoa. Some protozoa contain chlorophyll, and the majority are aerobic.

Disease Examples Caused by Protozoa

Amebic Dysentery. Amebic dysentery is an infection caused by the microorganism *Entamoeba histolytica.* The symptoms are severe diarrhea and, in extreme cases, abscesses develop in the liver. This disease is prevalent in countries where the drinking water is contaminated and overall poor hygiene conditions prevail. Drug treatment is necessary to effectively kill the parasite.

Periodontal Disease. Periodontal disease is caused by protozoa along with bacteria. Both microorganisms are found in the inflamed tissue around the tooth. Protozoa are located in the plaque in the periodontal pockets around the tooth. Treatment includes a thorough cleaning around the area to remove any plaque and diseased tissue and then impeccable oral hygiene maintenance.

Malaria. Malaria and sleeping sickness are two other diseases caused by protozoa. Both are prevalent throughout the tropics and have symptoms during the first two weeks, such as fever and soreness at the point of entry.

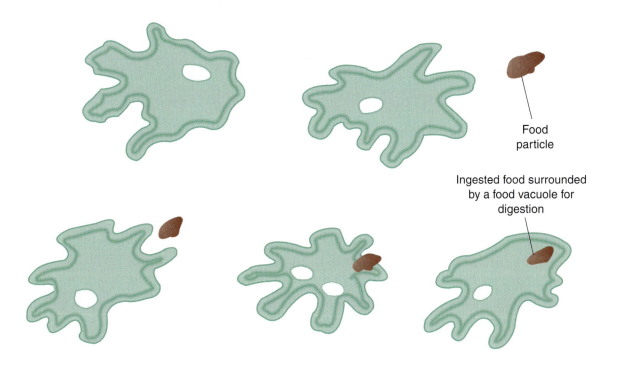

Food particle

Ingested food surrounded by a food vacuole for digestion

FIGURE 8-4 The protozoon changing shape as it travels to and engulfs its food.

Malaria is spread by the bites of mosquitoes, and sleeping sickness is spread by the bites of the tsetse fly. Both require drug therapy to kill the parasites in the blood.

RICKETTSIAE

Rickettsiae, other microorganisms, appear like tiny bacteria (Figure 8-5). They are parasites and cannot live outside a host. Often, lice, fleas, ticks, and mites are hosts to rickettsiae. They are able to multiply only by invading the cells of another life form. The hosts then transmit the disease to humans.

Disease Examples Caused by Rickettsiae

Rocky Mountain Spotted Fever. **Rocky Mountain Spotted Fever** is a rare disease. The symptoms occur

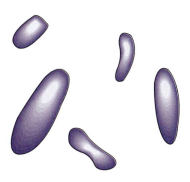

FIGURE 8-5 Rickettsiae as seen under an electron microscope.

about a week to ten days after transmitted from the host and are much like that of the flu. Two to six days after the symptoms have occurred, small pink spots appear on the ankles and wrists. The body is soon covered with these spots. Treatment with antibiotics normally cures the disease.

Typhus. **Typhus** is another fairly rare disease, similar to Rocky Mountain Spotted Fever. The microorganism is spread by a host, and symptoms appear rapidly. A severe headache, back and limb pain, constipation, and high fever develop suddenly. A rash similar to that of measles appears, confusion takes place, and the heart beats weakly. Typhus fever is treated with antibiotic drug therapy.

YEASTS AND MOLDS

Yeasts and molds (fungi) are smaller than protozoa and larger than bacteria (Figure 8-6). This group of microorganisms includes bread yeast, mushrooms, and bread molds. Yeasts and molds are a low form of plant life that lack chlorophyll. Some are sporulating, and they reproduce by budding. They cannot be killed by the antibiotics that kill bacteria (penicillin is made from mold but does not act upon fungi, from which it is made).

Disease Examples Caused by Yeast and Molds

Candidiasis. **Candidiasis** is an infection by the fungus *Candida albicans,* often on areas covered with mucous

FIGURE 8-6 Yeasts and molds.

membrane, like the inside of the mouth or the vaginal area. It is commonly called thrush, or moniliasis (Figure 8-7). It is kept at bay with **normal flora**, which is normal bacteria microorganisms in these areas. If antibiotics destroy too many of the bacteria, or if the body's immune system is in a lowered state, such as is the case with acquired immunodeficiency syndrome (AIDS), then the fungi multiply and overgrow. The disease causes thick white or creamy yellow ("cottage cheese") raised patches. These patches may become irritated and cause discomfort to the infected individual. Treatment for candidiasis is antifungal drug therapy.

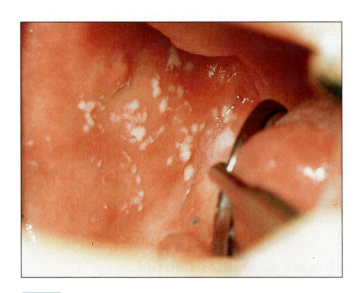

FIGURE 8-7 Patient presenting with thrush. *(Courtesy of Joseph L. Konzelman, Jr., DDS)*

Tinea. **Tinea** includes any group of common fungal infections. They are acquired from another infected person, animal, or inanimate object, such as a shower stall. The appearance is named according to the site infected. Tinea pedis, commonly called athlete's foot, causes itching and cracking between the toes and on the foot. Tinea corporis, commonly called ringworm, usually appears circular with a raised edge in red on the body. For most types of tinea, a treatment of antifungal drugs in the form of skin creams, ointments, or lotions is prescribed. Oral antifungal drugs may be necessary in persistent strains of the fungus.

VIRUSES

Viruses are the smallest microorganisms known to date (Figure 8-8). They are tiny particles, one one-hundredth the size of bacteria. An electron microscope must be used to visualize viruses. Like rickettsiae, they only are able to reproduce inside host cells. Viruses are difficult to grow in a culture, and their morphology is varied, like bacteria. Most are easy to kill by disinfecting or exposure to air, but the hepatitis B virus is very resistant. It can live on a dry surface for up to two weeks. Antibiotics will not kill any true virus. The outbreaks of viruses, like herpes simplex, can last from ten days to two weeks, whether treated or not. Treatment is primarily to ease the symptoms in order to make the patient more comfortable.

Disease Examples Caused by Viruses

Measles, Mumps, and Rubella. **Measles**, **mumps**, and **rubella** are some of the childhood illnesses caused by viruses. Measles cause a rash, and a fever is spread by airborne droplets of nasal secretions. An incubation period of nine to eleven days takes place before symptoms appear. With mumps, the main symptom is the swelling of the parotid (salivary) glands on one side or both sides. Mumps is spread by airborne droplets.

FIGURE 8-8 Viruses as seen under an electron microscope.

Rubella, also known as German measles, appears as a rash on the face and may spread to the trunk and limbs. This disease is only serious when it affects women in the early stages of pregnancy. The disease may infect the fetus and result in birth defects. The incubation period for both mumps and measles is two to three weeks long. The MMR (measles, mumps, and rubella) vaccine is highly effective in providing long-lasting immunity to the diseases and is given to all babies at about fifteen months of age. If an individual has the disease, the treatment is for the comfort of the patient only. An analgesic such as aspirin is given for fevers and lotion is applied for any itching in the area of the rash.

Poliomyelitis.
Poliomyelitis (poh-lee-oh-**my**-eh-**LYE**-tis), commonly called polio, invaded the United States in the 1950s. It attacked the central nervous system and in many cases led to extensive paralysis. Since the development of vaccines in the late 1950s, very few cases have developed. The virus IPV (inactivated polio vaccine), which contains dead virus, is given by injection; the IPV, however, is not used as much as OPV (oral poliovirus vaccine), which contains live but harmless virus and is given orally at the ages of two, four, and eighteen months. A booster dose at five years of age is also given.

Chicken Pox.
Chicken pox is a childhood disease caused by the varicella-zoster virus. It is characterized by a rash and slight fever. The virus remains dormant in the nerve tissue after the attack and may cause herpes zoster (shingles) later in life. Patients are contagious from about two days prior to the fever and five days after. The disease is spread through airborne droplets. The patient is treated for the fever but will heal totally within ten days. A varicella virus vaccine is recommended for this disease, but the longevity of the immunity is not known. It is best if the disease is contracted prior to the age of ten, because adults have much more severe symptoms, such as pneumonia.

Common Cold and Influenza.
The **common cold** and **influenza** are caused by viruses. Treatment is for fever, upset stomach, headache, and body ache. Anti-influenza vaccines are available and are highly recommended for the elderly and medically compromised. The vaccines are successful in sixty percent of the cases. Patients are contagious from twelve to seventy-two hours after the symptoms appear. Colds are spread through airborne droplets, contact with contaminated objects, or hand-to-hand contact. Flu is spread through airborne droplets.

DISEASES OF MAJOR CONCERN TO THE DENTAL ASSISTANT

Herpes Simplex

Herpes (**HER**-peez**) simplex** is a common and troublesome viral disease (Figure 8-9). **Herpes simplex virus**

FIGURE 8-9 Heptic labialis lesion. *(Courtesy of Joseph L. Konzelman, Jr., DDS)*

type 1 (HSV1) is usually associated with infections of the lips, mouth, and face, and herpes simplex virus type 2 (HSV2) is normally associated with the genital area. Type II can appear in the oral cavity. Both of these viruses are extremely contagious and spread by direct contact with a fluid-filled lesion, called a vesicle, or the fluid from this lesion.

Most adults have been infected by herpes simplex virus type 1. Initially, the infection may cause flu-like symptoms and a blister or sore in the mouth. It remains in the nerve cells within that area for life. HSV1 reactions are often due to a fever, prolonged exposure to sun, stress, or some foods high in acid being digested. These herpes simplex viruses (**cold sores** or **apthous ulcers**) reactivate and appear in the same general areas. The virus may infect the fingers if open sores are present, but this virus on the finger (**herpetic whitlow**) is rare and was more of a concern to dental personnel prior to the usage of latex gloves. The virus can be transferred to the eye and cause **conjunctivitis** or a **corneal ulcer**, which could result in blindness.

Treatment of HSV1 depends on its type, site, and severity. Dental teams may suggest to reschedule the patient if the sores are apparent at the time of scheduled treatment. This is primarily for the comfort of the patient, but it also may be office policy not to provide treatment when vesicles are present in the oral cavity. A number of topical treatments are available for patient comfort. Some people take L-Lysen, an amino acid, when they feel the symptoms coming on. Antiviral drugs such as acyclovir, generic for Zovirax, are sometimes helpful.

HSV2 is the sexually transmitted genital herpes. It displays the same vesicles, but they erupt on the sex organs or may erupt orally as well. As with type 1, they can recur occasionally.

Bloodborne Diseases.
Bloodborne diseases of concern to the dental assistant are viral hepatitis (HBV) and human immunodeficiency virus (HIV), which later develops into acquired immunodeficiency syndrome (AIDS). These diseases are transmitted directly through blood-contaminated body fluids.

High Risk Behavior for Acquiring Hepatitis B, HIV, and AIDS

▶ Injuries or sticks with sharp objects contaminated with blood or body fluid

▶ Multiple sexual partners, unprotected sex (homosexual, bisexual, or heterosexual)

▶ Sharing contaminated needles

▶ Exposure to non-intact skin or open wound with contaminated blood or body fluid

Viral Hepatitis

Viral hepatitis has five different types. **Hepatitis A** and **E** are transmitted by person-to-person contact or by ingestion of contaminated water or food. The symptoms, which appear from fifteen to forty days after contact, range from generally flu-like symptoms to acute liver injury. Hepatitis A (often called infectious hepatitis) is in the news when a fast-food provider has a number of customers become ill and the virus becomes identified. No long-term immunization has been available until recently. People who had possible contact with the contaminated food or water are given an injection of gamma globulin within fourteen days of exposure to provide short-term immunization. In 1995, a vaccine called *Havrix* was licensed by the U.S. Food and Drug Administration (FDA). A recent paper by the Centers for Disease Control and Prevention (CDC) stated the benefits of *Havrix* and, in 1997, *Havrix* was awarded the pediatric vaccine contract. Children in areas with a high rate of hepatitis A will be given the initial and booster dose of *Havrix* between the ages of two and eighteen years.

Hepatitis B is the major concern to dental personnel. This disease (commonly called serum hepatitis) has been recognized only since the early 1950s. It is primarily transmitted through contaminated needles and syringes. The incubation period is from fifty to 180 days, and only one-third of infected people have symptoms that can be easily identified; one-third have slight symptoms and one-third have no symptoms at all. The symptoms include loss of appetite, digestive upset, upper abdominal pain and tenderness, fever, weakness, muscle pain, and jaundice (yellowing of the skin). According to the CDC, about 300,000 people are infected each year; of that number, 300 will die from the disease, 10,000 will be hospitalized, and 20,000 will become chronic carriers. The CDC estimates that there are over a million carriers in the United States today.

In 1982, a plasma-derived Heptavax-B vaccine was introduced in the United States. Since that time, Recombivax HB and Energix B have been licensed for use in the United States and are shown to be effective against the hepatitis B virus.

Hepatitis C, often called non-A and non-B, reacts somewhat like hepatitis B but has no vaccine available currently. About 50 percent of those infected become chronic carriers.

Hepatitis D, also know as the Delta Agent, cannot replicate on its own and requires the presence of hepatitis B. The vaccination against hepatitis B should prevent hepatitis D from surviving.

Human Immunodeficiency Virus

Human immunodeficiency virus (HIV) belongs to the class of retroviruses and is the cause of acquired immunodeficiency syndrome (AIDS). It gains access to the body's blood stream via sexual intercourse, transfusions, and sticks with infected needles that break the skin. Also, a fetus can be infected by its mother. HIV attacks T-lymphocytes, part of the immune system, and multiplies. People in this stage pose no threat to the health-care worker if standard precautions are followed. People who have HIV but are unaware that they carry it are called asymptomatic carriers. Some have vague complaints, such as fever, weight loss, or unexplained diarrhea. These individuals are referred to as having AIDS-related complex (ARC).

In most cases, the disease progresses and the infected individual develops some brain damage in the form of dementia. If the individual is in this state for a long period of time, more severe brain damage may occur; normally, the infected individual most likely succumbs to AIDS before this happens.

Current treatment is for symptoms and not the disease itself. A great deal of research is being done currently to develop a vaccine to fight these retroviruses.

Acquired Immunodeficiency Syndrome

Acquired immunodeficiency syndrome (AIDS) is due to infection with HIV. A syndrome is a group of symptoms that characterize a disease. Not all individuals infected with HIV develop AIDS. In the United States, 100,000 cases of HIV were diagnosed in the 1980s. The first few cases were reported in 1981. The CDC was notified of a rare and unusual lung infection in young homosexual men. Also, a previously slow-growing skin tumor found in aging men, called Kaposi's sarcoma, was found to be growing aggressively in this same group of men. Individuals with these two symptoms reported with a number of opportunistic infections, such as pneumonia.

After much research, the virus was found to be transmitted in the semen and blood of infected individuals. "Casual" spreading of the disease does not seem to happen. For example, kissing does not spread the disease. A person with full-blown AIDS exhibits cancers, infections, diarrhea, or a number of other viral diseases. The prognosis is often fatal, but life may be sustained for a number of years with appropriate diet and health measures. Through June 1998, the cumulative number of AIDS cases reported to the CDC is 665,357. The total deaths of this same group are 401,028. The majority of these diagnosed cases are in the age group of thirty to forty.

There is no cure for AIDS. The complications are treated accordingly. Several antiviral drugs are used, such as zidovudine (AZT) and acyclovir. AZT has a number of side effects but has been shown to slow the progression of the disease. Research continues in an effort to find a vaccine for HIV, with several drugs showing promise.

HOW THE BODY RESISTS DISEASES

The body responds to diseases in a number of ways. A person may get a fever or chills or develop a localized inflammation. These are all ways the body uses to fight the disease. Before these symptoms occur, however, the pathogens must fight the body's other lines of defense.

Our bodies repel thousands of infections that come our way every day. Intact skin makes it impossible for a number of bacteria to get into our systems. If dust or some pathogen-laden particles get into the nose, a person sneezes. If something enters the throat, a person coughs. If spoiled food is swallowed, a person normally vomits or expels it through diarrhea.

If the pathogen gains access to the body, the second line of defense, the circulatory system, begins fighting the pathogen. The area becomes inflamed and swollen. Swelling and redness are due to the engorgement of the capillaries with blood. White cells in great numbers migrate to the area and engulf large numbers of bacteria. Many of these cells die and produce enzymes that digest the dead tissues. These mobile phagocytes or leukocytes engulf the invading pathogens and destroy them. The result of this process is **purulence** (pus). While this is going on, the body is building a dam around the infected area, called the **pyogenic membrane**. This membrane is a wall that contains the infection and does not allow it to spread to other parts of the body. If the infection can be controlled, the involved area fills in with connective tissue and is healed.

If the pathogens overcome the body's first and second lines of defense, the infection spreads to adjoining tissues and finally to the whole body. When this happens, the body utilizes its final defenses: **antibodies**. These antibodies produce immunity against any foreign substance or pathogen. Pathogens that stimulate the production of antibodies are called **antigens**.

There are a number of different groups of antibodies that perform different functions in response to an antigen. For instance, **antitoxin** neutralizes the toxins given off by certain bacteria.

Infection

Another way the body fights off infection or pathogens is with fever and inflammation. Few bacteria can survive a fever of 102 to 104 degrees for long. Inflammation, an increase in blood vessels in the injured area, is characterized by four signs: **erythema** (redness), heat, edema (swelling), and pain. An increase in blood supply in the area causes the redness and heat and the walls enlarge, allowing the antibodies into the area. The swelling causes pain and pressure on nerve endings.

Immunity

The person's ability to resist pathogens is called **immunity.** People differ in their abilities to resist disease, and this resistance is stronger at various times in a person's life. Two different general types of immunity are natural and acquired. Humans are born with **natural immunity.** Local inflammation and blood phagocytes are part of the natural immune system.

If immunity is developed as a result of exposure to a pathogen, it is called **acquired immunity**. This also can be a borrowed immunity, called **passive acquired immunity**. This occurs when antibodies from another animal or person are injected into an individual, giving protection to the individual from a specific disease. This immediate immunity normally only lasts up to six weeks. A fetus obtains temporary passive immunity from the mother through the placenta. While breastfeeding, the mother's milk also provides some passive immunity to the baby.

Lasting longer and preferred over passive acquired immunity is **active acquired immunity**. The two types of active acquired immunity are natural acquired immunity and artificial acquired immunity. **Natural acquired immunity** occurs when an individual has had a disease, the body has manufactured antibodies to the disease, and the person has recovered from the disease. Normally, the individual is then immune to the disease and does not contract the disease again. The second type of active acquired immunity is **artificial acquired immunity**. This is when the individual is vaccinated (inoculated) with a specific antigen. An **antigen** is a substance that is injected into the individual in order to stimulate production of specific antibodies. This antigen is often an expired or a weakened state of the pathogen. The process is used to increase an individual's resistance to a particular disease or to provide **immunization**.

The body itself may over-react to an antigen. If the antigen causes an allergic response, it is called an **allergen**. Individuals who are generally more sensitive to certain allergens than most people are called **hypersensitive**. In severe cases, a person's antigen-antibody stimulates a massive secretion of histamine. This severe reaction, called **anaphylactic shock** (anaphylaxis), is sometimes fatal. It is important to take a thorough health history in order to identify individuals who are hypersensitive to one or more substances.

Normal Routes of Microorganism Exposure in the Dental Office

Three normal routes of microorganism exposure take place in the dental office. Exposure occurs when a pathogen from an infected individual passes to a susceptible person.

Direct Contact

The dental caregiver touches the lesion or blood of an infected person while working in the oral cavity. This is direct contact. Standard precautions should be followed to prevent contact with microorganisms.

Indirect Contact

Indirect contact is when the dental caregiver obtains the disease from contaminated instruments, supplies, or equipment. Standard precautions should be followed to prevent cross-contamination.

Inhalation

Inhalation of microorganisms takes place during the utilization of the high-speed handpiece, which creates an aerosol spray during patient care. The dental caregiver inhales the pathogen, which is also considered direct contact from the carrier or the infected person. Standard precautions should be followed to prevent this.

CHAPTER SUMMARY

In order to safeguard against microorganism exposure in a dental office, one needs to understand how these pathogens pass from an infected person to a susceptible person. Therefore, within this chapter you will learn about pathogenic microorganisms along with the diseases they cause and how the body can defend them.

CASE STUDY

Darin Scott came down with flu-like symptoms. Two days after these symptoms occurred, he noticed spots on his ankles and wrists. Within a day, his body was covered with spots.

Case Study Review

1. What is one of the diseases you would consider?

2. Is this a common disease?

3. What treatment will most likely be prescribed?

4. What microorganism caused this disease?

 To complete your study of this chapter, work the review activities that follow. Also, refer to the software that accompanies this text.

REVIEW QUESTIONS

Multiple Choice

1. Who gave us the theory of the etiologic agent?
   a. Anton Van Leeuwenhoek.
   b. Louis Pasteur.
   c. Robert Koch.
   d. Joseph Lister.

2. Most bacteria is said to require air and is therefore called
   a. aerobic.
   b. anaerobic.
   c. facultative bacteria.
   d. gram positive.

3. Which bacteria has been implicated in dental caries?
   a. Staphylococcal.
   b. Mycobacterium tuberculosis.
   c. Bacillus corynebacterium diphtheria.
   d. Streptococcus mutans.

4. The herpes simplex virus that infects the finger and was a concern prior to the usage of latex gloves is called
   a. corneal ulcer.
   b. herpetic whitlow.
   c. tinea.
   d. candidiasis.

5. The name of the slow-growing skin tumor that develops from HIV is called
   a. Kaposi's sarcoma.
   b. pyogenic membrane.
   c. allergen.
   d. herpes zoster.

Critical Thinking

1. If two individuals kiss on the lips and neither has open sores around the mouth but one of the two has AIDS, is the probability high for the other individual to acquire AIDS because of this kiss?

2. Periodontal disease can be which microorganisms?

3. Which one of the hepatitis viruses is of greatest concern to the dental assistant and why?

Preclinical Dental Skills

Infection Control

OBJECTIVES

The student should strive to meet the following objectives and demonstrate an understanding of the facts and principles presented in this chapter:

1. Identify the rationale, regulations, recommendations, and training that govern infection control in the dental office.

2. Describe how pathogens travel from person to person in the dental office.

3. List the three primary routes of microbial transmission and the associated dental procedures that affect the dental assistant.

4. Demonstrate the principles of infection control, including medical history, handwashing, personal protective equipment, barriers, chemical disinfectants, ultrasonic cleaners, sterilizers, and instrument storage.

5. List various disinfectants and their applications as used in dentistry.

6. Identify and demonstrate the usage of different types of sterilizers.

7. Demonstrate the usage of several types of sterilization monitors, such as biological and process indicators.

8. Identify and show the proper usage of pre-procedure mouth rinses, high volume evacuation, dental dams, and disposable items.

9. Identify and demonstrate the correct protocol for disinfecting, cleaning, and sterilizing prior to seating the patient, as well as at the end of the dental treatment, in the dental radiography area, and in the dental laboratory.

KEY TERMS

American Dental Association (ADA) (p. 152)

antimicrobial (p. 155)

asepsis (p. 152)

aseptic technique (p. 152)

Bloodborne Pathogens Standard (p. 152)

Centers for Disease Control and Prevention (CDC) (p. 152)

contamination (p. 152)

direct contact (p. 155)

disinfect (p. 161)

Environmental Protection Agency (EPA) (p. 154)

Food and Drug Administration (FDA) (p. 153)

glutaraldehyde (p. 162)

indirect contact (p. 155)

infection control (p. 155)

inhalation (p. 155)

iodophor (p. 163)

Occupational Safety and Health Administration (OSHA) (p. 152)

other potentially infectious materials (OPIM) (p. 152)

pathogens (p. 152)

personal protective equipment (PPE) (p. 152)

polynitrile autoclavable gloves (p. 159)

standard precautions (p. 152)

sterilization (p. 162)

universal precautions (p. 152)

INTRODUCTION

The dentist is responsible for ensuring that the process of infection control is adequate. Compliance with all regulations must be accomplished on a continuing basis; staff must be trained at the time of initial employment or when job tasks change (before the employee is placed in a position where occupational exposure may occur) and annually thereafter. The records must be maintained for the duration of employment plus thirty years, in accordance with the regulations. Even though the dentist is ultimately responsible, often an employee (full time) is designated as the infection control and hazard waste coordinator. This person ensures that the office is in compliance with all regulations, reads updated information on infection control and hazard waste, and presents the information to the dental team for review. The infection control and hazard waste coordinator schedules staff training, oversees the entire process of infection control, and makes sure that procedures ensure complete **asepsis**. Asepsis means the creation of an environment free of **pathogens** (disease-causing microorganisms). It also includes the steps, or **aseptic technique**, used to provide this environment. Aseptic technique is needed for all procedures in which there is a danger of introducing infection or disease into a human's body.

RATIONALES AND REGULATIONS

Rationale of Infection Control

All efforts are made to stop infectious diseases from spreading. Routine practices eliminate mistakes from being made. **Universal precautions** mean that all patients are treated as if they are infectious. **Standard precautions** (universal precautions and body substance isolation techniques) are practiced prior to, during, and after each procedure in the dental office. Therefore, every precaution is taken to ensure that the **chain of asepsis** (aseptic procedures ensuring that no cross-contamination occurs) is not broken and that **contamination** does not occur.

Regulations and Recommendations for Infection Control in the Dental Office

A number of agencies have established guidelines for infection control in the dental office. These minimal standards change from time to time as more information is known about disease prevention. **Regulations** are made by government agencies (such as OSHA) and licensing boards that have the authority to enforce compliance. If compliance is not met, the dentist may be fined, lose his or her license to practice dentistry, or face imprisonment. **Recommendations** can be made by anyone, and no authority for enforcement is mandated. Most often, when the regulations are made, the profession has a specific time frame in which to comply. During this time, consultants, the dental association, and other groups make recommendations on the best means for compliance. See Appendix A for addresses and phone numbers for regulating and recommending agencies.

American Dental Association (ADA). The **American Dental Association (ADA)**, the parent organization for dentistry in the United States, makes recommendations through its **councils** (Chapter 1, Introduction to the Dental Profession) in the form of literature, videotapes, news broadcasts, manuals, brochures, the *Journal of the American Dental Association* (JADA), *ADA News,* and an Internet site (http:www.ada.org). The American Dental Assistants' Association (ADAA), the American Dental Hygienists' Association (ADHA), and the American Dental Laboratory Association (ADLA) also provide information to their members through support services and journals.

Centers for Disease Control and Prevention. The **Centers for Disease Control and Prevention (CDC)** is the basis for many of the regulations. This agency, part of the Public Health Service, a division of the United States Department of Human Health and Services, has established a number of recommendations that have been made by federal, state, and local agencies into regulations.

In 1996, the CDC and United States Public Health Department issued standard precautions, which augmented and synthesized universal precautions and **body substance isolation (BSI)** techniques. BSI is a system requiring **personal protective equipment (PPE)** to be worn in order to protect against contact with all body fluids, whether or not blood is visible. Standard precautions, adopted by numerous health-care industries, protect the health-care providers, patients, and others from infectious diseases.

Occupational Safety and Health Administration. The **Occupational Safety and Health Administration (OSHA)** is a regulating body that enforces the requirements that employers must protect their employees from exposure to blood and **other potentially infectious materials (OPIM)** during the time when employees are at work. This agency is part of the United States Department of Labor. Its overall mission is to protect the workers in the United States from physical, chemical, or infectious hazards while in the workplace. The OSHA **Bloodborne Pathogens Standard** became effective in 1992. This standard applies to any facility where employees can or have the potential to be exposed to body fluids, such as in hospitals, funeral homes, emergency medical services, medical and dental offices, and research laboratories.

Compliance with these standards is monitored through investigations of the facilities by OSHA compliance inspectors. If the facility fails to come into compliance, a citation resulting in a possible fine is given. If the facility continues to refuse to comply, the fine increases and additional steps are taken to ensure that the conditions are corrected.

When Investigations of Dental Offices for Compliance Are Done

▶ After an employee or a patient complaint is made

▶ In any office having eleven or more employees, on a random basis

▶ By invitation of the office when an inspection is requested

All states are regulated by the OSHA standard. Twenty-two states are regulated through state agency standards that run parallel to or are more demanding than the federal standard; the other states are administered through regional branches of the federal Occupational Safety and Health Administration.

Overview of the 1992 OSHA Bloodborne Pathogens Standard

Every facility must:

▶ Review the Bloodborne Pathogens Standard

▶ Prepare a written exposure control plan and means to protect and train employees

▶ Train all employees in a timely manner (initially, after a job task change, and annually)

▶ Provide employees with everything needed in order to meet standard regulations

▶ Provide personal protective equipment (PPE)

▶ Maintain and dispose of necessary PPE

▶ Establish standard operating procedures (SOP) in infection control

▶ Offer the hepatitis B vaccination series to all employees

▶ Establish a post-exposure plan, including medical evaluation and follow-up procedures (for example, occupational exposure needle stick)

▶ Provide communication on biohazards

▶ Establish standards for handling and disposing of hazardous waste

▶ Maintain records of training, hepatitis B vaccinations, and exposure incidents

Written Exposure Plan This plan documents the specific exposure determination for each employee and identifies a schedule of implementation (how and when the provisions of the standard will be implemented). This document must list how the situations surrounding an exposure will be evaluated and what measures will be taken to correct the situation (if necessary).

Exposure Determination To evaluate an employee's chances of having an occupational exposure to bloodborne pathogens, an exposure determination is made.

An **occupational exposure** is any reasonably anticipated eye, mucosa, skin, parenteral (cut, needlestick, puncture, abrasions, and so on), or any contact with blood or saliva that may be a result of employment tasks. The determination is made based on three categories:

Step 1. All employees make a list of tasks they perform in each job classification and then identify which category they fall under. Any employee who may have any occupational exposure at any time is covered under the standard.

▶ **Category 1** includes all tasks that involve exposure to blood, body fluids such as saliva, and body tissues. (This group includes the dentist, dental assistant, dental hygienists, and dental laboratory technician.)

▶ **Category 2** includes all tasks that involve no exposure to blood, body fluids such as saliva, or body tissues, but occasionally may involve unplanned tasks from Category 1. (This group includes the receptionist, coordinating assistant, and so on.)

▶ **Category 3** includes all tasks that involve no exposure to blood, body fluids such as saliva, or body tissues. (This group includes the accountant, insurance assistant, and so on.)

Step 2. The office must have a schedule for implementation. This schedule must designate how and when each provision of the standard will be implemented.

▶ How and when are the hepatitis B vaccinations being offered to employees?

▶ How and when is communication of hazards to employees being covered?

▶ How and when are the post-exposure evaluation and office follow-up procedures being accomplished?

▶ How and when is the recordkeeping being accomplished and updated?

Step 3. A manual and procedure plan must be written to cover methods of compliance for office PPE and safety issues. For instance, the office must have written information covering all aspects of the following:

▶ Personal protective equipment

▶ Engineering controls

▶ Housekeeping controls

▶ Work practice controls

Step 4. A written policy on how exposure incidents are evaluated is required. Included in this area are the circumstances that surround the incident and how they can be corrected. What type of evaluation will be done by the office if an exposure incident occurs?

The Food and Drug Administration. The Food and Drug Administration (FDA), which is a division of the

United States Department of Health and Human Services, regulates the manufacturing and labeling of medical devices and solutions. The FDA requires that certain performance standards be met prior to use by the public. It requires that general controls be used with the devices and solutions and that labeling give the appropriate information to the consumer. It holds the manufacturers responsible for problems that develop, unless the medical device or solution is misused by the consumer. In that instance, the liability lies with the user.

Items in the dental office regulated by the FDA are sterilizers; chemical and biologic indicators; cleaning solutions such as ultrasonic solution and cold chemicals; PPE such as gloves, masks, glasses, and disposable clothing; sterilizing solutions; and disinfectants.

Environmental Protection Agency. The **Environmental Protection Agency (EPA)** is another regulatory agency involved in the safety and effectiveness of disinfecting and sterilizing solutions. It also regulates the disposal of hazardous waste after it leaves the dental office. Each of the disinfecting and sterilizing solutions must be submitted by the manufacturer to the EPA for approval. If a solution meets all the claims listed and safety concerns are noted on the container, the EPA assigns an EPA number that must appear on the label of each of the approved solutions.

OSHA-Mandated Training for Employees in the Dental Office

All employers must ensure that employees (full time, part time, and temporary) who fall into Category 1 and/or 2, where tasks involve exposure to blood, body fluid such as saliva, and/or body tissues, have training. This training must be provided at no cost to the employee. The training must be given prior to placement in a position where bloodborne pathogens are a factor, to all new employees, and to all employees reclassifying into different positions.

Mandated OSHA Training for Dental Employees

The following must be available to all dental employees:

▶ A copy of the Bloodborne Pathogens Standard and specific information regarding the meaning of the standard
▶ Information about bloodborne pathogens, both the epidemiology and symptoms of the diseases
▶ Information about the cross-contamination pathways of bloodborne pathogens
▶ A written copy or means for employees to obtain the employer's/office's written exposure control plan
▶ Information on the tasks, category placement of employee classifications, and how each is identi-

fied in relation to bloodborne pathogens and other potentially infectious materials (OPIM)
▶ Information regarding the hepatitis B vaccine
▶ Information about exposure reduction, including PPE; work practices; standard precautions, including universal precautions; and engineering practices
▶ Information about the selection, placement, use, removal, disinfection, sterilization, and disposal of PPE
▶ Information about what to do and whom to contact if an emergency involving blood or OPIM arises
▶ Information about the procedure to follow if an incident of blood exposure occurs, how to report the incident, and what type of medical follow-up is available at no cost to the employee
▶ Information about the post-exposure evaluation and follow-up the employer provides
▶ A copy of the OSHA Hazard Communication Standard
▶ **Material Safety Data Sheets (MSDSs)** and information about labeling and hazardous waste
▶ Opportunity for employees to ask questions of the individual giving the information

The training cannot be accomplished by videos or interactive computer training programs alone. The training must be accomplished by an individual who has the background necessary to answer questions and to supplement the training with in-office (on-site), specific information. The information must be given in a manner for all to understand. If an employee is unable to understand the content due to a language barrier or a disability, the employer must provide an interpreter or convey this information in a manner for the employee to understand completely.

A record of the date of the training session, employees present, and qualifications of the trainer must be maintained.

CROSS-CONTAMINATION PATHWAYS

Pathogens can travel from patients to dentists, dental assistants, dental hygienists, dental laboratory technicians, and other patients. Pathogens can also travel from dental personnel to patients. The transfer then can go to the families and friends of the dental personnel. This cycle must be broken through aseptic techniques (Figure 9-1).

ROUTES OF MICROBIAL TRANSMISSION

In dentistry, three primary routes transmit most microorganisms: direct contact, indirect contact, and inhalation/aerosol. Microorganisms may be missed because they appear as a mist or dry clear on the

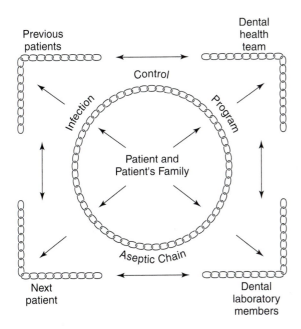

FIGURE 9-1 Pathways of cross-contamination.

surfaces that are touched. They are overlooked if careful, consistent aseptic procedures are not followed. The dental assistant is the primary caretaker of the infection control practices. Using the correct barriers, PPE, treating all patients as if they are infectious, using proper disinfection, and sterilization break the cycle of infection and eliminate cross-contamination (see also Chapter 8, Microbiology). The possible routes of microbial transmission are as follows:

1. **Direct contact**: An individual has direct contact with a lesion or microorganism while performing intraoral dental procedures.

2. **Indirect contact**: An individual contacts the microorganism through another means, such as contaminated instruments, supplies, or equipment.

3. **Inhalation/aerosol**: An individual contacts the microorganism through inhalation. This normally happens when the high speed handpiece or the ultrasonic cavitron is used in the dental office.

INFECTION CONTROL IN THE DENTAL OFFICE

A number of steps must be followed to accomplish the goal of **infection control**, or asepsis. The first step is for the dental assistant to maintain good health standards. Eating and sleeping properly aids in staying healthy. Proper exercise, along with maintaining a positive mental attitude, provides the energy to attain individual goals for good overall health.

Immunizations

The dental assistant should have the immunizations necessary to fight off pathogens that are encountered due to the close proximity to patients during dental treatment. If the dental assistant has not had the hepatitis B series, the employer must provide the information about immunizations and the available vaccine during initial training and is required to pay for the series. Review the initial part of this chapter for employee training information regarding the hepatitis B vaccine (see also Chapter 8, Microbiology, for additional information regarding immunizations).

Medical History

Taking the patient's medical history and updating it at each appointment is a good way to gather information but may not identify infectious diseases patients have. It is important to update this information both verbally and in writing. Patients are sometimes more willing to disclose information during conversation. The majority of individuals infected with HBV and HIV are **asymptomatic**, having no symptoms. Therefore, the medical history may give information to the health-care workers, but it cannot be used alone to identity patients who place dental personnel at high risk. Standard precautions incorporating universal precautions and practicing infection control standards with each and every patient is essential in infection control.

Handwashing

One of the most important ways to prevent the transfer of microorganisms from one person or object to another person is handwashing. Handwashing is the vigorous rubbing together of well-lathered soapy hands (ensuring friction on all surfaces), concluding with a thorough rinsing under a stream of water and proper drying. Handwashing is both a mechanical cleaning and chemical **antisepsis** (inhibiting the growth of causative microorganisms).

Hands contain resident and transient microflora (visible by use of microscope). The mechanical process of scrubbing removes transient microorganisms and some resident microorganisms. Transient microorganisms are fresh contaminants of brief duration. Transient microorganisms are of primary concern to the dental profession because they constitute the pathogen group that includes hepatitis. Resident microorganisms survive and multiply for a longer period of time primarily in the top layers of the skin but can be located in deeper layers of the skin. The chemical antisepsis is accomplished through the use of an antimicrobial soap. Applying the proper technique and using **antimicrobial** (microorganism growth inhibitor) handwashing products can add additional protection to ensure that microorganisms are removed each time the hands are washed.

Currently, antimicrobial handwashing agents that are the most beneficial include chlorhexidine digluconate, triclosan, and para-chlorometaxylenol. These handwashing agents exhibit prolonged antimicrobial effects.

At the beginning of each day, every member of the dental team should complete two consecutive thirty-second handwashes. It is important to use plenty of antimicrobial soap and water while rubbing all areas of the hands (Figure 9-2). Getting between the fingers, rubbing each finger and thumb, and cleaning beneath the fingernails is essential. Some offices provide brushes that aid in scrubbing. These brushes (often made of foam rubber pad and plastic bristles) must not be so hard that they abrade the tissue, allowing microorganisms access to the body. Remember, the skin is a barrier to microorganisms, and care should be taken to prevent cuts and lesions. A final rinse with cold water is used to close the pores in the skin. Dry the hands completely with paper towels, and use the paper towels to turn off the hand-controlled sink faucets and wipe the area clean. The brushes are sterilized or disposed of after each use.

A minimal thirty-second handwashing should be completed before and after patient care, donning and removing gloves, breaks, ending each day, and at any other time the hands become contaminated. Due to constant handwashing, the hands may show effects of skin irritation. Hand lotions help to prevent hands from chapping.

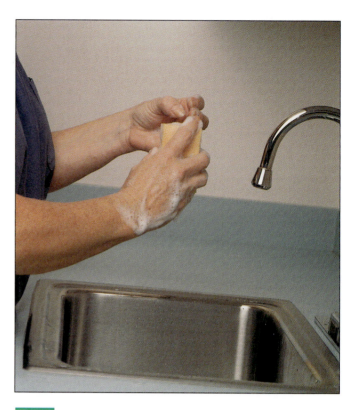

FIGURE 9-2 Dental assistant handwashing with antimicrobial soap and scrub brush/sponge.

P R O C E D U R E

9-1 Handwashing

The procedure is performed by all dental team members.

EQUIPMENT AND SUPPLIES

▶ Liquid antimicrobial handwashing agent

▶ Soft, sterile brush or sponge (optional)

▶ Sink with hot and cold running water

▶ Paper towels

PROCEDURE STEPS

At the beginning of each day (two consecutive thirty-second handwashes)

1. Remove jewelry (rings and watch).

2. Adjust water flow and wet hands thoroughly.

3. Apply antimicrobial handwashing agents with water; bring to a lather.

4. Scrub hands together or with a sterile brush or sponge, making sure to get between each finger, the surface of the palms and wrists, and under the finger nails.

5. Rinse and repeat Steps 3 and 4.

6. Final rinse with cool to lukewarm water for ten seconds to close the pores.

7. Dry with paper towels, the hands first and then the wrist area.

8. Use paper towels to turn off the hand-controlled faucets.

Routine Handwashing: Thirty-second handwash before and after patients, donning gloves, and taking breaks. Routine handwashing must be completed at the end of each day and any other time the hands become contaminated.

1. Complete the handwashing steps for the beginning of each day, except Step 5.

Artificial fingernails are not recommended for health professionals. Artificial fingernails have been found to exhibit high microbe counts under the nail, even after thorough handwashing.

The soap containers and the sink area become contaminated and should be disinfected routinely. Foot-operated soap dispensers prevent unnecessary hand contamination. The water controls should be foot or light sensor operated to cut down on contamination. Do not use reusable towels to dry hands; instead, use air or disposable towels.

Dental teams that are involved in oral surgery should perform a surgical scrub (see Chapter 19, Oral and Maxillofacial Surgery, for directions in performing a surgical scrub).

Personal Protective Equipment (PPE)

The dental assistant has constant exposure to saliva and blood during intraoral/invasive dental procedures. Even with the maintenance of good health and immunizations, it is essential for dental team members to ensure better protection from microorganisms through constant use of personal protective equipment (PPE). The employers must provide this equipment according to OSHA regulations. Barriers are used to prevent potential pathogens, encountered during patient care, from gaining access to dental personnel. Barriers such as protective eyewear, face masks, disposable gloves, and appropriate uniforms should be used routinely to minimize exposure.

Protective Eyewear. It is essential that dental team members wear protective eyewear during specific phases of dental treatment. The splatter of blood and saliva can transfer infectious diseases, such as hepatitis and herpes simplex viruses, to the mucous membranes of the eye. Aerosol droplets that contain microorganisms can cause an eye infection known as pink eye (conjunctivitis). Also, during some dental procedures, particles of gold, amalgam, and tooth fragments can be hurled into the eye, causing damage. Dental offices provide protective eyewear for patients to wear during dental treatment. These glasses, like the ones worn by the dental personnel, can be disposable or disinfected or sterilized after use.

Protective eyewear should provide front, top, and side protection; several choices are available. The American National Standards Institute developed a standard for the design and characteristics of occupational glasses. Dental team members who wear corrective lenses may choose to wear goggles that fit over their glasses or side shields that fit on their own eyewear (Figures 9-3A and B). Others wear glasses designed for dental personnel that incorporate top and side shields (Figure 9-3C). In addition, a face shield can be worn that covers the entire face (Figure 9-3D). A mask must still be worn with a face shield.

FIGURE 9-3 (A) Goggles. (B) Eyewear with protective side shields. (C) Dental protective eyewear with attached side shields. (D) Dental face shield.

Eyewear is also utilized to protect the eyes from high intensity lights used for curing dental materials. These glasses or shields are normally colored orange for protection.

At times, the eyewear becomes fogged due to warm breath coming from under the dental mask. Several antifog products are available to minimize fogging. Fog spray can be used, or the eyewear can be placed under warm water to reduce the fog problem.

Gloves. Gloves are used as a barrier to microorganisms. Any time a dental team member anticipates contact with saliva or blood, gloves should be worn. This includes saliva- or blood-contaminated surfaces, instruments, or mucous membranes. Numerous gloves are on the market that meet FDA regulations. The FDA regulates the gloves specific for the health-care industry. Five primary types of gloves are used in the dental office (FDA regulated*):

1. Latex gloves (nonsterile and sterile)*

2. Vinyl gloves (nonsterile and sterile)*

3. Overgloves (nonsterile)

4. Utility gloves (nonsterile)

5. Polynitrile, nitrile (autoclavable)

Choose the appropriate gloves according to comfort, tactile sensitivity required, and the procedure being completed. Obtaining the best quality for the greatest value is another factor in choosing gloves.

Both the **latex and vinyl gloves** are ambidextrous, used interchangeably for the right or left hand (Figures 9-4A and B). They are supplied in a variety of sizes to provide the proper fit for most individuals. Many individuals feel that latex gloves provide a better fit. Latex-sensitive individuals use vinyl gloves as an alternative to latex. The vinyl gloves, however, are more rigid, therefore tearing more easily and lacking the tactile sensitivity. But, due to increased use, vinyl gloves are being improved. The gloves (latex and vinyl) can be ordered with powder on the inside to aid in donning (placing the gloves on). Both types of gloves are supplied as nonsterile, referred to as examination gloves, and sterile, referred to as sterile surgical gloves. Most procedures in the dental office require only the use of the nonsterile gloves. They provide the minimal barrier protection needed for the dental personnel. Sterile surgical gloves are only used in specific surgical procedures requiring a sterile environment, such as oral, periodontal, and implant surgery.

Both the latex and the vinyl gloves need to be changed with each new patient. If, during the procedure, they become torn or punctured, they should be removed, the hands washed, and the gloves replaced with new gloves to complete the procedure. *Gloves should never be washed and reused.*

Harmful Reactions to Latex Gloves and Other Latex Products

Symptoms	Condition
Hands become dry, red, itchy, and sometimes cracked	Irritant contact dermatitis
Redness, initial itching, and vesicles appear in areas of contact within twenty-four to forty-eight hours, followed by dry skin with fissures and sores	Type IV hypersensitivity (delayed hypersensitivity)
Runny nose, sneezing, itchy eyes, scratchy throat, asthma, and, in rare cases, anaphylaxis	Type I hypersensitivity (immediate-type hypersensitivity)

Gloves in the Dental Office

▶ Use new gloves for each patient.
▶ Never wash gloves.
▶ If gloves become penetrated during treatment, remove gloves, wash and dry hands, and place new gloves on hands.

Overgloves, also known as food handlers' gloves, are placed over the latex or vinyl gloves during a procedure to prevent cross-contamination if the dental assistant has to reach inside a drawer, write on a chart, or touch an area that is not contaminated (Figure 9-5). Overgloves are big, loose gloves that do not have the tactile touch that the latex and vinyl gloves have, but they quickly fit over the gloves to obtain something in a sterile area. They are not to be used as examination gloves. Overgloves can be placed on rapidly to accomplish the

FIGURE 9-4 (A) Vinyl and (B) latex examination gloves.

FIGURE 9-5 Overgloves used for opening a drawer or writing on a chart. *(Courtesy of Biotrol International 1-800-822-8550)*

FIGURE 9-6 (A) Utility and (B) polynitrile gloves used during infection control procedures.

secondary task needed, such as opening a container. They should be discarded after each use.

Utility gloves are thicker gloves used during disinfection and cleanup procedures (Figure 9-6A). These are gloves used for "dishwashing" and they, like the overgloves, are not regulated by the FDA. An assistant carries the tray to the sterilization area, removes the latex or vinyl gloves, washes his or her hands, and dons the utility gloves to complete the cleanup. The utility gloves can be washed and reused. If they do become cracked or punctured, they should be discarded and new gloves used.

Polynitrile autoclavable gloves are much like utility gloves; however, an added benefit is that they can be sterilized in the autoclave after use (Figure 9-6B). Each dental member involved in cleanup and instrument recycling must have his or her own set of polynitrile gloves.

Masks. Masks are worn at any time the possibility for splatter or aerosol of saliva or blood can occur (Figure 9-7). The dental assistant must wear a mask to protect the mucous membranes of the nose and the mouth. The aerosol mist that remains suspended in the air may come from the use of the dental handpiece, the ultrasonic scaler, or the air-water syringe. At times, due to the use of the air-water syringe, splatter occurs where a concentrated amount of saliva or blood projects from the oral cavity to the dental health worker. Proper placement of the high volume evacuator and the air-water syringe (Chapter 14, Introduction to Chairside Assisting) aids in the reduction of splatter; however, it can still occur. Wearing a mask, covering the nose and mouth, protects dental personnel in such cases.

Utilization of the dental mask also protects the patient and the dental assistant from the transmission of communicable diseases.

FIGURE 9-7 Dental face masks used in dentistry.

Masks During Dental Treatment

▶ Use a new mask for each patient.
▶ Replace the mask if it becomes moist or wet.
▶ Never let the mask dangle around the neck or from the ear; remove and discard after use.

The mask should be placed along with the eyewear, prior to washing hands and donning gloves (Figure 9-8). It is important that the mask be placed properly so that it fits snugly against the face and stays in place during the procedure. Normally, the face mask has an outside and an inside (next to the face); place it according to the manufacturer's directions. Often, a color is on the outside surface for quick identification. Masks are also available in a variety of designs for a positive practice image. For example, cartoon images are available for a pediatric practice.

The mask are secured with elastic that goes around the head or over the ears, or with ties that are fastened behind the head. Some masks can be pinched above the nose to fit better and not allow the breath to fog the protective eyewear. Always adjust the mask to proper position prior to the procedure. Masks should be removed after the procedure by grasping the ties or attachments. Never reuse a mask; replace after every patient or during the procedure if the mask becomes moist. Never slip the mask down on the neck area or let it dangle from the ear after treatment is over. Remove the mask and dispose of it.

Protective Clothing. Special protective clothing worn only in the dental office is regulated by OSHA. Protective clothing includes uniforms, laboratory coats, gowns, and clinic jackets. The dentist must provide protective clothing that is worn and laundered in the office or by a commercial laundering service. One uniform for each staff member each day is appropriate. Dental personnel enter the office and change into uniforms or other PPE overgarments (Figure 9-9). The employer is required to clean, launder, and dispose of PPE at no cost to the employee. The uniforms or other PPE overgarments, such as laboratory coats, should be removed if the dental assistant is going out to lunch or going into the staff lounge for lunch.

Long isolation gowns are worn by the dental team members who fall in Category 1 or 2 (Figure 9-10). Gowns and uniforms cover the arms and fit closely around the neck and the wrists and provide the greatest protection if impermeable to fluids. During the time the gloves are on, the gloves fit over the cuffs of the uniform.

Protective clothing should be changed daily or immediately if splattered with body fluids. Special attention to the design of the protective clothing should be taken. Any buttons, zippers, and ornamental design should be kept to a minimum, because they can harbor pathogens. Disposable outer gowns are an option for dental personnel. The specific types of uniforms or gowns worn during patient care is a decision dictated by office policy.

FIGURE 9-8 Dental assistant putting on PPE prior to performing dental procedures.

FIGURE 9-9 Dental assistant in uniform.

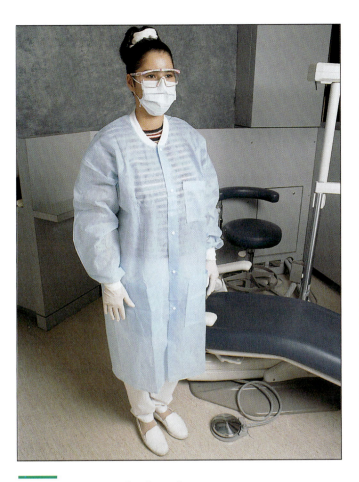

FIGURE 9-10 Dental assistant in treatment gown.

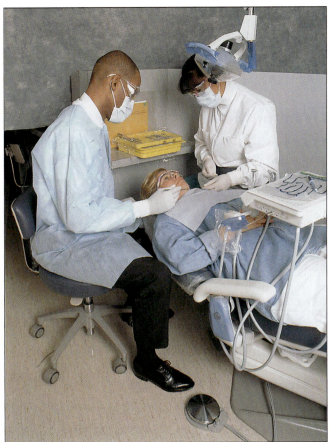

FIGURE 9-11 Barriers in place in a dental treatment room. Doctor, patient, and assistant with PPE.

Protective Clothing Worn in the Dental Office

▶ Worn only in the dental offices (not in staff lounges or lunch rooms)
▶ Must close tightly at neck and around cuff area
▶ During a high-risk procedure, must be knee length when sitting
▶ Must be removed at the end of the day, prior to going home
▶ Must be laundered in the office or sent to a laundry service

Barriers

Barriers are used in all aspects of the dental office, where possible. In the operatory, the patient dental chair, the light (handles and operating switch), the handpieces, air-water syringe, high volume evacuator, saliva ejector, tubing, writing utensils, and surfaces are covered with barriers (Figure 9-11). Any area that can be covered where contamination is possible during dental treatment should be covered. Barriers have been made specifically for areas that have been hard to disinfect or sterilize in the past, such as tubing and hoses for the handpieces. The patient should wear protective eyewear and a patient napkin or bib for protection from splatter and debris.

▶ Using disposable shower caps to cover the light and handles provides a barrier to the entire light. It allows light to pass through it but can be disposed of quickly.
▶ The dental chair can be covered with plastic dry-cleaning bags to shield them from contaminants. The dry-cleaning bags are fairly inexpensive and can be purchased on a roll. After the procedure is completed, the bag is turned inside out (contamination inside), and all disposable supplies are placed in the bag for easy cleanup.

DISINFECTION

Areas that do not lend themselves to the use of barriers in the dental office need to be disinfected if they cannot be sterilized. Some dental offices use barriers and also **disinfect**. As long as all surfaces are disinfected and/or protected by a barrier, the requirement of asepsis is met.

Using paper mixing pads makes proper disinfection difficult. However, the plastic ends in the dental x-ray film boxes can be used to mix some cements. These ends can be cleaned and placed in a submersion sterilization solution and reused.

Cleaning the Area

All areas where dental procedures are performed must be cleaned prior to disinfection and sterilization. **Cleaning** is the physical removal of organic matter, such as blood, tissue, and debris. The process of cleaning decreases the number of microorganisms in the area and removes substances that may hinder the processes of disinfection and sterilization. This process is much like washing off dishes prior to placing them in the dishwasher. If the substances stay on the instruments, they cannot be disinfected or sterilized properly.

If something is **sanitized**, the process is much like cleaning. Sanitization means that the area has been decontaminated, but it does not mean that all microorganisms in the area have been destroyed.

Environmental Protection Agency Approval

The EPA approves disinfection and sterilization solutions only after the products have undergone careful testing. The disinfecting and sterilization solutions must have EPA approval on their labels. Each product registered with the EPA must have determination as to whether a solution sterilizes or disinfects and what types of microorganisms it will destroy. **Sterilization** means that all forms of microorganisms are destroyed and disinfection occurs when *some* microorganisms are destroyed. The contact time needed for each product is also defined on the label. Some products disinfect after ten minutes but need to have ten hours of submersion to sterilize. The disinfection levels according to the EPA are rated as high, intermediate, and low.

▶ **High-level disinfection** is a tuberculocidal that kills most but not all bacterial spores. If it is extremely strong and can kill all the bacterial spores, it is noted as a sporicidal on the label.

▶ **Intermediate-level disinfection** is a tuberculocidal that normally does not kill bacterial spores.

▶ **Low-level disinfection** kills some viruses and fungi and most of the bacteria microorganisms. It does not kill tuberculosis or bacterial spores.

When choosing the products for disinfection and sterilization for the dental office, be aware that no one product meets all the needs. Each product has advantages and disadvantages for use with specific materials. Staining and corrosiveness to instruments and equipment, along with the toxicity of the material, should be considered when choosing solutions. Read labels carefully to gain information needed about product effectiveness. Reading the information recommended by the dental organizations or asking the dental supply representative assists dental personnel in choosing the proper solutions for the dental office.

Chemical Disinfectants

A universally accepted technique for cleaning and disinfecting surfaces is the **spray-wipe-spray-wipe technique**. First, the surface is sprayed then wiped to eliminate debris and to accomplish initial surface cleaning. The second spray, which must be a surface disinfectant, is left on the item and/or surfaces for the specific time indicated by the manufacturer (normally ten minutes) and then items and surfaces are wiped and items are put away (Table 9-1).

Chlorine Dioxide. Chlorine dioxide (EPA registered) is a high-level disinfection that should be used only on items not subject to corrosion. Any materials made of or having parts made of stainless steel, carbide steel, copper, or brass will corrode if chlorine dioxide is used. The solution should be stored only in glass or plastic containers. Follow the manufacturer's directions for dilution and contact time. Normally, disinfection is rapid, but sterilization takes six to ten hours. Proper ventilation is necessary when using this product.

Glutaraldehyde. **Glutaraldehyde** (EPA registered) is used for high-level disinfection and sterilization. Some of the solutions are corrosive to metals. Read the manufacturer's directions regarding the dilution and contact time for disinfection and sterilization. Times for disinfection are normally ten to ninety minutes and sterilization is normally six to ten hours. Any time additional instruments are added to the solution, the time must be started over. Therefore, most sterilization done with glutaraldehyde must be done overnight and is more efficiently done in a steam or an autoclave sterilizer. Some glutaraldehydes, after activated, are only effective for twenty-eight days. Fumes from glutaraldehyde are toxic and can irritate the skin and eyes, so proper ventilation is essential.

Sodium Hypochlorite. Sodium hypochlorite can be obtained in a number of different concentrations. The concentration referred to here is the same as "household bleach," which is 5.25 percent sodium hypochlorite. The desired concentrations for use in the dental office is 1:10 dilution. This is obtained by placing one cup of household bleach in one gallon of water. The mixed solution is ready for use. It is highly effective for an intermediate-level disinfection and is effective against a broad spectrum of microorganisms. A 1:100 dilution of ¼ cup bleach to one gallon of water is used for general purpose disinfection. Sodium hypochlorite works rapidly (within ten minutes) on surfaces. The solution is extremely unstable and has to be mixed daily. It is also extremely corrosive to metals. Sodium hypochlorite is irritating to the eyes and skin and can harm clothing. PPE should be worn while using all cleaning and disinfection solutions. Good ventilation is essential when using sodium hypochlorite, and caution should be used when mixing it with other cleaning agents because it can become extremely toxic.

Iodophor. **Iodophor** is used as an intermediate-level disinfection. Care should be used when diluting the solution to procure the correct concentration. One of the active ingredients in iodophor is iodine. The iodine in this solution can stain white countertops and light-colored vinyl with repeated use. Iodophor works rapidly, taking five to twenty-five minutes of surface contact to be effective. It is corrosive to some metals and has a short life span. Solutions should be changed every three days minimum to remain active. Iodophor can be irritating to skin; thus, utility gloves should be worn while disinfecting surfaces.

Phenolics. Phenolics are used for intermediate-level disinfection. They are irritating to the skin and eyes. Fol-

low manufacturer's directions when diluting the solution. The surface contact time is normally ten minutes. Many phenolics come premixed in spray or pump containers. They are destructive to plastic surfaces but are effective overall surface disinfectants.

Alcohol. Isopropyl alcohol was used routinely for disinfection prior to the 1980s. Essentially, it cleaned the areas and had some disinfecting qualities, but it provides limited properties. *Alcohol is no longer recommended for disinfection in the dental office.* Alcohol evaporates so quickly that it is difficult to have surface contact for the length of time necessary to be effective.

Ultrasonic Cleaning

If the dental assistant is not able to recycle the instruments immediately after the procedure, the instruments may be submerged in a holding bath (pre-cleaning), a solution that loosens hardened debris

TABLE 9-1 DISINFECTANT COMPARISON

Disinfectant	Level	Advantages	Disadvantages	Time Required for Effectiveness
Chlorine dioxide	high	Rapid disinfection	Corrosive to metals Requires ventilation Irritating to eyes and skin	5–10 minutes
Glutaraldehyde	high	Used to disinfect some impressions Instrument can be submerged Many have a twenty-eight-day useful life.	Some are corrosive to metal Requires ventilation Irritating to eyes and skin	10–90 minutes
Iodophors	intermediate	Used as holding solution for impressions	May discolor white or pastel vinyls Surface disinfectant or holding solution Irritating to eyes and skin	10 minutes on surfaces
Sodium hypochlorite	intermediate	Rapid disinfection	Corrosive to metals Irritating to skin and eyes Diluted solution unstable, must be mixed daily	5–10 minutes
Phenolics	intermediate	Available as sprays or liquids	Skin and mucous membrane irritation Cannot be used on plastics	10 minutes
Alcohol	cleaner only	NA	NA	NA

from the instruments prior to cleaning and sterilizing. It also prevents contamination from airborne bacteria and begins the process of disinfection. The instruments remain in the holding bath until the dental assistant is ready to proceed with the processing.

After the dental assistant has removed the treatment tray from the operatory and disinfected the area and/or placed the instruments in a holding bath, he or she returns to the sterilizing area to process the instruments. The utility gloves remain on during this procedure as the dental assistant takes the instruments from the tray or holding bath and places them in an ultrasonic cleaner. Metal or plastic containers sometimes are used to hold instruments as they pass from the tray to the different solutions for processing and then on to storage (Figure 9-12). In the past, the dental assistant hand scrubbed the instruments with soap, rinsed, and placed the instruments in containers for ultrasonic cleaning or in the sterilizer for processing. The chance of being punctured with a contaminated instrument was much greater than it is today, because the manual scrub was done without gloves or use of an ultrasonic unit. The use of the utility gloves, along with the containers and ultrasonic cleaning instead of hand cleaning significantly reduces the high risk to the dental assistant. The ultrasonic cleaning device uses sound waves that travel through glass and metal using a special solution to clean the debris from the instruments (Figure 9-13). This **cavitation** process (whereby bubbles are formed) takes three to ten minutes to complete. During that time, the bubbles implode (burst inward) and produce a cleaning effect on anything within the solution. When ultrasonic cleaning is complete, the instruments are

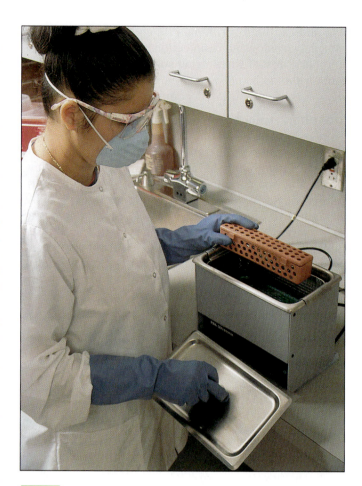

FIGURE 9-13 Dental assistant using the ultrasonic cleaning unit.

rinsed thoroughly and dried. All instruments, both loose and remaining in containers, are rinsed and dried prior to sterilization. They may be placed in an alcohol bath to aid the drying process. It does not matter which method is used to prepare the instruments for sterilization. What is important is that all the debris, blood, saliva, and tissue are removed from the instruments to ensure that the sterilization can be completed on all surfaces. The ultrasonic cleaner should be drained each night, rinsed out with water, and refilled with new ultrasonic solution each morning. It should be emptied and refilled any time the ultrasonic cleaning solution becomes exhausted, which varies depending on individual offices.

To determine whether the ultrasonic cleaner is working properly, take a small piece of aluminum foil and submerge it in the solution vertically and run the ultrasonic for thirty seconds. Remove the foil from the ultrasonic solution, and hold it up to the light for examination. It should have no area larger than a half square inch without holes in it. This indicates whether the cleaner is operating properly. If the ultrasonic unit is not operating properly, the assistant should have it tested and repaired.

FIGURE 9-12 Dental assistant using plastic instrument cassettes for ultrasonic cleaning procedure.

Packaging and Loading the Sterilizers

Most of the sterilizers can be loaded with loose instruments and obtain effective sterilization. Problems occur after the instruments come out of the sterilizer and are stored. There, they may become contaminated. If they are sterilized in a labeled bag, then after the sterilization cycle is completed the instruments can stay in the labeled and sealed bag until used, therefore maintaining the sterile condition. Labeling of the bag is normally done in pencil so that when moisture occurs (in the steam and chemical sterilizers), the information remains readable. Special pre-printed indicator tape is designed for identification of instrument setups in the sterilizing bag. Amalgam or prophy tape can be used.

Many dental offices use the cassette instrument sterilizing system (Figure 9-14). The instruments from a procedure are kept in a cassette during the ultrasonic cleaning, rinsing, and drying and then the cassette is wrapped in penetrable paper or biofilm/paper pouches, sealed, and sterilized. The bags are heat sealed or taped because staples or pins make holes, thereby allowing microorganisms to enter. This cassette, often labeled or color coded for the procedure, is removed after the sterilization cycle and is ready to be placed on a treatment tray to be opened at the chairside for use on the next dental procedure. This keeps the instruments in a sterile state, ready for immediate use at the dental chair.

The dental assistant must ensure that the sterilization bags are not overfilled, hampering proper sterilization to be accomplished throughout. It is important also that the sterilizing units are not overpacked for the cycle. Use **sterilization indicators** routinely to ensure that errors in this area are not happening.

STERILIZATION

All forms of microorganisms are destroyed in the process of **sterilization**. The dental assistant most often is the person who ensures that all items used in intraoral procedures are sterile. Any items that touch the skin or mucosa or are involved in invasive procedures must be sterilized. Several choices are available for sterilization. (Table 9-2, on page 167)

Liquid Chemical Disinfectant/Sterilization. Many of the disinfecting solutions can be used for immersion sterilization. The items are placed in the liquid for six to ten hours to ensure that all microorganisms are destroyed. The instruments are then rinsed off thoroughly, dried, and stored. Some of the items used in the dental office cannot endure heat sterilization and must be placed in a cold sterile solution. This is the primary reason for using cold sterilizing. The disadvantages to this type of sterilization is the time involved and the limited shelf life of the solution. Cold sterilizing is difficult to monitor for effectiveness and the solution may be toxic to skin and inhalation, therefore requiring proper ventilation. Another disadvan-

FIGURE 9-14 Cassette instrument sterilizing system. (A) Cassettes wrapped for sterilization. (B) Autoclave monitor tape. (C) Instrument Management System tape. *(Courtesy of Hu-Friedy Mfg. Co., Inc.)*

tage is that when the sterilizing procedure is complete, the instruments are rinsed with water that is not sterile and left unwrapped for storage; therefore, they are not maintained in a sterile state.

Ethylene Oxide Sterilization. Sterilization in the dental office can be accomplished by using an ethylene oxide sterilization unit (Figure 9-15). There are two different types: the heated unit, which is fairly expensive, and a unit that can be used at room temperature. Both units are reliable for sterilization, but with all equipment, always follow the manufacturer's directions for use. Most heated units sterilize at 120°F (49°C) for two to three hours. Plastics and other instruments can be sterilized in this low-temperature unit. The room-temperature unit takes twelve hours to complete sterilization. It is less expensive but not as efficient as the heated unit. One disadvantage, besides the long processing time, is the toxicity of the ethylene oxide gas. Adequate ventilation is required, and any porous materials require an additional twenty-four hours for the gas to dissipate from it prior to use.

Hot (Glass) Bead or Salt Sterilization. A small sterilizer positioned at the dental unit is the hot (glass) bead, or salt sterilizer (Figure 9-16). This unit operates at temperatures of approximately 450°F (234°C) and sterilizes burs and endodontic instruments immersed in the glass beads or salt for twenty seconds and larger instrument tips for thirty seconds. The electrically heated cup that contains numerous 2mm glass beads or salt conducts the high heat temperature. The disadvantage of this sterilizer is its size and limited use. The advantage is that contaminated root-canal instruments and burs can be quickly sterilized. Monitors for effectiveness are not yet available (see "Biological Monitors," page 168).

Dry Heat Sterilization. A sterilization unit that requires little maintenance and is easy to use is the dry heat sterilization unit (Figure 9-17). Other advantages are that dry instruments placed in the unit do not experience corrosion or rust. Instruments that are very delicate or have movable joints will not become rusty and lose their cutting edges as rapidly. After an initial preheat time of twenty minutes, this unit uses heat at 340°F (171°C) for one hour to sterilize. Several units are on the market, some using the long electromagnetic waves of

FIGURE 9-16 Glass bead sterilizer.

radiation, the heated moving air/convection, or conduction (direct contact with the source of heat). Be sure to follow the manufacturer's directions to ensure proper sterilization. This unit can be monitored for effectiveness and is very reliable.

The high heat of the dry heat sterilizer can be a disadvantage, because plastic items and some solder joints melt and fabric chars. Instruments can be placed in this unit loose or wrapped. It requires that loads be carefully organized in the unit to allow circulation of the air and complete sterilization.

Chemical Vapor Sterilization. The chemical vapor sterilizer uses gaseous vapor of formaldehyde and alco-

FIGURE 9-15 Ethylene oxide sterilizer. *(Courtesy of 3M Health Care, St. Paul, MN)*

FIGURE 9-17 Dry heat sterilizer.

FIGURE 9-18 Chemical vapor sterilizer. *(Courtesy of Barnstead/Thermolyne Harvey Chemiclave)*

FIGURE 9-19 Steam (flash) sterilizer—Statium. *(Courtesy of Sci-Can)*

hol under pressure to sterilize (Figure 9-18). The unit must be at 270°F (132°C) for twenty minutes to sterilize either loose or wrapped instruments. It is very reliable, and the effectiveness of the unit can be monitored. It is used frequently in the dental office due to the efficient sterilization time and because it causes very little rust and corrosion on metals. A special solution must be purchased for use in the unit, and it requires good ventilation. The high temperature does cause plastic and some other materials to be destroyed during the sterilization process. Like all sterilizers, the manufacturer's directions must be followed to ensure proper technique in the sterilization process.

Steam Autoclave (Flash) Sterilization. Most dental offices have a steam autoclave sterilizer (Figure 9-19). These units use steam under pressure to quickly sterilize items. The effectiveness of this unit can be monitored, and it is very reliable. Items can be loose or wrapped during the process. Items must be wrapped, bagged, or placed in pouches and sealed to remain sterile after removing them from the sterilizer. The unit

TABLE 9-2 METHODS OF STERILIZATION

Sterilization	Temperature/Time	Ability to Monitor	Special Considerations
Liquid chemical sterilization	Room temperature/ 6–10 hours	Difficult	Poper ventilation required Does not remain sterile after process
Ethylene oxide sterilization	Heated unit 120°F/ 2–3 hours Room temperature/ 12 hours	Difficult	Proper ventilation Additional 24 hours to dissipate gas after sterilization
Glass bead sterilizer	450°F/20–30 seconds	Not available	Limited size and use Special beads or salt required
Dry heat sterilization	340°F/1 hour	Easily monitored	Limited rust or corrosion of equipment
Chemical vapor sterilization	270°F/20 minutes	Easily monitored	Proper ventilation Special solution required
Steam under pressure sterilization	250°F/5 minutes wrapped	Easily monitored	Requires distilled water
Steam (flash) autoclave sterilization	270°F/3 minutes unwrapped	Easily monitored	Requires distilled water

takes fifteen minutes at 250°F (121°C) at fifteen pounds of steam pressure at sea level. Careful packing of the unit so that the steam can penetrate all areas is essential. The steam pressure, along with the temperature, allows for much more rapid sterilization to occur. When unwrapped at 270°F (132°C) at fifteen pounds of steam pressure, sterilization for immediate use can be accomplished in three minutes.

The high temperature, along with the steam, may cause plastics to melt, corrosion and rust to occur, and instruments to dull after repeated use. Most dental offices sterilize their dental handpieces exclusively in the steam sterilizer. The handpieces should be properly lubricated and wrapped prior to sterilization if they are going to be stored. Improper care of the dental handpiece diminishes its life span. Because dental equipment is relatively expensive, a rapid sterilization turnaround time is beneficial so that multiple handpieces do not need to be purchased. Many of the steam sterilization units require distilled water to be used in the machine. Always read the manufacturer's directions when using any sterilization equipment.

Equipment Maintenance

Sterilization equipment, like all equipment, must be maintained to function properly. The chambers should be cleaned out monthly, if not more frequently. Some sterilizers have special cleaners that must be used for this process. Other sterilizers require that the used solution be drained at the end of each day. A removable tray, or drainage hose, facilitates this process. Some sterilizers indicate when the solutions are low; others must be checked frequently to ensure that they are full. *Making sure the right solution is used in the appropriate machine is essential.* Using the wrong solution may cause the machine to break down, resulting in costly repair charges.

Many of the machines have gaskets around the door to seal the chamber during the sterilization process. If the machine is losing pressure and/or making a hissing sound, the dental assistant should check the gasket. This is an inexpensive item, and it can be replaced quite easily.

Continued maintenance allows the equipment to work at capacity for a greater amount of time. The dental assistant can set up a maintenance program so that each item is routinely checked.

Instrument Storage

The best way to store instruments is in the packages in which they were sterilized. Limit the amount of package handling after sterilization. If packages become torn, wet, or contaminated in any manner, they need to be reprocessed. It is also important that "clean" and "dirty" areas in the sterilization room be identified. To avoid contamination, nothing from the dirty side should be placed on the clean side. This will aid in the process of maintaining the integrity of the sterilization.

Sterile packs should be stored in an area that has protection from recontamination, is dry, and is away from heat. Normally, instruments used in dentistry have a quick turnaround time due to the expense and limited quantity of the instruments. The shelf life of the packages is indefinite as long as the packaging material remains intact and uncontaminated.

STERILIZATION MONITORING

The heat sterilizers are normally very reliable. It is important, however, that the sterilization process be monitored continually due to many factors that can diminish effectiveness. For example, the dental assistant could wrap instruments improperly, overload the unit, improperly set the time and temperature, or the sterilizer could malfunction.

Ongoing monitoring of the sterilization process is important to ensure proper technique and operation. Documentation reflecting the date monitoring was concluded and the outcome must be completed. Records for each sterilizer should be maintained. There are several types of monitors available for use: biological monitors, process indicators, and dosage indicators.

Biological Monitors

The biological monitors offer the most accurate way to assess that sterilization has actually occurred (Figure 9-20A). They are supplied as paper strips or sealed glass ampules of bacterial endospores. Biological monitors are placed in the sterilizer along with the instrument load being sterilized. After completion of the cycle, the spores are cultured to determine if any have survived. Many dental offices have incubators for culturing. If one is not available, the processed monitors can be sent out to a laboratory for culturing and result data. Both of the incubation processes will take several days to obtain the results, so this must be an ongoing procedure, normally done weekly.

Process Indicators

Process indicators are normally printed on packaging materials for sterilization or on the sterilization tape that can be placed on any packaging (Figure 9-20B). They contain dyes that change color upon quick exposure to sterilizing cycles. They identify whether the packages have been exposed to heat but do not indicate that sterilization has taken place. Process indicators should be used in conjunction with biological monitoring to ensure effectiveness of the sterilization process.

Dosage Indicators

Dosage indicators work in much the same manner as process indicators. They are dyes placed in the steril-

FIGURE 9-20 (A) Biological monitors. (B) Process indicators used for dental sterilizers.

ization packing, and they change color when exposed to dry heat, chemical vapor, or steam for a specific amount of time. They indicate whether the correct conditions were present for sterilization to take place. Dosage indicators also must be used in conjunction with biological monitoring.

Monitors for Liquid Disinfectants/Sterilizers. Monitors are not available to effectively determine whether proper sterilization was achieved in a liquid sterilizer. There are several strips that can be placed in the solution to test if the proper concentration is being used. Using this, along with an EPA-registered solution and closely following manufacturer's directions, ensures that the product is working.

TECHNIQUES AND AIDS FOR INFECTION CONTROL

Several techniques and aids are effective in infection control if practiced routinely. The dental office can continue to seek means to help reduce the exposure to microorganisms during invasive procedures. Staff training is essential to ensure that all procedure guidelines are followed.

Pre-Procedure Antiseptic Mouth Rinses

Using a pre-procedure antiseptic mouth rinse is not a regulation but a recommendation. A patient who rinses before treatment reduces the total number of microorganisms in the oral cavity. Reducing the microorganisms in the mouth leads to fewer microorganisms coming from the mouth during indirect contact through splatter and aerosols. Patient mouth rinse helps prevent diseases from passing from the patient to dental team members.

The antimicrobial rinse often used is 0.12 percent chlorhexidine gluconate, which has a lasting effect up to five hours. Some procedures benefit from the rinse more than others. For instance, the prophylaxis cleaning and ultrasonic scaling allow microorganisms to splatter mist in the air, unlike the restorative procedures in which a dental dam (which is a barrier) can be utilized.

High Volume Evacuation

The high volume evacuator (HVE) is an extremely effective way to minimize the spray coming from the high-speed rotary handpiece and the air-water syringe. (See Chapter 14, Introduction to Chairside Assisting, for correct placement of the HVE for maximum efficiency.) Evacuation systems use tips that are sterilizable or disposable. Most evacuation units have disposable traps that need to be cleaned routinely. Dental assistants must wear PPE while performing the cleaning procedure. Running water and specialized detergent deodorizers through the HVE at the end of each day aids in reducing the number of microorganisms in hoses and the trap.

Dental Dam Usage

The dental dam is used routinely as a barrier to the fluids and microorganisms in the oral cavity. If placed correctly, contact with saliva and oral debris is greatly reduced. However, the dental dam does not act as a perfect seal; thus, the use of gloves, glasses, and mask is required. Using the dental dam in conjunction with the HVE significantly minimizes dental splatter and aerosols during dental procedures.

Disposable Items

Many disposable items are available for use in the dental office. These items are manufactured for a single use. They are disposed of after one use to prevent microorganisms from transferring from one patient to another. These disposable items should not be reused under any circumstances. They are not designed to be sterilized and are often not tolerant of heat or chemicals. Disposable items are usually made from plastic, paper, or low-grade metals. From the infection-control standpoint, they are the most effective way to eliminate cross-contamination; however, functionally they may not be as efficient as reusable items, and they are more expensive overall.

CLINICAL ASEPSIS PROTOCOL

Routine steps should be followed in order for all treatment areas to maintain absolute clinical asepsis. Shortcuts should never be an option for asepsis in dentistry. The dental assistant must ensure that infectious diseases are not spread from patient to patient, health-care worker to patient, patient to health-care worker, or health-care worker to family.

Treatment Area Protocol for Disinfecting and Cleaning

As stated earlier, the surfaces in the treatment area can be protected with barriers, disinfected, or both. When a barrier becomes dislodged or torn, microorganisms are allowed to pass through to the surface beneath the barrier. Then, this surface must be disinfected.

Dental Radiography Room and Equipment

So much attention is paid to treatment rooms that often rooms such as separate radiography rooms and radiography darkrooms are missed during infection control. When dental assistants expose and process radiographs, infection control practices must be followed. The room first must be prepared, much like a treatment

P R O C E D U R E

9-2 Preparing the Dental Treatment Room

The procedure is performed by the dental assistant prior to seating the dental patient in the treatment room. By following a routine procedure that meets the regulations and the protocol set forth by the dentist and the regulatory agencies discussed earlier in the chapter, the dental assistant prepares the operatory and equipment.

EQUIPMENT AND SUPPLIES

▶ Patient's medical and dental history (including dental radiographs)

▶ Barriers for dental chair, hoses, counter, light switches, and controls

▶ PPE for dental assistant (protective eyewear, mask, gloves, and overgloves)

▶ Patient napkin, napkin chain, and protective eyewear

▶ Sterile procedure tray

PROCEDURE STEPS (Follow aseptic procedures)

1. Wash hands.

2. Review the patient's medical and dental history, place the radiographs on the viewbox, and identify the procedure to be completed at this visit. Patient's medical and dental history can be placed in a plastic envelope barrier or under a surface barrier.

3. Place new barriers on all potential possible surfaces that can be contaminated (for example, dental chair, hoses, counter, light switches and controls) (Figure 9-21).

4. Bring the instrument tray with packaged sterile instruments into the operatory with patient's napkin and protective eyewear.

5. Place on PPE (protective eyewear, mask, gloves, and overgloves).

FIGURE 9-21 Dental assistant placing barriers.

PROCEDURE

9-3 Completion of Dental Treatment

The procedure is performed by the dental assistant at the completion of the dental treatment. By following a routine procedure that meets the regulations and the protocol set forth by the dentist and the regulatory agencies discussed earlier in the chapter, the dental assistant completes the procedure and dismisses the patient.

EQUIPMENT AND SUPPLIES

▶ Patient's medical and dental history (including dental radiographs)

▶ Barriers for dental chair, hoses, counter, light switches, and controls

▶ Dental handpiece

▶ Air-water syringe tip (disposable)

▶ Patient napkin

▶ Contaminated instruments on tray, including HVE tip

PROCEDURE STEPS (Follow aseptic procedures)

1. Remove the handpieces, HVE tip, and air-water syringe tip and place on the treatment tray.

2. Place on overgloves to document information on the chart or on the computer and assemble radiographs and chart, preventing cross-contamination (Figure 9-22).

3. Remove patient napkin and place over the treatment tray prior to dismissing patient (see Chapter 14, Introduction to Chairside Assisting).

4. With glove in place, complete Steps 5 through 11.

5. Place the handpiece, HVE, and air-water syringe back on the unit and run for twenty to thirty seconds to clean the lines or flush the system. Remove handpiece and air-water syringe and place back on the treatment tray.

6. Place sharps into puncture-resistant sharps disposal container if sharps disposal containers are kept in the dental treatment room (waist high). Sharps should be discarded in the treatment room to prevent any possible mishaps or in the sterilization area.

7. Remove the chair cover from the patient dental chair, inverting it so that any splatter or debris remains on the inside of the bag.

8. Remove all the barriers and place them in the inverted bag. All disposables can be placed in the bag as well (Figure 9-23).

9. Carry the treatment tray with all items from the treatment area to the sterilizing area. Nothing that is to be sterilized is to be left in the operatory at this time.

10. Remove the treatment gloves and place them in the inverted bag. Dispose of the bag.

11. Wash hands.

FIGURE 9-22 Wearing overgloves while writing on a patient's chart.

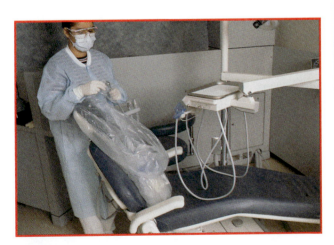

FIGURE 9-23 Post-dental treatment, barriers being removed and placed in inverted bag for disposal.

PROCEDURE

9-4 Final Treatment Room Disinfecting and Cleaning

The procedure is performed by the dental assistant after the treatment has been completed and the patient has been dismissed. By following a routine procedure that meets the regulations and the protocol set forth by the dentist and the regulatory agencies discussed earlier in the chapter, the dental assistant completes the procedure.

EQUIPMENT AND SUPPLIES

▶ Utility gloves

▶ Necessary disinfecting solutions (intermediate level)

▶ Wiping cloths

▶ 4 × 4 gauze

PROCEDURE STEPS (Follow aseptic procedures)

1. Wash hands, place on utility gloves.

2. Bring the necessary solutions and wiping cloths, including 4 × 4 gauze, to the operatory.

> Use a small utility carry tote to hold and transport items such as disinfecting solutions, HVE solution, 4 × 4 gauze, towels, and chair disinfectant.

3. Have a routine procedure established for disinfection to ensure that nothing is missed. All surfaces need to be sprayed and cleaned first, then wiped to remove debris (Figures 9-24A and B). The surfaces are then sprayed a second time and the solution is left on for a designated time according to the manufacturer's directions (normally this time is about ten minutes). After ten minutes, wipe the surfaces again.

4. Another method to accomplish the initial spray wipe is to use saturated "wiping devices." Lay out several pieces of 4 × 4 gauze on the counter, spray them with disinfectant, and wipe each surface carefully.

5. Spray on the disinfectant and leave for the correct time to accomplish disinfection (normally ten minutes).

6. Rewipe all surfaces.

7. It is critical that all surfaces that could have been contaminated are disinfected. Areas that are sometimes missed include the amalgam cradle (holding device for amalgam capsule in the triturator), the chair adjustments, the curing light, and the radiographic viewbox switch. (Take care when spraying disinfectants near switches.)

Disinfecting Procedure

▶ Spray.

▶ Wipe. (The "Spray and Wipe" technique also can be accomplished by wiping with a disinfectant-saturated "wiping device.")

▶ Spray and leave (normally ten minutes).

▶ Rewipe.

 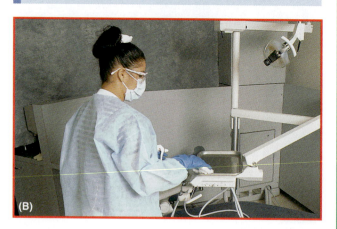

FIGURE 9-24 (A) Spraying the area. (B) Wiping and spraying the area with disinfectant again.

9-5 Treatment of Contaminated Tray in the Sterilization Center

The procedure is performed by the dental assistant in the sterilization center. By following a routine procedure that meets the regulations and the protocol set forth by the dentist and OSHA regulatory agencies discussed earlier in the chapter, the dental assistant completes the procedure.

EQUIPMENT AND SUPPLIES

▶ Utility gloves

▶ Necessary disinfecting solutions

▶ Wiping cloths

▶ 4 × 4 gauze

▶ Contaminated procedure tray

PROCEDURE STEPS (Follow aseptic procedures)

1. Place the treatment tray in the contaminated area of the sterilization center immediately following dental treatment by the dental assistant. Sterilization can be taken care of immediately or after the operatory is disinfected and prepared for another patient.

2. If it is going to be a long time before the tray is taken care of, immerse the instruments in a disinfecting holding solution. This prevents debris from drying, begins the process of killing the microorganisms, and prevents any airborne microorganisms from being transmitted.

3. Wear utility gloves during the entire procedure of caring for a contaminated instrument tray.

4. Sharps are disposed of in a sharps container if not already done while in the dental operatory (Figure 9-25).

5. All disposable items are discarded. If they are biohazard waste, they must be placed in an appropriately labeled waste container. (See Chapter 10, Management of Hazardous Materials, for further information.)

6. Place the instruments in the ultrasonic cleaner either open method or in a cassette. A small strainer is used for items that may become lost.

FIGURE 9-25 Dental assistant placing the sharps in a sharps container.

Normally, burs, dental dam clamps, and other such items are placed in this small container. After the timed cleaning is accomplished in the ultrasonic unit (three to ten minutes), rinse the items off thoroughly.

7. After the instruments are rinsed, towel dry, bag, and place in the appropriate sterilizer (Figure 9-26). Remember that if they are in a cassette, they can be dipped in an alcohol bath and left to air dry before being placed in a sealed bag and in the sterilizer.

8. Rinse off or wipe off the dental high-speed handpiece with isopropyl alcohol. Then, it must be lubricated, bagged in an instrument pouch with indicator tape, and placed in the sterilizer (follow manufacturer's directions). The sterilizer used is normally the steam under pressure sterilizer due to the quick turnaround time.

9. The tray and other items on the tray need to be spray wiped, sprayed again, left for ten minutes or a time designated by the manufacturer of the

(continued)

P R O C E D U R E   **9 - 5** *continued*

disinfectant, and wiped again before assembling them for another tray setup.

10. Clean up the area, wash and dry the utility gloves, remove them, and wash and dry hands.

11. After the sterilizer indicates that the time has lapsed and that the instruments are sterile, they can be removed from the sterilizer with forceps.

PPE for a Contaminated Tray

▶ Utility gloves are required when handling contaminated trays.

▶ Protective eyewear is required when handling contaminated trays.

▶ Masks are only required if cleaning causes splash, aerosols, and/or splatter to occur.

FIGURE 9-26 (A) Dental assistant placing the bagged instruments in the sterilizer. (B) Sliding tray with bagged instruments into sterilizer.

room with appropriate barriers. Upon completion of the procedure, the radiography room must be disinfected in the same manner, disinfecting all surfaces that were contaminated. (See Chapter 17, Dental Radiology, for further information). The radiographs that have been placed in the mouth must be cared for properly and all the equipment must be disinfected.

Dental Laboratory

The dental laboratory should be disinfected in the same manner as other rooms. Use the spray-wipe-spray-wipe technique on all the surfaces. If the dental assistant is polishing with pumice on the rag wheel, PPE should be worn. Extra care should be used when wearing gloves while using the rotary equipment for polishing, because gloves easily can become caught in the wheels or motors.

After polishing, discard the pumice and disinfect the pan. (Some dental offices mix the pumice with disinfectant.) Rinse off the rag wheel and cycle it through the autoclave. Many disposable buffing wheels are now available as an alternative and can be discarded after use.

Thoroughly disinfect any contaminated dental laboratory cases before being handled in the office or sent

to an outside laboratory. One effective way to achieve this is to place all acrylic appliances in a diluted sodium hypochlorite disinfection solution. Cases with any metal parts need to be placed in another solution, such as glutaraldehyde. Check the manufacturer's directions to identify solutions that will meet the criteria for this process.

Dental impressions also must be disinfected prior to sending them out. Check the manufacturer's directions regarding the correct procedure to accomplish this task. Alginate impressions cannot be immersed in any solution, because this can cause distortion. Alginate impressions must be sprayed and then placed in a sealed bag.

Final impression materials such as polysulfide and silicone can be immersed in most disinfecting solutions according to the manufacturer's directions without distortion. Procedures for disinfecting polyether and polysiloxane impression materials vary. Some of the polyether impressions cannot go through the disinfecting procedure until a final set time of thirty minutes has elapsed. If the impression has not been disinfected prior to sending it to the dental laboratory, place it in a leak-proof bag to transport and identify that it has not been disinfected by a biohazard label on the bag.

P R O C E D U R E

9-6 Dental Radiology Infection Control Protocol

The procedure is performed by the dental assistant in the dental radiography room if it is a separate area or at the dental unit if the radiographs are taken in the same location as the dental treatment. By following a routine procedure that meets the regulations and the protocol set forth by the dentist and the regulatory agencies discussed earlier in the chapter, the dental assistant completes the procedure.

EQUIPMENT AND SUPPLIES

▶ Utility gloves

▶ Barriers

▶ Necessary disinfecting solutions

▶ Wiping cloths

▶ 4 × 4 gauze

PROCEDURE STEPS (Follow aseptic procedures)

1. Wash hands and place the barriers. The x-ray head fits in one of the dental chair bags. Using this type of barrier is much easier than trying to get into all areas to disinfect. It will also not be as hard on the equipment (spraying the disinfecting solution can destroy electrical equipment over time).

2. The x-ray room must have a lead-lined door and walls. Both sides of the door handle need barriers. Sandwich bags work well for this type of barrier. If the switches for use of the dental radiography machine are located in another area, place a barrier over them. The chair can be covered, although no splatter or spray is anticipated (unless the patient vomits).

3. Dental x-rays can be placed in barriers at this time. (See Chapter 17, Dental Radiology, for more information about dental x-ray barriers.)

4. Place PPE as the patient is seated. Place the lead apron on the patient.

5. After each of the x-rays is taken, place it in a disposable cup outside the x-ray room.

6. After the procedure is completed and the patient is dismissed, remove the barriers and dispose of them, along with the treatment gloves. If the x-rays have been in a barrier, remove the barrier carefully while allowing the untouched x-rays to fall into a clean disposable cup. Then, remove the treatment gloves.

7. Disinfect any areas not covered by the barriers.

   NOTE: The lead apron is often missed during disinfection.

8. X-rays are then processed. If barriers on the dental x-ray packets have not been used, special attention should be taken not to cross-contaminate. Either new gloves must be donned as the x-rays are removed from the infected packets or a two-cup method must be used. Careful attention in aseptic techniques will ensure that x-rays are not recontaminated prior to putting them through the processor.

9. One area that is often contaminated is the sleeves of the daylight processor. Place two cups inside the processor (one with contaminated x-rays in it and one with nothing in it). Don new gloves prior to placing hands through the sleeves of the processor. Open the contaminated x-rays and place them in the clean cup. Remove the gloves and place them in the contaminated cup before using clean hands to place the uncontaminated dental film through the processor. Take the clean hands out of the sleeves of the daylight processor and lift the lid. Remove the two cups from the daylight loader, touching only the outside of each cup. There are a number of other ways to accomplish this task without cross-contaminating, such as using overgloves and packet barriers.

CHAPTER SUMMARY

Staff must be trained for a safe workplace. Compliance with all regulations must be accomplished to ensure that the process of infection control will be adequate. Training will occur at initial employment, when job tasks change, and annually thereafter.

CASE STUDY

Lisa Scott, a dental assistant, received a personal telephone call during patient dental care. She left the dental treatment room, removed her latex gloves, and answered the telephone in the sterilization area. While in the area, she looked up another telephone number in the phone book, put instruments from the ultrasonic unit under water to rinse and then into the sterilizer, and then returned to the treatment room. Knowing that leaving the treatment area during patient care is not advocated and focusing on asepsis, answer the following questions:

Case Study Review

1. From the information gathered, what (if any) areas were contaminated?

2. What procedures should have been followed to prevent cross-contamination?

3. Identify the gloves(s) that should have been utilized during each procedure.

 To complete your study of this chapter, work the review activities that follow. Also, refer to the software that accompanies this text.

REVIEW QUESTIONS

Multiple Choice

1. Ultimately, the responsibility for infection control lies with the
   a. patient.
   b. dentist.
   c. dental hygienist.
   d. dental assistant.

2. A regulating body that enforces that employers protect their employees from exposure to blood and OPIM is the
   a. Centers for Disease Control.
   b. Environmental Protection Agency.
   c. Food and Drug Administration.
   d. Occupational Safety and Health Agency.

3. Dental assistants fall into which category of job classification for exposure determination?
   a. 1
   b. 2
   c. 3
   d. 4

4. Personal protective equipment includes all the following *except*
   a. face masks.
   b. eyewear.
   c. ear plugs.
   d. uniforms.

5. Gloves that are primarily utilized during dental patient care are
   a. latex gloves.
   b. overgloves.
   c. utility gloves.
   d. rubber gloves.

Critical Thinking

1. If a small dental office with only four employees routinely follows infection control guidelines, would a surprise OSHA inspection be anticipated?
2. If a problem develops after a dental assistant misuses a dental solution, where does the liability lie?
3. During the use of the high-speed handpiece, the dental assistant would be concerned with what primary route of microbial transmission?

Management of Hazardous Materials

OBJECTIVES

The student should strive to meet the following objectives and demonstrate an understanding of the facts and principles presented in this chapter:

1. Identify the scope of the OSHA Bloodborne/Hazardous Materials Standard.

2. Identify physical equipment and mechanical devices provided to safeguard employees.

3. Demonstrate safe disposal of sharps.

4. Describe MSDS manuals.

5. Demonstrate the use of the colors and numbers used for hazardous chemical identification.

6. Describe employee training required to meet the OSHA standard for hazardous chemicals.

KEY TERMS

material safety data sheets (MSDS) (p. 178)

National Fire Protection Association's color and number method (p. 185)

Occupational Safety and Health Administration (OSHA) (p. 178)

other potentially infectious material (OPIM) (p. 182)

parenteral (p. 182)

pericardial (p. 182)

peritoneal (p. 182)

pleural (p. 182)

synovial (p. 182)

INTRODUCTION

Infection control and the standards that relate to it are discussed in Chapter 9, Infection Control. This chapter discusses the requirements of the **Occupational Safety and Health Administration (OSHA)** Bloodborne/Hazardous Materials Standard, such as engineering controls, labeling, **material safety data sheets (MSDS)**, housekeeping, laundry, and the disposal of hazardous materials. Dental assistants must understand the complete standard and how compliance is accomplished (Figure 10-1). Dental assisting students do not fall under OSHA guidelines because they are not employees; however, following the same safety standards that are practiced in the workplace is preparation for employment. The scope of the standard covers:

▸ Employee training, safety, and documentation requirements

▸ Exposure determination

▸ Infection control, universal precautions, and standard measures used to control possible exposures

▸ Post-exposure follow-up

▸ Labeling/material safety data sheets (MSDS)

▸ Housekeeping/laundry

▸ Disposal of biohazardous waste

Scope and Application

- The Standard applies to all occupational exposure to blood and other potentially infectious materials (OPIM) and includes part-time employees, designated first aiders, and mental health workers, as well as exposed medical personnel.
- OPIM includes saliva in dental procedures, cerebrospinal fluid, unfixed tissue, semen, vaginal secretions, and body fluids visibly contaminated with blood.

Methods of Compliance

- General—Standard precautions.
- Engineering and work practice controls.
- Personal protective equipment.
- Housekeeping.

Standard Precautions

- *All* human blood and OPIM are considered to be infectious.
- The *same* precautions must be taken with all blood and OPIM.

Engineering Controls

- Whenever feasible, engineering controls must be the primary method used to control exposure.
- Examples include needleless IVs, self-sheathing needles, sharps disposal containers, covered centrifuge buckets, aerosol-free tubes, and leak-proof containers.
- Engineering controls must be evaluated and documented on a regular basis.

Sharps Containers

- Readily accessible and as close as practical to work area.
- Puncture resistant.
- Labeled or color coded.
- Leak proof.
- Closeable.
- *Routinely replaced* so there is no overflow.

FIGURE 10-1 Understanding OSHA's Bloodborne/Hazardous Materials Standard.

(continued on following pages)

Work Practice Controls

- Handwashing following glove removal.
- No recapping, breaking, or bending of needles.
- No eating, drinking, smoking, and so on in work area.
- No storage of food or drink where blood or OPIM are stored.
- Minimize splashing, splattering of blood, and OPIM.
- No mouth pipetting.
- Specimens must be transported in leak-proof, labeled containers. They must be placed in a secondary container if outside contamination of primary container occurs.
- Equipment must be decontaminated prior to servicing or shipping. Areas that cannot be decontaminated must be labeled.

Personal Protective Equipment (PPE)

- Includes eye protection, gloves, protective clothing, and resuscitation equipment.
- Must be readily accessible and employers must require their use.
- Must be stored at work site.

Eye Protection

- Is required whenever there is potential for splashing, spraying, or splattering to the eyes or mucous membranes.
- If necessary, use eye protection in conjunction with a mask or use a chin-length face shield.
- Prescription glasses may be fitted with solid side shields.
- Decontamination procedures must be developed.

Gloves

- Must be worn whenever hand contact with blood, OPIM, mucous membranes, nonintact skin, or contaminated surfaces/items or when performing vascular access procedures (phlebotomy).
- Type required—Vinyl or latex for general use.
    —Alternatives must be available if employee has allergic reactions (e.g., powderless).
    —Utility gloves for surface disinfection.
    —Puncture resistant when handling sharps (e.g., Central Supply).

Protective Clothing

- Must be worn whenever splashing or splattering to skin or clothing may occur.
- Type required depends on exposure. Prevention of contamination of skin and clothes is the key.
- Examples—Low-level-exposure lab coats.
    —Moderate-level-exposure, fluid-resistant gown.
    —High-level-exposure, fluid-proof apron, head and foot covering.
- *Note:* If PPE is considered protective clothing, then the *employer must* launder it.

Housekeeping

- There must be a written schedule for cleaning and disinfection.
- Contaminated equipment and surfaces must be cleaned as soon as feasible for obvious contamination or at end of work shift if no contamination has occurred.
- Protective coverings may be used over equipment.

FIGURE 10-1 (continued)

Regulated Waste Containers (Non-Sharp)

- Closeable.
- Leak proof.
- Labeled or color coded.
- Placed in secondary container if outside of container is contaminated.

Laundry

- Handled as little as possible.
- Bagged at location of use.
- Labeled or color coded.
- Transported in bags that prevent soak-through or leakage.

Laundry Facility

- Two options:
  1. Standard precautions for all laundry (alternative color coding allowed if recognized).
  2. Precautions only for contaminated laundry (must be red bags or biohazard labels).
- Laundry personnel must use PPE and have a sharps container accessible.

Hepatitis B Vaccination

- Made available within ten days to all employees with occupational exposure.
- At no cost to employees.
- May be required for student to be admitted to college health program as well as for externship.
- Given in accordance with United States Public Health Service guidelines.
- Employee must first be evaluated by health-care professional.
- Health-care professional gives a written opinion.
- If the vaccine is refused, the employee signs a declination form.
- Vaccine must be available at a future date if initially refused.

Post-Exposure Follow-Up

- Document exposure incident.
- Identify source individual (if possible).
- Attempt to test source if consent obtained.
- Provide results to exposed employee.

Labels

- Biohazard symbol and word Biohazard must be visible.
- Fluorescent orange/orange-red with contrasting letters may also be used.
- Red bags/containers may be substituted for labels.
- Labels required on—Regulated waste.
             —Refrigerators/freezers with blood of OPIM.
             —Transport/storage containers.
             —Contaminated equipment.

Information and Training

- Required for all employees with occupational exposure.
- Training required initially, annually, and if there are new procedures.
- Training material must be appropriate for literacy and education level of employee.
- Training must be interactive and allow for questions and answers.

FIGURE 10-1 (continued)

Training Components

- Explanation of bloodborne standard.
- Epidemiology and symptoms of bloodborne disease.
- Modes of HIV/HBV transmission.
- Explanation of exposure control plan.
- Explanation of engineering, work practice controls.
- How to select the proper PPE.
- How to decontaminate equipment, surfaces, and so on.
- Information about hepatitis B vaccine.
- Post-exposure follow-up procedures.
- Label/color code system.

Medical Records

Records must be kept for each employee with occupational exposure and include:
- A copy of employee's vaccination status and date.
- A copy of post-exposure follow-up evaluation procedures.
- Health-care professional's written opinions.
- Confidentiality must be maintained.
- Records must be maintained for thirty years plus the duration of employment.

Training Records

Records are kept for three years from date of training and include:
- Date of training.
- Summary of contents of training program.
- Name and qualifications of trainer.
- Names and job titles of all persons attending.

Exposure Control Plan Components

- A written plan for each workplace with occupational exposure.
- Written policies/procedures for complying with the standard.
- A cohesive document or a guiding document referencing existing policies/procedures.

Exposure Control Plan

- A list of job classifications where occupational exposure control occurs (e.g., medical assistant, clinical laboratory scientist, dental hygienist).
- A list of tasks where exposure occurs (e.g., medical assistant who performs venipuncture).
- Methods/policies/procedures for compliance.
- Procedures for sharps disposal.
- Disinfection policies/procedures.
- Procedures for selection of PPE.
- Regulated waste disposal procedures.
- Laundry procedures.
- Hepatitis B vaccination procedures.
- Post-exposure follow-up procedures.
- Training procedures.
- Plan must be accessible to employees and be updated annually.

FIGURE 10-1 *(continued)*

Employee Responsibilities

- Go through training and cooperate.
- Obey policies.
- Use universal precaution techniques.
- Use PPE.
- Use safe work practices.
- Use engineering controls.
- Report unsafe work conditions to employer.
- Maintain clean work areas.

Cooperation between employer and employees regarding *The Bloodborne Pathogen Standard* will facilitate understanding of the law, thereby benefiting all persons who are exposed to HIV, HBV, and OPIM by minimizing the risk of exposure to the pathogens.

Meeting the OSHA standard is not optional, and failure to comply can result in a fine that may total $10,000 for each employee.

FIGURE 10-1

ENGINEERING/WORK PRACTICE CONTROLS

The physical equipment and mechanical devices that employers provide to safeguard and protect the employees at work is known as the engineering and work practice controls. Examples of these would be the splash guards on model trimmers, puncture-resistant sharps containers, and ventilation hoods for hazardous fumes. The employer must provide this equipment in order to meet OSHA standards and provide a safe environment for employees. The employer must ensure that employees wash their hands immediately after gloves are removed and flush their eyes with water at an eye-wash station if contact with microorganisms or hazardous materials is suspected (Figure 10-2). The employer must ensure that employees flush any mucous membranes immediately if there has been possible contact with blood or **other potentially infectious material (OPIM)** in the office.

The employer sets up work practice controls to diminish harmful occupational exposure. OSHA defines occupational exposure as reasonably anticipated eye, skin, mucous membrane, or parenteral contact with blood or other OPIM that may result from the performance of an employee's duties. It further defines **parenteral** as a means of piercing mucous membranes or the skin barrier through such events as needlesticks, cuts, and abrasions.

OSHA and the Centers for Disease Control and Prevention define the following human fluids as blood and OPIM according to the standard:

- ▶ Blood and anything that is visually contaminated with blood
- ▶ Saliva in dental oral procedures
- ▶ Cerebrospinal fluid (brain and spinal fluid)
- ▶ Amniotic fluid (fluid around the fetus)

- ▶ **Synovial** fluid (joint and tendon fluid)
- ▶ **Pleural** (lung fluid)/**peritoneal** fluid (abdominal fluid)/ **pericardial** fluid (heart fluid)
- ▶ Semen and vaginal secretions
- ▶ Unfixed tissue or organ (other than intact skin) from a human (living or dead)
- ▶ HIV-containing cell or tissue cultures, organ cultures, and HIV- or HBV-containing culture medium or other solutions
- ▶ Blood, organs, or other tissues from experimental animals infected with HIV or HBV

FIGURE 10-2 Flushing eyes at an eye-wash station.

SHARPS

The dentist may purchase needle guards for dental needles to protect employees from unnecessary sticks. There are a number of different types available. Needles should never be recapped using the two-hand technique, because it is easy to stick the opposing hand or the other individual's hand. Instead, a scoop method using one hand must be followed during the recapping procedure (see Chapter 16, Management of Pain and Anxiety).

Upon completion of a procedure, contaminated sharps and needles must be placed immediately in a labeled, leak-proof, puncture-resistant container (Figure 10-3). Other sharps that are placed routinely in the sharps disposal container are blades from knives used in surgery, broken glass, anesthetic capsules, and orthodontic wires. When the sharps disposal containers are full, they are sealed, sterilized using an autoclave if possible, and sent to an outside biohazard agency for safe disposal.

Occupational Exposure to Bloodborne Pathogens

Any employee who has an occupational exposure incident must report it immediately (Figure 10-4). The employer must make available immediately to the exposed employee a confidential medical evaluation and follow-up. The medical evaluation and follow-up is made available to the employee at no cost. The dentist refers the exposed employee to a licensed health-care professional to have the most current medical evaluation and procedures performed that are in accordance with the United States Public Health Service. OSHA standards do not dictate the procedures to be performed but allow for the most current recommendations to be applied. Reporting the incident immediately allows the dentist to carefully evaluate the circumstances surrounding the incident and to find ways to prevent the situation and exposure incident from happening again.

FIGURE 10-3 Puncture-resistant sharps containers.

Documentation of the Exposure Incident. The dentist documents the information of the exposure incident on a report. This report includes the route(s) of exposure, the circumstances that surrounded the exposure incident, and (if known) the identity of the source patient. The exposure incident report is placed in the employee's confidential medical record and a copy of this report is provided to the health-care professional who is providing the evaluation.

The employer is required to provide the licensed health-care professional with a description of the employee's job duties and their relation to the incident; information about the route of the exposure; the circumstances surrounding the incident; relevant employee medical records, including vaccination status; a copy of the bloodborne pathogen standard; and the results of the source patient's blood testing (if available).

If the employer has eleven or more employees, the employer may be required to complete the OSHA forms 200 (Log and Summary of Occupational Injuries and Illnesses) and 101 (Supplemental Record of Occupational Injuries and Illnesses) to meet the "recordable occupation injury" requirement.

In a bloodborne pathogen exposure, the dentist must identify and document in writing the source patient, if known. Further, the dentist must contact the source patient and request his or her consent to be tested for HBV and HIV and then further to disclose the results of these tests to the exposed employee. If the source patient does not give consent for the testing, the dentist must document this on the report of the exposure incident. If the source patient agrees to be tested, the tests should be completed as soon as feasible. When the results are disclosed to the exposed employee, information regarding the source patient's rights to disclosure must be discussed.

Exposed Employee Blood (Collection and Testing). The employee has the right to decline testing after an exposure incident or to delay the testing for up to ninety days. The employee may consent to have a baseline blood test that will determine the HBV and HIV serological status. The employee may choose to be tested only for HBV and not give consent for HIV testing at that time. The employee's blood sample must be saved for ninety days in case the employee elects to consent to the HIV testing. All tests must be performed by an accredited laboratory at no cost to the employee. The health-care professional will notify the employee directly of all test results.

Post-Exposure Follow-Up Procedures. The employer must provide to the exposed employee counseling, prophylaxis to prevent sexual transmission of any possible infection, and evaluation of reported illnesses. The counseling provided will aid the employee in interpretation of all tests and discussions about the potential risk of infection and the need for further post-exposure prophylaxis. The employee should also be counseled on the necessary use of protection during sexual contact.

The post-exposure prophylaxis is provided according to the current recommendations of the United States Public Health Service. OSHA did not define this procedure in the bloodborne standard due to the ongoing changes that have developed in this area.

Treatment may include, but is not limited to, HBV vaccine if the employee has not had it or chemoprophylaxis for high risk cases of HIV transmission.

The health-care professional also evaluates any reported illnesses that the exposed employee develops. The health-care professional can evaluate the symptoms in relation to the HBV and HIV infection. This allows the exposed employee to have immediate medical evaluation and referral for medical treatment to take place so that the treatment can be started as soon as possible. This does not mean that the employer is responsible for any costs associated with the treatment of the disease.

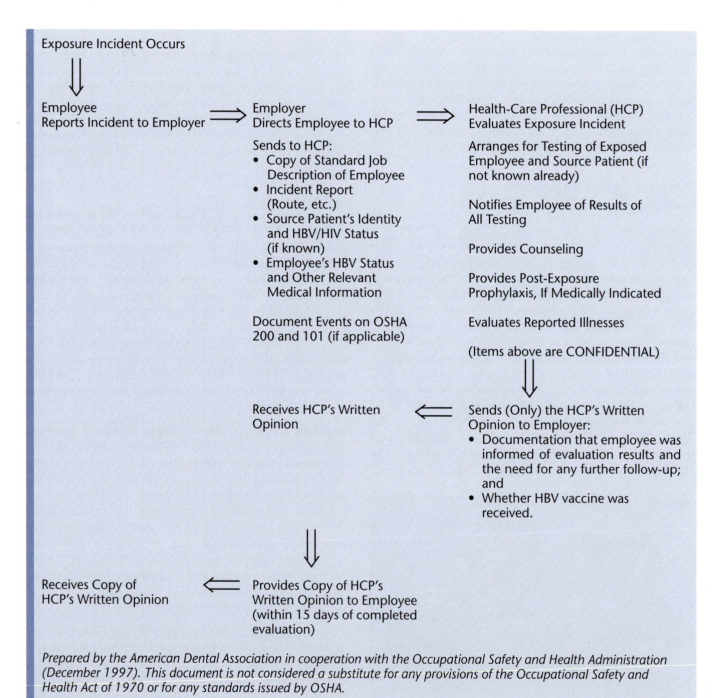

Prepared by the American Dental Association in cooperation with the Occupational Safety and Health Administration (December 1997). This document is not considered a substitute for any provisions of the Occupational Safety and Health Act of 1970 or for any standards issued by OSHA.

FIGURE 10-4 Flow chart for occupational exposure to bloodborne pathogens. *(Courtesy of the American Dental Association)*

The health-care professional sends the dental employer a written opinion about the evaluation and notification that the employee was informed of the test results of the evaluation and of the further follow-up. The dentist provides the employee with a copy of this written opinion and evaluation of the exposed employee within fifteen days of the completion of the evaluation. The original document is placed in the employee's confidential record. The employer must maintain employee records in a confidential manner for the duration of employment plus thirty years in accordance with OSHA's standard on Access to Employee Exposure and Medical Records, 29 CFR 1910.20.

Employee Work Site

The employer must provide a work site that is clean and sanitary. Each office must have a written schedule for infection control and decontaminating procedures for each area. Wastepaper baskets, floors, and all other surfaces that may have been contaminated with blood or OPIM must be included. The assistant must wear utility gloves while cleaning contaminated surfaces. All disposable items that are contaminated, including gloves, must be discarded in a biohazard container.

Broken Glass. Broken glass must be cleaned up with a broom (or brush) and dust pan (or cardboard). Dental assistants must never touch broken glass with hands or gloved hands, therefore risking a puncture. Broken glass must be placed in a leak-proof sharps container, labeled biohazard.

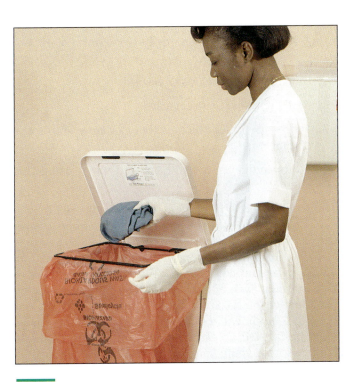

FIGURE 10-5 Proper disposal of contaminated laundry.

Laundry. Contaminated laundry must be handled as little as possible. Gloves must be used when placing it in a biohazard container or a red bag that is labeled with a biohazard symbol (Figure 10-5). If the laundry is damp or wet, it must first be placed in a plastic bag to prevent blood or OPIM from seeping through it.

Laundry that is sent off site for cleaning is placed in a red biohazard bag for transportation. Dental assistants should take special care when removing the protective clothing, especially items that are taken over the head. The chance for contamination of the face can take place if the outside surface of the clothing makes contact with it.

HAZARDOUS CHEMICALS

The OSHA hazard communication standard is set up so that employees receive training about the risks of using hazardous chemicals and the safety precautions required when handling them. Employees must be trained in identification of hazardous chemicals and personal protective equipment to be utilized for each chemical. This training must occur within thirty days of employment or prior to the employee using any chemicals, and annually thereafter (Figure 10-6).

Employees must have a certificate available or in their personnel files that shows they have had the proper training. The certificate must identify that the employer has trained the employee in the proper handling of hazardous substances in the dental office (Figure 10-7).

As with the bloodborne pathogen standard, a written plan identifying employee training and detailing specific control measures used in the workplace must be compiled for hazardous chemicals. If the office is not in compliance, penalties may be imposed on the employer.

All hazardous chemicals must be identified on a written form, such as a chemical inventory form (Figure 10-8). Other information required about the chemicals includes the quantity stored (each month or year), the physical state of the substance (liquid, solid, or gas), the hazardous class (health problem, fire hazard, reactive), what PPE is required, and the manufacturer's name, address, and phone number.

Material Safety Data Sheets

Each office must have a material safety data manual that is alphabetized, indexed, and available to all employees. These manuals can be in hard copy or on a computer. The manual contains the MSDS (Figure 10-9). These sheets come from the manufacturer. If the MSDS is unavailable, the employer or a designated employee (the safety assistant) must request it from the manufacturer. The National Fire Protection Association's color and number method is used to easily identify information

SAFETY TRAINING FORM

Safety training will be offered to all employees within 30 days of employment or before the employee assumes responsibilities that involve exposure to body fluids or chemicals.

Items to be covered in training session:

- General explanation of OSHA laws
- General explanation of the epidemiology and symptoms of HBV and HIV
- Who is at risk in office
- Modes of transmission of HBV and HIV
- Method of control in workplace
- Universal precautions
- Handwashing
- Personal protective equipment
- How to clean up spills
- What to do after a needlestick injury
- Medical follow-up after an exposure
- Cleaning protocol for office
- Hazardous Communication Standard
- Types of chemical labels
- How to read MSDS and NFPA signs
- Warning signs
- How to get MSDS
- Location of MSDS
- How to store chemicals
- How to record chemical inventory
- Hazardous waste laws
- How to comply with laws
- How to use and label bio-bins and sharps containers
- How to keep records
- Who keeps the records
- Medical consent forms
- HBV forms
- Safety training certificate
- Engineering control records

FIGURE 10-6 Safety training form. *(Courtesy of POL Consultants)*

SAMPLE

CERTIFICATE OF TRAINING

_____

First Name   Middle Initial   Last Name

has completed the

OSHA HAZARD COMMUNICATION
INFORMATION TRAINING PROGRAM

This certificate indicates your successful participation in a program instructing you of your rights as a worker and the proper handling of hazardous substances in the workplace.

_____   _____

Date   Employee Signature

_____

Instructor's Signature

_____

Employer's Signature

FIGURE 10-7 Sample certificate of training. *(Courtesy of POL Consultants)*

about various hazardous ingredients on the MSDS and product labels.

Chemical Warning Label Determination. The National Fire Protection Association's color and number method is used to signify a warning to employees using the chemicals (Figure 10-10). Four colors are used:

1. Blue identifies the health hazard.
2. Red identifies the fire hazard.
3. Yellow identifies the reactivity or how stable the chemical is.
4. White indicates the PPE needed when using this chemical.

The level of risk for each category is indicated by the use of numbers 0–4. The higher the number, the greater the danger. Letters are used to identify the PPE needed.

A chemical warning label, a diamond-shaped symbol, displays the four colors with a place for the numbers to be written on each (Figure 10-11). The employee quickly can identify the hazard category, the risk for each, and the PPE equipment required. All hazardous chemicals must be labeled unless they are poured into separate containers for *immediate use* (Figure 10-12).

SAMPLE

CHEMICAL INVENTORY FORM

Office of _____

Date _____

Chemical Name	Catalog #	Quantity Stores L./gm. (monthly)	Physical State	Hazard Class				Manufacturer	Comments
				H	F	R	P		

(H) Health
0 - Minimal
1 - Slightly
2 - Moderate
3 - Serious
4 - Extreme

(F) Fire Hazard
0 - Will not burn
1 - Slight
2 - Moderate
3 - Serious
4 - Extreme

(R) Reactivity
0 - Stable, is not reactive
   with water
1 - Slight
2 - Moderate
3 - Serious
4 - Extreme

(P) Protection
A - Goggles
B - Goggles/Gloves
C - Goggles/Gloves/Apron
D - Face Shield/Gloves/Apron
E - Goggles/Gloves/Mask
F - Goggles/Gloves/Apron/Mask
X - Gloves

FIGURE 10-8 Sample chemical inventory form. *(Courtesy of POL Consultants)*

MATERIAL SAFETY DATA SHEET

I—PRODUCT IDENTIFICATION

COMPANY NAME: We Wash Inc.

ADDRESS: 5035 Manchester Avenue
        Freedom, Texas 79430

PRODUCT NAME: Spotfree

Synonyms: Warewashing Detergent

Tel. No: (314) 621-1818
Nights: (314) 621-1399
CHEMTREC: (800) 424-9343

Product No.: 2190

II—HAZARDOUS INGREDIENTS OF MIXTURES

MATERIAL:	(CAS#)	% by Wt.	TLV	PEL
According to the OSHA Hazard Communication Standard, 29 CFR 1910.1200, this product contains no hazardous ingredients.		N/A	N/A	N/A

FIGURE 10-9 Sample MSDS.

(continued next page)

III—PHYSICAL DATA

Vapor Pressure, mm Hg: N/A
Evaporation Rate (ether=1): N/A
Solubility in H_2O: Complete
Freezing point F: N/A
Boiling Point F: N/A
Specific Gravity H_2O=1 @25C: N/A

Vapor Density (Air=1) 60–90F: N/A
% Volatile by Wt. N/A
pH @ 1%   Solution 9.3–9.8
pH as Distributed: N/A
Appearance: Off-white granular powder
Odor: Mild chemical odor

IV—FIRE AND EXPLOSION

Flash Point F: N/AV

Flammable Limits: N/A

Extinguishing Media: The product is not flammable or combustible. Use media appropriate for the primary source of fire.

Special Fire Fighting Procedures: Use caution when fighting any fire involving chemicals. A self-contained breathing apparatus is essential.

Unusual Fire and Explosion Hazards: None known

V—REACTIVITY DATA

Stability—Conditions to Avoid: None known

Incompatibility: Contact of carbonates or bicarbonates with acids can release large quantities of carbon dioxide and heat.

Hazardous Decomposition Products: In fire situations, heat decomposition may result in the release of sulfur oxides.

Conditions Contributing to Hazardous Polymerization: N/A

Spotfree
VI—HEALTH HAZARD DATA

EFFECTS OF OVEREXPOSURE (Medical Conditions Aggravated/Target Organ Effects,
A. ACUTE (Primary Route of Exposure)   EYES: Product granules may cause mechanical irritation to eyes.
   SKIN (Primary Route of Exposure): Prolonged, repeated contact with skin may result in drying of skin.
   INGESTION: Not expected to be toxic if swallowed; however, gastrointestinal discomfort may occur.
B. SUBCHRONIC, CHRONIC, OTHER: None known

VII—EMERGENCY AND FIRST AID PROCEDURES

EYES: In case of contact, flush thoroughly with water for fifteen minutes. Get medical attention if irritation persists.
SKIN: Flush and dry Spotfree from skin with flowing water. Always wash hands after use.
INGESTION: If swallowed, drink large quantities of water and call a physician.

VIII—SPILL OR LEAK PROCEDURES

Spill Management: Sweep up material and repackage, if possible.
Spill residue may be flushed to the sewer with water.

Waste Disposal Methods: Dispose of in accordance with federal, state, and local regulations.

IX—PROTECTION INFORMATION/CONTROL MEASURES

Respiratory: None needed   Eye: Safety glasses   Glove: Not required

Other Clothing and Equipment: None required

Ventilation: Normal

FIGURE 10-9 (continued)

X—SPECIAL PRECAUTIONS

Precautions to Be Taken in Handling and Storing: Avoid contact with eyes. Avoid prolonged or repeated contact with skin. Wash thoroughly after handling. Keep container closed when not in use.
Additional Information: Store away from acids.

Prepared by: D. Martinez   Revision Date: 04/11/__

Seller makes no warranty, expressed or implied, concerning the use of this product other than indicated on the label. Buyer assumes all risk of use and/or handling of this material when such use and/or handling is contrary to label instructions.

While Seller believes that the information contained herein is accurate, such information is offered solely for its customers' consideration and verification under their specific use conditions. This information is not to be deemed a warranty or representation of any kind for which Seller assumes legal responsibility.

FIGURE 10-9

RED: FIRE HAZARD

4 = Danger: Flammable gas or extremely flammable liquid

3 = Warning: Flammable liquid

2 = Caution: Combustible liquid

1 = Caution: Combustible if heated

0 = Non-combustible

YELLOW: REACTIVITY

4 = Danger: Explosive at room temperature

3 = Danger: May be explosive if spark occurs or if heated under confinement

2 = Warning: Unstable or may react if mixed with water

1 = Caution: May react if heated or mixed with water

0 = Stable: Non-reactive when mixed with water

BLUE: HEALTH HAZARD

4 = Danger: May be fatal

3 = Warning: Corrosive or toxic

2 = Warning: Harmful if inhaled

1 = Caution: May cause irritation

0 = No unusual hazard

WHITE: PPE

A   Goggles

B   Goggles, gloves

C   Goggles, gloves, apron

D   Face shields, gloves, apron

E   Goggles, gloves, mask

F   Goggles, gloves, apron, mask

X   Gloves

FIGURE 10-10 The National Fire Protection Association's color and number method.

CHEMICAL WARNING LABEL DETERMINATION

The Hazard Communication Act contains specific labeling requirements. Labels must be on all hazardous chemicals that are shipped to and used in the workplace. Labels must not be removed. Material safety data sheets for all chemicals will be available to employees.

Manufacturer Requirements: Chemical manufacturers are required to evaluate chemicals, determine status as hazards, provide material safety data sheets (MSDS), and label all shipped chemicals properly. Manufacturer labels must never be removed. The best way to determine the hazards of the chemical is to read the MSDS, obtain an OSHA designated list or State Hazardous Substance list. For most mixed chemicals, it is necessary to contact the manufacturer for MSDS.

Office Chemicals: Search through your office and write down all chemicals you have in the office. Most pharmaceuticals and common household products do not come under this standard. Ingredients can then be compared to a list of regulated substances or MSDS sheets will provide necessary information.

Employer's Responsibility: Any hazardous chemical used in the workplace that is not in its original container **must** be labeled with the identity of the chemical and hazards. "Target Organ" chemical labels may be used. The label must include the chemical and common name, warnings about physical and health hazards, and the name and address of the manufacturer. The employer is to compile a chemical inventory list that is to be updated as needed. MSDS information should be located in a place where it is accessible to all employees. Label and MSDS information should be provided during the safety training program.

Identity: The term *identity* can refer to any chemical or common name designation for the individual chemical or mixture, as long as the term used is also used on the list of hazardous chemicals and the MSDS.

NOTE: If a chemical is poured into another container for immediate use, it does not need to be labeled.

Chemical Name

Common Name

Manufacturer

FIGURE 10-11 A chemical warning label.

FIGURE 10-12 Containers with chemical warning labels.

CHAPTER SUMMARY

The Occupational Safety and Health Administration regulations, including the hazard communication standard, are intended to require the employer to provide a safe work environment for all employees. The dental assistant must understand the complete standard and how compliance is accomplished. Staff must be trained for a safe workplace. Compliance with all standards must be accomplished to ensure a safe workplace.

CASE STUDY

Rebecca Thomas, a twenty-five-year-old, is a newly hired employee in the office of Dr. Charles. She is working as a chairside dental assistant. She will be completing her first month of employment. A fellow employee is discussing a case with Rebecca and accidentally knocks over a glass container. It breaks into several pieces.

Case Study Review

1. What training should Rebecca have completed?

2. What records of the incident must be kept by Rebecca's employer? For how long must they be kept?

3. What must be used to clean up the broken glass?

4. Where should the pieces of broken glass be disposed of?

 To complete your study of this chapter, work the review activities that follow. Also, refer to the software that accompanies this text.

REVIEW QUESTIONS

Multiple Choice

1. The Bloodborne/Hazardous Materials Standard covers all the following except
   a. housekeeping.
   b. laundry.
   c. hours of employment.
   d. material safety data sheets.

2. An example(s) of engineering/work practice controls is (are)
   a. personal protective equipment.
   b. splash guards on model trimmers.
   c. gloves, masks, glasses.
   d. dental uniform.

3. All the following are OPIM except
   a. saliva.
   b. intact skin.
   c. pleural fluid.
   d. pericardial fluid.

4. The color and number method often used to label various chemicals was developed by the
   a. Occupational Safety and Health Administration.
   b. American Dental Association.
   c. Environmental Protection Agency.
   d. National Fire Protection Association.

5. The color blue on the chemical warning label indicates
   a. health hazard.
   b. fire hazard.
   c. reactivity or stability of chemical.
   d. PPE needed.

Critical Thinking

1. Would the scope of the OSHA Bloodborne/Hazardous Materials Standard cover the employee while traveling to the place of employment?

2. Employees have a lunch room that becomes untidy and disorderly. The dentist never uses the lunch room. If one of the employees has an accident in the room, who is responsible?

3. Standard precautions are issued by whom? To protect whom?

Preparation for Patient Care [CDA]

OBJECTIVES

The student should strive to meet the following objectives and demonstrate an understanding of the facts and principles presented in this chapter:

1. Assist the patient in completing the patient history.

2. Review the medical and dental history. Alert the dentist to any areas of concern.

3. Perform or assist the dentist in an oral evaluation including lips, tongue, glands, and oral cavity.

4. Perform vital signs on the patient, including temperature, pulse, respiration, and blood pressure.

5. Read the vital signs. Alert the dentist if they are abnormal.

KEY TERMS

antipyretic (p. 197)

asymmetric (p. 195)

baseline vital signs (p. 197)

brachial artery (p. 200)

bradycardia (p. 200)

bradypnea (p. 200)

Celsius (p. 197)

commissures (p. 195)

diastolic blood pressure (p. 201)

exhalation (p. 200)

Fahrenheit (p. 197)

fever (p. 197)

hypothermic (p. 197)

inhalation (p. 200)

palpates (p. 195)

smile line (p. 195)

sphygmomanometer (p. 200)

stethoscope (p. 200)

symmetric (p. 195)

systolic blood pressure (p. 200)

tachycardia (p. 200)

tachypnea (p. 200)

vermilion border (p. 195)

vital signs (p. 197)

INTRODUCTION

Preparation for patient care is an important part of providing quality dental service to each patient. The dental assistant can begin the process of patient preparation by obtaining personal, medical, and dental history from each patient. After history forms are completed, the dental assistant reviews the information and alerts the dentist to any areas of concern.

Once the patient is in the treatment room, the dental assistant performs or assists the dentist in an evaluation of the patient. This clinical evaluation includes obtaining vital signs and performing both an internal and an external evaluation.

PATIENT HISTORY

The dental team members must thoroughly review a patient's medical history in order to treat the patient effectively. The information must be reviewed and updated at each visit. Most dental offices have a broad questionnaire for patients to complete. The information is confidential and should be as thorough as possible so that the best possible care is rendered. Sensitive topics may be discussed, such as medications being taken, medical treatment, and other factors contributing to the patient's health.

Personal Information

One of the first steps in caring for patients is to have them complete a patient history. The patient is requested to fill out a personal history that includes the following: full name, address, phone number, Social Security number, insurance, emergency contacts, and physician's name and his or her phone number (Figure 11-1).

FIGURE 11-1 Health and medical history.

Medical Information

The patient also is requested to fill out a medical history. The medical history contains questions about past surgeries, systemic diseases, injuries, and/or allergies. It is critical for the dental team to know about any allergies that may affect treatment. Normally, the allergies of concern are related to anesthetics, latex, and/or antibiotics. The patient also should disclose any medical concerns such as epilepsy, diabetes, or a heart condition. Allergies and medical alerts are to be noted on the chart and highlighted to bring them to the attention of dental team members. Any drugs the patient has taken recently or is currently taking should be recorded on the medical history. Often, a variety of questions are asked to gain the information needed. The assistant should tactfully question any abnormalities. Usually, any "yes" answers on a questionnaire require further inquiry.

Dental Information

Questions regarding the patient's dental history are included in the patient's history. This information alerts the dental assistant to any concerns the patient has regarding his or her current dental health. It also gives insight into any concerns the patient may have had regarding previous dental care. The last dental examination is noted, as well as the patient's last dental appointment and how often the patient seeks dental treatment. Some questions are asked regarding the patient's attitude toward dentistry and how he or she maintains his or her own personal oral health care.

Upon completion of the patient history, the patient signs and dates the form. This record provides the dentist and staff with useful information so that they may provide better care for the patient. The dentist and/or dental assistant will review the answers prior to initiation of treatment. The personal and medical history should be reviewed prior to each treatment series. It is the dentist's ethical and legal responsibility to gain information about the patient's medical history prior to dental treatment. The highest degree of confidentiality must be maintained by the dental team regarding the patient's history.

After thoroughly reviewing the patient's personal and medical/dental history and collecting the appropriate data, the patient is seated.

Clinical Observation

The dental assistant observes patients as they are escorted into the treatment room. If the patient displays any deviation from the normal, such as walking with an abnormal gait, further probing into the health history may be required. The assistant may notice speech or behavior problems that should be brought to the dentist's attention. Looking at the patient's face for symmetry is the first step in the oral inspection. Although most individuals do not have faces that are totally **symmetric** (meaning that if the face was divided in half, the other half would be a mirror image), each side of the face should look fairly similar. If one eyelid droops, for example, or if the face is **asymmetric**, this should be noted on the patient's chart. The dental assistant also evaluates the patient's eyes and facial skin for any scars or abnormalities in color or texture.

CLINICAL EVALUATION

Examine the lips for cracking and dryness. The dental assistant also observes the **smile line** (where the lips are when the patient smiles), the **vermilion border** (the line around the lip), and the **commissures** (the corners of the lips) (Figure 11-2). Any deviations from normal are noted on the patient's chart.

The assistant may place a lip lubricant (petroleum jelly) on the patient's lips prior to the examination to ensure the patient's comfort.

The next area to be examined is the external floor of the mouth and the cervical lymph nodes. The floor of the mouth is examined with the patient's mouth closed. The dental assistant palpates the soft tissues in the area with the fingers, checking for any abnormalities (Figure 11-3).

The cervical lymph nodes are examined by having the patient turn his or her head to the side. The dental assistant gently feels the chain of lymph nodes from the ear to the collar bone. This is done on the opposite side of the neck as well (Figure 11-4).

The last external area to be examined is the temporomandibular joint (TMJ). The dental assistant sits behind the patient's head and **palpates** the joint as the patient opens and closes his or her mouth. Also, the dental assistant places a finger from each hand just anterior to

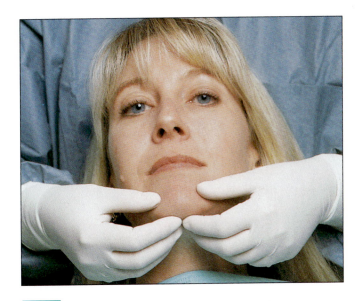

FIGURE 11-3 Examining the external tissues of the mandible and the floor of the mouth.

the tragus of each ear and has the patient open and close his or her mouth (Figure 11-5). The operator listens for any noise in the TMJ, such as clicking, and feels for any catching as the patient's mouth opens. Any symptoms, pains or tenderness are noted on the patient's chart.

At the beginning of the internal oral examination, the operator first does a quick visual assessment, looking for any obvious problems. Problems could include lesions in the mouth, abscessed teeth, or any color changes in the oral mucosa. The operator examines the tissues of the floor of the mouth. This is accomplished by supporting the mandible with one hand while gently palpating with the fingers of the other hand on the ventral sides of the tongue and the floor of the mouth (Figure 11-6). The mucosa and the frena of the upper

FIGURE 11-2 Visually examining the (A) smile line, the (B) vermilion border, and the (C) commissures of the lip.

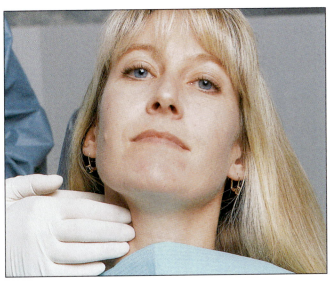

FIGURE 11-4 Examining the cervical lymph nodes.

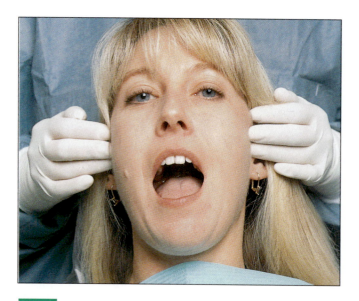

FIGURE 11-5 Examining the temporal mandibular joint as the patient opens and closes her mouth.

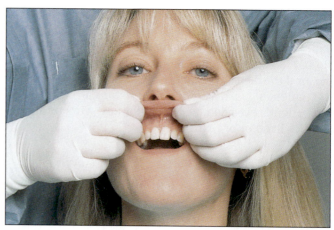

FIGURE 11-7 Examining the oral mucosa and the frenum.

and lower lips are examined by gently pulling the lips out and inspecting the area (Figure 11-7). The mouth mirror is used in the maxillary and mandibular buccal area. Using the mirror, the palate and the posterior of the tongue are examined visually (Figure 11-8).

The last area in the oral cavity to be examined is the tongue. A gauze sponge is needed to grasp the tongue. Placing the gauze around the tip of the tongue, the operator pulls to the side to visually inspect the posterior area on each side, then lifts to examine the underportion of the tongue (Figure 11-9). During this time, the patient is asked to say "ah-ah," therefore allowing the operator to examine the uvula and the tissues of the oropharynx.

FIGURE 11-8 Examining the palate and the posterior of the tongue using a mouth mirror.

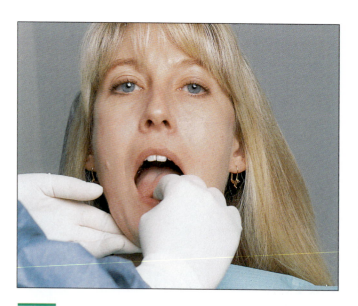

FIGURE 11-6 Operator (dentist or dental assistant) performing an intraoral examination of the floor of the mouth.

FIGURE 11-9 Examining the tongue using a gauze sponge on the tip of the tongue.

VITAL SIGNS

The measuring and recording of vital signs is an important part of the health evaluation, and it should be done with every patient before starting any dental treatment. After the patient's history is completed and the patient is seated, the dental assistant can obtain vital signs. Vital signs give the dental operator specific information about the physical and emotional condition of the patient. They may point out previously undetected abnormalities. Vital signs aid in the planning of the patient's dental treatment and are essential during emergency treatment.

Vital signs are the basic signs of life. They include body temperature, pulse, blood pressure, and respiration rate. **Baseline vital signs** are the initial measurements of vital signs. Baseline vital signs help the dentist compare subsequent measurements with the initial measurements.

Body Temperature

Measurement of body temperature is an essential component of every patient's health evaluation (Figure 11-10). Body temperature is compared to the normal body temperature range and, if higher or lower, it should be further investigated. A range is used when identifying the normal body temperature, because temperature varies from person to person and at different times of the day. It is well known that after exercise, emotional excitement, and even eating, the temperature increases. A person's face may turn red and blush due to excite-

ment, increasing the body temperature. Temperature in young children and young infants will vary more than in adults. Normal temperature ranges are as follows:

▶ Normal range in Fahrenheit   99.5°
                                              98.6° (Average)
                                              96.0°

▶ Normal range in Celsius   37.5°
                                              37.0° (Average)
                                              35.5°

Fahrenheit is the measure of temperature where the freezing point of water is 32°F and the boiling point of water is 212°F. **Celsius** is the centigrade measure of temperature where the freezing point of water is 0°C and the boiling point of water is 100°C.

The patient has a **fever** if he or she is above the normal range. An **antipyretic** is often used to reduce fever. An antipyretic could include cold packs, alcohol rubs, or an aspirin. A patient is said to be **hypothermic** if the body temperature is below normal. Hypothermia could be caused from prolonged exposure to cold and/or an overdose of antipyretic drugs, such as aspirin.

TECH   There are a number of new digital thermometers on the market for measuring temperature in an expedient manner. If the manual thermometer is used, place it under the tongue to remain in place with the lips closed for five minutes. The manual thermometer is mercury filled, which is a hazardous chemical, and if breakage occurs, it must be disposed of properly. If a digital thermometer is used to obtain temperature, dispose of the probe cover in a biohazard waste container.

FIGURE 11-10 Fahrenheit and Celsius thermometers with the normal range indicated.

P R O C E D U R E

11-1 Taking an Oral Temperature Using a Digital Thermometer

This procedure is performed by the dental assistant in order to obtain the patient's body temperature.

EQUIPMENT AND SUPPLIES

▶ Digital thermometer

▶ Probe covers

▶ Biohazard waste container

PROCEDURE STEPS (Follow standard precautions)

1. Wash hands.

2. Assemble the thermometer and probe cover.

3. Seat patient in the dental treatment room and position him or her comfortably in an upright position.

4. Verify that the patient has not had a hot or cold drink or smoked within the last half hour. (This may give a false temperature reading.)

5. Explain the procedure to the patient.

6. Position the new probe cover on the digital thermometer (Figure 11-11).

7. Insert the probe under the tongue to either side of the patient's mouth.

8. Instruct the patient to carefully close his or her lips around the probe without biting down on it (Figure 11-12).

9. Leave the probe in position until the digital thermometer beeps.

10. Remove the probe from the patient's mouth.

11. Read the results from the digital thermometer display window.

12. Dispose of the probe cover in a hazardous waste container.

13. Wash hands.

14. Document the procedure and record the results on the patient's chart.

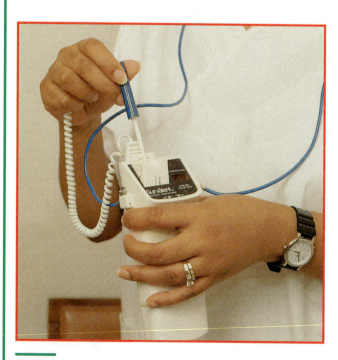

FIGURE 11-11 Slide the probe into the disposable cover, adjusting if necessary.

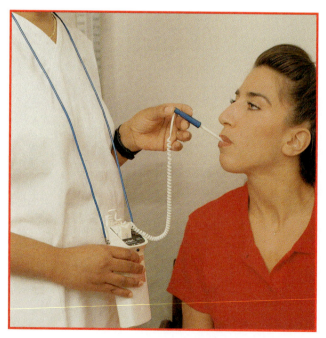

FIGURE 11-12 Insert thermometer under tongue to enter side of mouth.

Pulse

The pulse is the intermittent beating sensation felt when the fingers are pressed against an artery. A pulse rate is determined by **palpation** (feeling with the fingers or hand). Do not use the thumb to palpate, because it has a pulse of its own and could throw off the readings. Pulse may be palpated on one of several arteries: radial, carotid, or temporal. The dental assistant most commonly uses the radial artery.

Radial Pulse Site. The radial pulse site is located on the radial artery, on the thumb side of the wrist (Figure 11-13). It can be found approximately one inch above the base of the thumb. This is the most common site used for obtaining pulses in the dental office.

Carotid Pulse Site. The carotid pulse site is located on the carotid artery in the neck just below the angle of the mandible (Figure 11-14). It is normally large and therefore easy to locate.

Temporal Pulse Site. The temporal pulse site is over the smaller temporal artery located in the temporal fossa, which is a slight depression located about the level of the eyebrow just in front of the ear (Figure 11-15). The temporal pulse is more difficult to locate than the radial of the carotid.

After locating the pulse site, the dental assistant determines the number of beats per minute. This varies depending on the patient's age, sex, and physical and

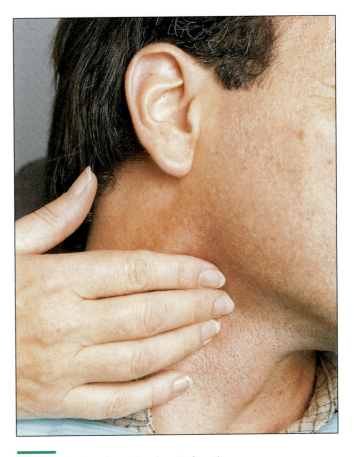

FIGURE 11-14 Carotid pulse site location.

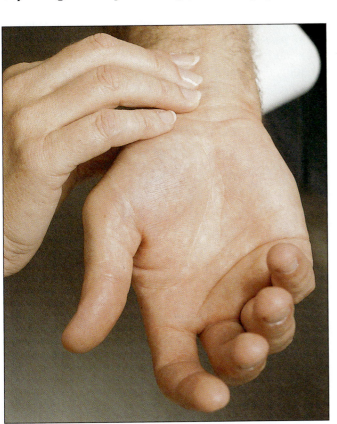

FIGURE 11-13 Radial pulse site location.

FIGURE 11-15 Temporal pulse site location.

mental conditions. It is expressed in a range without an absolute number. **Tachycardia** is an abnormally rapid resting pulse rate, and **bradycardia** is an abnormally slow resting heart rate. Normal pulse rates are as follows:

▶ Normal pulse rate for adults   Sixty to ninety beats per minute

▶ Normal pulse rate for children   Ninety to one hundred and twenty beats per minute

Respiration

Respiration is one breath taken in (**inhalation**) and one breath let out (**exhalation**). To ensure an accurate reading—where the patient is unaware that the respiration is being measured—take it after obtaining the pulse rate. Leave the fingers over the pulse site and count the breaths in and out for one minute. The patient will assume that the pulse is still being taken. **Tachypnea** is an abnormally rapid resting respiratory rate and, **bradypnea** is an abnormally slow resting respiratory rate. There are similarities in respiration and pulse rates. Children have a more rapid respiration rate; generally, as with the pulse rate, the younger the child, the faster the rate.

Normal respiration rates are as follows:

▶ Normal respiration rate in adults   Twelve to eighteen respirations per minute

▶ Normal respiration rate in children   Twenty to forty respirations per minute

Blood Pressure

Blood pressure is an important indicator of the health of a patient's cardiovascular system. A patient may have heart disease and still feel good and look outwardly healthy. However, the fear of dental treatment may be stressful enough to induce a heart attack. Therefore, taking and recording a patient's blood pressure is very important. It is not done in all offices today, because often the dental assistants have not been trained to perform this skill. Take time to learn this skill!

Blood pressure is measured by placing a **sphygmomanometer**, a "blood pressure apparatus," around the **brachial artery** (Figure 11-16). This apparatus is a cloth-covered inflatable rubber bladder used to control the flow of blood in the artery. There is a rubber hand bulb and pressure control valve attached to one tube and a pressure gauge attached to the other tube. The brachial artery is palpated. It is located at the inside of the elbow in the **antecubital space**, the indented area, as the arm is stretched out straight.

Position the arm at the patient's heart height. After the brachial artery is located, the cuff of the sphygmomanometer can be placed one inch above the bend in the elbow and secured. The dental assistant then uses the **stethoscope**, an instrument used to hear and amplify

FIGURE 11-16 Aneroid sphygmomanometer.

the sounds produced by the heart (Figure 11-17). The stethoscope has two earpieces that must be placed in the ears in a forward position. At the end piece of the stethoscope is a diaphragm, which does the amplification and sends the sounds up the tubing to the ears. The dental assistant pumps up the cuff and closes off the blood in the artery and then slowly lets the air escape.

During this time, the assistant listens to the first pulsation sound and notes where the needle is indicating on the pressure gauge. This first sound indicates the **systolic blood pressure**, which is created when the heart contracts and forces blood through the arteries. Listening carefully, the dental assistant then watches the pressure gauge until the pulsation sound disappears. This reading

FIGURE 11-17 A single-head stethoscope. Used with a sphygmomanometer to measure blood pressure.

11-2 Taking a Radial Pulse and Measuring the Respiration Rate

This procedure is performed by the dental assistant in order to obtain the patient's pulse and respiration rate.

EQUIPMENT AND SUPPLIES

▶ Watch with a second hand

PROCEDURE STEPS *(Follow standard precautions)*

1. Wash hands.

2. Position the patient in a comfortable position, upright in the dental chair (same position used for taking the temperature).

3. Explain the procedure.

4. Have the patient position the wrist resting on the arm of the dental chair or counter.

5. Locate the radial pulse by placing the pads of the first three fingers over the patient's wrist.

6. Gently compress the radial artery so that the pulse can be felt.

7. Using the watch with the second hand, count the number of pulsations for one full minute (Figure 11-18).

8. Record the number of pulsations.

9. Note any irregular rhythm patterns.

10. While still keeping the finger pads placed on the radial pulse, count the rise and fall of the chest wall for one minute. This allows the patient to

FIGURE 11-18 Taking patient's radial pulse and respiration.

breath normally due to the fact that he or she believes the pulse is still being recorded.

11. Record the number of respirations. Note any irregularities in the breathing.

12. Wash hands.

13. Document the procedure and the pulse and respiration rates on the patient's chart.

---

is noted on the gauge as the **diastolic blood pressure**. The diastolic blood pressure is created as the arteries return to their original state when the heart relaxes between contractions. Two measurements are always recorded when taking blood pressure. They are recorded as a fraction: The systolic pressure is the upper figure and the diastolic pressure is the lower figure. They are always recorded in even numbers (the gauge has indications for even numbers only). There is no absolute number for the normal blood pressure; it is recorded in ranges, much like other vital signs. Children normally have lower pressure and, as adults age, the blood pressure goes up. Some, however,

use 120 over 80 as an average for an adult. This means 120 systolic over 80 diastolic pressure, shown as 120/80. Normal blood pressure range is as follows:

▶ Normal systolic pressure   100 to 140 mm Hg

▶ Normal diastolic pressure   60 to 90 mm Hg

A higher-than-normal blood pressure is called **hypertension,** and lower-than-normal blood pressure is **hypotention**. An increase in the diastolic pressure is more significant than an increase in the systolic pressure, because it indicates that the heart is working harder.

P R O C E D U R E

11-3 Measuring Blood Pressure

This procedure is performed by the dental assistant in order to obtain the patient's blood pressure.

EQUIPMENT AND SUPPLIES

▶ Stethoscope

▶ Sphygmomanometer

▶ Disinfectant and gauze

PROCEDURE STEPS *(Follow standard precautions)*

1. Wash hands.

2. Assemble the stethoscope and sphygmomanometer and disinfect the earpieces of the stethoscope.

3. Position the patient in a comfortable position, upright in the dental chair (same position used for taking the temperature).

4. Explain the procedure.

5. Have the patient position the arm resting at heart level on the counter or the arm of the dental chair.

6. Have the patient remove any outer clothing that is restrictive to the upper arm. Bare the upper arm and palpate the brachial artery (Figure 11-19).

7. Center the bladder of the cuff securely, about two inches above the bend of the elbow.

8. Position the earpieces of the stethoscope in a forward manner, into the ears.

9. Place the diaphragm of the stethoscope over the brachial artery and hold it in place with a thumb. Place other fingers under the elbow to hyperextend the artery. (By extending the elbow, the artery can be accessed more easily and enable better reading of the blood pressure.)

10. Inflate the cuff using the bulb and the control valve on the sphygmomanometer. If the cuff is not inflating, recheck the control valve on the sphygmomanometer to ensure that it is closed. Air should not be escaping. The inflation should be to a level of 160 for a normal adult.

11. Deflate the cuff at a rate of two to four millimeters of mercury per second by rotating the control valve just slightly (Figure 11-20).

12. Listen for the first sound and note its measurement on the scale.

13. Continue to deflate the cuff and listen to the pulsing sounds. Note when all sounds disappear. Continue deflating for another ten millimeters to ensure that the last sound has been heard.

14. The cuff can then be deflated rapidly and removed from the patient's arm.

15. Disinfect the earpieces of the stethoscope.

16. Wash hands and record the procedure and the measurement on the patient's chart. (Remember that blood pressure is recorded in even numbers in a fraction format with the systolic measurement on top.)

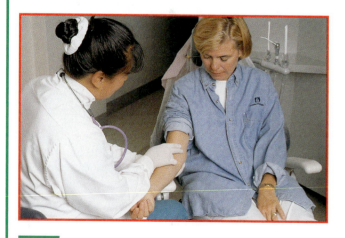

FIGURE 11-19 Palpating patient's brachial artery.

FIGURE 11-20 Taking patient's blood pressure.

Normal Blood Pressure Readings	
Child 10 years of age	100/66
Adolescent 16 years of age	118/76
Adult	Systolic below 140
	Diastolic below 90

CHAPTER SUMMARY

The health condition of a dental patient must be private, confidential, and updated at each visit. To treat a patient effectively, the patient's chart should include personal history, medical information, dental history, clinical observation, clinical evaluation, and vital signs.

CASE STUDY

Dwayne Allen, a fifty-year-old male, was in the dental office for a dental examination. Upon taking his blood pressure, the dental assistant documented that Dwayne had a systolic pressure of 150 and a diastolic pressure of 90.

Case Study Review

1. Is Dwayne's blood pressure within the normal range?

2. Should the blood pressure be retaken to ensure that it was completed accurately?

3. Should this reading be brought to the attention of the dentist?

To complete your study of this chapter, work the review activities that follow. Also, refer to the software that accompanies this text.

REVIEW QUESTIONS

Multiple Choice

1. The line around the lip is called the
   a. commissure.
   b. smile line.
   c. vermilion border.
   d. frenum.

2. The corners of the lips are called the
   a. commissures.
   b. smile lines.
   c. vermilion borders.
   d. frena.

3. The initial measurements of vital signs are the
   a. pulse.
   b. respiration.
   c. fever.
   d. baseline.

4. The normal range in body temperature, in Fahrenheit, is
   a. 95–100°.
   b. 96–99.5°.
   c. 97–99°.
   d. 96.5–98.5°.

5. An average range for a child's pulse rate is
   a. 60 to 90 beats per minute.
   b. 70 to 100 beats per minute.
   c. 80 to 110 beats per minute.
   d. 90 to 120 beats per minute.

Critical Thinking

1. What temperature would constitute a fever for a child? What effects on the dental treatment would a fever pose?

2. A patient has had a negative experience with his or her teeth in the past. What impact could this have on the current treatment? What role can the dental assistant play in making this a positive experience for the patient?

3. If a dental assistant observes a patient walking with an unsteady gait to the dental treatment room but finds no indication of this symptom in the patient's medical and dental history, what should the assistant do?

Pharmacology

OBJECTIVES

The student should strive to meet the following objectives and demonstrate an understanding of the facts and principles presented in this chapter:

1. Identify the terms related to drugs, pharmacology, and medicines.
2. Identify the difference between drug brand names and generic names.
3. Identify the parts of a written prescription.
4. Identify the texts pertinent to pharmacology.
5. Give the English meanings of the Latin abbreviations used for prescriptions.
6. Specify the drug laws and who enforces them.
7. Identify the schedules for the Comprehensive Drug Abuse Prevention and Control Act of 1970.
8. Identify the routes in which drugs can be administered.
9. Summarize the uses and effects of tobacco, caffeine, alcohol, marijuana, and cocaine.
10. Summarize information about heroin, morphine, and codeine.
11. Supply information about amphetamines.
12. Demonstrate an understanding of hallucinogenic drugs such as LSD, PCP, and mescaline.
13. Demonstrate an understanding of barbiturates.
14. Demonstrate an understanding of the drugs used in dentistry and the ways in which they are used.

KEY TERMS

addiction (p. 206)

analgesic (p. 213)

anesthesia (p. 213)

brand names (p. 206)

broad spectrum (p. 213)

closing (p. 208)

Comprehensive Drug Abuse Prevention and Control Act of 1970 (p. 208)

Council on Dental Therapeutics (p. 207)

drug (p. 206)

Drug Enforcement Agency (DEA) number (p. 206)

drug interaction (p. 206)

Food and Drug Administration (FDA) (p. 208)

generic names (p. 206)

habit forming (p. 206)

hallucinate (p. 212)

heading (p. 207)

inhalation (p. 209)

inscription (p. 206)

intradermal (p. 209)

intramuscular (p. 209)

intravenous (p. 209)

medicines (p. 206)

oral (p. 209)

over-the-counter (OTC) drugs (p. 206)

pharmacology (p. 206)

Physician's Desk Reference (PDR) (p. 207)

prescription (p. 206)

psychologically dependent (p. 206)

The Pure Food and Drug Act (p. 208)

The Pure Food, Drug, and Cosmetic Act (p. 208)

rectal (p. 209)

side effect (p. 206)

subcutaneous (p. 209)

sublingual (p. 209)

subscription (p. 207)

superscription (p. 207)

topically (p. 209)

withdrawal (p. 206)

INTRODUCTION

The terms pharmacology and drugs are normally associated with treating a disease, but in reality they cover a much broader aspect of chemically induced changes in the body. **Pharmacology** is the study of all drugs, their properties, how they react with each other, and the actions of the drugs within the body. Pharmacology is constantly changing due to the constant information and knowledge gained about drugs, new drugs being created, and drugs being altered. A **drug** is a substance that can change life processes within the body. **Medicines** are drugs that are used to treat diseases.

Drugs have never been as widely used/misused as they are today. The dental assistant needs to pay attention to patient's medical and dental histories and carefully document the drugs used by each patient. The dental assistant must have knowledge about pharmacology, the side effects of drugs, and the interactions that take place when more than one drug is used. When a drug causes an unintended result, this result is called a **side effect**. For example, if a patient is taking antihistamines and decongestants to clear up the symptoms of a cold and the patient becomes tired, fatigue is a side effect.

At times, it is necessary to take more than one drug at a time. This can be dangerous and should be avoided if the patient taking the drugs is unknowledgeable about the interaction. **Drug interaction** occurs when one drug changes the effect of another drug by increasing or decreasing the intended result. The risk of combining the drugs (synergistic effect) is much greater to the person than the risk of taking either one of the drugs alone.

Some drugs are addictive. When a person has an **addiction**, he or she is physically dependent on a drug. Being physical dependent means that the addict must continue to take the drug in order to avoid withdrawal symptoms. The symptoms that occur when the person addicted to the drug stops taking it are called **withdrawal**. Nervousness, stomach cramps, diarrhea, shaking, and depression are symptoms of withdrawal.

Some people become **psychologically dependent** on a drug. This means that the person taking the drug has developed a strong emotional need to take that drug. It is similar to a craving. This person may not have any physical need for the drug but becomes psychologically dependent on it. The drugs that cause psychological dependence are referred to as **habit forming**.

Legal drugs are classified according to their availability to the public and their potential for abuse. A person can purchase drugs that do not have the **inscription** "Federal law prohibits dispensing without prescription"; these drugs are referred to as **over-the-counter (OTC) drugs**. When drugs carry this inscription, they must be prescribed by a licensed medical professional and dispensed by a pharmacist.

DRUG NAMES

Drug Brand and Generic Names

When filling a **prescription** for a dentist, the pharmacy identifies whether the drug is to be filled with a drug brand or with a generic substance. The generic substance has a similar composition to the drug brand and often does not affect the outcome for the patient.

Brand Names of Drugs. **Brand names** of drugs are assigned to the drug by the manufacturer. These brand names, often referred to as trade names, are always capitalized and have registered trademarks. These names are controlled by the manufacturer. For example, Bayer™ is a brand name for aspirin.

Generic Names of Drugs. **Generic names** of drugs are not capitalized and are unprotected, allowing any business to use them. They refer to the chemical composition of the drug. They are less expensive than the brand-name drugs. For example, aspirin, which is composed of acetylsalicylic acid, is a generic name.

PRESCRIPTIONS

Only physicians, dentists, and physician assistants are legally allowed to write prescriptions. This limits the dispensing of controlled substances to those trained and licensed to provide patients with drugs. The drugs are dispensed only when a customer gives the pharmacist a correctly written prescription signed by a doctor with his or her **Drug Enforcement Agency (DEA) number** on it. In the past, a prescription had a form of recipe for the drug needed on it. Today's medicines are packaged in correct dosage amounts preformulated for dispensing. Therefore, the doctor can simplify the prescription, asking for the number of tablets, pills, capsules, or liquid amount and not indicating the dosage amounts (Figure 12-1). This

FIGURE 12-1 Solid preparations are manufactured in various forms, such as the caplet, tablet, and capsule.

ensures that the patient receives the proper dosage each time the drug is taken, and the correct packaging saves time for the doctor and the patient.

All dentists have the legal obligation to utilize "due care" while treating their patients. They must have a complete health history on the patient and must be knowledgeable about the drug that they prescribe to the patient. The American Dental Association **Council on Dental Therapeutics** gathers information about the drugs used in dentistry, and this information is given to the dentist to assist him or her in gaining necessary information about the use of new therapeutic agents. A recent publication of accepted dental therapeutics can be obtained from the American Dental Association (ADA). The dentists can call the ADA with questions concerning accepted dental therapeutics or if questions arise regarding any drug or chemical used in the office. Dentists can also obtain information about drugs from several texts. The most commonly used in the dental office is the ***Physician's Desk Reference* (PDR)**. The PDR is printed annually and has the drugs listed by trade or product name, generic and chemical names, and by category. Information about the drug includes the chemical description, indications and use of the drug, contraindications of using the drug, warnings and precautions related to the use of the drug, and adverse drug reactions. Information about the recommended drug dosages and how the drug is supplied is also listed in the PDR (Figure 12-2). Many of the drugs are packaged with inserts that list the same information contained in the PDR about the drug. These inserts usually are not given to the patient but are retained by the pharmacist. Many drugs now have inserts that give clear instructions to the patient and identify warnings. These are given to the patient with the prescription unless the doctor specifies on the written prescription not to do so. Pharmacists use two main references that have detailed information about each drug. These are the *United States Pharmacopoeia* (USP) and the *National Formulary* (NF).

Parts of a Prescription

A prescription is written in several parts (Figure 12-3). All information must be completed to ensure that the correct drug is being dispensed in the correct manner according to the directions of the dentist. Being thorough and writing clearly will assist in accuracy and quality control. It is recommended that a copy of the prescription be placed in the patient's chart for future reference.

Heading. The **heading** includes the doctor's name and degrees, office address, and phone number. The dentist's Drug Enforcement Agency (DEA) number must be printed in this area or near the signature. This number was assigned to the doctor and must be used every time a controlled substance is prescribed.

Superscription. The **superscription** is directly below the heading. This area has blank lines where the dentist

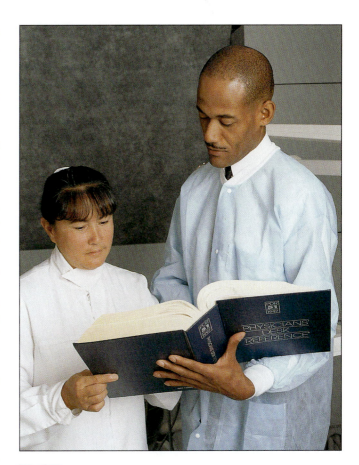

FIGURE 12-2 Dentist and dental assistant using the *Physician's Desk Reference* (PDR) to obtain information about a specific medication.

can fill in the name and address of the patient. Included in this area is a space for the date that the prescription was written. Other information, such as the patient's phone number, age, and gender, is also helpful to the pharmacist. Patients do not always fill the prescriptions immediately and may in fact not need them at a later date. Having the date filled in aids the pharmacist in obtaining pertinent information about the need for the drug. The age and gender gives further information as to the dosage amount needed by the patient. The pharmacist has extensive training about each drug and is a helpful member of the health-care team. The pharmacist may call the dentist and consult about a prescription or about a patient obtaining prescriptions from numerous offices. Health-care providers must work together in discouraging drug abuse.

The Body of the Prescription. The **body of the prescription** is labeled with the **Rx symbol** and has both the **inscription** area and the **subscription** area. In this area, the doctor inscribes or writes the name and strength of the drug being prescribed, the dose, and in what form the drug is to be dispensed. He or she subscribes or specifies the number of doses and directions on how the drug should be taken. Special directions to the pharmacist are written in this area as well. The writing of the body of the

Parts of a Prescription

1. The dentist's name, address, telephone number, and registration number.

2. The patient's name, address, and the date on which the prescription is written.

3. The *subscription* that includes the symbol Rx ("take thou").

4. The *inscription* that states the names and quantities of ingredients to be included in the medication.

5. The *subscription* that gives directions to the pharmacist for filling the prescription.

6. The *signature* (Sig) that gives the directions for the patient.

7. The dentist's signature blanks. Where signed, indicates if a generic substitute is allowed or if the medication is to be dispensed as written.

8. REPETATUR 0 1 2 3 p.r.n. This is where the dentist indicates whether or not the prescription can be refilled.

9. ☐ LABEL Direction to the pharmacist to label the medication appropriately.

[1] LEWIS & KING, DDS
2501 CENTER STREET
NORTHBOROUGH, OH 12345

[2] Name _Juanita Hansen_
Address _143 Gregory Lane, Apt. 43_ Date _4/7/--_

[3] Rx

[4] _Amoxicillin   500 mg_

[5] _Disp. #40_

[6] _Sig   1 cap quid x 10 days_

[7] Generic Substitution Allowed _Susan Rice_
D.D.S.

Dispense As Written _____
[8] REPETATUR 0 1 2 3 p.r.n.   D.D.S.

[9] ☐ LABEL

FIGURE 12-3 Prescription with parts identified.

prescription is often done in abbreviated format. Many Latin abbreviations are used for this. For example, the prescription might read as follows: Sig: 1 tab qid for 2 wks. This means take one tablet four times a day for two weeks. When the prescription is dispensed by the pharmacist, it is a law that the name of the drug and directions be put on the label of the drug container.

The Closing of the Prescription. The **closing** of the prescription is where the dentist signs his or her name, authorizes whether the prescription can be refilled and how many times, and checks whether a generic brand of this medication can be dispensed in place of the one written.

Latin Abbreviations and English Meanings Used for Prescriptions

Latin Abbreviations	English Meaning of Latin Abbreviation
a.a.	Of each
a.c.	Before meals
q.d.	Daily
b.i.d.	Twice a day
t.i.d.	Three times a day
q.i.d.	Four times a day
q.h.	Every hour
q.4.h.	Every four hours
q.8.h.	Every eight hours
Sig	Take
p.c.	After meals
p.r.n	When necessary or as needed

Many offices have prescription pads that are numbered sequentially and the information regarding the office and doctor's name and address is preprinted on them. They may have them printed in triplicate so that a copy of each written prescription can be kept in the corresponding patient's chart or on the pad according to the number. Either way, a notation should be written on the patient's chart about the prescription and instructions given. The prescription pads must be kept in a secure place so that they cannot be stolen.

DRUG LAWS

In 1906, the United States government passed **The Pure Food and Drug Act**. This law was enacted to control and regulate the composition, sale, and distribution of drugs. Prior to 1906, drugs were not regulated and drugs of varying compositions and purity were sold. Many of these drugs were harmful for human consumption.

Other laws were passed to control the sale of narcotic drugs in the early twentieth century. **The Pure Food, Drug, and Cosmetic Act** was passed in 1938. This allowed only the United States **Food and Drug Administration (FDA)** to have control of all food, cosmetics, and drugs sold. The drugs and cosmetics must pass standards set by the FDA and obtain approval prior to sale. The FDA also controls the advertising for all food, drugs, and cosmetics. Products may note, on their packaging, that they have met the rigid standards set by the FDA.

The **Comprehensive Drug Abuse Prevention and Control Act of 1970** was established to identify drugs according to five schedules of abuse potential. Title II of this act deals with the control and enforcement of drugs. The **Controlled Substance Act** gives the power of enforcement of this act to the DEA, which is part of the United States Department of Justice. Individuals who dispense drugs must have DEA-issued numbers to prescribe drugs. Dentists who dispense controlled substances improperly can have their offices closed and their licenses revoked. The dental assistants and the dentist must carefully check the patient's medical and dental histories prior to writing the prescription.

Drug Schedule for the Comprehensive Abuse Prevention and Control Act of 1970

▶ **Schedule I** drugs have a high potential for abuse and no accepted medical use. Drugs in this schedule include marijuana, heroin, and hallucinogens, such as LSD.

▶ **Schedule II** drugs have a high potential for abuse but also have accepted medical uses. These drugs lead to physical and psychological dependence. Drugs in this schedule include narcotics such as morphine, heroin, and cocaine; barbiturates such as tranquilizers; and amphetamines. Prescriptions in this schedule cannot be refilled.

▶ **Schedule III** drugs have a lower potential for abuse than those in Schedule II and have accepted medical uses. Compounds from this category are used in several of the drugs routinely prescribed in the dental office. The drugs in this category may lead to chemical dependency. Drugs in this schedule include barbiturates, stimulants, and depressants not in Schedule II and a number of compounds such as Tylenol III.

▶ **Schedule IV** drugs have less potential for abuse than those in Schedule III and also have acceptable medical uses. Schedule IV drugs have limited dependency. Drugs in this schedule include depressants, anti-anxiety drugs, and sedative drugs not included in the first three schedules.

▶ **Schedule V** drugs have the least potential for abuse and may consist of a compound from other schedules in small amounts. The drugs in this schedule may be anti-diarrhea medicines or cough medicines. The drugs in this group are also called "over-the-counter" drugs.

▌ DRUG ADMINISTRATION ROUTES

Drugs can be administered in a number of ways. The dentist will evaluate and decide the most beneficial route for the patient to take the drug.

▶ **Oral** administration is the most common method of taking medications. Tablets, capsules, pills, and liquids are taken in this manner. The patient swallows the dispensed amount of the drug with a glass of water.

▶ The ointment, lotion, gel, or cream is applied **topically** to the skin surface or mucosa. Dentistry uses a topical drug during local anesthetics. It is applied on the oral mucous membrane to numb the area prior to the injection.

▶ **Inhalation** means to breathe in the gas or aerosol. This allows the drug to be taken quickly into the lungs. One of the drugs used in dentistry by inhalation is nitrous oxide.

▶ **Sublingual** administration involves placing the medication under the tongue until it dissolves. For example, if a patient is experiencing angina pectoris, a nitroglycerin pill or spray is administered sublingually. Drugs are seldom administered by this route in the dental office.

▶ **Rectal** route of administration for drugs used in the dental office is nonexistent. Patients are able to administer enemas or suppositories in this manner to obtain the effects of drugs in this class. This route is used when an oral route is not recommended.

▶ **Intravenous** route of administration means to inject the substance directly into the vein. This route is used for immediate drug response.

▶ **Intramuscular** route of administration means to inject the substance into the muscle tissue. This route gives a slower response than intravenous administration but has a longer-lasting effect.

▶ **Subcutaneous** route of administration means to inject the substance just under the skin, above the muscle.

▶ **Intradermal** route of administration means to inject the substance under the epidermis (top layer of skin).

▶ Transdermal route of administration means to deliver medications from a drug reservoir from a patch applied to the skin in a consistent, controlled manner (Figure 12-4).

FIGURE 12-4 Nitro-Dur® is a transdermal system of delivering medication (nitroglycerin) for the management of angina pectoris.

DRUGS

The following section covers both illegal and prescription drugs. Dental assistants are concerned with the drugs that are prescribed but must have knowledge about illegal drugs that patients may be involved in and must understand what can happen if the drugs interact. It is also important to know the signs and symptoms that individuals may experience if under the influence of drugs. Having background knowledge about drugs and their effects helps the dental assistant provide better patient care.

Tobacco

People often do not associate tobacco with drugs, but tobacco does contain nicotine. Nicotine is a **stimulant**; it speeds up body activities. The drug nicotine is not used for any useful purpose to treat disease and therefore is not a medicine. It has been shown that tobacco is harmful to the health of smokers as well as to others who may breathe in the secondary smoke. Cancer, lung, and heart disease are much more prevalent in smokers than non-smokers. A smoker has ten times the risk of developing lung cancer than non-smokers have. Tobacco smoke contains carbon monoxide (the same gas found in car exhaust). This gas does not allow the blood to obtain the correct amount of oxygen in the cells and therefore the heart and circulatory system have to work harder. This leads to heart disease, the number one cause of death in the United States today. Federal law requires that every package of cigarettes carry a warning indicating the health hazards of smoking.

Smokeless tobacco (chewing tobacco) causes some of the same problems that smoking does. Chewing tobacco adds a high risk factor for oral cancer. Both smoking and chewing tobacco are causative factors in tooth staining, periodontal disease, and halitosis.

Many dental offices are reluctant to hire a dental assistant who smokes. The dental office is a health facility where the promotion of good health habits is essential. Dental assistants should seriously consider stopping the habit of smoking. A number of measures are currently available to aid in smoking cessation.

Caffeine

Caffeine is a habit-forming stimulant. It can be found in a number of sources, including coffee, espresso, tea, soft drinks, chocolate, and cocoa. This habit-forming drug also has side effects that may be harmful. Because it is a stimulant, caffeine causes the heart to work harder and may affect the nervous system. It may cause or irritate open sores (**ulcers**) in the wall of the stomach. Teeth are often stained by caffeine use. Too much caffeine can be toxic. If an individual were to drink thirty double "shots" of espresso or seventy to 100 cups of coffee, the result could be fatal. However, under normal use, coffee and espresso are safe to drink.

Count of Caffeine	
Source	**Mg of Caffeine**
Cocoa (1 cup)	13
Tea (1 cup)	30–45
Coffee (1 cup)	40–150
Espresso (1 shot)	60–175
Carbonated diet soft drink (1 8-oz glass)	30–50
Carbonated regular soft drink (1 8-oz glass)	35–65

Alcohol

One of the oldest known drugs is ethyl alcohol. Ethyl alcohol is found in alcoholic beverages such as wine, beer, and whiskey. Alcohol is a **depressant**, a drug that slows down body processes. This habit-forming drug has the opposite effect of stimulants. It affects the body functions rapidly because it is absorbed directly into the blood and then carried throughout the body. A 0.1 percent alcohol level is considered legal intoxication in most states. At 0.5 percent, an individual experiences a loss in judgment and coordination and exhibits slowed reactions and slurred speech. More than 20,000 people are killed each year by drunken drivers unable to respond to situations while behind the wheel of a car. This statistic represents about one-half of the driving accidents.

A person can become both physically and psychologically dependent on alcohol. Some people cannot stop at one drink and become alcoholics, unable to control their drinking. Some people are more likely to experience this disorder than others. Genetics, body weight, and size play a role in the likelihood of experiencing this disease. Alcoholics also suffer from withdrawal and symptoms of convulsions and delusions. Other side effects of this drug are liver deterioration, called **cirrhosis**. The liver eventually stops working and death results. A pregnant woman who drinks large amounts of alcohol may cause birth defects in the fetus. Patients may take alcohol to overcome the fear of dentistry. Dental assistants must be alert to this because of possible ill effects of the alcohol and other drugs used in dentistry. Alcoholics feel full and satisfied and do not seek a well-balanced diet, often resulting in poor nutrition.

Marijuana

A number of illegal drugs may be taken by patients prior to their visits to the dentist. Assistants should watch for signs of drug abuse. An assistant must have a basic knowledge of drugs and how they act on the function of the body in order to help if an emergency situation should arise. One illegal drug that is both a stimulant and a depressant is marijuana. Marijuana contains a number of drugs, one of the most active being tetrahydrocanaabinol (THC). Some of the side effects of marijuana use include increase in heart rate (as much as a fifty percent increase), lung tissue damage due to the smoking, and reproductive system disorders (abnormal hormonal levels, abnormal sperm production, and, in some cases, defects in the developing fetus).

The nervous system of regular marijuana users is affected. They are not able to speak and think as clearly, coordination is deteriorated, and they seem to lose the motivation to be productive without the marijuana use. Individuals who use the drug daily have ten percent more THC in their body tissues than monthly users have. A person is unlikely to become physically dependent on marijuana but often becomes psychologically dependent.

Marijuana derivitive is used as a medicine to treat patients taking other drug therapy for cancer. It seems to decrease nausea and regurgitation. Another application of marijuana is as a medicine to treat eye conditions such as glaucoma.

Cocaine

Cocaine is a very habit-forming drug. It makes the user feel in control, as if he or she has tremendous power. This feeling only lasts for a short time and then the user desires to obtain that feeling again. This drug is often referred to as the "rich man's drug" because a day's usage can cost hundreds or thousands of dollars. Side effects of this stimulant are heart problems, mental disorders, violent behavior, and death. Long-term users have great anxiety and are restless and irritable.

Cocaine is often mixed with other drugs to allow the user to get even higher. Sometimes, a mixture of heroin and cocaine (called a speedball) is injected intravenously. The result can be fatal. Purified cocaine that appears like a crystalline rock is called crack. This substance is smoked in a pipe or sprinkled on tobacco and smoked. The powder form of cocaine is inhaled into the nose or rubbed into the mucosa. Intraorally, this may appear much like toothbrush abrasion but over a wider area, because the substance is abrasive and wears on the tooth structure as it is rubbed back and forth into the tissue. If the person inhales cocaine, permanent damage occurs to the nasal mucosa over time.

Due to the abuse of this drug, its use as a medical treatment has been reduced. Cocaine causes both a physical and a psychological dependency. The physical dependency may happen after only one use or after varying uses. This dependency varies with each individual according the quantity used, the frequency, and the sensitivity of the person to the drug. If the person tries to stop usage, withdrawal symptoms such as craving the drug, intense anxiety, and mental illness such as depression will be experienced.

NARCOTICS

Narcotics are addictive depressants used to relieve pain. They have been used over the past 7,000 years. For most of these years, they were the most useful pain killers that physicians had available. Morphine and codeine are made from the opium poppy plant. Heroin is made from morphine. All drugs in this classification cause strong psychological and physical dependency and have been replaced for medical use by drugs less addictive.

Heroin

An individual who uses heroin regularly and tries to stop will become sick within twelve hours. Symptoms include hot and cold flashes with goose bumps, stomach cramps, vomiting, diarrhea, nervousness, shaking, muscle and bone pain, and an intense craving for the drug. The intensity of the withdrawal is dependent upon how much the individual has been taking. It does not take long for a person who uses heroin to develop a **tolerance** to the drug. This tolerance causes the person to need larger amounts of the drug in order to produce the same effect. The desired effect is loss of pain, highness, or a feeling of euphoria and drowsiness.

The side effects are addiction, loss of appetite, constipation, and decreased respiratory and heart rates. The drug can be taken intravenously, injected subcutaneously, or inhaled. Drug users who share their needles run the risk of contacting contagious diseases such as hepatitis B and HIV (human immunodeficiency virus).

Heroin is the most addicting of the narcotic drugs. A person can become addicted the first time he or she uses the drug. Overdoses cause the user to vomit and experience diarrhea and decreased respiratory and heart rates. This may follow with symptoms of shock and possible coma. The patient should be taken immediately to a hospital for treatment. If heroin overdose is diagnosed, the narcotic antagonist will be given to reverse the effects of the heroin. Not treating an overdose can be fatal. Newborns of addicted heroin mothers show symptoms of addiction and will die if not treated properly.

Morphine

Morphine is one of the best known narcotic **analgesic** (pain killer) drugs. Medically, it is given intravenously to relieve severe pain caused by myocardial infarction (heart attack). It is administered intramuscularly to control post-operative pain. It also can be given orally to patients who are terminally ill. Possible side effects include constipation, nausea, vomiting, and confusion. Long-term use leads to addiction and an increased level of tolerance. Due to physical dependence, if the drug is stopped suddenly, the person experiences symptoms of withdrawal, such as sweating, stomach and body cramping, and flu-like manifestations.

Codeine

Used since the early 1900s, codeine is an effective analgesic drug (pain killer). Dentistry uses it in combination with other drugs to relieve mild to moderate pain. Other medical uses for codeine are as a cough suppressant (because it suppresses the part of the brain that triggers coughing) and as an antidiarrheal drug (one that acts in the intestinal wall to slow down muscle contractions).

Codeine induces drowsiness, especially if taken with alcohol. Other side effects are constipation if taken over a long period of time and physical and psychological dependence.

AMPHETAMINES

Amphetamines are a group of stimulant drugs that increase the heart and respiratory rates and blood pressure. They were used in the past to treat obesity because they cause a loss of appetite along with the side effects of nervousness and restlessness. The street name for these drugs is "uppers." Taking amphetamines leads to violent behavior and poor judgment. Prolonged use causes physical dependence and a tolerance to the drug.

Medically, amphetamines are used to treat narcolepsy (abnormal daytime sleeping) and children with attention deficit disorder (ADD). Amphetamines have an opposite effect on hyperactive children. Rather than causing restlessness, the drug has a calming effect. This stimulant, together with the stimulated behavior of the child, slows down hyperactive behavior. There are very few other medical uses for amphetamines.

HALLUCINOGENS

Hallucinogens are drugs that cause people to see and hear images and sounds (**hallucinate**) that do not exist. An individual taking an hallucinogen may experience a mild hallucination where colors may change or have a hallucination that is extremely frightening. Sometimes, a person under the influence of a hallucinogen becomes so frightened that he or she reacts in an extreme manner—doing anything to "escape" the hallucination. This loss of control over emotions or actions is due to a change in the brain activity. Hallucination is a major symptom of schizophrenia. The symptom may also be caused by the illness manic depression.

Hallucinogenic drugs of abuse, also called psychedelic drugs, are LSD, PCP, mescaline, and psilocybin. Marijuana and alcohol taken in large amounts have also been reported to cause symptoms of hallucinogenic drugs.

Lysergic Acid Ciethylamide (LSD)

LSD is a synthetic drug made from ergot, a fungus that is grown on rye and wheat. LSD has a high potential for abuse and no medical role. Minute amounts of LSD can produce a "bad trip," where the user has a serious personality breakdown (including violence), which may last up to twelve hours. Flashbacks from these bad trips may occur up to several years after the user has taken LSD. There is no scientific evidence proving that LSD causes mental illness, but it is thought that it may induce psychosis and be a predisposition to mental illness. A user becomes both physically and psychologically addicted to the drug. Psilocybin is a hallucinogenic drug similar to LSD that originates from mushrooms.

Phencyclidine (PCP)

One of the most dangerous hallucinogenic drugs is phencyclidine, called PCP. This drug is often given the name of "angel dust" because users often think they can fly when under its influence. It is ingested by eating, smoking, and sniffing and is either a stimulant or a depressant. As it scrambles the brain's messages, it causes the user to become violent. Adverse side effects include violent behavior, respiratory depression, agitation, nausea, vomiting, and convulsions. A loss of memory that can last for weeks often transpires from PCP drug use.

Mescaline

The hallucinogenic drug mescaline is obtained from the peyote cactus. It produces psychosis and effects similar to LSD that last for four to eight hours. The likelihood of "bad trips" is not as prevalent with mescaline. However, this additive drug may leave the user with permanent psychosis and a constant craving for the drug.

BARBITURATES

Barbiturates are sedative drugs that depress the brain activity. If used over a long period of time, a physiological and physical dependency develops, along with a tolerance for the drug. If withdrawal occurs after four weeks of use, the user experiences stomach cramps, nausea, vomiting, twitching, convulsions, weakness, and sleeplessness. An overdose of the drug can result in delirium and a comatose state; it can also be fatal. If barbiturates are used with alcohol, the outcome is particularly harsh.

Barbiturates such as amobarbital, pentobarbital, and secobarbital are used today to treat sleeplessness and anxiety. Phenobarbital sometimes is given to dental patients who exhibit severe anxiety to dental treatment. This is especially true with the treatment of children. It is dispensed in a liquid and taken orally. Pentobarbital also is used in the treatment of epilepsy because it reduces the sensitivity of the brain to the abnormal electrical activity that brings on the seizures.

DRUGS PRESCRIBED

Dentists take great care in administering drugs. After discussing the condition with the patient, the dentist may prescribe or administer certain medications to alleviate treatment anxiety and discomfort. The dental assistant must record all prescriptions given to the patient, the route administered, and the information the doctor gave orally to the patient at the time of dispensing. A copy of the prescription should be placed in the patient's record indicating the dosage amount. Any other OTC drugs the dentist recommended to the patient should be noted on the patient's record as well.

Analgesics

Analgesic drugs (**anesthesia**) cause a loss of pain but not a loss of all sensation. Drugs that relieve pain can be non-narcotic, such as aspirin and acetaminophen, or narcotic, such as codeine and morphine. The non-narcotic analgesics are useful in the treatment of mild or moderate pain. If severe pain persists, a stronger narcotic analgesia is prescribed. Aspirin normally is not prescribed after a dental extraction because of its ability to thin blood and inhibit clotting. This effect is a contraindication for healing of the socket area following an extraction. Other side effects of aspirin are stomach irritation and nausea. Patients must be instructed to take aspirin with a large glass of water to ensure that the pill dissolves and does not irritate the stomach lining in a condensed form.

Side effects of the narcotic analgesics, such as nausea, vomiting, constipation, and breathing difficulties, are minimal but may still occur.

Tranquilizers

Drugs that provide a sedative effect fall in the category of tranquilizers. Tranquilizers relieve anxiety and allow the patient to undergo the procedure with reduced tension. Valium (diazepam) is often given to the patient orally a half-hour before the procedure to calm and relax the patient.

Antibiotics

A group of aminoglycosides, cephalosporins, penicillins, tetracyclines, and others are given to patients to treat infection. These drugs are derived from fungi and molds or are manufactured synthetically. Some of the antibiotics are **broad spectrum**, meaning they are effective against a wide range of bacteria, while some treat only one type of bacteria. At times, more than one type of antibiotic is prescribed in order to increase the probability of success in treatment of the disease. A culture can be taken to further identify the specific type of bacteria to be treated. The antibiotics are ineffective against viruses.

Normally, antibiotics are taken to treat infections, but they are often prescribed as a prophylactic measure to prevent infection. Any patient who has had rheumatic fever, joint replacement, heart valve replacement, or a heart murmur should take a dose of antibiotics prior to dental treatment to reduce the risk of endocarditis (inflammation of the lining of the heart).

Resistance to antibiotics can develop. This often occurs when the user fails to take the antibiotic drug as directed. The patient begins to feel better and stops taking the antibiotic before all the disease-causing bacteria have been killed. The bacteria then return stronger and more resistant to the antibiotic.

Adverse side effects of antibiotics include nausea, diarrhea, and an allergic rash. Patients can also kill normal body flora, causing oral, intestinal, or vaginal candidiasis (thrush). Some people also have severe allergic reactions with a rash, itching, swelling, and difficulty in breathing. If this happens, an antihistamine is used to counteract the reaction of the allergen.

Penicillin. **Penicillin** was the first group of antibiotic drugs to be discovered. It is still used in the treatment of many diseases, including tonsillitis, bronchitis, and pneumonia. Side effects of the drugs in this category are allergic reactions. If an individual becomes allergic to one type of penicillin, others in this group or any derivatives must be administered with great caution.

Erythromycin. **Erythromycin** is an antibiotic much like penicillin that can be used by individuals who are allergic to penicillin and given to children in place of tetracycline. It is a coated tablet so that it is not destroyed by the acid in the stomach when taken orally. It can be given in capsule or liquid form, injected, and by ointment. Side effects include stomach pain, nausea, vomiting, and diarrhea. It can produce a rash if the individual becomes hypersensitive to the substance.

Tetracycline. **Tetracycline** is a broad-spectrum drug, killing a wide range of bacterial microorganisms. It must be taken with care, taking one tablet one hour before meals or two hours after a meal. The drugs become useless if taken with some foods or dairy products. Tetracycline must not be given to children under twelve or to pregnant women because it discolors developing teeth. People with poor kidney function should not take tetracycline antibiotics, because they may cause kidney failure.

Side effects of tetracycline are much like those of the other antibiotics: nausea, vomiting, diarrhea, and possible rash, if allergic.

Antifungal Agents

A group of drugs prescribed to treat infections caused by fungi are antifungal agents. They are available in a number of forms, such as tablets, suspension, creams, injections, and vaginal suppositories. Preparations applied to the skin may show adverse reactions by increasing the irritation. Preparations taken orally may, in remote instances, show serious side effects of liver or kidney damage.

Nystatin. **Nystatin** is an antifungal drug used in dentistry to treat candidiasis (oral thrush). The suspension administered orally is held in the mouth prior to swallowing. It is safely taken during pregnancy. An individual should continue to take it forty-eight hours after the last sign of infection is apparent. Extremely high doses taken orally may cause nausea, vomiting, and diarrhea.

Anticholinergic

Anticholinergic drugs are used as pre-medications before general anesthesia to reduce secretion from the lungs and as emergency drugs to treat people with abnormally slow heart rates (bradycardia). They are also used to dilate the eyes during an ophthalmology examination.

Atropine. Atropine, an anticholinergic drug, is used in dentistry to inhibit the flow of saliva. A patient who produces excessive saliva may make it difficult for the dental team to obtain a good impression for crown or bridge treatment. If atropine is taken a couple of hours prior to treatment, the patient will have a dry mouth, which allows for a clearly defined impression to be obtained. This effect will disappear in four to six hours after the drug is administered.

CHAPTER SUMMARY

At no other time have drugs been so widely used/misused as they are today. The dental assistant will need to pay attention to the medical and dental history and carefully document the drugs used by the patient. The dental assistant will have to become knowledgeable about pharmacology, the side effects of drugs, and the interactions that take place when more than one drug is used. Dental assistants are concerned with the drugs that are prescribed, but they must also have knowledge about illegal drugs that patients may be involved in and what will happen if the two types of drugs interact. It also important to know the signs and symptoms that individuals may experience if under the influence of drugs. Background knowledge about drugs and their effects aids the dental assistant in providing better patient care.

CASE STUDY

Jordan Taylor, a twenty-year-old male, comes in because an upper anterior tooth is abscessed. He is a smoker and has just had a four shots of espresso (coffee) in a drink. He seems nervous about the upcoming treatment. Further information obtained from Jordan is that he also had two regular soft drinks and a candy bar within the past two hours.

Case Study Review

1. What reaction should the dental team expect from Jordan Taylor due to the drugs he has had recently?

2. Are these drugs stimulants or depressants?

3. Would giving other drugs to Jordan be a problem?

 To complete your study of this chapter, work the review activities that follow. Also, refer to the software that accompanies this text.

REVIEW QUESTIONS

Multiple Choice

1. The most commonly used resource to obtain information about drugs in the dental office is the
   a. *United States Pharmacopoeia.*
   b. *National Formulary.*
   c. *Dental Therapeutics.*
   d. *Physician's Desk Reference.*

2. Dental ointment that is placed on the mucosal surface is administered by which route?
   a. Sublingual.
   b. Oral.
   c. Topical.
   d. Intravenous.

3. A form of addictive depressants used to relieve pain are
   a. narcotics.
   b. amphetamines.
   c. hallucinogens.
   d. barbiturates.

4. The act that was established to identify drugs according to five schedules of abuse potential is
   a. Pure Food, Drug, and Cosmetic Act.
   b. Comprehensive Drug Abuse Prevention and Control Act of 1970.
   c. Occupational Safety Health Act.
   d. Controlled Substance Act.

5. If an antibiotic is said to be broad spectrum, it means that
   a. a culture can be taken to identify the type of microorganism.
   b. many microorganisms are resistant to it.
   c. it causes side effects such as nausea or an allergic rash.
   d. it is effective against a wide range of bacteria.

Critical Thinking

1. How does knowledge of illegal drugs assist the dental assistant in his or her career?

2. What are some of the side effects of tetracycline and when is it contraindicated?

3. If a patient has a heavy flow of saliva, what drug classification and what drug may be used during the impression phase of a crown preparation procedure?

Emergency Management CDA

OBJECTIVES

The student should strive to meet the following objectives and demonstrate an understanding of the facts and principles presented in this chapter:

1. Describe several emergency situations that may take place in the dental office. Explain how dental assistants can be prepared for these possibilities.

2. Describe the ABCs of CPR and demonstrate the skills associated with it.

3. Define the terms and anatomy used in the delivery of CPR. Determine if the patient is unconscious and demonstrate knowledge of opening the airway and when and how to deliver chest compressions.

4. Identify several causes of airway obstructions in the dental office. Demonstrate the ability to open the airway and to perform the Heimlich maneuver, manual and chest thrusts, and the finger sweep.

5. Identify the causes, signs, and treatments of the emergencies of syncope, asthma, allergic reactions, anaphylactic reaction, hyperventilation, epilepsy, diabetes mellitus, hypoglycemia, angina pectoris, myocardial infarction, congestive heart failure, and the stroke/cerebrovascular accident.

6. Identify several dental emergencies that a patient may have, such as abscessed tooth, alveolitis, avulsed tooth, broken prosthesis, soft tissue injury, broken tooth, and loose crown.

KEY TERMS

abscessed tooth (p. 234)

alkalosis (p. 229)

allergens (p. 228)

allergic reactions (p. 229)

allergy (p. 228)

alveolitis (p. 234)

anaphylactic shock (p. 229)

angina pectoris (p. 231)

angioedema (p. 229)

antibodies (p. 228)

antigens (p. 228)

antihistamines (p. 228)

arteriosclerosis (p. 231)

bronchioles (p. 228)

cardiopulmonary resuscitation (CPR) (p. 220)

cerebral embolism (p. 232)

cerebral hemorrhage (p. 232)

cerebral infarction (p. 232)

congestive heart failure (p. 232)

diabetes mellitus (p. 230)

edema (p. 229)

epilepsy (p. 229)

erythema (p. 229)

foreign body airway obstruction (FBAO) (p. 224)

gingival hyperplasia (p. 230)

grand mal seizure (p. 230)

hemiplegia (p. 233)

hyperventilation (p. 229)

inhaler (p. 228)

Jacksonian epilepsy (p. 230)

myocardial infarction (p. 232)

oral hypoglycemics (p. 231)

partial seizures (p. 230)

petit mal seizure (p. 230)

status epilepticus (p. 230)

sternum (p. 220)

stroke (p. 232)

sublingually (p. 231)

syncope (p. 227)

transient ischemic attacks (p. 233)

Trendelenburg position (p. 220)

unconscious (p. 227)

universal distress signal (p. 225)

urticaria (p. 229)

INTRODUCTION

Emergencies can happen at any place at any time. Even though members of the dental profession try to make dentistry as comfortable as possible, patients feel stress about dental care, and this can increase the possibility of an emergency occurring in the dental office. Other factors that did not exist in the past to the same degree that may increase the incidence of an emergency are advancements in medical care, increase in drug therapy, increase in street drugs, elderly patients seeking dental treatment, and longer dental appointments.

Advancements in medical care have allowed treatments that were not available in the past. A patient seeking dental treatment may have a heart or liver transplant or pacemaker or be taking any number of drug therapies. Many patients, especially elderly patients, take more than one drug. Other patients take one or more street drugs prior to dental treatment. Any drugs given in the dental office for treatment may interact with the drug therapy or street drugs taken by the patient, therefore causing an emergency situation. Another contributing factor to the increased likelihood of emergencies is the length of appointments. Most patients would rather sit for longer appointments and have more complex dentistry completed at one time to accommodate their busy schedules. The dental offices are also more productive when longer appointments are scheduled, because less time is wasted removing barriers and practicing aseptic techniques before and after several shorter appointments. These lengthy appointments may overtax the patient's ability to remain comfortable, therefore causing more anxiety and stress, leading to an emergency situation.

Even though the number of emergencies is not great in a dental office, the dental assistant must always be observant of the patient and be prepared to deal with emergencies. Additionally, emergencies may happen to the dentist and to other dental assistants and staff.

Routine Preparedness for Dental Team Members

When an emergency arises, the dental team must react with an automatic response. Any hesitation at such a time could cost a life. A routine response should be established. Details such as who should call for emergency help and written directions on how to locate the office should be predetermined and posted close to the phone. Providing medical response teams with specific directions regarding the office location, including which door to enter, will save valuable time during the emergency response.

The Dental Assistant's Role in Emergency Care

The dental assistant has a vital role in prevention of emergencies and emergency care. First, the assistant closely observes the patient while escorting him or her from the waiting room to the dental treatment room. Does the patient have difficulty moving? Do the patient's eyes respond to light? Is the patient's speech slurred? Does the patient indicate anxiety about the dental treatment? Look for signs of concern. Many of these signs will be covered up after the patient is seated, the anesthetic is given, and the dental dam is placed. Any areas of concern should be reported to the dentist prior to starting dental care. The patient's medical history should be reviewed as a matter of routine procedure. It is crucial that the dental team have knowledge of any changes in the patient's health. The dental assistant must be alert to any area of concern, because he or she will more than likely be the first one to suspect a possible emergency.

Another role of the dental assistant is to stay well trained for an emergency. Ideally, the dentist and dental assistants will establish a definitive plan to render treatment in an emergency situation. Often, this training takes place in a staff meeting or at a seminar. All members of the dental team should have current cardiopulmonary resuscitation (CPR) cards and have continuing training and updated knowledge of emergency situations. The dental assistant should know the answers to the following questions in order to ensure competency in dealing with emergencies:

▶ Where is the emergency kit and who will retrieve it?

▶ Who will take and monitor vital signs?

▶ Who will retrieve and administer oxygen?

▶ When will the call for help be placed and by whom?

▶ Who will perform basic life support, if needed?

▶ Who will review the medical history of the individual?

If any of these questions cannot be answered quickly by the dental team, training is needed. Once the emergency takes place, the attention to the patient's condition will take precedence. All personnel must perform their tasks in a timely manner to ensure that the best treatment is administered.

DENTAL OFFICE EMERGENCY KIT

Every dental office should have an up-to-date emergency kit (Figure 13-1). A dentist may choose to design his or her own. This kit must be arranged for the specific needs of the practice. Other kits are manufactured for use in dental offices and can be obtained from a dental supply company. These are normally color coded for easy equipment and drug access. All dental emergency kits should include:

▶ Sterile syringes, tourniquets, tracheotomy needle, barrier devices for delivery of CPR, and several oral airway devices.

FIGURE 13-1 Example of a dental office emergency kit.

▶ Oxygen inhalation equipment, if office does not have nitrous/oxygen equipment in each treatment room (Figure 13-2).

▶ Stimulants (ammonia inhalants, thin glass vials of ammonia covered with a strong gauze fabric that can be broken easily).

▶ Vasodilators that will increase oxygenated blood supply to heart (such as nitroglycerin, translingual nitroglycerin, or amyl-nitrite inhalants).

▶ Antihistamine drugs (such as adrenaline-epinephrine, Benadryl-antihistamine, solu-corticosteroid, or aminophyline-bronchodilator). An epi-pin (a two-dose syringe of epinephrine) is recommended for quick and easy delivery.

▶ Vasopressor to increase blood pressure (such as Wyamine™).

▶ Analgesics for pain (such as Talwin™).

▶ Depressants for convulsions (such as Diazepam™).

▶ Vagal blockers to increase pulse rate (such as Atropine™).

This kit should be labeled and located in an easily accessible place so that it can be quickly obtained. A crash cart with oxygen and emergency equipment can be utilized for quick access. Time is an extremely important factor in treating emergencies. The kit should be well organized so that the assistant or dentist can find the necessary items at a glance. All items should be labeled with information pertinent to their uses and dosages. A periodic inspection of the emergency items is essential. Many of the drugs have shelf lives and need to be replaced annually. A sphygmomanometer and stethoscope are essential parts of the emergency kit to monitor the vital signs.

Oxygen inhalation equipment must be readily available as well. The oxygen tanks are green and must be stored upright and secure. Administration of oxygen may be the most important factor in caring for the patient until medical help arrives. Even though the dental team is well trained in emergencies, a medical response team should be contacted immediately if the patient becomes unconscious.

FIGURE 13-2 Oxygen inhalation equipment for use in dental emergency. *(Courtesy of Mada Medical Products, Inc.)*

13-1 Administration of Oxygen

Many dental assistants may routinely administer oxygen in conjunction with the nitrous oxide gas under the supervision of the dentist. This system is most often brought into the dental treatment room through a wall-piped system. In some instances, the tanks may be on a mobile unit that is brought into the treatment area. The dental assistant should know where the system is located and how to administer oxygen during an emergency.

EQUIPMENT AND SUPPLIES

▶ Oxygen tank with gauge at top or gauge in the dental treatment area

▶ Oxygen mask and tubing

PROCEDURE STEPS (*Follow aseptic procedures*)

1. Position the patient comfortably in a supine or **Trendelenburg position**.

NOTE: The Trendelenburg position is a supine position with the feet elevated above chest level.

2. Explain the procedure to the patient and reassure the patient that everything is being taken care of (if an emergency should occur).

3. Place the oxygen mask over the patient's nose and drape the tubing on either side of the face. The mask may need to be adjusted so that it is secure over the nose.

4. Start the flow of oxygen immediately. It should flow at two to four liters per minute.

5. Instruct the patient to breath through his or her nose and have the mouth remain closed.

6. Continue to calm the patient by talking softly in reassuring tones.

CARDIOPULMONARY RESUSCITATION (CPR)

If the patient has a sudden cardiac arrest or progresses to this condition, **cardiopulmonary resuscitation (CPR)** is necessary to help the person survive. If the patient becomes unconscious, the first step is to immediately call for emergency medical care. ***Phone first and phone fast!*** After calling for help, start CPR. The technique of CPR is easy to remember if you follow the ABCs.

The ABCs of CPR

"A" stands for **airway**. After determining that the patient is unconscious and calling for help, the airway must be opened. If the patient is in a supine position on a firm surface, CPR can be administered more effectively. If the patient is in the dental chair, adjust the chair so that the operator has the access needed (clear pathway and correct height). Tilt the head backward and lift the chin. This process lifts the tongue and epiglottis from the back of the throat and opens the airway.

The rescuer places his or her ear and face close to the adult patient's mouth while looking for the patient's chest to rise and fall. The rescuer *looks* for the chest to rise and fall, *listens* for air exchange, and *feels* for any breath. **"B"** stands for **breathing**. The patient may begin breathing, but, if not, the rescuer administers two slow breaths (one-and-one-half to two seconds per breath for an adult and one to one-and-one-half seconds per breath for a child).

The rescuer watches for the chest to rise and waits for the exhalation between breaths.

"C" is for **circulation**, which is the next step in CPR. The rescuer checks the carotid pulse. If the patient has a pulse, the rescuer continues breathing at a rate of one breath every five seconds or about twelve breaths per minute (one breath every three seconds or about twenty per minute for a child one to eight years of age). If the patient does not have a pulse, a cycle of fifteen chest compressions are given at a rate of eighty to 100 per minute (about 100 per minute for a child one to eight years of age). The lower third of the **sternum** (breastbone) is located, the heels of the rescuer's hands (one on top of the other with the fingers interlocked) are placed on the lower third of the sternum and compressions begin. The breastbone must be compressed downward about one-and-one-half to two inches (one or one-and-one-half inches for a child aged one to eight). Counting one and, two and, three and, etc. helps establish a rhythm and a total count. After every fifteen compressions, deliver two more slow breaths. Repeat this cycle four times and then check the pulse. If no pulse is found, continue another four cycles of fifteen compressions and two breaths and then recheck the pulse. This process continues until medical help arrives.

With the advances in technology, a "D" is being added to the ABCs of CPR. **"D"** stands for **defibrillation** and requires additional equipment (Figure 13-5). If the site has an automated defibrillator, it increases the chances of survival for patients who have cardiac arrest. The equipment guides the user. The equipment's voice system indicates

P R O C E D U R E

13-2 Rescue Breathing for Adults

If an emergency occurs, the dental assistant must be prepared to respond to a patient who ceases breathing and/or to assist the dentist in rescue breathing for a patient.

EQUIPMENT AND SUPPLIES

▶ Resuscitation mouthpiece

▶ Gloves (latex or vinyl–optional)

PROCEDURE STEPS *(Follow aseptic procedures)*

1. Determine if the patient is responding. Ask, "Are you okay?"

2. If the patient gives no response, have someone call emergency services. (If alone, call quickly and return to the patient.)

3. Don gloves (if possible). Look, listen, and feel for breathing.

4. If the patient is not breathing, tilt back the head, lift the chin, position the resuscitation mouthpiece, and close the nose by pinching it together (Figure 13-3A).

5. Give two slow breaths. Watch the chest gently rise while the breaths are being given. Turn your face to the side and listen and watch for air to return.

6. Check the pulse on the carotid artery, the side closest to you. Use the forefinger and the middle finger to palpate the pulse (Figure 13-3B).

7. If a pulse is present but the patient is not breathing, give one slow breath every five seconds. Continue to do this for one minute (twelve times).

8. Recheck the pulse and breathing after each twelve breaths or each minute.

9. Continue rescue breathing for as long as the pulse remains. If the pulse ceases, begin CPR. If the pulse remains, continue rescue breathing until breathing is restored or until someone else arrives and takes over.

10. Dispose of the resuscitation mouthpiece in a biohazard container. Remove gloves and wash hands.

11. Document what was done on the patient's chart.

 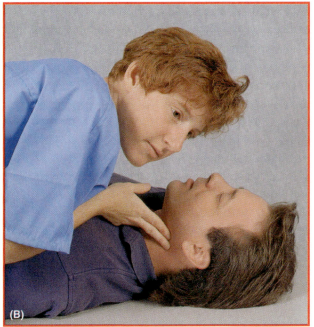

FIGURE 13-3 (A) Tilt head back, lift chin, and pinch nose closed. (B) Use the forefinger and middle finger to check the pulse at the carotid artery.

13-3 CPR for an Adult, One Rescuer

If an emergency occurs, the dental assistant must be prepared to respond to breathing and/or cardiac arrest and perform CPR or to assist the dentist in performing CPR.

EQUIPMENT AND SUPPLIES

▶ Recuscitation mouthpiece

▶ Gloves (latex or vinyl)

PROCEDURE STEPS *(Follow aseptic procedures)*

1. Assess the patient's condition. Ask the patient, "Are you okay?"

2. If he or she gives no response, have someone call emergency services. (If no one is available, call for emergency services immediately and return to the patient.)

3. Wash hands (if possible). Place on gloves (if possible).

4. Look, listen, and feel for breathing. If the patient is not breathing, continue to Step 5.

5. Tilt the head back and lift the chin. Insert the mouthpiece and pinch the nose closed (Figure 13-3A).

6. Give two breaths and watch the chest rise.

7. Check the pulse (for ten to fifteen seconds) at the carotid artery (Figure 13-3B).

8. If the patient does not have a pulse, start chest compressions.

9. Locate the area on the chest, two inches above the xiphoid process (Figure 13-4A).

10. Position hands on top of each other and position your shoulders over your hands. Compress the chest fifteen times at a rate of eighty to 100 per minute (Figure 13-4B).

11. Follow with two slow breaths (Figure 13-4C).

12. Continue for four cycles of breaths and compressions.

13. Check the pulse at the carotid artery. If no pulse is apparent, continue for four cycles and then repeat.

14. Continue until the patient is revived or another person takes over.

15. Dispose of the resuscitation mouthpiece.

16. Document the emergency information and procedure on the patient's chart.

(A)

(B)

(C)

FIGURE 13-4 (A) Locate the area on the breastbone two inches below the xiphoid process. (B) Position hands on top of each other and position shoulders over your hands. Compress the chest fifteen times. (C) Follow with two slow breaths.

PROCEDURE

13-4 Operating an Automated External Defibrillation (AED) Unit

Health professionals may have a defibrillator available within the facility for emergencies.

EQUIPMENT AND SUPPLIES

▶ Gloves (latex or vinyl–optional)

▶ Automated external defibrillation (AED) unit (Figure 13-5)

PROCEDURE STEPS *(Follow aseptic procedures)*

▶ If there is no pulse, follow the ABCs of CPR.

▶ Perform CPR until the defibrillator is attached.

1. Press "analyze" on the defibrillation unit.

2. Follow each step as the unit instructs.

3. Attach the AED to the patient as indicated by instructions on the lip of the unit.

4. State loudly, "Everybody clear of the patient!" Verify that everyone is clear of the patient and press the analysis control switch on the AED. The assessment takes ten to twenty seconds depending on the brand of AED. Everyone should remain clear during this time.

5. If the device indicates that a shock is not advised, resume CPR.

6. Once the unit begins charging, a synthesized voice message or light indicator indicates that it is charging. Assume that ventricular fibrillation (VF/VT) is present and that the AED will indicate the need to deliver a shock.

7. Verify that everyone is clear of the unit. The AED delivers shocks without additional actions from the operator. It may indicate "shock now."

8. Give three consecutive shocks.

9. Check the pulse.

10. If a pulse is present, assess the vital signs, support airway, and breathing.

11. If no pulse is present, give CPR for one minute.

12. Check the pulse. If it is not present, press "analyze" on the AED.

13. Defibrillate up to three times.

14. If VF persists after nine shocks, repeat sets of three stacked shocks with one minute of CPR between each set until the "no shock indicated" message is received on the AED or until the patient is revived.

FIGURE 13-5 An automated defibrillator increases the chances of survival for patients who have cardiac arrest. (A) Transportable defibrillator. (B) Machine with electrodes ready for placement. *(Courtesy of Medtronic Physio-Control)*

when and where the electrodes are to be placed. The electrodes are only placed if the patient is unconscious, not breathing, and has no pulse.

FOREIGN BODY AIRWAY OBSTRUCTION (FBAO)

The body depends on oxygen availability to function. Oxygen is an odorless, tasteless, and colorless gas that is essential for life. In the dental office, incidents of airway obstruction are greater than other possible emergencies. The patient is lying in a supine position, therefore allowing objects to be propelled naturally down the throat. The moisture from saliva and blood makes objects more slippery and harder to hold. Also, the use of a number of items and materials in the mouth allows for a greater possibility of foreign body airway obstruction (FBAO). A patient may take a breath at a time when a tooth is being removed, thereby dislodging it from the forceps and allowing it to fall directly into the airway. Other items causing FBAO are crowns, amalgam, composite, cotton

PROCEDURE

13-5 Heimlich Maneuver for a Conscious Adult

If an adult is conscious and has a blocked airway, the rescuer can talk to him or her and perform the Heimlich maneuver to open up the blocked airway.

EQUIPMENT AND SUPPLIES

▶ No equipment required

PROCEDURE STEPS (*Follow aseptic procedures*)

1. Verify that the patient is choking. Ask, "Are you choking?"

2. If the patient is standing, tell him or her what the procedure is going to be, position yourself behind the patient, and proceed to wrap arms around the patient's abdomen.

3. Place the thumb side of a fisted hand against the middle of the abdomen, just above the umbilicus (Figure 13-6).

4. Grasp hands together, keeping one hand fisted and the other wrapped on top of it.

5. Give quick, upward thrusts with hands against the abdomen (Figure 13-7).

6. Repeat the procedure until the patient expels the object or until the patient becomes unconscious.

7. Wash hands.

8. Document the procedure.

FIGURE 13-6 The thumb side of your fist is placed against the middle of the abdomen, just above the umbilicus.

FIGURE 13-7 Quick, upward thrusts are given against the abdomen.

rolls, gauze, endodontic instruments, and impression material. The person may begin choking and clutch the throat with the hands, which is the **universal distress signal** (Figure 13-8). Ask, "Are you choking?" The first action is to stop treatment, sit the patient upright, and encourage him or her to cough. If the patient cannot expel the foreign body, the rescuer goes behind the patient and wraps his or her arms around the patient's waist. Tightly wrap one hand over the other, fisted hand and, with a quick movement, give upward thrusts into the patient's abdomen. This procedure is referred to as the **Heimlich maneuver**. If the patient is in the final stages of pregnancy or obese, the rescuer stands behind, wraps his or her arms under the patient's armpits, and gives quick, inward chest thrusts. If the rescuer is unable to do this technique and the patient is still conscious, have the patient lie over a chair back to force air from the abdomen and help him or her expel the foreign body.

If the patient becomes unconscious, lay the patient on the floor and immediately activate emergency medical services (EMS). Look into the oral cavity of the patient and, with a hooked finger, sweep deeply from one side to the other in order to remove the foreign body. Attempt to give the patient two slow breaths. If unable to do this, reposition the head and chin to see if rescue breathing can be accomplished. If the airway remains obstructed, perform the chest thrust maneuver on the patient by

FIGURE 13-8 Holding hands to the throat is the universal distress signal for choking.

P R O C E D U R E

13-6 Abdominal Thrusts for an Unconscious Adult with Airway Obstruction

If an adult is unconscious and has a blocked airway, the rescuer performs abdominal thrusts to open up the blocked airway.

EQUIPMENT AND SUPPLIES

▶ Gloves

▶ Resuscitation device

PROCEDURE STEPS *(Follow aseptic procedures)*

1. If the patient is unconscious, activate EMS immediately.

2. Lay the person on his or her back.

3. Perform the tongue-jaw lift followed by a finger sweep to remove the object (Figure 13-9A).

(A)

FIGURE 13-9 (A) Perform the tongue-jaw lift followed by a finger sweep to remove the object.

(continued)

4. Open the airway, place the resuscitation device, and try to ventilate (Figures 13-9B and C). If the airway is still obstructed, reposition the patient's head and try to ventilate again.

5. Place the heel of hand against the person's abdomen (Figure 13-9D).

6. Kneel astride the patient's thighs. Give up to five abdominal thrusts in a motion toward the diaphragm (Figure 13-9E).

7. Repeat Steps 3 through 6 until effective or help arrives.

FIGURE 13-9 (B) Open the airway. (C) Attempt to ventilate. (D) Place the heel of your hand against the person's abdomen. (E) Apply five abdominal thrusts.

straddling the patient's thighs and pressing into the abdomen with quick, upward thrusts. Place hands below the tip of the xiphoid notch (lowest portion of the sternum) and above the patient's navel. Place the heel of one hand on the victim's abdomen and the second hand on top of the first to deliver the thrusts. If this is not successful after three to five thrusts, repeat the sequence.

CAUSES, SIGNS, AND TREATMENT OF EMERGENCIES

If an anxious or a fearful patient has heart problems, his or her heart may be beating rapidly and working harder, precipitating a heart attack. Patients may become lightheaded as they see instruments in the dental treatment room and anticipate the procedures. These patients may react by **syncope** (fainting) (see Table 13-1 on page 233).

Syncope

The most common and least life-threatening emergency that may occur in the dental office is the vasodepressor syncope, commonly known as fainting. This loss of consciousness is caused by a decrease in blood flow to the brain. Syncope is normally caused by some form of stress, either emotional, physical, or both. When a patient experiences stress, the body reacts by pumping large amounts of blood to the arms and legs. This response (often referred to as the "fight or flight syndrome") is so that the patients can quickly respond by moving their bodies. Dental patients often remain motionless, so their blood pools in the arms and legs and the cerebral blood flow is diminished. As a result, the brain is deprived of oxygenated blood and the patient becomes **unconscious** (unable to respond to any sensory stimulation).

The patient may feel dizzy, nauseated, or extremely weak prior to syncope. The patient appears pale and clammy and breathes in shallow gasps. If the patient indicates that he or she is feeling faint, remain calm, quickly sit the patient down, and lean his or her head forward and place it between the knees. If a fainting person is unconscious and breathing normally, lay him or her down in the Trendelenburg position (Figure 13-10). This position allows the blood to flow back to the head. If the patient is not breathing normally, establish an airway by tipping the head back and performing a chin lift. At this

P R O C E D U R E

13-7 Treatment of a Patient with Syncope

Dental assistants must be prepared to treat syncope in the dental office. Often, patients will have syncope in the treatment room while in the dental chair, but it may happen anywhere in the office. The dental assistant should keep the patient in the Trendelenburg position.

EQUIPMENT AND SUPPLIES

▶ Oxygen tank with gauge at top or gauge in the dental treatment area

▶ Oxygen mask and tubing

▶ Spirits of ammonia

PROCEDURE STEPS (*Follow aseptic procedures*)

1. Position the patient in a supine or Trendelenburg position (supine with feet elevated to increase blood flow to the brain). If the patient is wearing a dress or other garments that are misplaced during the syncope, attend to modesty issues as soon as possible.

2. Establish that the airway is open. If it is not, perform the head-tilt, chin-lift to open the airway.

3. Breathing normally begins spontaneously within the first ten to fifteen seconds.

4. Administer oxygen as a precaution treatment only.

5. If the patient has not revived within the first fifteen seconds, remove the oxygen mask (if one has been placed) and pass a broken ammonia gauze sponge under the patient's nose for one or two seconds only. (Holding the ammonia for a long period of time under the patient's nose may cause undue irritation.)

6. The patient will normally respond rapidly to the pungent odor of the ammonia and take in a breath of air, therefore receiving oxygen.

7. Full revival of the patient should occur within a minute or two.

8. If revival of the patient does not occur, follow the guidelines of CPR.

9. Postpone dental treatment and call for patient transportation.

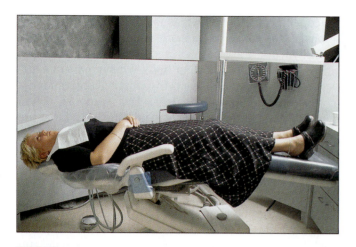

FIGURE 13-10 The Trendelenburg position (supine position with the feet elevated slightly).

time, any tight, constricting clothing or jewelry can be loosened or removed around the neck area.

Administer oxygen and monitor vital signs. The patient will normally resume breathing in less than ten seconds. If the patient becomes unconscious, break a vial of **spirits of ammonia** and pass it under the patient's nose. The strong odor of the ammonia causes the patient to quickly inhale, which stimulates breathing. This gauze-covered ammonia vial is very strong, so only pass it under the patient's nostrils a couple of times and *do not* leave it in a place where it can cause irritation to the nasal passage membranes. The patient normally will revive totally within a couple of minutes but may remain weak. It is best to reschedule dental treatment and contact someone to drive the patient home. If the patient does not revive from the unconscious state, call for emergency help, closely monitor breathing, and begin CPR, if necessary, until help arrives.

Asthma

Recurrent attacks of breathlessness accompanied by wheezing while breathing out and often a dry cough are symptoms of asthma. The wheezing and breathlessness are due to the narrowing of small airways in the lungs (**bronchioles**). When a patient with asthma exhales, the lungs collapse to expel the air, causing the bronchioles to further narrow and making it more difficult to breathe. If the lining of the bronchioles is inflamed, sputum (phlegm) is produced, making the bronchioles further obstructed, increasing the difficulty of breathing.

Asthma is becoming more prevalent. Normally, the disease occurs during childhood, but the symptoms improve in adulthood. Approximately one in ten children in the United States have asthma. Heredity is a major factor in the development of the disease. Asthma may be caused by an allergy to a substance. An **allergy** is an exaggerated reaction of the immune system to an offending agent. Upon the first contact with the agent,

the body becomes sensitized to it and develops **antibodies** (also called immunoglobulins) to fight these **antigens** (foreign bodies). The second or subsequent time that the body has contact with these offending agents, it overreacts in a **hypersensitive** manner. The most common **allergens** (the antigens that trigger the allergic reaction) responsible for asthma are animal fur, house dust, pollens, tobacco smoke, feathers, food, and drugs.

Asthma attacks are more frequent in the morning and vary from slight breathlessness to respiratory failure. There is no cure for asthma, but tests are available to identify what causes the most severe reactions in an individual so the individual can avoid it. **Immunotherapy** (injection of the allergen) can be a treatment choice, and corticosteroid drugs also provide successful therapy.

Antihistamines are often used to treat the physical symptoms produced by the antigen. These drugs counteract the body's production of histamine. They are administered with an **inhaler**, a pressurized canister with a mouthpiece (Figures 13-11A and B). The patient carries an inhaler and, when an asthma attack is anticipated, the drug can be dispensed. The patient should bring an inhaler to any dental treatment appointment. If the patient has an attack and an inhaler is unavailable, the dentist may use the bronchodilator from the emergency kit. The drug of choice in this bronchodilator (inhaler) is *albuterol,* because it widens the bronchioles and improves air flow but does not stimulate the cardiovascular system like the drug epinephrine would. To use the bronchodilator, the patient exhales first, then takes a slow, deep breath while releasing the drug as the canister is depressed. After two dispensed amounts are taken, breathing should improve within fifteen minutes. If the patient does not improve, the inhaler is used

Exhale first

Inhale slowly while depressing the canister

(A) (B)

FIGURE 13-11 (A) Inhaler or nebulizer. (B) Inhalation of bronchodilator drug from inhaler.

again. If this does not alleviate the condition, emergency services should be deployed to take the patient to the hospital. While waiting for the emergency services, the dental office team should administer oxygen and reassure and calm the patient. The patient should also be instructed to see his or her general physician.

Allergic Reactions

A number of other **allergic reactions** may take place in the dental office. The body may react to drugs, toothpaste, latex protein, or a number of the dental materials. Keep in mind that these exaggerated reactions of the immune system occur only subsequent to exposures to the offending antigen. The hypersensitive reaction may vary in symptoms and severity. It may be localized or cover the entire body. It could occur immediately or several hours after exposure to the antigen. Dermatitis, or skin reaction, may occur. If a skin reaction is apparent, dental treatment ceases until the irritant is removed.

Examples of skin reactions include:

▶ **Edema** (eh-**DEE**-mah), or swelling

▶ **Erythema (**er-ih-**THEE**-mah), or redness

▶ Vesicle formation

▶ **Urticaria** (ur-tih-**KAY**-ree-ah), or hives

▶ Giant urticaria, or **angioedema** (**an**-jee-oh-eh-**DEE**-muh), poorly defined, single swelling areas

Treatment for both urticaria and angioedema is to remove the irritant. In some cases, the dentist will administer an antihistamine to reduce the edema.

Anaphylactic Reaction

Anaphylactic shock is a severe allergic reaction that is life threatening. It occurs in people who are extremely sensitive to a particular allergen. This may happen to a patient who has been administered local anesthetic or has taken penicillin. Once the allergen is in the blood stream, the body produces large amounts of histamine and other chemicals. The blood pressure drops, bronchospasm (constriction of the airways in the lungs) occurs, the tongue and throat swell, and the person experiences stomach pain. All of these symptoms come on rapidly and a injection of epinephrine must be administered immediately to save the patient's life. Patients who know they are extremely sensitive to some allergens (bee sting venom, for example) may carry antihistamine drugs and take immunotherapy treatment to desensitize for the allergen.

Hyperventilation

Dealing with the patient's anxiety prior to treatment alleviates fear and distress and, hopefully, reduces the chance of **hyperventilation**. Children normally do not experience hyperventilation because they can more readily express their concerns about dentistry. However, because adult patients may try to hide their fears, their anxiety can result in hyperventilation. They start to breathe deeply and rapidly, not realizing that they are breathing differently. When they continue in this manner, they experience a numbness in the extremities, faintness, and a sense of inability to take a full breath. A loss of carbon dioxide from the blood, causing **alkalosis** (increase in blood alkalinity), occurs. The patient panics and breathing speeds up. This is hyperventilation.

To treat the patient, first stop all dental treatment. Sit the patient upright to allow easier breathing and then calm him or her. Tell the patient what is happening and encourage him or her to breathe in and hold it several seconds before exhaling. This process allows more carbon dioxide to get into the blood. If the patient is too agitated to follow instructions, instruct the patient to breathe into cupped hands or a paper sack (Figure 13-12). This allows the correct levels of carbon dioxide and oxygen to return to normal.

Epilepsy/Seizure Disorder

Human emotions and thoughts normally occur in an organized, methodical, electrical excitation of nerve cells in the brain. With **epilepsy**, an unorganized and chaotic electrical discharge occurs. Seizures may appear spontaneously or as a result of a stimuli, such as a flashing light. The symptoms of the seizures may range from insignificant to severe. It is estimated that one person in every 200 suffers from epilepsy. Many

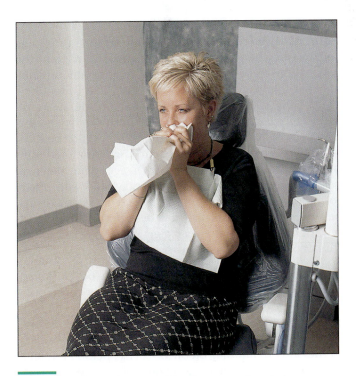

FIGURE 13-12 Patient breathing in a paper bag to increase carbon dioxide in body.

wear bracelets or carry identification cards. Epileptics should advise colleagues what to do in the case of a seizure.

The dentist will utilize fixed appliances, if feasible, when treating patients who experience seizures due to epilepsy. During an epileptic seizure, the muscles tighten and the person has no control over movements. A loose dental appliance may become dislodged or broken, obstructing the airway during a seizure.

Some identified causes of epilepsy are head injury, infections, fever, brain tumor, strokes, metabolic imbalance, and drug and alcohol withdrawal states. However, the causes of the majority of cases are unknown. Heredity is known to play a factor. Types of seizures are classified in three general categories: grand mal, petit mal, and partial seizures.

Grand Mal Seizure.

The **grand mal seizure** (tonic clonic seizure) is the most common. During this seizure, which lasts two to five minutes, the person becomes unconscious and the body jerks, twitches, and stiffens. Breathing is often irregular. Once the seizure subsides, bladder and bowel control may be lost as the muscles relax. The person may be disoriented and exhausted, normally with no memory of the seizure. He or she may want to sleep. After the seizure, reassure the patient. If the patient experiences one seizure after another, called **status epilepticus** (continuous seizures), emergency services should be summoned.

> **NOTE:** About 10 percent of patients experiencing status epilepticus will die due to the body's inability to deal with this overexertion.

Petit Mal Seizure.

The **petit mal seizure** (absence seizure) is where a person experiences a momentary loss of consciousness. The patient may exhibit a blank stare or blinking of the eyes that lasts five to ten seconds. Others around the person may not be aware of the seizure because of the lack of abnormal movements. The person may appear inattentive or seem to be daydreaming. Absence seizures occur in children and normally decrease in frequency with age. The absence seizure may occur several times a day and with other forms of seizures. Often, prior to having a grand mal seizure, a petit mal seizure may be experienced first, as a warning. A person then can alert someone prior to the loss of consciousness.

Partial Seizure.

Partial seizures can be classified into two categories: simple (person remains conscious) and complex (person becomes unconscious). The simple partial seizure is referred to as **Jacksonian epilepsy**. As a twitching occurs and spreads slowly from one part of the body to another on one side, the person remains conscious and is able to recall details of the event. During a complex seizure, a person remembers very little and exhibits involuntary actions, such as lip smacking, as the twitching spreads from one part of the body to another on one side. If the seizure develops into total body, it is then referred to as a grand mal seizure.

To prevent seizures, a person should try to eliminate times of extreme stress and fatigue. Anti-convulsant drugs are the first line of treatment for epilepsy and may minimize the seizures. Side effects of the drugs are fatigue and loss of concentration. Some of the drugs (such as dilantin) cause **gingival hyperplasia**, or overgrowth of gingiva tissue. This thick, granular tissue may cover the teeth and have to be surgically removed.

Treatment for Patients Who Experience Seizures.

When patients experience seizures, stop dental treatment and remove everything from the oral cavity. Also, remove items from the area that could harm the person. Normally, no further action is necessary. The seizure runs its course. Do not restrain the person or place anything in the patient's mouth. Once the seizures have ceased, place the patient in the recovery position (on the right side with the airway open). Always be cognizant of the person's dignity and treat him or her in a considerate manner. The patient may feel embarrassed and reassurance is important. If the seizures continue for more than five minutes or continue one after another, summon emergency help and reassure the patient.

Diabetes Mellitus

The cause of **diabetes mellitus** was discovered in the 1920s: The pancreas produced an insufficient amount of or no **insulin** (the hormone responsible for absorbing glucose into the cells for energy and into the liver and fat cells for storage). Therefore, the level of glucose in the blood becomes high, which causes thirst and excessive urination. In addition, the body cannot store glucose for the vast number of cells in the body that need glucose to survive. The body normally experiences weight loss and fatigue. Diabetes mellitus is classified in two categories: Type I and Type II.

Type I Diabetes Mellitus.

Type I diabetes mellitus, the more severe, normally occurs in people between the ages of ten and sixteen. Type I is often termed juvenile diabetes due to the age at which it commonly affects people. However, the condition also can occur in older people. It is known that heredity is a factor in the disease. It can pass from one generation to another or miss a generation. There is a theory that the mumps virus may damage the cells of the pancreas, thereby bringing on diabetes. Insulin-dependent diabetes mellitus (Type I) develops rapidly when the insulin-secreting cells in the pancreas become ineffective. If the person does not have regular injections of insulin, he or she could lapse into a coma. Individuals with Type I diabetes mellitus (about ten percent of diabetes cases) experience the most medical complications because they have the disease for such long periods of time. Thus, the disease has to be monitored very carefully.

Type II Diabetes Mellitus. **Type II diabetes mellitus** was first referred to as adult-onset diabetes until it also was identified in the younger population. Type II, making up ninety percent of diabetes mellitus cases, normally is diagnosed in obese, middle-aged people. It can be controlled with diet and **oral hypoglycemics** (medications that lower blood sugar levels) and does not require insulin injections.

Disturbances in the balance of glucose intake and insulin can result in hyperglycemia (too much glucose in the blood). The onset is slow and the person experiences early symptoms days prior to the onset, such as increased thirst, increased urination, nausea/vomiting with abdominal pains, loss of appetite, fatigue, and pain. If these patients (possibly undiagnosed diabetics) are having dental treatment, they could go into diabetic comas. If a patient reacts in this manner, stop dental treatment; if the patient is conscious, have him or her administer an insulin shot. If the patient becomes unconscious, call for emergency help and transfer him or her to a medical facility as soon as possible. One of the most serious consequences of hyperglycemia, a condition in which the patient goes into a coma and dies if not treated, is **diabetic acidosis**. This condition occurs when the patient has too much sugar (glucose) and not enough insulin. The body in this condition produces acids, and the body's pH is lowered. The body's pH range is 7.35 to 7.45. If the body's pH drops below 7.0, diabetic acidosis may occur.

Today, more is known about diabetics, and patients are diagnosed more readily and therefore deal with the symptoms before the diabetes gets to the later stage, such as diabetic coma. Some patients have insulin pens or portable pumps that inject insulin if needed (Figure 13-13). Individuals can test their urine and blood for glucose levels.

Hypoglycemia

Too little glucose or sugar causes a person to experience **hypoglycemia**. This condition comes on rapidly and the

FIGURE 13-13 (A) Insulin pen. (B) Portable insulin pump.

patient becomes nervous, shows signs of trembling and weakness, and has cold sweats. The patient becomes hungry and shows signs of a personality change. If the person remains conscious, stop dental treatment and give him or her a sugar source, such as orange juice. If the person becomes unconscious, terminate dental treatment, summon medical assistance, perform basic life support, and if necessary, give him or her an injection of glucagon or a sugar source such as cake icing gel placed in the buccal mucosa. If this condition happens frequently, the individual's physician may prescribe anti-diabetic drugs to stimulate the pancreas to produce more insulin. Normally, however, the condition arises only when the person misses a meal, is overexerted, or is in a situation that causes emotional stress. Due to the stress patients have regarding dentistry and the long appointment times, most dental offices have orange juice or other sources of sugar available for patients feeling changes in their blood sugar levels. Severe hypoglycemia causes **insulin shock**, manifested by tremors, sweating, and nervousness, and is soon followed by delirium, seizure-like jerkings, and collapse. Treatment requires glucose intravenously.

Cardiovascular Emergencies

An emergency involving the heart may occur in the dental office, so it is important to understand the anatomy of the heart. (Refer to Chapter 3, under the circulatory system, to review the heart.) The heart can be required to work harder due to physical and emotional stress. If the heart is healthy, the vessels dilate and pump more oxygen-rich blood into it. If the heart is diseased and unhealthy, this process cannot take place. **Arteriosclerosis** (commonly referred to as hardening of the arteries) is one condition that will not allow the heart to get more oxygenated blood. This condition evolves over a number of years. The arteries build up plaque deposits on the inside of the artery wall (Figure 13-14). This narrows the diameter of the artery, therefore restricting blood flow. In the later stages, a patient may experience angina pectoris and, if the vessel is totally occluded, the patient may experience a myocardial infarction.

Angina Pectoris

A Latin phrase meaning "strangling the chest," **angina pectoris** causes a pain in the chest area. This pain may radiate into the jaw area from the base of the neck; this continuous jaw pain may be the first indication of heart disease. The chest pain normally lasts for five minutes. During that time, the person wants to remain motionless and stop all activity. The person may experience an increase in blood pressure and pulse rate, have a feeling of impending doom, and become pale and clammy. If this is not the first indication of the disease, the patient may be under the care of a physician. If the patient is under the care of a physician, he or she has nitroglycerin pills or spray. The small nitroglycerin pills are placed **sublingually** (under the tongue) to allow them

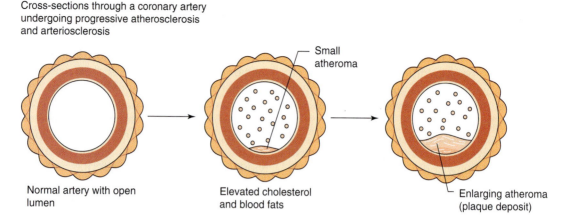

Cross-sections through a coronary artery undergoing progressive atherosclerosis and arteriosclerosis

Small atheroma

Normal artery with open lumen

Elevated cholesterol and blood fats

Enlarging atheroma (plaque deposit)

FIGURE 13-14 The progression of coronary heart disease.

to dissolve and be absorbed rapidly. Nitroglycerin spray (sprayed translingually into the oral cavity) also can be used. Nitroglycerin helps dilate the coronary arteries, allowing the heart to receive more oxygenated blood. This rapid-action drug is the accepted remedy for angina pectoris. Each patient is given a very specific dosage, because some individuals are more susceptible to the drug. If the condition arises in a dental office, all dental treatment stops. The dental team remains calm and reassures the patient. Any items that may increase stress for the patient are removed from sight. Oxygen can be administered while the patient takes the first dosage of nitroglycerin. A second dose can be administered within three to five minutes if the patient is feeling no relief while at rest. A final, third dose can be administered three to five minutes following the second dose. If the pain is not alleviated, the dental team can assume that the patient is experiencing myocardial infarction and emergency help should be summoned to transport the patient to a medical facility.

Myocardial Infarction

A condition known as **myocardial infarction**, commonly known as a heart attack, occurs when the coronary arteries are blocked or severely narrowed (Figure 13-14). It causes sudden death of part of the heart tissue and may be precipitated by angina pectoris or may occur in a person who never had any prior symptoms. In about one-third of the cases, the person will die from myocardial infarction. The signs of a heart attack are similar to those of angina pectoris, but the pain may be increased and is not alleviated by the nitroglycerin pills. A number of risk factors for the disease can be identified:

▶ Males are more likely to exhibit heart attacks than females.

▶ Smokers have a higher incident of heart attacks than non-smokers.

▶ Increased age, specific diseases such as diabetes mellitus, and heredity are uncontrollable factors.

▶ Diet, stress level, high blood pressure, and exercise levels are controllable factors.

The dental team should remain calm, stop all dental treatment, reassure and reposition the patient in a comfortable position (normally the head is elevated slightly), and remove any items that may increase stress. Administer oxygen and nitroglycerin pills or spray and summon medical emergency help immediately.

Congestive Heart Failure

As the heart weakens, the person may experience **congestive heart failure**. The weakened heart is not able to pump the fluids around the body as it should. When the person stands or sits for long periods, this fluid collects around the ankles and legs. The person may appear with swollen ankles and legs and report indigestion and difficulty breathing. Many older patients show signs of the heart getting weaker. When they lie in bed, these patients report difficulty breathing and need to have large pillows to keep the head and heart elevated. This occurs because the fluids from the feet, legs, and other parts of the body gravitate toward the heart and lungs. The medical treatment for this patient is diuretic drugs to rid the body of excess fluid by increasing the output of urine. In some cases, these patients take other drugs to strengthen the contractions of the heart beat. In the dental office, be sure that these patients are seated with their heads elevated to eliminate discomfort, and reduce undue stress. Allow them to visit the restroom as needed.

Stroke/Cerebrovascular Accident (CVA)

Stroke is a leading cause of disability and death for Americans. This condition has a sudden onset and is caused by the blood supply to the brain having a **cerebral infarction**, or being interrupted by a blockage such as a **cerebral embolism** (blood clot), or a **cerebral hemorrhage** (rupture of a blood vessel). Strokes happen to people of all ages but occur primarily in older people. The person may have an intense headache, loss of speech, unexplained dizziness, hemiplegia (weakness, numbness, or paralysis on one side of the body), and loss of consciousness. An average of 200 people per 100,000 suffer strokes annually in the United States and Canada, according to the Centers for Disease Control (CDC). This figure rises with age; men have more strokes than women, and African Americans suffer more strokes than Caucasian Americans. If the person has diabetes mellitus or if the person has had a prior stroke, the risk is greater. Heredity is also a risk factor. Controllable risk factors are cigarette smoking, high blood pressure, heart disease, and a high red blood cell count. Some people experience transient ischemic attacks (stroke-like symptoms that disappear within twenty-four hours). They should seek medical attention, because these are strong predictors of an

TABLE 13-1 **EMERGENCY CONDITIONS, SYMPTOMS, AND TREATMENTS**

Condition	Symptoms	Treatment
Syncope	Loss of consciousness	Lower the head to increase blood flow to the brain
Asthma	Breathlessness	Administer patient's bronchodilator (inhaler)
Allergic reaction	Edema, erythema, urticaria	Remove irritant, administer an antihistamine, if needed
Anaphylactic reaction	Blood pressure drops, airways constricted	Injection of epinephrine
Hyperventilation	Quick breathing, nervousness, faintness	Calm patient, have patient breathe in paper bag or cupped hands
Epilepsy Grand mal	Seizure lasting two to five minutes, body jerking, twitching	Remove items that harm patient, make patient comfortable after seizure
Status epilepticus	Continuous seizures	Summon emergency services
Petit mal seizure	Blank stare	No treatment necessary
Partial seizures	Simple/patient conscious, complex/patient unconscious, involuntary twitching	No treatment necessary
Type I diabetes mellitus	Thirst, frequent urination, disorientation, nausea/vomiting, abdominal pain	Administer patient's insulin
Type II diabetes mellitus	Same symptoms as Type I but not as severe	Normally controlled by diet, may need to administer oral hypoglycemics
Hypoglycemia	Nervousness, trembling, weakness, cold sweats	Administer orange juice or other source of sugar, such as cake icing gel, in buccal mucosa or administer injection of glucagon
Angina pectoris	Pain in chest/base of neck	Administer nitroglycerin pills or spray
Myocardial infarction	Possible pain in chest, ashen color, diaphoresis (sweating profusely)	Position patient with head slightly elevated, administer oxygen and nitroglycerin pills, summon medical services
Congestive heart failure	Difficulty breathing, swollen ankles and legs	Elevate the head and heart, allow frequent restroom breaks
Stroke	Loss of speech, dizziness, weakness on one side of body	Administer oxygen, take vital signs, summon medical services

impending stroke. A person may be given blood thinner to prevent blood clots from forming and the onset of a stroke.

If a patient has a stroke in the dental office, stop all dental treatment and remove any items from the patient's mouth. Position the patient so that his or her head is slightly elevated. Administer oxygen and monitor vital signs while emergency medical help is summoned. Calm the patient and provide CPR as needed.

▌ Dental Emergencies

Patients may call the office about any number of dental emergencies. Most offices will reserve time in the schedule for emergencies. Some emergencies require rescheduling other patients and giving specific instructions for the patient seeking dental treatment. Several of the possible patient emergency situations have been mentioned here. After the dentist sees each patient, a diagnosis is made and treatment rendered.

Abscessed Tooth

One of the most common emergencies for which patients seek dental care is an **abscessed tooth**. The patient's symptoms include pain from pressure, swelling, and severe responses to heat. The tooth has become infected, and as it grows, it places a great deal of pressure in the area because it has no place to escape in the bone. If the abscessed tooth goes untreated long enough in this painful state, the infection process may create a fistula in the bone and through the oral mucosa near the root end of the tooth. This **fistula**, an abnormal, tube-like passage at the end of the tooth to the outside surface in the oral cavity, allows the fluid to be discharged and the pressure to be released slightly. The fistula normally closes after the tooth is treated and the infection is relieved.

Alveolitis

Alveolitis (al-vee-o-**LIGH**-tis; alveolar osteitis), a condition commonly known as a dry socket, happens after a tooth has been removed. This condition occurs when a blood clot does not form or is washed out of the socket, allowing the nerve endings over the bone to become exposed. This condition increases the chance of infection in the area. Alveolitis causes great discomfort. It is treated by gently rinsing the socket with saline solution to remove any debris and packing a medicated iodoform gauze strip that is cut in a sufficient length into the socket. The medicated iodoform gauze treatment, which is only palliative, may have to be repeated every day or two until the pain diminishes. The patient may be given analgesics to relieve additional discomfort.

Avulsed Tooth

A patient may call the dental office and report that one tooth has been forcibly misplaced (avulsed). This **avulsed tooth** (also spelled evulsed) can be replanted into the socket and have a fairly high success rate if the emergency is handled quickly. The patient should immediately wrap the tooth in clean, wet gauze, place it in the mucosa between the teeth and the lip, or place it in milk while transporting it to the office. The area where the tooth came out of can be packed with gauze and pressure applied to control the bleeding. The outcome correlates greatly to the time that is lapsed. Getting the patient to the office and under the dentist's care quickly is essential. The dentist replants the tooth in the socket and secures it to the adjacent teeth. The dentist may perform immediate root canal therapy on the avulsed tooth prior to replanting it in the socket or complete the endodontic treatment six to eight weeks after reimplantation. Follow-up care is necessary until the tooth is reattached. There are individual emergency tooth avulsion kits available through dental suppliers and pharmacies.

Broken Prosthesis

A patient may call with a **broken prosthesis**. Normally, the patients are not in any physical pain but need help due to appearance concerns and loss of function. The broken prosthesis can be repaired in the office by the dentist or sent to the dental laboratory. Additional treatment is scheduled at a convenient time for the patient and dental office. The length of time for repair of the prosthesis varies. It may be necessary to perform temporary repairs in the interim, until the permanent treatment can be completed.

Soft Tissue Injury

Patients experience a number of **soft tissue injuries**. Running with sharp or blunt objects or falling down with something in their mouths may cause a number of oralfacial injuries. Electrical burns in the oral cavity can result from an individual biting into an electrical cord. Children can also fall and push newly erupted teeth back down/up into the sockets, called **traumatic intrusion**. Sports injuries result in soft tissue damage. The dental office should be contacted if any of these soft tissue injuries occur.

Soft tissue injury can occur in the dental office during any intraoral dental procedure. The oral cavity is moist and slippery, the patient may move quickly, and dental instruments and equipment can easily become displaced, causing injury.

Broken Tooth

A patient may call with a broken tooth. Anterior teeth are commonly fractured at drinking faucets, on steering wheels, or on diving boards. The dental receptionist discerns whether the patient needs to be scheduled immediately by gaining information from the patient as to the level of discomfort, whether there are sharp edges, and how extensive the broken area is. In most offices, the patient is seen for an initial appointment on an emergency basis to determine the treatment needed.

Loose Permanent or Temporary Crown

A patient's crown may become loose or come off, requiring recementation. The patient may be in discomfort if the pulp is exposed or if the restoration has sharp edges. If the patient is out of town and unable to get dental care, petroleum jelly or orthodontic wax can be used to temporarily keep the crown in place. The patient will have to exercise extreme care while eating. If the patient can get to the dental office, treatment is to recement the crown with either temporary or permanent cement, as indicated.

CHAPTER SUMMARY

Even though the number of emergencies is not great in a dental office, the dental assistant must always be observant of the patient and prepared to deal with emergencies. Emergencies may also happen to the dentist and to other dental auxiliaries.

When an emergency arises, the dental team must react with an automatic response. Any hesitation at such a time may cost a life. It is best if a routine is established so everyone can ensure everything is taken care of. The assistant has a vital role in the prevention of emergencies and emergency care. Patient observation at all times assists in the prevention evaluation.

CASE STUDY

Thelma Lynd, a forty-six-year-old female, is seated in the dental treatment room. She indicates that recently she has not been feeling well. As she continues to talk, she has loss of speech, dizziness, and weakness on one side of her body. Her vital signs are elevated and she cannot respond.

Case Study Review

1. What probable condition is Thelma experiencing?

2. What should the dental assistant do in this situation?

3. Is reassurance for the patient important in this case? Why?

To complete your study of this chapter, work the review activities that follow. Also, refer to the software that accompanies this text.

REVIEW QUESTIONS

Multiple Choice

1. An exaggerated reaction of the immune system is called an
  a. allergy.
  b. antibody.
  c. antigen.
  d. allergen.

2. Asthma attacks are more frequent in the
  a. late evening.
  b. afternoon.
  c. morning.
  d. night.

3. A medical term for giant hives is
  a. edema.
  b. erythema.
  c. urticaria.
  d. angioedema.

4. A seizure in which a person experiences a momentary loss of consciousness is called a
  a. grand mal seizure.
  b. petit mal seizure.
  c. partial seizure.
  d. status epilepticus.

5. The type of diabetes mellitus that is more severe is
   a. Type I.
   b. Type II.
   c. Type III.
   d. Type IV.

Critical Thinking

1. A patient is having extensive dental work completed. The patient's health history indicates a history of epilepsy. The patient becomes nervous and then unconscious as the body begins to jerk, twitch and stiffen. How should the dental team respond?

2. The disease in which an individual has too little glucose or sugar is called hypoglycemia. What are the steps for treating a patient experiencing hypoglycemic symptoms?

3. A patient has heart disease that continues to progress over the years. He has a condition that will not allow the heart to receive the oxygenated blood that it needs. What is the condition and what is it commonly called?

Clinical Dental Procedures

Introduction to Chairside Assisting

OBJECTIVES

The student should strive to meet the following objectives and demonstrate an understanding of the facts and principles presented in this chapter:

1. Describe the design of a dental office, explaining the purpose of each area.

2. Explain basic concepts of chairside assisting.

3. Describe the necessary steps to prepare a patient for treatment.

4. Explain the necessary steps to seat the patient for treatment.

5. Describe the position of the operator and the assistant at chairside.

6. Describe the necessary steps to dismiss the patient after treatment is concluded.

7. Identify the special needs of certain patients.

8. Describe the grasps, positions, and transfer of instruments for a procedure.

9. Define and demonstrate how to maintain the oral cavity and the equipment utilized in treatment of the oral cavity.

KEY TERMS

activity zones (p. 253)
air compressor (p. 251)
air-water syringe (p. 246)
amalgamator (p. 250)
central vacuum system (p. 251)
classifications of motion (p. 254)
curing light (p. 249)
delivery systems (p. 253)
dental unit (p. 245)
four-handed dentistry (p. 253)
fulcrum (p. 259)
handpieces (p. 246)

high volume evacuation (HVE) (p. 248)
intraoral camera (p. 250)
laboratory (p. 242)
lumbar (p. 248)
mobile carts (p. 245)
modified pen grasp (p. 260)
operating light (p. 249)
palm grasp (p. 260)
palm-thumb grasp (p. 261)
patient records (p. 254)
pen grasp (p. 260)

reception room (p. 240)
reverse palm-thumb grasp (p. 261)
rheostat (p. 246)
saliva ejector (p. 247)
six-handed dentistry (p. 253)
sterilizing area (p. 241)
subsupine position (p. 245)
supine position (p. 245)
treatment rooms (p. 241)
triturates (p. 250)
ultrasonic scaler (p. 247)

INTRODUCTION

Dental offices have numerous designs, including a single building, a medical/dental complex of individual units, a remodeled home, a suite in an office building, or space in a mall. Dental professionals go to great lengths to ensure that their offices are clean, convenient, and offer pleasant settings for patients. The dentist's vision and expectations are reflected in the office design, which should always consider the patients the dentist will be serving. The practice may serve families, primarily children, or primarily adults and may be located in a rural or an urban setting. The most successful practices encompass all relative facets into a welcoming atmosphere where dental treatment can be provided.

The appearance of the dental office makes a statement about the dentist, the dental staff, and the quality of the dental care. The following information describes the rooms in the dental office, the specific equipment used by dental professionals, and the concept of chairside assisting.

THE DENTAL OFFICE DESIGN

The dental office is composed of several basic components designed to meet the individual dentist's preferences and needs. The office may be small with two or three treatment rooms or may have a clinic setting with any number of treatment rooms (Figure 14-1). Most offices are designed with a reception area, a business area, treatment rooms, a sterilizing area, a laboratory, an x-ray processing room, a restroom, and the dentist's office. The sizes and numbers of these rooms varies (Figure 14-2). Dental offices may also include the following: consultation rooms/areas, staff lounge, prevention and/or patient education area, storage area, office for the office manager, space for panoramic radiograph machine, shower/change room, and laundry room. OSHA requirements have changed the office by requiring a room for staff to change and store uniforms. Some offices have added laundry facilities. In addition, dental offices are requiring more space in the business office to accommodate high technology equipment and to facilitate increased dental insurance processing.

New innovations in dental offices include more open designs with partial walls and greater access to the treatment rooms, sterilizing area, and so on. Higher ceilings, open doorways, and more windows also create the feeling of openness for the patient and the dental team. The office should have a climate-control system that remains at a comfortable temperature throughout the year, regardless of the weather conditions. Architects and decorators often work together with dental professionals to achieve the look the dentist desires.

The Reception Room

The **reception room** is the area the patient initially enters and therefore gives the first impression of the

FIGURE 14-1 Small dental office blueprint. *(Courtesy of Burkhart Dental Supply)*

FIGURE 14-2 Large office blueprint. *(Courtesy of Burkhart Dental Supply)*

office. It is important that this room be pleasing and comfortable as well as neat and clean (Figure 14-3). The dental staff should tidy this room on a regular basis. Magazines should be current and appropriate for the dentist's clientele. Often, there is an area designed specifically for children with a table, chairs, and activities to keep them occupied while they wait.

The reception room is an excellent place to provide patient education materials for all age groups. The decor of this room should be changed as often as needed to keep the atmosphere friendly and positive for the patients as they enter the dental office.

The Reception Desk and Business Office

The reception desk and business office is often part of or adjacent to the reception room, so patients can be greeted as they enter the office. This area is where ap-

pointments are made, telephone calls are received, and patient records are updated and stored (Figure 14-4). This area includes counter space, desk space, adequate lighting, accessible filing system, access to computer terminals, and telecommunication systems. The counter space allows some privacy for the business office staff and provides a space for patients to pay bills and schedule appointments. Often there is a conference room or an area somewhere close to the business office for private conversations with patients. Because this area is where the staff makes the first and last contact with the patient, it should reflect a positive image of the qualities of the dental practice.

Sterilizing Area

The **sterilizing area** should be located near the **treatment rooms** and should be neat and clean at all times (Figure 14-5). The sterilizing room should have good air

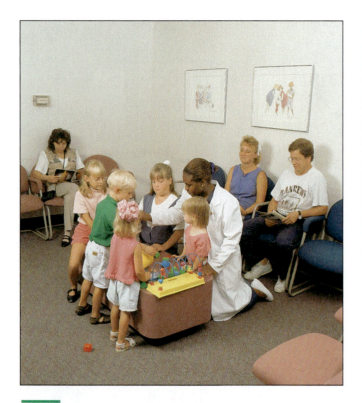

FIGURE 14-3 Reception and play area for children.

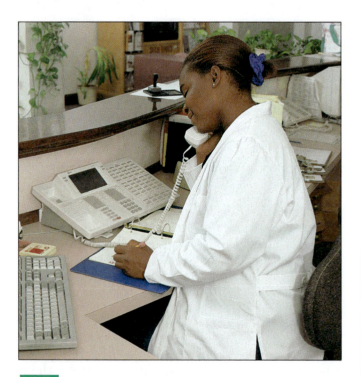

FIGURE 14-4 Business area.

circulation to protect everyone from the chemical fumes and exhaust from the sterilizers. In this area, there is a sink, counter space for the ultrasonic equipment, and sterilizing units. Infection control protocol is accomplished in the sterilizing area for the patient

FIGURE 14-5 Sterilizing area with sink, counter space, storage, ultrasonic unit, and sterilizing unit.

treatment tray and equipment. Upon completion of sterilization, trays are set up and stored in this area. Infection control, procedure supplies, and hazardous waste supplies are stored in the sterilization area. (The sterilizing equipment is discussed in Chapter 9, Infection Control.)

Dental Office Laboratory

The dental office **laboratory** is a separate area that is also well vented (Figure 14-6). The amount of lab work done in the office depends on the dentist's preference. If the dentist's practice includes a number of patients needing prosthodontic treatment, a lab technician and a lab is set up in the office. In other offices, the dental lab may be used for finishing or adjusting crowns, bridges, partials, or dentures and for pouring impressions, trimming models, polishing removable appliances, and making custom trays.

The dental laboratory may contain a vibrator, a model trimmer, a laboratory handpiece, a vacuum former, a

FIGURE 14-6 Laboratory area. *(Courtesy of Drs. Rodney Braun and Chris Chaffin)*

sink, an exhaust fan, plaster and stone storage bins, a heat source, and a dental lathe. Cupboards provide storage for instruments such as lab knives, spatulas, and rubber bowls. All aseptic precautions must be followed when working in this setting, because often the materials have been in the patient's mouth before coming to the lab. The staff should wear protective glasses and masks to prevent dust and debris from causing injuries when working on the equipment.

X-Ray Processing Room

The x-ray processing room or **darkroom** is a small room near the treatment rooms (Figure 14-7). This room contains a sink, a manual processing tank, drying racks, space for storage, safelights, and counter space for processing and mounting radiographs. With the use of automatic processors with daylight loading, the need for this space has changed. The automatic processor may be located in the processing room or in treatment rooms, the sterilizing area, or an open area in a hall space. (This room and the equipment are described in detail in Chapter 17, Dental Radiography.)

Radiography Room

In most dental offices, radiograph machines are located in each treatment room for intraoral x-rays. The extraoral radiographic equipment is located in a radiography room. This room must provide occupational safety from ionizing radiation and be large enough to house this equipment. Guidelines come from the state health department, and periodic inspections may be required by state agencies (Figure 14-8).

Optional Rooms in the Dental Office

Optional rooms in the dental office are dictated by the dentist's preference, patient usage, amount of space

FIGURE 14-8 Panoramic machine area.

available, and practice budget. Any or all of the following rooms may be included in the dental office design. Often the office is built with additional rooms available for later growth in the practice.

Dentist's Private Office. The dentist's private office is designed according to the individual taste of the doctor. The dentist's private office is where the dentist conducts personal and professional business. This office may be used to consult with patients privately or for staff meetings.

Staff Lounge. A staff lounge is a place for staff to have lunch, meet, and relax. Located in the staff lounge is a sink, refrigerator, microwave, coffee machine, table and chairs, storage cupboards, and countertop space.

Patient Education Area. A patient education area is a very functional and diverse area in the dental office. With each type of practice, the use may vary; for example, in the orthodontic office, the space may be furnished with mirrors and sinks where patients can practice home-care techniques. The patient education area may be an information center containing a variety

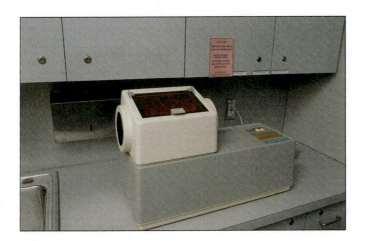

FIGURE 14-7 X-ray processing area with sink, counter space, storage, and automatic processing unit with daylight loader.

of information on dental care and treatments available to patients, such as bleaching treatments or dental implants.

Often this room has a sink, a counter or table with chairs, and multimedia equipment including a television and VCR. This area also is used for consultations with the patient or for the patient to wait, if necessary.

THE TREATMENT ROOMS

Dental treatment rooms are also called **operatories** (Figures 14-9 and 14-10). Each dentist has a minimum of three treatment rooms. The type and size of practice also dictate the number of operatories. The treatment rooms in a general practice are usually designated for either operative dentistry or hygiene and are equipped accordingly. They can be individual rooms or open spaces divided by walls and/or equipment. The rooms need to be large enough to contain the necessary equipment while still allowing for easy access to it. The treatment rooms should be designed for maximum efficiency.

A dental treatment room contains a dental chair, dental unit, operating stools, cabinets, sinks, x-ray machine, x-ray viewbox, and mobile carts. There are many manufacturers and designs of equipment to choose from in order to meet the requirements of the office. Dental equipment is expensive and, with careful maintenance,

FIGURE 14-9 Dentral treatment area: counter space and storage, patient chair, operator and assistant chairs, dental light, dental unit with handpieces, air-water syringe, high volume evacuator, rheostat.

it is meant to last for years. Someone in the office often is assigned to perform the routine maintenance of the equipment. A dental equipment technician is called when more substantial problems occur.

FIGURE 14-10 Two operatories with the open concept. *(Courtesy of A-dec, Inc., Newberg, Oregon, USA)*

The Dental Chair

The dental chair is the center of all clinical activity (Figures 14-11 and 14-12). The chair is designed for the operator and the assistant to work on the patient in a comfortable and efficient manner. The dental chair supports the patient's entire body, in either an upright, **supine position** (reclined position with the nose and knees on the same plane) or a **subsupine position** (reclined position with the head lower than the feet). The dental chair is designed to accommodate both children and adults. The head rest is narrow to allow the dentist and the assistant to be positioned close to the patient's head and is adjustable to provide support. The dental chair has arm rests designed to lift or move out of the way when the patient is being seated or dismissed.

It also has controls to move the chair up and down, recline the back rest, and raise the seat and a combination button that automatically reclines or raises the patient. The controls are either on the sides of the chair back or on the floor (the floor controls are becoming more popular because they eliminate the need for barriers). The chair also has a control on the floor that allows it to be rotated left and right. To prevent cross-contamination, the head rest and controls located on the chair are covered with barriers.

The dental chair is upholstered in a material that is comfortable, easy to clean, and coordinates with the office color theme. The base of the chair is secured to the floor. The chair base should be cleaned and disinfected routinely.

The Dental Unit

The **dental unit** consists of handpieces, an air-water syringe, a saliva ejector, an oral evacuator (HVE), an

FIGURE 14-12 Dental chair with foot controls for adjusting the chair.

ultrasonic scaling unit, and numerous other options. The dental unit may be fixed to the wall, the cabinets, or on mobile carts. The unit is positioned according to the preference of the dentist, whether the dentist is left- or right-handed, if he or she routinely works with an assistant, and according to the design of the treatment room. The dental unit is available in three basic modes of delivery:

1. The **rear delivery system** is designed with the equipment located behind the patient's head (Figure 14-13).

2. The **side delivery system** is designed with the equipment located on the dentist's side. The unit is mounted to a moveable arm or a mobile cart (Figure 14-14).

3. The **front delivery system** is designed so that it can be pulled over the patient's chest and is located between the dentist and the assistant (Figure 14-15).

Mobile Carts. Sometimes, **mobile carts** are used to hold delivery systems, including the air-water syringe, oral evacuator, handpieces, and saliva ejector (Figure 14-16). One cart may be used by both the operator and the dental assistant with the instrumentation on the

FIGURE 14-11 Dental chair with side controls for adjusting the chair.

FIGURE 14-13 Rear delivery system. *(Courtesy of A-dec, Inc., Newberg, Oregon, USA)*

FIGURE 14-14 Side delivery system. *(Courtesy of A-dec, Inc., Newberg, Oregon, USA)*

FIGURE 14-15 Front delivery system. *(Courtesy of A-dec, Inc., Newberg, Oregon, USA)*

appropriate side. Two carts, one on each side of the dental chair, may be equipped and used. The **operator's cart** is usually set up for two or three dental handpieces plus an air-water syringe (Figure 14-16A). The **assistant's cart** is usually set up with the air-water syringe, saliva ejector, and HVE (Figure 14-16B). Carts are designed to be moved easily, provide a work space and some storage, and hold basic instruments.

Air-Water Syringe. The air-water syringe provides air, water, or a combination spray of air and water (Figure 14-17). The tip of the syringe is removable and made of either disposable plastic or autoclavable metal. New barriers are placed on the syringe handle and the tubing for each patient. The controls for the syringe are on the handle and should be easy to operate with the thumb of

one hand. Air, water, and the combination spray help keep the oral cavity clean and dry and protect the tooth from the heat produced by the handpieces. For easier use, the syringe tips come in several lengths and are slightly angled. To reduce the risk of retaining oral fluids, flush the air-water syringe with water between patients and at the beginning and end of the day.

Dental Handpieces. There are usually two dental handpieces: low and high speed (Figure 14-18A). The handpieces are attached to hoses that are part of the dental unit. It is important that these hoses are not bent or tangled. Each handpiece has two controls. First, the hose attachment has an on/off switch to prevent more than one handpiece from running at once. Second, the speed of the handpiece is controlled by a foot pedal called a **rheostat** (**REE**-oh-stat). The dental handpieces are removed after each patient's treatment and are sterilized. (Prior to removal from the unit, like the air-water syringe, caution should be taken to flush oral fluids from the handpieces.) There are ways to test handpieces to see whether they retract fluids when they stop running and manufacturers are designing means to prevent this from occurring. At the beginning and end of the day, the handpiece should be run for several minutes. Between patients, run the handpieces for at least one minute to flush the system. Some dental

(A)

FIGURE 14-17 Air-water syringe. (A) Handle. (B) Air-water controls. (C) Removable and disposable tips.

(B)

FIGURE 14-16 (A) Operator's cart with dental handpieces and air-water syringe. (B) Assistant's cart with saliva ejector, HVE, and air-water syringe. *(Courtesy of A-dec, Inc., Newberg, Oregon, USA)*

manufacturers provide a water reservoir for the handpieces and air-water syringe on the unit.

Ultrasonic Scaler. The **ultrasonic scaler** is attached to the dental unit. The scaler is used during prophylaxis and periodontal procedures. Small tips attach to the ultrasonic scaler. The scaler has a vibrating action that

removes hard deposits, such as calculus, and other debris from the teeth.

Saliva Ejector. The **saliva ejector** is used to remove saliva and fluids from the patient's mouth slowly. It has a low volume suction that is used during certain procedures, such as fluoride treatments and under rubber dams. The saliva ejector tip is a thin, flexible, plastic tube that is disposed of after each patient's treatment. This plastic tip slides into the opening of the saliva ejector hose that is part of the dental unit. There is a small

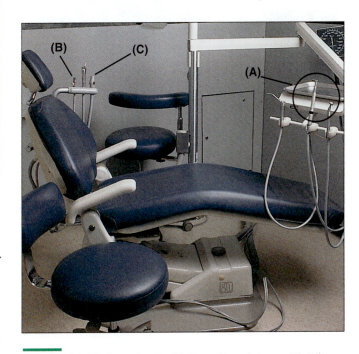

FIGURE 14-18 Dental unit. (A) Dental handpieces. (B) Saliva ejector. (C) HVE.

trap located in the saliva ejector that needs to be cleaned routinely (Figure 14-18B).

High Volume Evacuation (HVE). The **high volume evacuation (HVE)** is also called the oral evacuator. It is used by the assistant to remove fluids from the patient's mouth. Evacuation tips are wider tubes that are often beveled at both ends. Some of the tips are metal and can be sterilized, but most offices use plastic tips that can be sterilized or disposed of. The evacuation tips fit into the handle of the hose, which is covered with a protective barrier during procedures. The on/off control for the HVE is on the handle. Each unit has a trap that collects debris from the evacuator. This trap must be changed or cleaned weekly or as needed. There are cleaning systems available to flush the HVE at the end of the day and week (Figure 14-18C).

Dental Stools

Dental stools are required by the operator and the assistant during most procedures. Ergonomic studies have resulted in the improved design of dental stools to provide comfort and prevent fatigue during dental procedures. When selecting stools, the dentist and staff should try a variety of stools to find the one that meets their requirements, provides good support, and is comfortable. The operator's and assistant's stools have some similarities but also have several differences (Figures 14-19 and 14-20).

FIGURE 14-20 Assistant's stool with front arm support, seat, broad base, and foot rest and casters.

FIGURE 14-19 Operator's stool with back support, broad base, and seat and casters.

Operator's Stool. The operator's stool has the following characteristics:

▶ **Adjustable height**—The stool should have adjustment for height so that the operator's feet can be flat on the floor and the thighs can be parallel to the floor when seated.

▶ **Adjustable back rest**—The stool should have a back rest that is adjustable, both vertically and horizontally, to provide support and comfort. The back rest should support the **lumbar** region (lower region of the back) of the operator's back.

▶ **Comfortable seat**—The stool seat should be broad with firm padding and have no seams or edges to restrict circulation in the legs and feet. The seat also should be covered with a material that is easy to clean.

▶ **Mobility**—The stool should move easily on four to five casters and freely, even on floors with carpet.

▶ **Broad base**—The stool should have a broad, heavy base to prevent tipping, especially during movement. The base stabilizes the stool for the operator.

Dental Assistant's Stool. The dental assistant's stool has the following characteristics:

- **Adjustable height**—The stool should adjust to a variety of different levels to accommodate the height of the assistant. The assistant is positioned four to eight inches higher than the operator, with feet resting on the foot ring and thighs parallel to the floor.

- **Adjustable back rest**—The stool back rest should provide support for the lumbar region and be easily adjustable. Some stools have an extended arm for support of the abdomen or side areas. The arm moves easily into place and locks to stabilize the assistant when leaning or reaching.

- **Comfortable seat**—The seat of the stool has the same criteria as the operator's stool: a broad, flat surface with no seams or hard edges.

- **Mobility**—The assistant's chair should be designed to move freely. Usually, five casters are recommended in order to provide stability.

- **Broad base**—The base of the stool should be broad and well balanced. It should be heavy and stable to prevent tipping.

- **Foot rest**—The assistant is usually positioned higher than the operator, so it is difficult to sit correctly on the stool and rest feet flat on the floor. The foot rest gives the assistant support so that good circulation is maintained.

- **Easy to adjust**—All parts of the assistant's stool should be easy to adjust. Adjustments should be made quickly between patients.

Operating Light

The operating light is attached to the dental chair or mounted to the ceiling (Figures 14-13, 14-14, and 14-18). Both the operator and the assistant should be able to adjust the position of the light. Operating lights have improved in many ways: They are easier to move, more flexible, and direct less heat on the patient. The light has a control switch for high and low intensities, an on/off switch, and handles on both sides. The light is attached to extension arms for positioning over the patient's face in order to view either the maxillary or mandibular arch.

The handles and on/off switch are covered with barriers during procedures. The barriers are changed between each patient. Maintenance includes changing the lightbulb occasionally and keeping the heat shield clean. It is important to follow the manufacturer's instructions for both of these procedures.

Cabinetry

Most treatment rooms have some type of cabinetry for storage of supplies and materials used during treatment. Some dental units are designed in **fixed cabinets** that surround the patient, operator, and assistant. These units include cupboards that open from the front and

the back for treatment trays, drawers for materials frequently used, and sinks for both the operator and the assistant (Figures 14-13 and 14-14). The amount of cabinetry depends on the size of the room and the dentist's preference.

Mobile cabinets are also used in the treatment room. These cabinets come in a variety of designs and are used for storage and as a work space. The mobile cabinet is stored against the wall and then pulled into position after the patient is seated.

Sink

The treatment room should be designed with sinks in convenient locations for the dentist and the assistants. Some treatment rooms have two sinks, one on each side of the dental chair. Other treatment rooms have one sink that is located centrally behind the dental unit for both the dentist and assistant to use.

The water controls on the sink should be operated by wrist, foot, or knee controls (this prevents the hands from becoming contaminated after handwashing by turning off the water controls). There are light and motion sensor devices that turn the water on and off automatically when standing in front of the sink.

The sinks should be easy to clean and have an area nearby for soap and towel dispensers.

Dental X-Ray Unit

A dental x-ray unit used to expose intraoral radiographs is part of most treatment rooms. Sometimes the x-ray tubehead is housed between two rooms with doors on both sides for the x-ray tubehead to slide out into either room. The controls are found outside the room so that the dental assistant is not exposed to radiation. (Further information about the x-ray unit can be found in Chapter 17, Dental Radiography.) The panoramic machine for exposing extraoral radiographs is usually located in a separate area outside the treatment room.

Small Equipment Found in the Treatment Room

There may be a variety of equipment in the treatment room depending on the primary use of the room. Most rooms have an x-ray viewbox, curing light, amalgamator, communication system, computerized intraoral dental camera, and a satellite computer.

X-ray Viewbox. The x-ray viewbox is used to read and diagnose radiographs (Figure 14-21). The viewbox may sit on a counter or be placed in a wall or cabinet. It consists of a bright light source covered with a frosted surface. X-rays are placed on the frosted surface for clear viewing.

Dental Curing Light. A dental curing light is used to "cure" or "set" light-cured materials (Figure 14-22A). Many dental products are now light cured. The curing

FIGURE 14-21 X-ray viewbox.

light has a small motor that produces the high intensity light, a wand, a protective shield, a handle, and a trigger to turn the light on and off. To determine if the light is working at full capacity, the curing light should be tested periodically. A small, hand-held instrument will test the light and give a reading to determine the strength of the light. The curing light uses halogen bulbs. Follow the manufacturer's instructions when changing the bulb.

High intensity curing units are competing with conventional light curing. The lasers and plasma arc (pac) lights offer the high intensity curing (Figure 14-22B). The lasers and pac units decrease the curing time, increase the depth of the cure, and show some reduction in post-operative sensitivity. These lights have small tips that allow light to be delivered into interproximal areas and other hard-to-reach areas. The tips can also be used in orthodontics. Curing time is as little as five seconds.

Disadvantages include the high cost, the large size of the unit (but can be placed on a cart for mobility), and a foot control.

Amalgamator. The **amalgamator** is a small machine that mixes (**triturates**) dental amalgam and some dental cements. It is placed near the assistant, either on the counter or in a drawer (Figure 14-23). (The amalgamator is discussed further in Chapter 26, Chairside Restorative Materials.)

Communication System. The communication system is a color-coded light system or intercom system that the office uses as a method for the staff and the dentist to communicate with each other. Usually, the system is found on the walls in the treatment rooms, sterilization area, laboratory, and staff lounge. It is made up of a series of colored buttons that light up when pushed or an intercom/phone system. (Refer to Figure 14-2, the layout of the dental treatment room.) The system can designate a specific message or call a member of the dental team. For example, the hygienist lets the dentist know the patient is ready for examination or tells everyone that the next patient has arrived.

FIGURE 14-22 (A) Dental curing light. (B) Laser curing light. *(Courtesy of Lasermed, Inc., Salt Lake City, Utah)*

These systems can be customized for the individual needs of an office.

Computerized Equipment. Computerized equipment includes an **intraoral camera** and a **computer terminal**.

FIGURE 14-23 Amalgamator.

The intraoral wand contains a small camera that transmits to the television monitor (Figure 14-24). The wand is placed in the patient's mouth, and the image is displayed on the monitor. The computer freezes a picture on the screen or prints it out. The intraoral computer allows the

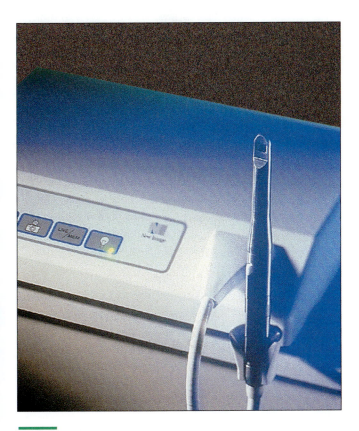

FIGURE 14-24 Intraoral camera. *(Courtesy of Midwest Dental Products Corporation, a Division of DENTSPLY International)*

patient to see areas and conditions in their mouths while the dentist is discussing them.

Many offices are computerized with terminals in the treatment rooms as well as the business office. Computer systems allow the office to be "paperless" and to more efficiently complete specific tasks, such as billing. Some systems allow the dentist and staff to enter treatment plans, chart the condition of the patient's mouth, make the patient's next appointment, bill the insurance company, and give information and instructions. The number of computers and the programs/systems used in the office are the choice of the dentist. In order to use the computers efficiently and effectively, additional training and cooperation of all staff members is required.

Digital radiography equipment is also part of the technology found in the dental office. (Digital radiography equipment is discussed in Chapter 17, Dental Radiography.)

Dental Air Compressor and Central Vacuum System

The **air compressor** provides compressed air for the handpieces and air for the air-water syringes. The size of the air compressor depends on the number of dental units utilized by the office. Usually, the compressor is stored away from the main office because of its size and noise level.

The **central vacuum system** provides suction for saliva ejectors and oral evacuators at each dental unit. The filters or traps must be cleaned regularly to keep this system working to capacity. This system is also stored away from the main office.

Dental office staff and dental service companies must follow the manufacturer's instructions for maintenance and repairs on the air compressor and the vacuum system. Both units may be set up on time clocks to run only when the office is open and operating.

▌ROUTINE OFFICE CARE

With the amount of equipment being operated in the dental office, a routine schedule needs to be in place to ensure proper maintenance control. Often this responsibility is given to the dental assistants. Usually, the office is cleaned professionally, but the assistant should periodically check the overall appearance of the office.

Weekly or monthly maintenance tasks might include the following: changing x-ray processing solutions, cleaning the inside of the sterilizers, changing ultrasonic solutions, performing monitoring activities to check the effectiveness of the sterilizers, and making miscellaneous repairs. It is necessary to keep replacement parts on hand for equipment that needs routine care (for example, the O-rings in the air-water syringe, which need to be changed when leaking of air or water occurs).

PROCEDURE

14-1 Daily Routine to Open the Office

These tasks are done by the assistant each morning. The assistant arrives to the office early to open the office and prepare for the day's schedule.

PROCEDURE STEPS

1. Turn on master switches to lights, each dental unit, vacuum system, and air compressor.

2. Check the reception room, turn on lights, straighten the magazines and the children's area, and unlock the patients' door to the office.

3. Turn on the communication system, check the answering machine or the answering system, start up the computers, unlock the files, and organize the business area.

4. Post copies of patient schedules in designated areas throughout the office.

5. Turn on all equipment in the x-ray processing area. Change the water in the processing tanks and replenish solutions, if necessary.

6. Change into appropriate clinical clothing, following OSHA guidelines.

7. Review the daily patient schedule.

8. Prepare the treatment rooms for the first patients. Check supplies, place barriers, and review patient records. Then, prepare the appropriate trays and lab work for the first patients.

9. Turn on any sterilizing equipment and check solutions levels. Prepare new ultrasonic and disinfecting solutions. Complete overnight sterilization procedures.

10. Replenish supplies needed for the day.

PROCEDURE

14-2 Daily Routine to Close the Office

These tasks are done by the assistant at the end of the day. The office evening routine includes closing the office down for the evening and preparing for the next day. As with the opening routine, the assistants usually share the responsibility of closing the office. Each office has specific details, but the following are general tasks.

PROCEDURE STEPS

1. Clean the treatment rooms. This may include an in-depth cleaning of the dental chair and dental unit. Flush the handpieces and air-water syringes, run solutions through the evacuation hoses, and clean traps/filters.

2. Position the dental chair for evening housekeeping.

3. Turn off all master switches.

4. Process, mount, and file any x-rays. Follow manufacturer's instructions to shut down automatic processors. Turn off water supply to manual processing tanks.

5. Wipe counters and turn off the safe light.

6. Sterilize all instruments and set up trays for the next day. Empty ultrasonic solutions and turn off all equipment. Restock supplies.

7. Make sure all laboratory cases have been sent to the lab and early-morning cases have been received from the lab.

8. Confirm and complete appointment schedule for the next day, insurance forms, and daily bookkeeping responsibilities. Pull charts for the next day.

9. Turn off business office equipment and turn on the answering machine or service. Lock patient and business office files.

10. Straighten the reception room. For the security of the office, all doors and windows should be locked.

11. Change from uniform to street clothes, following OSHA guidelines.

12. Turn off machines in the staff lounge and clean up tables and counters.

CONCEPTS OF DENTAL ASSISTING

Originally, the dentist and the dental assistant worked standing on either side of the dental chair. Although some dentists still may stand occasionally, both the dentist and assistant now sit during procedures the majority of time. Many studies and research in ergonomics found that sit-down dentistry was the best for both the dentist and the assistant, creating less strain and increasing efficiency. When both the dentist and assistant are working at the dental chair together, it is called **four-handed dentistry**. The assistant assists the dentist throughout the entire procedure, passing instruments, mixing materials, and watching the patient. Sometimes, an additional assistant is needed to bring items to the treatment room, assist the assistant in mixing materials, or help with a patient. This is called **six-handed dentistry**. Four- and six-handed dentistry have proven to be efficient and effective in providing patients with quality care.

Activity Zones

When the dentist and the assistant are positioning themselves around the patient, it is vital that there is:

▶ Good visibility of the patient's mouth

▶ Easy access to all areas of the patient's mouth

▶ Easy access to dental equipment, instruments, and materials

▶ Safety and comfort for the patient, the operator, and the assistant

The area around the patient's mouth is divided into four **activity zones**: **operating zone**, **assisting zone**, **static zone**, and **transfer zone**. These activity zones are determined by visualizing the patient's head as the center of a clock (Figure 14-25).

The operating zone is the area where the operator is positioned to access the oral cavity and have the best visibility. For right-handed operators, this area extends from the 7 to 12 o'clock position. For left-handed operators, this area extends from the 12 to 5 o'clock position. The operator moves within the zone depending on which arch, quadrant, or surface of the patient's teeth the operator is working on.

The assisting zone is the area where the assistant is positioned to easily assist the dentist and have access to instruments, the evacuator, and so on on the dental unit or cart without interference. The assistant's zone for a right-handed operator is 2 to 4 o'clock and for a left-handed operator it is 8 to 10 o'clock.

The static zone extends from 12 to 2 o'clock for a right-handed operator and from 10 to 12 o'clock for a left-handed operator. Rear **delivery systems** are found in the static zone, along with dental instruments and equipment used at the chair.

The transfer zone is the area below the patient's nose where instruments and materials are passed and

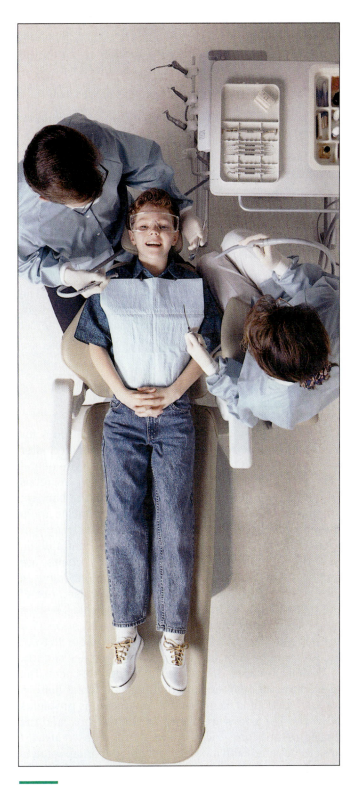

FIGURE 14-25 Activity zones for a right-handed operator and assistant. *(Courtesy of A-dec, Inc., Newberg, Oregon, USA)*

received. Usually, the operator and the assistant transfer instruments between the area that is below the patient's nose and above the upper chest. To follow the clock concept, this would be between 4 and 7 o'clock for a right-handed operator and 5 and 8 o'clock for a left-handed operator.

Classifications of Motion

There are five **classifications of motion** to show the amount of motion the dental team is involved with:

1. **Class I motion** involves only finger movement.

2. **Class II motion** involves movement of the fingers and wrist.

3. **Class III motion** involves finger, wrist, and elbow movement.

4. **Class IV motion** involves movement of the entire arm and shoulder.

5. **Class V motion** involves movement of the arm and twisting of the body.

Ideally, the operator and the assistant should be positioned to stay in Class I, II, and III motion ranges. The dental unit, counter space, instruments, and equipment should all be close enough to avoid Classes IV and V.

PREPARING TO SEAT THE PATIENT

Preparing the Treatment Room

The dental assistant prepares the treatment room for each patient. The room is cleaned and disinfected after each patient, and new barriers are placed on the dental unit, dental chair, counters, and dental light switches (see Chapter 9, Infection Control). After all the barriers are placed, the room is tidied so that no obstacles are in the patient's path when he or she enters the treatment room. The rheostat is placed behind the dental chair, and the operator and dental assistant's chairs are moved out of the way. Any mobile carts are pulled out of the patient's path, and the dental light is raised out of the patient's way as he or she sits in the chair. The arm of the dental chair is raised or turned for easy access for the patient. The dental chair is positioned about 15 to 18 inches from the floor, and the chair is tilted back slightly.

Patient records are reviewed to double-check the procedures to be done, and the medical/dental history for each patient is examined for any previous problems or alerts. The x-rays are placed on the viewbox, and the charts/records are located away from the treatment area or covered with a barrier. Any model or lab work is brought into the treatment room. The tray is set up, and accessory items for specific procedures are prepared.

SEATING THE DENTAL PATIENT

Greet and Escort the Patient

Greet the patient by stepping into the reception area and identifying him or her by name. Then, tell the patient that you are ready for him or her now. If you have not met the patient before, introduce yourself and, before leaving the reception area, ask the patient if he or she wants to hang up his or her coat. Then, ask the patient to follow you into the treatment room.

When escorting the patient back to the treatment room, it is a good idea to identify the room by number, color, or location. Make sure that all obstacles are out of the way, and offer assistance if the patient appears to need it. For example, patients who have trouble getting up out of chairs or patients who walk with canes or walkers may need assistance.

Once in the treatment room, as a courtesy to the patient and for infection control, ask the patient if he or she would like to rinse his or her mouth with mouthwash before he or she sits down. Then, offer to store any personal items, such as a purse or briefcase, on a counter or shelf. These items should be placed where they are in the patient's view but not interfering with the treatment.

It is important to establish rapport with the patients and make them feel welcome and at ease. Remember to talk to the patients and show an interest in what they have to say. Ask them about subjects they are involved with and are comfortable discussing. People like to talk about themselves, their families, work, vacations, and hobbies. Note points of interest on the treatment chart so continued reference can be made. Often, patients will ask questions about dental concerns. General information can be given by the dental assistant. The dentist can answer specifically when he or she comes into the treatment room. Communication with patients begins when they walk into the office and should continue until they leave.

Seat and Prepare the Patient

Ask the patient to be seated in the dental chair. The patient's back should be against the back rest and his or her legs completely supported. Once the patient is in the chair, lower the arm of the chair and offer a drink of water, tissue to remove lipstick, or lip lubricant. Place the **napkin** or **bib** on the patient and secure it with the napkin chain (bib clips). Make sure more of the napkin/bib is on the operator's side of the patient. Give the patient **safety glasses** for protection during the procedure.

Before reclining the patient, review the medical history and ask if the patient has any questions. Then, inform the patient that you are going to recline the chair. Recline the patient to the **supine position**, with the patient's nose and knees at about the same level. Sometimes the chair height will need to be adjusted so the patient is at the height of the operator's elbow; this is about eight inches above the seat of the operator's chair. Adjust the head rest and ask the patient if he or she is comfortable (Figure 14-26).

Position the dental light for maximum illumination of the area where the dental procedure is being performed. This is accomplished by bringing the light three to five feet from the patient's mouth and tilting the light downward toward the patient napkin. Then, turn the light on (this is to avoid shining the light in the patient's

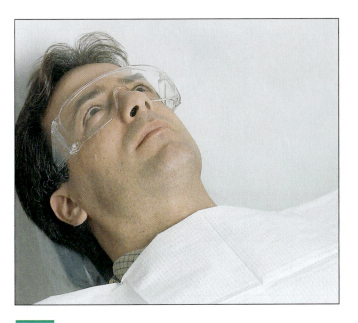

FIGURE 14-26 Patient prepared for treatment with protective glasses and bib.

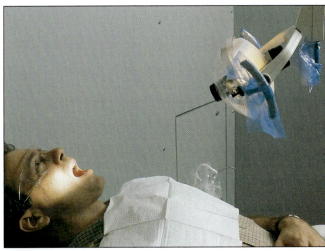

FIGURE 14-28 Patient seated and light adjusted for maxillary arch.

FIGURE 14-27 Patient seated and light adjusted for mandibular arch.

eyes). After the light is on, slowly raise it to the arch being treated:

▶ For the **mandibular teeth**, the light is raised and the beam is directed downward (Figure 14-27).

▶ For the **maxillary teeth**, the light is lowered and the beam is directed upward (Figure 14-28).

After the light is adjusted, the assistant turns the light off until the operator is seated. During the procedure, the light may need to be adjusted periodically. The assistant must be observant to keep the field of operation well lit.

POSITIONING THE OPERATOR AND THE ASSISTANT

Correct positioning of the operator and the assistant can save time and prevent muscle strain and fatigue. In four-handed, sit-down dentistry, it is ideal if the equipment and materials are as close as possible to the operator and the assistant. This will allow the dental team to function as a coordinated and organized unit. Both the operator and the assistant are seated according to the operating zones previously discussed.

Position of the Operator

The operator's position is key to the arrangement of the patient, assistant, and equipment. The operator must be seated in a comfortable position to perform the dental procedure efficiently, with easy access to the oral cavity and clear vision of the operating field. The following are characteristics of proper positioning of the operator:

1. The operator is positioned squarely on the seat of the operator's stool, with his or her weight evenly distributed.

2. The operator's thighs are parallel to the floor and his or her feet are flat on the floor. The stool should be adjustable to accommodate varying heights.

3. The operator's back is supported in the lumbar region. The back and neck are in an upright position with the top of the shoulders parallel to the floor.

4. The operator's elbows are close to the body.

5. The patient's chair is lowered over the operator's thighs, to about the same level as the operator's elbow.

6. The distance between the operator's face and the patient's oral cavity is approximately fourteen to eighteen inches.

7. The operator moves freely in the operator's zone (Figure 14-29).

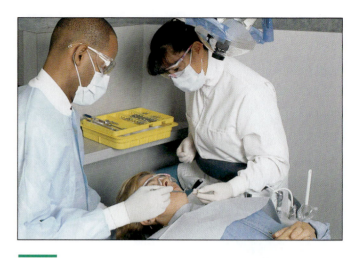

FIGURE 14-29 Operator and assistant positioned correctly with patient reclined and ready for treatment.

P R O C E D U R E

14-3 Seating the Dental Patient

This procedure is performed by the dental assistant in order to prepare the patient for the dental treatment. The dental assistant has reviewed the patient's medical and dental records, cleaned and prepared the treatment room with appropriate barriers, readied the tray setup, and removed any possible obstacles from the patient's pathway. After being greeted by name in the reception area, the patient is escorted to the treatment room by the dental assistant.

EQUIPMENT AND SUPPLIES

▶ Patient's medical and dental records

▶ Basic setup: mouth mirror, explorer, and cotton pliers

▶ Saliva ejector, evacuator (HVE), and air-water syringe tip

▶ Cotton rolls, cotton-tip applicator, and gauze sponges

▶ Lip lubricant

▶ Patient bib and bib clip

▶ Tissue

▶ Safety glasses

PROCEDURE STEPS *(Follow aseptic procedures)*

1. Greet and escort the patient to the treatment room. Show the patient where to place his or her personal items, such as a purse, backpack, or coat. Some offices offer mouth wash to the patient at this time.

2. Seat the patient in the dental chair. Have the patient sit all the way back in the chair. (At this time, the dental assistant may offer the patient a tissue to remove lipstick and ask if he or she would like lubricant for his or her lips.)

3. Place the bib on the patient, and give the patient safety glasses to wear during the procedure.

4. Review the patient's medical history for any changes since his or her last visit. Ask the patient if he or she has any questions, and give a brief explanation or confirmation of the dental treatment to be completed at this appointment. Place x-rays in viewbox.

5. Position the patient for treatment, adjust the head rest, and adjust the dental light for the appropriate arch.

6. Position the operator's stool and the rheostat.

7. Position the assistant's stool. Put on mask and protective eyewear, then wash hands and place on gloves before being seated at chairside.

8. Position the tray setup. Prepare the saliva ejector, evacuator tip, air-water (three-way) syringe tip, and dental handpieces.

Position of the Assistant

The assistant is positioned across from the operator on the opposite side of the patient. The assistant must also have good visibility and easy access to the oral cavity. The tray setup and other necessary instruments should be close at hand. The following are characteristics of proper positioning of the dental assistant:

1. The assistant's stool is positioned 4 to 6 inches above the operator's for good visibility (Figure 14-29).

2. The assistant is positioned on the stool so that his or her weight is distributed evenly over the seat.

3. The front edge of the assistant's stool is even with the patient's mouth.

4. The assistant's feet are resting on a flat ring around the base of the stool and his or her thighs are parallel to the floor.

5. The assistant is positioned as close as possible to the side of the patient.

6. The assistant's back is straight, with support in the lumbar region; on some assistant's chairs there is an arm support that extends around in front of the assistant. This arm supports the assistant when he or she leans forward slightly or when reaching. The arm is adjusted to fit the assistant at the level of the abdomen.

7. After the assistant is correctly positioned on the chair, the cabinet top or mobile cart is placed over the thighs as close as possible for convenience and efficiency.

DISMISSING THE PATIENT

After the treatment is completed, the light is turned off and moved out of the way. The dentist leaves and the assistant begins the process of dismissing the patient. The assistant raises the dental chair to an upright position. The patient is asked to remain seated for a minute,

P R O C E D U R E

14-4 Dismissing the Dental Patient

This procedure is performed by the dental assistant after the dental procedure has been completed.

EQUIPMENT AND SUPPLIES

The following items were set-up for the procedure and now need to be handled as the assistant dismisses the patient.

▶ Patient's medical and dental records

▶ Basic setup: mouth mirror, explorer, and cotton pliers

▶ Saliva ejector, evacuator (HVE), and air-water syringe tip

▶ Cotton rolls, cotton-tip applicator, and gauze sponges

▶ Lip lubricant

▶ Patient bib and bib clip

▶ Tissue

▶ Safety glasses

PROCEDURE STEPS (*Follow aseptic procedures*)

1. When the operator is finished with the procedure, rinse and evacuate the patient's mouth thoroughly. The dental light is positioned out of the patient's way.

2. The patient is positioned in an upright position and he or she is asked to remain seated. Remove any debris from the patient's face. (The patient can double-check in a mirror before leaving the office.)

3. The bib is removed from the patient and is placed over the tray setup.

4. The evacuator (HVE) tip, saliva ejector, and air-water syringe tip are removed.

5. The dental light is positioned out of the patient's way. The operator's stool and the rheostat are moved out of the patient's way.

6. After removing treatment gloves and washing hands or donning overgloves, the procedure is documented on the patient's chart or in the computer terminal. The patient's chart and x-rays are gathered.

7. Post-operative instructions are given to the patient.

8. The patient's personal items are returned and the patient is escorted to the reception area.

in case he or she is a little dizzy from being in the supine or subsupine position during treatment.

The HVE tip, saliva ejector, and syringe tip are removed and placed on the tray. During this time, the assistant wipes any debris from the patient's face and removes the bib. The tray can be covered with the patient's bib.

The dental assistant should place on overgloves or remove treatment gloves and wash hands before documenting the procedure and escorting the patient to the reception area.

The rheostat and the operator's chair should be moved out of the patient's way. The right arm of the chair is raised so that the patient can stand up easily. Ask the patient if he or she has any questions, and give post-operative instructions at the dentist's directions. Return any personal items to the patient, and escort him or her to the reception area.

The dental assistant gathers the patient's records, including the x-rays, to give to the receptionist. The receptionist can make future appointments and complete financial arrangements.

PATIENTS WITH SPECIAL NEEDS

Although most patients can be seated in a routine manner, some patients need special considerations. With most of these patients, planning and preparing before their appointments will eliminate any problems.

Child Patients

Many of the skills in seating a child patient are the same as when seating an adult. However, some changes are needed to adapt to the child's size, maturity, and age. Preparing the patient's records are the same, except the child's parent or guardian should be consulted when reviewing the medical history. The dental chair is lowered to accommodate the size of the child. A booster chair, pillow, or cushion may be used to elevate the child in the chair. If the child is too small to reach the head rest, some operators will just remove or reposition it so that it does not interfere with treatment or the patient's comfort. To prevent the child from sliding down in the dental chair, have him or her sit with legs crossed (Figure 14-30).

When the dental assistant steps into the reception room, it is important to greet both the parent and the child, but the focus should be on the child. Kneel down to the same level as the child and greet him or her. Escort the child to the treatment room, and assist him or her into the dental chair, if necessary. Answer questions the child has, using language appropriate to his or her level of understanding.

Once the procedure is completed and the child is dismissed, escort him or her to the reception area and inform the parent/guardian what treatment was per-

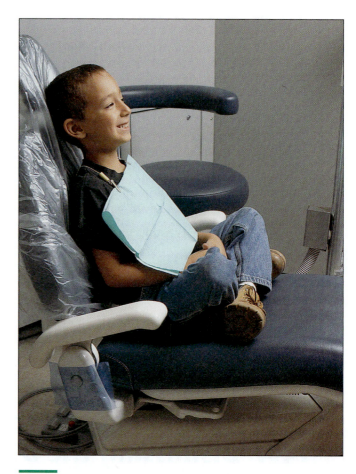

FIGURE 14-30 Child patient seated with legs crossed to prevent sliding down in the chair.

formed. Post-operative instructions for the child should be repeated to the parent/guardian.

Senior Patients

With senior patients, assistance may be needed. The dental assistant should be careful not to offend these patients and their abilities to take care of themselves. Usually, the older patient will ask for help if it is needed. Review the medical history for any changes in health or in medications the patient is taking. Treatment can be broken into shorter segments to accommodate restroom and stretching breaks. The senior patient may not be comfortable in the reclined position for long periods of time, so the dental assistant should position the patient upright whenever possible.

Pregnant Patients

When a pregnant woman is sitting in a reclined position, it may be difficult for her to breath. The dental assistant can allow her to sit in an upright position until the dentist is ready to begin the procedure. During the first trimester of pregnancy, women may find it uncomfortable to have dentistry performed because of symptoms of nausea.

The safest and most comfortable time to schedule dental appointments is during the second trimester of pregnancy. Restroom breaks may become more necessary for women in the third trimester of pregnancy.

Hearing Impaired or Blind Patients

When a patient has hearing difficulties, the dental assistant must be in a position where the patient can observe lip movement and facial expression. Remove the mask and speak normally but slowly; make eye contact and ask questions to be sure that the patient understands. To make the patient feel comfortable and show that the assistant really cares about him or her, the assistant may consider learning a few words in sign language.

The patient who is blind is usually escorted by someone, but he or she is often very independent. Good communication will gain information about his or her abilities and concerns. Talk to the blind patient throughout the procedure, explaining what is happening or what is about to be done.

Patients with Wheelchairs or Walkers

If a patient comes into the office in a wheelchair or using a walker, he or she may need some assistance getting into the dental chair. The pathway to the treatment room needs to be cleared as much as possible. If the patient is using a walker, give assistance when needed. Usually, the patient has a routine and will tell you if help is needed. The wheelchair patient often needs someone to lift or move him or her from the wheelchair to the dental chair (Figure 14-31).

Patients with difficulties know their abilities. Communicate with them to gain an understanding of their needs and treat them in the same manner as all patients who come into the office.

▌ INSTRUMENT TRANSFER

Instrument transfer or exchange is one of the basic functions in **four-handed**, **sit-down dentistry**. The assistant must learn to pass and receive instruments to the operator with confidence and skill. Efficient instrument transfer allows the operator to keep his or her eyes focused on the oral cavity and requires little movement of the operator's hand. A smooth transfer of instruments and materials occurs when the assistant is able to anticipate the operator's needs. This takes practice and cooperation between the operator and the assistant. Once the transfer skills are accomplished, the operator and assistant work as one. The following occurs when proper instrument transfer is accomplished:

▶ The operator's view remains on the oral cavity.

▶ Stress and fatigue for the operator and the assistant are reduced.

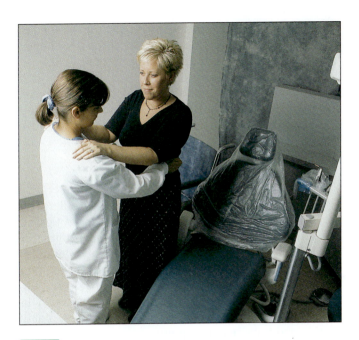

FIGURE 14-31 Patient being transferred from wheelchair to the dental chair.

▶ Safety and comfort are maintained for the patient.

▶ Production is increased in less time and with less motion.

The transfer of instruments between operator and assistant takes place in the **transfer zone**, the area just below the patient's nose, near the chin. The assistant brings the instrument to the operator so the operator will not have to move his or her hand from the established **fulcrum** to exchange the instrument. The **tactile** sensation allows the operator to know the exchange has taken place without his or her eyes moving from the area. The assistant should pass the instrument with pressure firm enough for the operator to feel the instrument in his or her hand.

Fulcrum

A fulcrum is a point of rest on which the fingers are stabilized and can pivot from. For example, when working on the mandibular first molar, the fingers rest on the occlusal surface of the mandibular bicuspids, providing the fulcrum.

Tactile Sensation

Tactile sensation is the feeling sensed by touch. For example, the pressure of the instrument exchanged during an instrument transfer is tactile sensation.

Transfer Hand

To aid the assistant in the delivery of instruments, the fingers and thumb of the hand are identified as follows: the thumb, the index finger or the first finger, the middle finger or the second finger, the ring finger or the third finger, and the little finger or the fourth finger (Figure 14-32).

The assistant passes and receives instruments with the **left hand** when working with a right-handed dentist and with the right hand when assisting a left-handed operator. Using one hand for instrument transfer frees the other hand for evacuation and retraction.

Instrument Grasps

The way an instrument is held influences how efficiently the instrument can be used. Selecting the correct grasp allows the operator control of the instrument, greater tactile sensitivity, and reduces fatigue to the operator's fingers and hand. The way an instrument is grasped also dictates how it is exchanged. There are several different instrument grasps that are commonly used in operative dentistry: pen, modified pen, palm, palm-thumb, and reverse palm-thumb.

Pen Grasp. The **pen grasp**, as the name indicates, is when an instrument is grasped in the same manner as a pen or pencil (Figure 14-33). The instrument is held between the pad of the thumb and the pad of the index finger, with the side of the middle finger on the opposite side of the thumb. With the pen grasp, the instrument is held at the junction of the shank and handle of the instrument (see Chapter 15, Chairside Instruments). The pen grasp is used to hold instruments that have angled shanks.

Modified Pen Grasp. The **modified pen grasp** is similar to the pen grasp. The instrument is held with the same fingers as the pen grasp, except the pad of the middle finger is placed on the top of the instrument with the index finger (Figure 14-34). The modified pen grasp

FIGURE 14-33 Pen grasp.

FIGURE 14-34 Modified pen grasp.

is preferred by some operators and provides more control and strength in some procedures. This grasp also lessens operator fatigue. The modified pen grasp is used with the same instruments as the pen grasp—those with angled shanks.

Palm Grasp. With the **palm grasp**, the operator holds the instrument in the palm of the hand and fingers grasp the handle of the instrument (Figure 14-35). The palm grasp is used with surgical pliers, rubber dam forceps, and other forceps. In some procedures, the palm is up when the operator is working on the maxillary teeth and the working end of the instrument is pointed upward. The palm is down when working on the lower teeth and

T Thumb
1 Index finger
2 Middle finger
3 Ring finger
4 Little finger

FIGURE 14-32 Fingers of the hand.

FIGURE 14-35 Palm grasp.

the working end of the instrument is pointed downward.

Palm-Thumb Grasp. For the **palm-thumb grasp**, the operator grasps the handle of the instrument in the palm of the hand with the four fingers wrapped around the handle while the thumb is extended upward from the palm (Figure 14-36). The palm-thumb grasp is used with instruments having straight shanks and blades, such as the straight chisel or the Wedelstaedt chisel.

Reverse Palm-Thumb Grasp. The **reverse palm-thumb grasp** is a variation of the palm-thumb grasp that is frequently used to hold the evacuator tip in the patient's mouth. The reverse palm-thumb grasp is sometimes called the **thumb-to-nose grasp**. With this grasp, the evacuator tip is held in the palm of the hand with the thumb directed toward the assistant instead of toward the patient, as with the palm-thumb grasp (Figure 14-37).

Instrument Transfer Methods

The assistant selects the next instrument and holds it ready for transfer until the operator signals for the exchange. Usually, this signal occurs when the operator tilts the instrument back away from the patient while still maintaining the fulcrum. The assistant removes the used instrument from the operator's hand and places the new instrument in it.

Eight Basic Rules for Instrument Transfer.

1. With angled-shank instruments, the primary working end should be placed *away* from the assistant on the tray.

2. With straight-shank instruments, the primary working end should be placed *toward* the assistant on the tray.

3. With hinged instruments, the beaks are placed toward the assistant, with the beaks up for the maxillary arch and down for the mandibular arch.

4. Hold the instrument between the thumb and the index finger and the middle finger (Figure 14-38).

5. Pick up the instrument from the tray near the end closest to the assistant. This is the end opposite from the one that the operator uses.

6. The assistant's hand is placed on the instrument opposite from the end the operator uses to allow the operator to receive the instrument (Figure 14-38).

7. Rotate the working end of the instrument until it is directed toward the dental arch being treated, positioned upward for maxillary and downward for mandibular.

FIGURE 14-36 Palm-thumb grasp.

FIGURE 14-37 Reverse palm-thumb grasp.

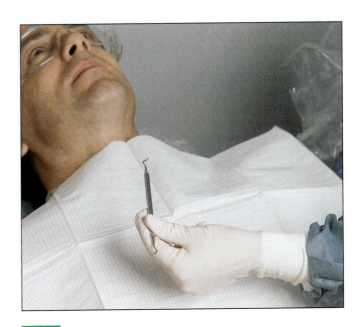

FIGURE 14-38 Instrument correctly held for transfer.

8. Hold the instrument to be passed parallel to the instrument held by the operator. Instruments are held as close to one another as possible, without becoming tangled during the transfer.

One-Handed Transfer. The one-handed transfer is the most common transfer. It saves time and allows the assistant to use the evacuator or the air-water syringe at the same time. With the one-handed transfer, the assistant picks up the next instrument to be transferred with one hand and with the same hand receives the instrument the operator is finished using. Immediately after receiving the used instrument, the dental assistant rotates the new instrument into the operator's hand.

With the one-handed transfer, the assistant can also receive an instrument from the operator and then rotate the instrument for use with the opposite working end. A sequence for instrument transfer includes the following movements: the approach, the retrieval, and the delivery.

Two-Handed Transfer. With the two-handed transfer, the assistant uses both hands for the transfer. One hand receives the instrument from the operator and the other passes the next instrument. This transfer is used most commonly for surgical forceps or when both hands are free. For the two-handed pass, the assistant picks up the instrument from the tray and positions it for delivery with one hand. When the operator signals for an exchange, the assistant retrieves the instrument from the operator with one hand and delivers the new instrument with the other hand. This transfer is also used for dental handpieces and the air-water syringe.

The two-handed exchange follows the same steps as the one-handed exchange: the approach, followed by the retrieval, and then the delivery (Figure 14-39). The two-handed transfer requires the assistant to use both hands

for the exchange—one to receive the used instrument and one to pass the new instrument to the operator.

Instrument Transfer Modifications

There are times when the transfer must be modified. The operator may have to come away from the mouth to receive some instruments, or the size or weight of some instruments may require the transfer to be modified.

The Mirror and Explorer Transfer. At the beginning of the procedure, the operator needs the mirror and the explorer to examine the area to be treated. The assistant picks up the mirror in the right hand and the explorer in the left hand to transfer to a right-handed operator. The operator signals readiness by putting his or her hands in position. The assistant then simultaneously places both instruments in the operator's hands (Figure 14-40).

The Cotton Pliers Transfer. When non-locking cotton pliers are used to transfer small items, a one-handed transfer can be accomplished with slight modifications. The assistant must hold the pliers closer to the working end; this way, the item remains secure in the pliers during the transfer. When the pliers are returned to the assistant, he or she receives them at the working end to avoid dropping any materials (Figure 14-45).

Scissors Transfer. Modifications are required of both the assistant and the operator when transferring scissors. The assistant picks up the scissors, slightly open, at the hinge near the working end. The operator's hand is moved away from the oral cavity and positioned with thumb and fingers apart to receive the scissors. The operator's hand comes away from the oral cavity. When finished with the scissors, the assistant receives the scissors near the hinge and the working area (Figure 14-46).

FIGURE 14-39 Two-handed pass. Assistant uses one hand to receive instrument from the operator and the other hand to pass a new instrument.

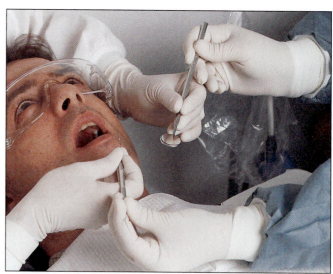

FIGURE 14-40 Mirror and explorer being transferred to the operator at the same time.

PROCEDURE

14-5 One-Handed Instrument Transfer

This procedure is performed at the dental unit by the dental assistant and the operator. In this procedure, the dental asistant uses his or her left hand to transfer instruments for a right-handed dentist. This is reversed for a left-handed operator. The dental assistant's free hand may hold the evacuator or retract oral tissues.

EQUIPMENT AND SUPPLIES

▶ Basic setup: mouth mirror, explorer, and cotton pliers

▶ Spoon excavator (for pen or modified pen grasp)*

▶ Straight chisel, forceps, or elevators (for palm grasp)*

*Any instrument combination can be used to provide a variety of instrument grasps and transfers.

PROCEDURE STEPS *(Follow aseptic procedures)*

Approach
1. Lift the instrument from the tray using the thumb, index finger, and second finger, holding it near the non-working end (Figure 14-41).

2. Turn palm upward into passing position, rotating the nib toward the correct arch (Figure 14-42).

FIGURE 14-42 Assistant carries the instrument and approaches the operator for the exchange.

3. Move toward the operator's hand.

Retrieval
4. Extend the little finger and close around the handle of the instrument the operator is holding (Figure 14-43).

FIGURE 14-41 Instruments on tray in order of the sequence of the procedure. Assistant picks up the instrument at the end closest to the edge of the tray.

FIGURE 14-43 Operator signals he or she is ready for an exchange. Assistant retrieves the instrument.

P R O C E D U R E **14 - 5** *continued*

5. Lift the instrument out of the operator's hand and pull this instrument toward the assistant's palm and wrist.

Delivery

6. Rotate the hand toward the operator and place the instrument in the operator's fingers (Figure 14-44).

7. Once the operator has the new instrument, rotate it to the delivery position for use again or return it to the tray.

FIGURE 14-44 Assistant places new instrument into operator's hand.

(A)

(B)

(C)

FIGURE 14-45 (A) Cotton roll in non-locking cotton pliers ready for transfer. (B) Operator receiving cotton pliers. (C) Operator returning cotton pliers to the assistant.

(A)

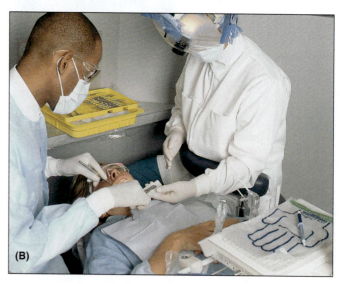

(B)

FIGURE 14-46 (A) Operator receives the scissors. (B) Operator comes away from the oral cavity to return the scissors to the assistant.

Dental Handpieces. Dental handpieces are bulky, but they can be transferred with the one-handed pass. The assistant picks up the handpiece near the hose attachment, away from the working end. Handpieces are heavier and, with the hose attachment, are difficult to transfer, but with time and practice the transfer will be smooth and manageable. If both hands are free, use the two-handed pass to transfer the handpieces (Figure 14-47).

Air-Water Syringe Transfer. To pass the air-water syringe, the assistant holds the end of the syringe covering the nozzle and tip with the palm of the hand. The handle of the syringe is projected toward the operator for easier grasping. The operator receives the syringe at the handle. For the return transfer, the assistant receives the syringe in the same manner it was passed, by covering the nozzle and tip with the palm of the hand. This process can be accomplished with both the one- and two-handed exchange (Figure 14-48).

(A)

(B)

FIGURE 14-48 (A) Assistant holds the air-water syringe near the handle in position for transfer. (B) Operator receives the syringe handle with the tip in position for use.

(A)

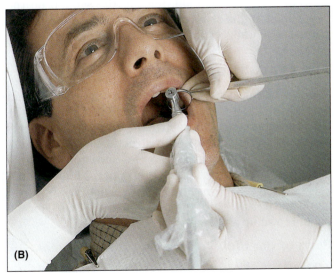
(B)

FIGURE 14-47 (A) Dental handpiece is prepared for transfer. (B) Operator receives the handpiece.

Miscellaneous Items. The dental assistant transfers dental materials close to the operator's reach, usually near the patient's chin. If the material is on a paper pad, the assistant holds the pad near the patient's chin and also holds a gauze for the removal of any excess material (Figure 14-49).

Materials that come in a syringe are passed like scissors, with the assistant holding the syringe near the working end. The operator grasps the handle to complete the transfer.

Any time the operator passes an instrument or material back to the assistant with blood and debris on the working end, the assistant should have a gauze ready to place over the working end as the instrument is received (Figure 14-50). This prevents the patient from viewing the blood and debris and contains it to one area.

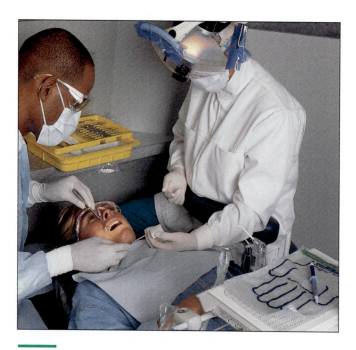

FIGURE 14-49 Dental assistant holds paper pad with mixed cement close to the patient's chin, ready for the operator's use.

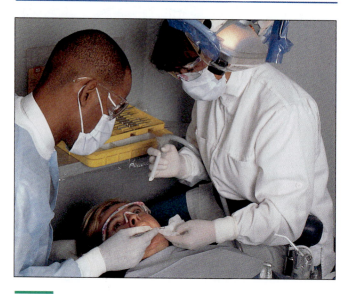

FIGURE 14-50 Assistant holds 2 × 2 gauze open to receive instrument with debris on the working ends.

MAINTAINING THE OPERATING FIELD

Maintaining the operating field is the process of keeping the area directly involved in the treatment clean, visible, as accessible as possible, and comfortable for the patient. A well-maintained field is essential for the procedure to be performed safely.

The requirements of maintaining the operating field are determined by the type of procedure, the tooth or teeth being treated, the oral anatomy of the patient, and the preferences of the operator. The dental assistant is primarily responsible to ensure that:

- The operator's vision and access are not obscured by the oral tissues, moisture, or debris

- Fluids do not interfere with the application of dental materials

- There are no fluids or materials for the patient to swallow or aspirate

- There is no interference with the manipulation of the handpiece and the instruments being used by the operator

Maintaining the operating field is accomplished by a combination of the following techniques:

- Use of the dental dam or cotton rolls to isolate the field

- Use of high volume evacuation and the air-water syringe to rinse and clean the oral cavity

- Retraction of oral tissues for clear vision

The following items are used by the dental team for maintaining the operating field:

- Dental light

- High volume evacuator

- Low volume saliva ejector

- Air-water syringe

- Retractors and mouth props

Lighting

The operator must be able to see the area of the oral cavity that is receiving treatment. Part of the dental assistant's responsibility is maintaining the operating field by positioning the dental light throughout the procedure. The dental light and the fiber optics on the dental handpiece provide the light needed to illuminate the oral cavity. (For more information, refer to the section on the dental light in this chapter and the fiber optic handpiece discussed in Chapter 15, Chairside Instruments.)

The Evacuation System

The evacuation system is designed to remove fluids and debris from the oral cavity. Dental handpieces require the use of a water coolant to reduce the frictional heat that is produced while cutting tooth structure. Because there is a considerable amount of water released from the handpiece during this phase of the procedure, a **high volume evacuator (HVE)** is used to remove the water, saliva, blood and debris. This system eliminates the need for the patient to sit up and empty his or her mouth.

Parts of the High Volume Evacuation System.

- **Hose**—The hose is flexible tubing that connects to the unit at one end and to the handle at the other end. The hose must be long enough for the assistant to reach the patient's oral cavity without any restrictions.

▶ **Evacuation tip**—The evacuation tip is a plastic or metal tip that fits into the handle/hose of the evacuation system. These tips come in a variety of lengths and shapes and can have beveled ends. They may be straight or slightly bent, and they are either disposable or can be sterilized (Figure 14-51A). Some procedures require a tip that is very narrow on one end. These are used during surgical procedures to allow evacuation in a restricted area.

▶ **Handle**—The handle is where the evacuation tip is inserted and the on/off controls are located. The control switch may be a dial, switch, or button—There are many variations. The assistant should be able to operate the control switch with the hand that holds the evacuator (Figure 14-51B).

In Which Hand Is the Evacuator Positioned?

The evacuator is held in the assistant's right hand when assisting a right-handed operator and in the left hand when assisting a left-handed operator.

Grasps for Oral Evacuation.

There are several ways to grasp an evacuator tip. Which grasp to use is determined by where the tip is placed, whether it is used to evacuate fluids or retract tissue or both, and how comfortable the assistant feels with the grasp. The grasps most commonly used are the pen, modified pen grasp, thumb-to-nose, or the reverse palm-thumb. The pen grasp or the modified pen grasp are used when working on the anterior maxillary and mandibular teeth or when using the narrow surgical tip. The thumb-to-nose grasp is used for the maxillary and mandibular posterior teeth. When using the thumb-to-nose grasp, the assistant has

greater control and better retraction of the cheeks and tongue and causes less strain on the assistant's hand.

General Guidelines for Oral Evacuation Tip Placement.

▶ Carefully place the evacuator tip in the patient's mouth. Avoid bumping the teeth, lips, or gingiva.

▶ Place the evacuator tip in the mouth, and position it before the operator positions the handpiece or an instrument.

▶ Place the evacuator tip approximately one tooth distal to the tooth being worked on.

▶ Hold the bevel of the evacuator tip parallel to the buccal or lingual surface of the teeth.

▶ The middle of the evacuator tip opening should be even with the occlusal surface. Position the tip far enough away from the handpiece so that it does not draw the water coolant away from the bur.

▶ Hold the evacuator tip still while the handpiece or instrument is being used. Any movement may startle the operator or the patient and may cause the handpiece or instrument to be bumped.

▶ Rest the tip on cotton rolls, not the gingival tissue. Cotton rolls are placed in the vestibular area near the tooth being worked on before the evacuator tip is placed.

▶ Avoid placing the evacuator tip on the soft palate, the back of the tongue, or the anterior pillar/tonsilar area. Allowing the tip to contact any of these areas could cause the patient to gag.

▶ Keep the evacuator tip far enough away from the mucosal tissue to prevent it from being sucked into the tip and making a noise. If this does occur, either turn it off or rotate the tip to break the seal, and avoid saying "Oops" or "I'm sorry." Just go on with the procedure.

Saliva Ejector

The saliva ejector is the low volume evacuation system. It is a flexible, plastic tube about one-third the size of the high volume evacuation tube. The saliva ejector is bent and then positioned between the tongue and the mandibular teeth or between the cheek and the mandibular teeth.

Parts of the Saliva Ejector.

▶ **Plastic tube** or a metal "shepherd's hook" tube—The plastic tube is the most common, although the stainless-steel tubes are available. The plastic saliva ejectors are less expensive and are disposable. The end that is placed in the patient's mouth has a guard cover to prevent large particles of debris from becoming lodged in the tube.

(A)

(B)

FIGURE 14-51 (A) Several types of evacuator tips (straight, curved, metal, and plastic). (B) Evacuator handle. *(Courtesy of A-dec, Inc., Newberg, Oregon, USA)*

P R O C E D U R E

14-6 Specific Tip Placements for Evacuation of the Oral Cavity

This procedure is performed by the dental assistant during dental treatment. The oral cavity is maintained to keep the area clear and clean for the operator and for the comfort of the patient. Each area of the mouth requires different evacuator tip positioning. The following illustrates how to position the tip for each quadrant when assisting a right-handed operator.

EQUIPMENT AND SUPPLIES

▶ Basic setup: mouth mirror, cotton pliers, and explorer

▶ HVE tip and air-water syringe tip

▶ Cotton rolls

▶ Dental handpiece

PROCEDURE STEPS *(Follow aseptic procedures)*

1. Maxillary right posterior tip placement (Figure 14-52).

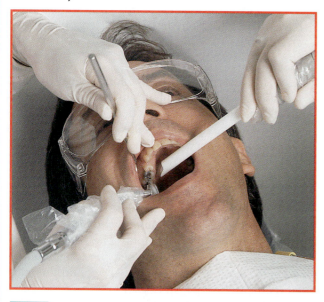

FIGURE 14-52 The tip is placed near the lingual surface just distal to the tooth being worked on. The bevel of the tip is parallel to the lingual surface of the teeth. Notice that the tip is resting on the teeth in the maxillary left quadrant.

2. Maxillary left posterior tip placement (Figure 14-53).

FIGURE 14-53 Evacuator tip in position with cotton rolls. Also, the handpiece and mouth mirror in position with the air-water syringe tip. The evacuator tip is positioned parallel to the buccal surface of the teeth and is resting on a cotton roll.

3. Mandibular right posterior tip placement (Figure 14-54).

FIGURE 14-54 Evacuator tip in position with handpiece and mouth mirror. The tip comes across the mandibular left teeth and is positioned between the lingual surface of the teeth and the tongue. The tip is parallel to the lingual surface of the teeth. A cotton roll is used for retraction of the tongue.

PROCEDURE 14-6 *continued*

4. Mandibular left posterior tip placement (Figure 14-55).

FIGURE 14-55 Evacuator tip placed and handpiece in position. The tip of the bevel of the evacuator tip is positioned parallel to the buccal surface of the teeth.

5. Maxillary anterior facial tip placement (Figure 14-56).

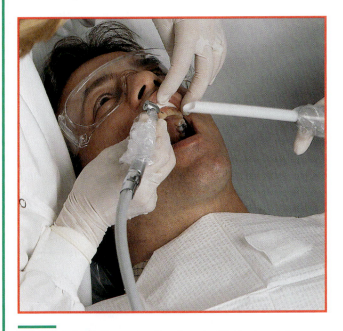

FIGURE 14-56 Evacuator tip placed with the handpiece positioned. For the anterior facial tip placement, the operator is positioned on the facial. The evacuator tip is placed out of the operator's vision. Optional tip placement from the lingual surface.

6. Maxillary anterior lingual tip placement (Figure 14-57).

FIGURE 14-57 Evacuator tip placed with handpiece, mouth mirror, and air-water syringe tip. The tip is placed on the lingual, out of the operator's way. Optional tip placement from the facial surface.

7. Mandibular anterior facial tip placement (Figure 14-58).

FIGURE 14-58 Tip placed and the handpiece in position. The evacuator tip is positioned on a cotton roll near the facial surface of the teeth. The lip is retracted and the bevel is parallel to the facial surface.

8. Mandibular anterior lingual tip placement (Figure 14-59).

FIGURE 14-59 Tip placed and the handpiece and the mouth mirror positioned. The evacuator tip is positioned with the bevel parallel to the lingual surface of the teeth.

▶ **Handle**—The plastic tube is inserted in the handle, which is connected to the hose. The handle has an on/off control and also a small screen that acts as a filter, located near the tube end of the handle.

▶ **Hose**—The hose end attaches to a low volume vacuum source in the unit.

The saliva ejector is used during procedures that do not require removal of large amounts of fluids, such as during fluoride treatments, under the rubber dam, or during a coronal polish (Figure 14-60).

The Air-Water Syringe

The air-water syringe, also referred to as the three-way syringe, emits water, air, or a combination of both in a spray. The patient's mouth is rinsed with the air-water syringe and simultaneously evacuated. The assistant can dry an area or keep the mirror clean with air for the operator to have clear vision. The air-water syringe is held in the assistant's left hand for a right-handed operator and in the right hand for a left-handed operator.

Parts of the Air-Water Syringe.

▶ **Handle**—The handle is connected to a hose that is connected to the unit. The top of the handle is called the nozzle area and has buttons for the *water* and the *air*. If the buttons are pressed simultaneously, a spray of water and air is released (Figure 14-61A). In the handle, there are O-rings that may have to be changed if the syringe begins to leak.

▶ **Syringe tip**—The syringe tip directs the air, water, or spray. The tips are either metal and can be removed and sterilized or plastic and disposable. The tips can be rotated for positioning toward the maxillary or mandibular teeth (Figure 14-61B).

Guidelines for Use of the Air-Water Syringe.

1. The most effective way to use the air-water syringe is with the air-water spray. A spray is effective and easier to control (Figure 14-62A).

2. When rinsing a patient's mouth, use the evacuator tip to follow the spray. The patient's mouth is rinsed in quadrants, and the evacuator tip and the air-water syringe tip are rotated for correct placement (Figure 14-62B). Rinsing and evacuating the patient's mouth requires practice to achieve efficiency and control.

3. When the operator is using the handpiece and a mirror for indirect vision, water from the handpiece falls onto the mirror and distorts the operator's view. The assistant will be expected to keep the mirror surface dry and free from debris. To accomplish this, the assistant places the tip of the air-water syringe tip *close to the edge* of the mouth mirror and directs air across the surface of the mirror without interfering with the operator's view.

(A)

(B)

FIGURE 14-60 (A) Saliva ejector hose, control, and several different types of saliva ejectors. (B) Saliva ejector in the patient's mouth. Notice the handle control on the hose and the flexibility of the saliva ejector, bent to stay in the patient's mouth.

4. When the operator stops the handpiece, the assistant completes a quick "rinse and dry" to give the operator a clean, dry mirror for good vision. This is accomplished by first using the spray, followed by the air.

Retraction of Tissues

Retraction of the tongue, cheeks, lips, and tissue is used to increase the field of vision in the oral cavity. There are several types of retractors used, including the

(A)

(B)

FIGURE 14-61 Parts of air-water syringe: (A) handle and (B) syringe tip. *(Courtesy of A-dec, Inc., Newberg, Oregon, USA)*

FIGURE 14-62 (A) Assistant using the air-water syringe. (B) Assistant using the HVE and the air-water syringe.

FIGURE 14-63 (A) Retraction using a mouth mirror. (B) Retraction using a cotton gauze.

mouth mirror, the rubber dam, the evacuator tip, cotton rolls, cotton gauze, and specially designed tissue retractors. Retractors are used during any procedure to allow for better access and lighting and to prevent injury to the tissues (Figures 14-63A and B).

Mouth Props. Mouth props are used to assist the patient in keeping his or her mouth open during treatment (Figure 14-64A). Mouth props are available in sev-

eral different wedge-shaped designs and materials such as rubber, plastic, and styrofoam. Another distinctive type of mouth prop is a metal adjustable prop, with rubber tubing over the area where the teeth rest and a handle to adjust the opening. To place the prop between the maxillary and mandibular teeth, ask the patient to open wide, insert the prop, and instruct the patient to close on the prop. After placing the prop, ask if the patient is comfortable and adjust the prop, if necessary (Figure 14-64B).

FIGURE 14-64 (A) Examples of mouth props. (B) Mouth prop in patient's mouth.

CHAPTER SUMMARY

Dental health professionals go to great lengths to ensure patient and employee safety. It is therefore extremely important to understand the dental setting by facility design, employee role responsibility, and specific job description by procedure.

CASE STUDY

Mrs. Maxine Rose, age 77, had several restorations completed during her hour-long appointment. She is in good health but was in the supine position for most of her appointment.

Case Study Review

1. What can the dental assistant expect to occur once the procedure is complete and the patient is again seated in an upright position?

2. How can the assistant aid Mrs. Rose before escorting her to the reception area?

3. Is there anything the dental assistant can do to prevent patients from experiencing discomfort resulting from positioning during treatment?

 To complete your study of this chapter, work the review activities that follow. Also, refer to the software that accompanies this text.

REVIEW QUESTIONS

Multiple Choice

1. In which of the following areas would a dental unit be located?
   a. Reception area.
   c. Sterilizing area.
   b. Dental treatment room.
   d. Processing room.

2. There are four activity zones. Which zone extends from 12 to 2 o'clock for a right-handed operator?
   a. Operating zone.
   c. Static zone.
   b. Assisting zone.
   d. Transfer zone.

3. When seating a dental patient, where does the dental assistant place the patient's personal items?
   a. In the reception area.
   b. In the treatment room where the patient can see them.
   c. In the lounge.
   d. In the dentist's office.

4. All of the following are instrument grasps *except*
   a. pen grasp.
   c. palm grasp.
   b. modified pen grasp.
   d. palm-index finger grasp.

5. Which of the following is used to remove small amounts of fluid and debris from the oral cavity?
   a. The saliva ejector.
   b. The oral evacuator.
   c. The HVE.
   d. The air-water syringe.

Critical Thinking

1. List ways that a dental assistant can create an atmosphere that would put patients at ease and give them the impression that this office is competent and provides quality dentistry.

2. How could contamination buildup in the evacuator and ai-water syringe be prevented?

3. Identify methods to ensure comfort for a patient having dental treatment while in the third trimester of pregnancy.

Chairside Instruments and Tray Systems

OBJECTIVES

The student should strive to meet the following objectives and demonstrate an understanding of the facts and principles presented in this chapter:

1. Identify the parts of an instrument and describe how instruments are identified.

2. Identify the categories and functions of dental burs.

3. Describe the types and functions of abrasives.

4. Explain the various handpieces and attachments.

5. Describe the types of tray systems and color-coding systems.

KEY TERMS

abrasives (p. 287)

air abrasion (p. 289)

bevel (p. 274)

binangle (p. 274)

Black's formula (p. 276)

blade (p. 274)

burs (p. 284)

chuck (p. 289)

contra-angle (p. 289)

cutting edge (p. 274)

fiberoptic light sources (p. 290)

frictional heat (p. 288)

high-speed handpieces (p. 289)

low-speed handpieces (p. 289)

mandrels (p. 287)

manufacturer's number (p. 276)

monangle (p. 274)

non-cutting (p. 275)

revolutions per minute (rpm) (p. 289)

rotary instruments (p. 284)

shaft (p. 274)

shank (p. 274)

working end (p. 274)

INTRODUCTION

Dental instruments are continually developing as technology changes and dental materials require instruments of specific designs or materials. Most instruments are constructed of stainless steel, and a few are a high-tech plastic/resin or anodized aluminum. Manufacturers of dental instruments provide many designs and sizes and make improvements as new materials become available. The dentist selects the instruments that he or she feels the most confident and comfortable using. Each procedure requires special instruments to accomplish the task; for example, when examining the pits and grooves of the teeth, the dentist uses an explorer. The ends of all explorers are pointed and sharp but designed with different angles to reach all surfaces of the tooth.

It is the dental assistant's responsibility to keep the instruments sterilized and in working condition. The dental assistant orders new instruments as needed and keeps the instruments in sequence while assisting during the procedure.

Instruments are generally categorized into hand instruments and rotary instruments. The hand instruments are manually operated and are categorized according to the specific procedure. In this chapter, the basic instruments used in general dental procedures are discussed, including common cutting and non-cutting instruments. Specialty instruments are covered in the related specialty chapters.

INSTRUMENTS FOR BASIC CHAIRSIDE PROCEDURES

Basic Structural Parts of Dental Hand Instruments

The dental instrument is generally six inches long and is single or double ended. The parts of the dental hand instrument include the working end, the shank, and the handle (Figure 15-1).

The Working End of an Instrument. The **working end** actually performs the specific function of the instrument. The working end may be a point, blade, or nib. A point is sharp and is used to explore, detect, and reflect materials. The **blade** may be flat or curved and have a rounded edge or a cutting edge. The **cutting edge** is formed by a **bevel** (slanted edge or side) on the working end of the instrument. The blade may also be **bi-beveled** (beveled on both sides of the blade). A nib is a blunt end that is either serrated or smooth (Figures 15-2A–C).

The working end of an instrument may also be beaks or rounded ends. The beaks may be smooth, serrated, or grooved, depending on their functions. The rounded ends come in different sizes and shapes and are used to smooth surfaces.

FIGURE 15-1 Parts of the single-ended dental instrument. *(Courtesy of Miltex Instrument Co., Inc., Lake Success, NY)*

Handle (Shaft). The handle, or **shaft**, of an instrument is where the instrument is held by the operator. The handle may be serrated or smooth. It is usually hexagonal (six sided), which provides for a better grip. Some handles are covered with a rubberized material that comes in different colors. These handles are easy to grip and identify. A few instruments are designed with **cone socket handles**, which allow the working ends to be replaced (Figures 15-3A and B).

Shank. The **shank** connects the handle to the working end. It narrows or tapers from the handle to the working end. The shank may be angled to reach different areas of the mouth. Usually, instruments that are used in the posterior areas of the oral cavity have more angles, while instruments with fewer angles are used in anterior areas. Shanks of dental instruments are formed in the following ways: **straight** (no angles), **curved** (slightly bent), **monangle** (one angle), **binangle** (two angles), or **triple angle** (three angles) (Figures 15-4A-E).

Basic Classification of Dental Instruments

Dental instruments are classified in many ways, including by number of working ends, function, manufacturer's name and number, and Black's number formula.

FIGURE 15-4 Instrument shanks. (A) Straight. (B) Curved. (C) Monangle. (D) Binangle. (E) Triple angle.

FIGURE 15-2 Various working ends. (A) Point. (B) Blade. (C) Nib. *(Courtesy of Miltex Instrument Co., Inc., Lake Success, NY)*

Number of Working Ends. The number of working ends an instrument has falls into two categories: single-ended and double-ended instruments. Single-ended instruments have only one working end and long handles. Double-ended instruments have two working ends in the following combinations (Figure 15-5):

▶ The two ends have similar functions, but one end is larger than the other (for example, an amalgam condenser).

▶ The two ends are paired right and left for preparing the right or the left side of the cavity preparation (for example, a gingival margin trimmer).

▶ The two ends have a combined function in which the ends are used for the same procedure but each end has a different use (for example, a plastic filling instrument).

Instruments Classified by Function. Instruments are classified by function to describe the specific usage. Operative hand instruments are divided into cutting and **non-cutting** for functional classification. Other instruments are classified according to a specialty, use with a specific material, or a procedure.

FIGURE 15-3 (A) Various instrument handle styles. (B) Serrated: cone socket. *(Courtesy of Miltex Instrument Co., Inc., Lake Success, NY)*

Cutting and Non-Cutting Instruments

Cutting Instruments

▶ Angle formers	▶ Gingival margin trimmers
▶ Chisels	▶ Hatchets
▶ Excavators	▶ Hoes

(A)   **(B)**

FIGURE 15-5 Working ends of (A) cotton pliers for transporting materials and (B) burnishers for smoothing materials. *(Courtesy of Miltex Instrument Co., Inc., Lake Success, NY)*

Non-Cutting Instruments

- Basic instruments (mouth mirror, explorer, and cotton pliers)
- Burnishers
- Carriers
- Carvers
- Composite instruments
- Condensers
- Files
- Finishing knives
- Plastic filling instruments

Manufacturer's Number. The **manufacturer's number** is a number found on the handle of the instrument. The number is used when ordering the instrument and indicates the instrument's placement in a set of instruments. Some instruments are named or classified by the name of the individual who designed the instrument.

Black's Formula. **Black's formula** was developed by G.V. Black to standardize the exact size and angulation of an instrument. This formula minimizes discrepancies in the production of instruments from one manufacturer to another and simplifies the ordering of these instruments. Black's formula for hand cutting instruments includes the size of the blade and the angle at which it is positioned to the handle. Some instruments such as chisels, hatchets, and hoes, have series of three numbers and some, such as angle formers and gingival margin trimmers, have four numbers.

Black's Three Number Formula (Figure 15-6)

1. The *first number* is the width of the blade in tenths of a millimeter. In the formula 20 9 14, the first number (20) indicates that the blade is 2.0 mm wide.
2. The *second number* is the measurement of the length of the blade in millimeters. In the formula 20 9 14, the second number (9) indicates that the length of the blade is 9 mm.
3. The *third number* gives the measurement of the angle of the blade to the long axis of the handle, in degrees centigrade. In the formula 20 9 14, the third number (14) indicates that the instrument has a blade at an angle of 14/100 of a circle.

Black's Four-Number Formula (Figure 15-7)

1. The *first number* is the same as that in the three-number formula, representing the width of the blade, in tenths of a millimeter. In the formula 15 85 8 12, the first number (15) indicates that the blade is 1.5 mm long.
2. The *second number* is different from that in the three-number formula, representing the degree of the angle of the cutting edge of the blade to the handle of the instrument. In the formula 15 85 8 12, the second number (85) indicates that the cutting edge forms a 95° C angle with the handle.
3. The *third number* is the same as the second number in the three-number formula. Using the formula 15 85 8 12, the third number (8) indicates that the blade is 8 mm long.
4. The *fourth number* is the same as the third number in the three-number formula. Using the formula 15 85 8 12, the fourth number (12) indicates that the blade forms a 12° C angle with the handle of the instrument.

FIGURE 15-6 Instrument with Black's three-number formula.

FIGURE 15-7 Instrument with Black's four-number formula.

Cutting Instruments

Hand cutting instruments are used to assist in the design of the cavity preparation. They refine and define the cavity walls and margins. There are six hand cutting instruments: chisels, hatchets, hoes, gingival margin trimmers, angle formers, and excavators.

Chisels. Chisels are used to shape and plane enamel and dentin walls of the cavity preparation. The blade of the chisel is straight and has a cutting edge with a one-sided beveled. The chisel is usually a double-ended instrument: one end with a standard bevel on the blade and one end with a reversed bevel on the end of the blade (Figure 15-8). Chisels have several different shanks, which is where they get their names.

▶ **Straight chisels** have no angle in the shank and are used on maxillary and mandibular teeth in Class III or IV cavity preparations (Figure 15-9A). Straight chisels are used in conjunction with a mallet to remove fixed prosthetics.

▶ **Wedelstaedt chisels** have slightly curved shanks and are used for Class III and IV cavity preparations (Figure 15-9B).

▶ **Binangle chisels** have two angles in the shanks of the instruments and are used in Class II cavity preparations (Figure 15-9C).

FIGURE 15-8 Chisel with standard and reverse bevel. *(Courtesy of Hu-Friedy Mfg. Co., Inc.)*

(B)

(A) (C)

(D)

FIGURE 15-9 Chisels. (A) Straight. (B) Wedelstaed. (C) Binangle. (D) Chisel being used to prepare cavity. *(Courtesy of Hu-Friedy Mfg. Co., Inc.)*

Hatchets. Hatchets, sometimes called enamel hatchets, are similar to wooden hatchets. There is an angle in the shank of a hatchet and the blade is flat. Hatchets are paired left and right, with a bevel on one side of the blade on one end of the instrument and the reverse side of the blade on the other end. The hatchet is used in a downward motion to refine the cavity walls and to obtain retention in the cavity preparation (Figure 15-10). Sometimes, hatchets are marked with rings on the handles to indicate left and right ends.

Hoes. A hoe is an instrument that is used in a pulling motion to smooth and shape the floor of the cavity preparation. A hoe is shaped similar to a garden hoe, with straight and angled shanks. All hoes have blades that form cutting edges (Figure 15-11A and B).

Gingival Margin Trimmers. The gingival margin trimmer (GMT) is similar to the hatchet in regard to the position of the blade to the handle, but there are two distinctive differences. First, the blade on the GMT is curved, not flat like the hatchet. Second, the cutting edge is at an angle, not straight across like the hatchet. The GMT is a double-ended and paired instrument. With the double ends of the instrument, one end curves toward the left and the other end curves toward the right. A pair of gingival margin trimmers is used during the cavity preparation, because one instrument is for the distal surfaces and another is for the mesial surface (Figures 15-12A and B). The GMTs are used to bevel the gingival margin wall of the cavity preparation.

> ### Gingival Margin Trimmers Identification
>
> To distinguish between the mesial and the distal GMT, consider the following:
> 1. The number on the handle. This is a Black's, four-numbered instrument, so the second number in the series on the handle indicates the angle of the blade. If this number is 90 or above, it is used on the distal surface of the cavity preparation; if it is 85 or below, it is used on the mesial surface.
> 2. Hold the instrument upright. If the cutting edge forms a line that is parallel to the handle, it is used on the distal (down for distal). If the cutting edge does not form this line, it is used on the mesial.

Angle Formers. The angle former is used in a downward pushing motion to form and define point angles and to sharpen line angles. The angle former is similar to the hoe, except the cutting edge is angled like the gingival margin trimmer. Therefore, this also is a four-numbered instrument. This instrument is double ended, so it can be used on either the left or the right surfaces of a cavity preparation (Figure 15-13).

Excavators. Excavators, also known as "spoon excavators," are used to remove carious material and debris from the teeth. This instrument is also used for numer-

FIGURE 15-10 Hatchet. *(Courtesy of Hu-Friedy Mfg. Co., Inc.)*

FIGURE 15-11 (A) Hoe. (B) Fracturing away the undermined enamel with a hoe. *(Courtesy of Hu-Friedy Mfg. Co., Inc.)*

FIGURE 15-12 Gingival margin trimmers. (A) Distal. (B) Mesial. *(Courtesy of Hu-Friedy Mfg. Co., Inc.)*

FIGURE 15-13 Angle former. *(Courtesy of Hu-Friedy Mfg. Co., Inc.)*

FIGURE 15-14 Excavators. (A) Blade. (B) Spoon. *(Courtesy of Miltex Instrument Co., Inc., Lake Success, NY)*

ous other tasks, including removing excess dental cement, tucking rubber dam material, and packing gingival retraction cord. The excavator is similar to the gingival margin trimmer with the curved blade, but the difference is that the cutting edge of the excavator is rounded all the way around the periphery of the blade (Figures 15-14A and B).

Non-Cutting Instruments

Non-cutting instruments include the basic examination instruments and instruments used to insert and finish amalgam and composite restorative materials. Examples of non-cutting instruments include basic examination setup, plastic instruments, amalgam carriers, condensers, carvers, burnishers, files, and finishing knives.

Basic Examination Instruments

The basic examination setup instruments are used for examination of the teeth but are also common to all tray setups. All procedures begin with the operator examining the teeth, so the mouth mirror, explorer, and cotton pliers are the first three instruments on a procedure tray setup. The periodontal probe is an optional instrument in the basic examination setup.

Mouth Mirrors. The mouth mirror is a single-ended instrument made of metal or plastic. It may have a handle with a "cone socket" for easy replacement of the mirror head or come in one piece. Mirrors are available in different sizes and types. The mirror sizes are identified by number, and the most commonly used are numbers 4 and 5. The mouth mirror may be sterilized (by autoclaving, dry heat, or cold chemical sterilizing) or may be disposable. The types of mirrors are the plane surface, front surface, and concave surface.

▶ **Plane or regular surface mirrors** have reflective surfaces (silver coatings) on the backs of the glass (Figure 15-15A). This gives the image a "ghost image" as the light reflects from the glass and the silver layer.

▶ **Front surface mirrors** have reflective coatings (rhodium) on top of the glass. This coating eliminates the "ghost image"; it reflects only once to give a clear view free of distortion (Figure 15-15B).

▶ **Concave surface mirrors** magnify the image.

FIGURE 15-15 (A) Plane (regular) surface mirror. (B) Front surface mirror. (C) Cone socket mirror. *(Courtesy of Miltex Instrument Co., Inc., Lake Success, NY)*

Uses of the Mouth Mirror

▶ **Indirect vision**—When the operator uses a mirror to view areas of the oral cavity not seen with direct vision

▶ **Reflection of light**—Illumination of an area being examined or treated

▶ **Retraction**—When the cheeks or tongue are retracted for better visibility and for protection of the tissues

▶ **Transillumination**—Reflection of light through the tooth surface to detect fractures

Explorers. Explorers are single- or double-ended instruments. The working end is a thin, sharp point of flexible steel. This allows the operator to examine surfaces of the teeth in order to detect any irregularity. There are a variety of angles of explorers, and often the ends are different so the operator can access various areas of the mouth. Several common shapes include the pig tail, the shepherd's hook, the right angle, and the #17 (Figures 15-16A and B).

Uses of Explorers

▶ **Examination** of the tooth structure for any defects or areas of decay

▶ **Examination** of restorations to check for faulty margins or fractures

▶ **Removal of excess materials** from around the margins of restorations or from bases and liners in the cavity preparation

Cotton Pliers. Cotton pliers are shaped like large tweezers with either smooth surfaces or serrations on the ends of the beaks. They are available in locking or non-locking handles, and the tips may be straight or angled. They are made of stainless steel and can be sterilized. They are used frequently during a procedure by the operator and the dental assistant to transport and manipulate various materials (Figure 15-17).

Uses of Cotton Pliers

▶ **To place** and remove items from the oral cavity, such as cotton rolls, cotton pellets, wedges, and large pieces of debris

FIGURE 15-17 Cotton pliers. *(Courtesy of Miltex Instrument Co., Inc., Lake Success, NY)*

▶ **To grasp** and transfer materials to and from the oral cavity

▶ **To retrieve** materials from drawers, cupboards, and so on in order to avoid contamination

Periodontal Probes. Periodontal probes are used to measure the depth of the gingival sulcus. It may be a single- or double-ended instrument. The working end of the probe is a blade that is rounded or blunted and is marked in millimeters (mm). There are variations in the indication of calibrations, including color coding. A combination instrument that has an explorer tip on one end and a periodontal probe on the other end is known as an **Expro**. It is very functional and reduces the number of instruments on the tray (Figure 15-18) (also see Chapter 23, Periodontics).

Plastic Filling Instruments/ Composite Instruments

Plastic Filling Instruments. Plastic filling instruments are used to place and condense pliable restorative materials and to place cement bases in the cavity preparation. These instruments are made of plastic or metal and are usually double ended. One of the most common plastic instruments has a paddle on one end and a small condenser on the other end (Figure 15-19A).

Composite Instruments. Composite instruments are very similar to plastic filling instruments in use and shape. They are also double ended. The main difference is that the composite instruments are made of a high-grade thermoplastic material or an anodized aluminum

FIGURE 15-16 Types of explorers. (A) Pigtail. (B) Shepherd's hook and #17. *(Courtesy of Miltex Instrument Co., Inc., Lake Success, NY)*

FIGURE 15-18 Expro with (A) explorer and (B) periodontal probe. *(Courtesy of Miltex Instrument Co., Inc., Lake Success, NY)*

to prevent discoloration of the composite or glass ionomer restoration materials (Figure 15-19B).

Amalgam Carriers

The amalgam carrier is designed to carry and dispense amalgam or composite into the cavity preparation. The carriers may be single or double ended with small and large ends. Most carriers are made of stainless steel, and some have Teflon or coated barrels to prevent clogging. The dental assistant loads both ends of the carrier with the restorative material and either passes it to the operator or places the amalgam in the cavity preparation and then refills the carrier as needed (Figure 15-20A).

A spring-action **amalgam gun** is used to carry and place composites, glass ionomers, and amalgam alloys. It is single ended and made of high-grade plastic (Figure 15-20B).

Amalgam Condensers (Pluggers)

The amalgam condensers, or pluggers, are used to pack amalgam into the cavity preparation. There are hand condensers and mechanical condensers. The hand condensers are usually double ended and have a wide variety of working ends. The locations and designs of cavity preparations have required condensers to be diverse in design. The working ends may be plain (smooth) or serrated. They may be round, ovoid, rectangular, diamond, or cone shaped (Figure 15-21). The shanks of condensers may be monangled, binangled, or triple angled.

The mechanical condensers, sometimes called amalgam packers or vibrators, are used to pack and condense amalgam through vibrations into the cavity preparation. The mechanical condensers are attached to the dental unit and operated with condensed air. The packing points come in a variety of shapes and sizes. The action of the condenser is like a woodpecker, with short, quick movements.

FIGURE 15-20 (A) Double-ended amalgam carrier. *(Courtesy of Miltex Instrument Co., Inc., Lake Success, NY)* (B) Amalgam gun. *(Courtesy of Hu-Friedy Mfg. Co., Inc.)*

FIGURE 15-19 (A) Plastic instruments. (B) Composite instruments.

FIGURE 15-21 Condenser. *(Courtesy of Hu-Friedy Mfg. Co., Inc.)*

Carvers

Carvers are used to remove excess restorative material and carve tooth anatomy in the restoration before the material hardens. Carvers are also used to carve wax inlays, onlays, and crowns. There are a wide variety of working ends on carvers, including long-bladed pointed ends and rounded and oval shapes. Usually, carvers are double ended, with some ends having sharp edges and others rounded blades similar to excavators. The operator usually has several favorite carvers; often these include the Hollenback and the cleoid-discoid. The Hollenback is a long-bladed carver used to shape the restoration. The cleoid-discoid carver is used to shape amalgam restorations. The cleoid end looks like a claw, and the discoid end is shaped like a round disc (Figures 15-22A through D).

Burnishers

Burnishers are used to smooth rough margins of the restoration and to shape metal matrix bands. Burnishers are blunt, rounded instruments that come in a variety of shapes, including the beavertail, the egg or football shape, the ball shape, and the T-ball. Burnishers may be single- or double-ended instruments (Figure 15-23).

Files

Files are used to trim excess filling material and to smooth the restoration, especially the margins. They come in a variety of shapes, with a serrated surface on one side of the blade. The working end is often thin and small enough to reach interproximal spaces. Files are available as either single- or double-ended instruments (Figure 15-24).

Finishing Knives

Finishing knives are used to trim excess filling material. The working ends of the finishing knives have sharp, knife-like blades. Finishing knives come in a variety of shapes and angles in order to access the margins of the restoration (Figure 15-25).

Miscellaneous Instruments

Additional instruments found on restorative trays include spatulas, articulating forceps, and scissors.

Spatulas. During restorative procedures, **cement spatulas** may be used. These spatulas are single ended and made of stainless steel. They come in a variety of sizes and strengths. Spatulas are used to mix cements, bases, and liners (Figure 15-26). **Plastic spatulas** are used to mix composite resin materials. These spatulas are usually double ended and may be disposable. **Laboratory spatulas** are used to mix impression materials and plaster. These spatulas are larger in size and have longer, wider blades. Laboratory spatulas are made entirely of plastic or with metal blades and wooden handles.

Articulating Forceps. Articulating forceps are used to hold articulation paper, which is a colored paper used to check the patient's occlusion after the filling material has been placed. The forceps are made of stain-

FIGURE 15-22 Carvers. (A) Hollenback. (B) 1. Cleoid/ 2. discoid. (C) Ward's. (D) Frahm. *(Courtesy of Hu-Friedy Mfg. Co., Inc.)*

FIGURE 15-23 Beaver tail burnisher. *(Courtesy of Hu-Friedy Mfg. Co., Inc.)*

FIGURE 15-24 File. *(Courtesy of Hu-Friedy Mfg. Co., Inc.)*

FIGURE 15-25 Finishing knife. *(Courtesy of Hu-Friedy Mfg. Co., Inc.)*

FIGURE 15-26 Cement spatulas. *(Courtesy of Miltex Instrument Co., Inc., Lake Success, NY)*

less steel or disposable plastic and are opened and closed by placing pressure on the handle (Figure 15-27). Sometimes, cotton pliers, especially locking cotton pliers, are used in place of articulating forceps.

Scissors. The scissors used most commonly with restorative procedures are **crown and collar scissors**. These scissors have short blades that may be either straight or curved. Crown and collar scissors are used to trim matrix bands and cut retraction cord and in a variety of other ways (Figure 15-28).

FIGURE 15-27 Articulating forceps. *(Courtesy of Miltex Instrument Co., Inc., Lake Success, NY)*

FIGURE 15-28 Straight crown and collar scissors. *(Courtesy of Miltex Instrument Co., Inc., Lake Success, NY)*

DENTAL ROTARY INSTRUMENTS

Dental **burs** are part of a group of instruments referred to as **rotary instruments**. Rotary instruments include disks and stones and are designed to be used with dental handpieces. They are used in differently speeded handpieces, both at chairside and in the dental laboratory. Burs are used for cavity preparations, finish and polish restorations, surgical procedures, and dental appliance adjustments.

Burs are made of either steel or tungsten carbide materials. The steel burs are not used as often as the carbide burs because they become dull very fast. Bur groups include cutting burs, diamond burs, surgical burs, laboratory burs, and finishing burs.

Parts of the Bur

All burs have three basic parts: the shank, the neck, and the head (Figure 15-29A).

Shank. The shank of the bur is inserted into the handpiece. To accommodate the dental handpieces, there are three styles of bur shanks (Figure 15-29B). The **straight shank** (designated HP when ordering), or long shank, functions with the straight, low-speed handpiece. The **latch-type shank** (designated RA) is shorter than the straight-shanked burs. On the latch-type shank there is a notch that fits into the contra-angle/right-angle handpiece and latches securely in place. The **friction-grip shank** (designated FG) is short, small, and smooth. These burs are used in friction-grip, high-speed handpieces.

Neck. The neck of the bur is the tapered connection of the shank to the head.

Head. The head is the working end of the bur. There are many shapes and sizes of heads on dental burs. A

FIGURE 15-29 (A) Parts of a bur. (B) Different shanks: straight, latch type, and friction grip.

variety of burs are needed to perform the multiple tasks in restoring teeth and specialty procedures.

Cutting Burs

There are nine basic cutting bur shapes, including round, inverted cone, plain fissure straight, plain fissure cross-cut, tapered fissure straight, tapered fissure cross-cut, end cutting, wheel, and pear. These burs are identified by number ranges. The bur numbers describe the shape, size, and variation of the bur. It is important to know the number ranges, because dentists often will ask for a bur by its number. Cutting burs have six to eight cutting blades or surfaces (Table 15-1 and Figure 15-30).

Burs have variations in both head and shank design. An example of a change in the head (working end) of the bur is on the fissure burs. Normally, the fissure burs are flat on the end, but there are some fissure burs that have rounded or dome-shaped working ends. The number range for these burs is different from that for the regular fissure burs.

TABLE 15-1 BURS AND THEIR SPECIFIC FUNCTIONS AND NUMBER RANGES (Figure 15-30)

Name	Function
Round bur	Used first to open the cavity and remove carious tooth structure.
Inverted cone bur	Removes caries and makes undercuts in the preparation.
Plain fissure straight bur and Plain fissure cross-cut bur	Forms the cavity walls of the preparation.
Tapered fissure straight bur and Tapered fissure cross-cut bur	Forms divergent walls of the cavity preparation.
End cutting bur	Forms the shoulder for crown preparations.
Wheel bur	Forms retention in preparations.
Pear bur	Opens and extends the cavity preparation.

FIGURE 15-30 Bur shapes and number ranges. *(Courtesy of Miltex Instrument Co., Inc., Lake Success, NY)*

The lengths of the three bur shanks vary and are designated by an "L" for longer length, an "S" for short shanks, or "P" for pedodontic shanks. The letter designation follows the number of the bur.

Diamond Burs

Diamond rotary instruments are categorized as diamond burs or stones. They are used for rapid reduction of tooth structure during cavity preparation, polishing and finishing composite restorations, and occlusal adjustment. Diamond burs are also used for bone and gingival contouring during surgical procedures.

Diamond burs come in a wide variety of shapes, sizes, and grits. Diamond particles are embedded in the bur head through an electroplating or a bonding process. The burs either are color coded for easy grit identification or have letters following the bur numbers to indicate the grit (Figures 15-31A and B). These burs may be specifically designed for a certain procedure, such as finishing, trimming, and composite restorations.

Finishing Burs

Finishing burs smooth, trim, and finish metal restorations and natural-tooth-colored materials. Finishing burs have thirty or more blades for ultra-fine finishing. These burs come in a variety of shapes and sizes, similar to the cutting burs. They are identified by the manufacturer's number (Figure 15-32).

Surgical Burs

Surgical burs are used in a low-speed handpiece to reduce and contour the alveolar bone and tooth structure. The heads of surgical burs come in various sizes and shapes and have long shanks (Figure 15-33).

Laboratory Burs

Laboratory burs are used to make adjustments on acrylic materials, such as partials, dentures, and custom trays. They are also used on plaster, stone, and metal materials. Laboratory burs have long shanks and large working ends. These burs come in a variety of sizes and shapes. Sometimes they are referred to as **vulcanite burs** (Figure 15-34).

FIGURE 15-32 Finishing burs. (*Courtesy of Midwest Dental Products Corporation, a division of DENTSPLY International*)

FIGURE 15-33 Surgical bur.

FIGURE 15-31 (A) Diamond bur with color coding for size of grit. (B) Various shaped diamond burs: course, fine, and extra fine. (*Courtesy of Miltex Instrument Co., Inc., Lake Success, NY*)

FIGURE 15-34 Laboratory burs. (*Courtesy of Miltex Instrument Co., Inc., Lake Success, NY*)

ABRASIVES

Abrasives are non-bladed instruments used to finish and polish restorations and appliances. Some abrasives also are used for cutting purposes. Abrasives come in a wide variety and are categorized by their shapes, such as discs, points, and wheels. Abrasives also are categorized by the materials they are made of, such as rubber, stone, and sandpaper. Some restorative materials come with selected abrasives that are designed to give the restoration a premium finish.

Mandrels

Mandrels are rods of various lengths that are used in low-speed handpieces. They are used with different abrasives. The abrasives are either permanently attached (mounted) to a mandrel or come separate and are placed on a mandrel (unmounted). Mandrels are available in three shanks: latch, friction grip, or straight. The head of the mandrel, where the abrasives attach, is available in snap on, screw on, or pin (Figure 15-35).

Discs

Discs are used to polish, smooth, and adjust restorative materials and dental appliances. Discs are circular, abrasive instruments that are usually designed to be mounted to mandrels. The abrasive agents are bonded on one or both sides of paper, metal, or plastic. The discs may be rigid or flexible and are available in a variety of sizes and grits. The abrasive material may be made of several different elements, such as garnet, diamond, quartz, sand, and carborundum. When ordering abrasives, size, grit, abrasiveness, and type of mandrel must be specified.

Sandpaper Discs.
Sandpaper discs are used to finish and polish all types of restorations and appliances. They come in a wide variety of sizes, grits, and abrasive materials. The abrasive materials include garnet, sand, emery, and cuttlefish. These materials are mounted to one side of the paper disc. Sandpaper discs are flexible and polish on one surface. They come with metal or pinhole centers (Figure 15-36).

Diamond Discs.
Diamond discs have diamond particles or chips bonded to both sides of steel discs. They are used for rapid cutting.

Carborundum Discs.
Carborundum discs, also known as **Jo-dandy discs** and **separating discs,** are thin, brittle discs that break easily. They are double sided and used primarily in the dental laboratory to cut and finish gold restorations, but they can be used intraorally as well (Figure 15-37A).

Stones

Stones are available in many sizes, shapes, and grits, similar to discs. They are used for cutting, polishing,

FIGURE 15-36 Sandpaper discs in various sizes, types, and grits.

FIGURE 15-35 Mandrels with different heads and shanks. (A) Screw-type mandrels. (B) Snap-on mandrels. *(Courtesy of Miltex Instrument Co., Inc., Lake Success, NY)*

FIGURE 15-37 (A) Carborundum discs. (B) Rubber wheel.

and finishing amalgam, gold, composite, and porcelain restorations. Stones are used in the laboratory to adjust and polish appliances and custom trays. The type of abrasive material and the grit control the cutting or polishing action of the stone. The abrasive materials include silicon carbide, garnet, and aluminum oxide. Stones may be mounted or unmounted. Some stones are considered heatless, thereby allowing the operator to polish a restoration without creating **frictional heat** (Figure 15-38).

Rubber Wheels

Wheels are made of rubber material impregnated with an abrasive agent (Figure 15-37B and 15-39). They come mounted and unmounted and are available in various grits. They are used for finishing and polishing.

Rubber Points

Rubber points come in a variety of sizes and grits. They are made of rubber material impregnated with abrasive agents. Points are used to polish and are especially adaptable for defining anatomy in the restoration (Figure 15-39).

FIGURE 15-38 Various types and grits of stones, wheels, and points.

FIGURE 15-39 Wheel and points.

FIGURE 15-40 Bur block with covers, magnetized, metal. *(Courtesy of Hu-Friedy Mfg. Co., Inc.)*

Sterilization and Storage

Rotary instruments are sterilized or disposed of after each use in the oral cavity. Burs that are sterilized are first scrubbed or placed in an ultrasonic unit to remove debris from the blades; if debris remains between the blades, a wire brush is used to remove embedded materials. The burs are then rinsed and sterilized according to manufacturer's instructions.

Bur Blocks. Rotary instruments are stored in a **bur block**. There are many variations and designs, such as round or rectangular shapes. Bur blocks come with covers and may be magnetic. Both friction-grip and latch-type burs can be stored in bur blocks. They are made of metal or plastic (Figure 15-40).

Some bur blocks can be sterilized with the burs they hold. If the bur blocks cannot be sterilized, the burs are placed in a mesh holder that looks like a tea strainer. The burs are placed in this holder, run through the ultrasonic cleaner, and then placed in the sterilizer.

▮ DENTAL HANDPIECES

There are a wide variety of dental handpieces available to meet the needs of dental procedures, both in the oral cavity and in a laboratory. Handpieces are used to remove dental decay and to prepare the tooth for a restoration; to polish the teeth; to polish and finish dental restorations; and to cut, finish, and polish dental appliances, models, and trays.

The Parts of the Dental Handpiece

All dental handpieces have the following basic parts (Figures 15-41A and B):

▶ **Working end (head)**—Where burs, discs, stones, and other rotary instruments and attachments are held and the cutting and polishing are accomplished.

▶ **Shank**—The handle portion of the handpiece.

▶ **Connection end**—Where the handpiece attaches to the power source. The forward and reverse controls may be located here.

(B)

(A)

(C)

FIGURE 15-41 (A) High-speed handpiece. (B) Low-speed handpiece. *(Courtesy of A-dec, Inc., Newberg, Oregon, USA)* (C) Air abrasion unit. *(Courtesy of Midwest Dental Products Corporation, a Division of DENTSPLY International)*

Dental handpieces are often divided into two categories: **high-speed handpieces** and **low-speed handpieces**. The high-speed handpieces operate at 400,000 **revolutions per minute (rpm)** and higher (Figure 15-41A). The low-speed handpieces operate under 30,000 rpm (Figure 15-41B).

Air abrasion technology is becoming increasingly popular. Air abrasion reduces or eliminates the use of anesthetics and drilling with dental handpieces. This shortens and/or reduces appointments for the patient. The technology allows various types of cavities to be prepared for restoration, special repairs in restorations to be accomplished, and the insides of restorations to be roughened before bonding.

Air abrasion base units (Figure 15-41C) come in movable floor models or small, countertop units. They consist of the base unit, control panel, foot switch, air pressure gradient (varies the pressure in small increments), handpiece and handpiece nozzler, abrasive flow control, and external suction device. Each unit requires an air pressure source (most can use air lines to the dental unit) and the abrasive. The abrasive used is aluminum oxide. The particle size varies, with 27 or 50 microns most commonly used, but more variations are being developed for specific tasks.

During use, the dental team and the patient should wear protective eyewear. The dental assistant uses the HVE in addition to the external suction to remove the debris.

Routine maintenance is important and manufacturer's directions should be followed.

High-Speed Handpiece

The high-speed handpiece is used for rapid cutting of tooth structure and finishing of restorations. Because of the high speed of this handpiece, **frictional heat** is produced. Frictional heat can cause pulpal damage to the tooth, so in order to reduce the frictional heat of the handpiece, a coolant such as air, water, or an air-water spray is used.

The high-speed handpiece design is a smooth, one-piece design, usually a **contra-angle**, with the head slightly angled to the shank of the handpiece (Figure 15-42A). The high-speed handpiece does not hold any attachments but does hold burs and other rotary instruments. To hold these rotary instruments, the head of the handpiece has a small, metal cylinder called a **chuck**. The chuck holds the shank portion of the bur in place. To tighten or loosen the chuck, either a bur tool/wrench or a button/release lever on the back of the head of the handpiece is used. The manufacturer provides the specific bur tool with the handpiece. The head of the handpiece comes in standard and pediatric sizes. The pediatric handpiece is used for easier access with children and adults with small mouth openings.

The power source for the dental handpiece comes from the unit. The compressed air drives the turbines

FIGURE 15-42 (A) High-speed handpieces with fiberoptics. *(Courtesy of Midwest Dental Products Corporation, a division of DENTSPLY International)* (B) Handpiece cleaner and lubricant maintenance unit. *(Courtesy of A-dec, Inc., Newberg, Oregon, USA)*

within the handpiece. To activate and control the speed of the handpiece, a **rheostat** (foot control) is operated, much like the accelerator on a car.

High-speed handpieces are available with **fiberoptic light sources**. Fiberoptic systems greatly improve visibility of the treatment area for the operator (Figure 15-42A). The fiberoptic light is carried along optical bundles within the tubing of the handpiece. The light source is either a separate control box or a bulb behind the handpiece in the dental unit.

Low-Speed Handpiece

The low-speed handpiece is often referred to as the straight handpiece because the shank and head are in a straight line. The low-speed handpiece is used both in the dental operatory and the laboratory. At the dental

unit, the low-speed handpiece is used to polish teeth and restorations, remove soft carious material, and define cavity margins and walls.

In the dental laboratory, this handpiece is used to adjust, finish, and polish appliances. Usually, the low-speed handpiece does not have or need a water supply, but in some procedures the dental assistant periodically applies air or water to the tooth or restoration to prevent any heating of the tooth.

The low-speed handpiece design is a little bulkier than the high-speed handpiece. The straight handpiece is used with long-shank rotary instruments, such as burs, discs and stones, and attachment heads such as the contra-angle and the right-angle (Figure 15-43).

▶ The contra-angles are usually latch type, but they also come in friction grip. The contra-angles hold burs, discs, stones, rubber cups, and brushes for intraoral and extraoral procedures.

▶ The right-angles or prophy angles are used to polish the teeth with rubber cups or brushes.

On the shank of the low-speed handpiece is a mechanism to lock the rotary instrument or the attachment onto the handpiece. This may be a tightening knob or a snap-on apparatus. Also on the shank near the connecting end there may be a reverse and forward control (Figure 15-43). The power source for controlling the speed of the low-speed handpiece is the rheostat.

Maintenance and Sterilization of Dental Handpieces

Manufacturer's directions for maintaining and sterilizing the handpiece should be followed carefully. Handpieces

FIGURE 15-43 A low-speed handpiece with attachments. (A) Contra-angle with and without a disk, (B) right-angle, (C) long bur with rubber cup.

that are used for patient treatment must be sterilizible; disinfecting handpieces is not acceptable. General guidelines include:

▶ While the handpiece is attached to the tubing and a bur is still in the handpiece, flush the handpiece by running it for twenty to thirty seconds. Follow the manufacturer's instructions for specific flushing and for the use and maintenance of water lines and check valves.

▶ Scrub the handpiece to remove debris. Rinse and dry it if manufacturer instructions include this step.

▶ Lubricate the handpiece if it is not lube free. This must be done before the handpiece is sterilized.

▶ Sterilize the handpiece as directed.

▶ Lubricate if instructed.

There are units available that both clean and lubricate handpieces. The maintenance units (Figure 15-42B) are located in the sterilizing area and require electrical and air pressure connections and water. Some of the units also sterilize the handpiece.

TRAY SYSTEMS

A **preset tray system** is most commonly used in dental offices. It provides an efficient means of transporting instruments to the treatment room, saving time for the dental assistant. With this system, instruments and auxiliary items are placed on a tray in the order of their use during the procedure. Then the tray is covered and carried to the treatment room when the patient is seated. There are many varieties of systems to choose from, including plastic or metal trays, tubs, or cassettes; trays, tubs, and accessories that are color coded; and systems that can be placed in the ultrasonic and then sterilized in the same cassette or tray (Figure 15-44).

Positioning on Trays

Every operator has certain preferences on the instrumentation for a procedure. However, there are some basic considerations:

▶ Instruments are placed in order of use, beginning on the left and moving to the right.

▶ The basic tray setup (mouth mirror, explorer, cotton pliers) is placed first on the left side.

▶ Instruments should be grouped according to functions; for example, all the carvers are placed together.

▶ Cotton supplies usually are arranged across the top of the tray.

▶ Scissors, hemostats, or other hinged instruments are placed on the far right of the tray for easy access.

▶ Return instruments to their original positions after receiving them from the operator. This ensures that an instrument can be found easily if the operator needs to use it again.

▶ Keep instruments clean and free of debris before returning them to the tray. Gauze sponges on the tray aid with immediate removal of cement, blood, or debris that will harden on the instrument after use.

Color-Coding Systems

 Color coding is a method used to easily identify instruments and trays (Figure 14-45). The color coding may be set up to indicate:

▶ Procedures, such as amalgam or composite.

▶ Treatment rooms, where the instruments are stored or used.

▶ Additional sets of instruments (there may be four composite setups, each marked for the procedure and then a second color for the set).

FIGURE 15-44 Variety of trays and tubs.

FIGURE 15-45 Tub, tray, and instruments, all color coded.

▶ Individual operators. The dentist may have two tray setups for prophylaxis and the hygienist may have four additional prophylaxis tray setups. Color coding keeps the dentist and the hygienist tray setups separated.

▶ Sequence. Instruments can be color coded diagonally to indicate the sequence of use.

▶ Any combination of these.

CHAPTER SUMMARY

The basic instruments used in general dental procedures include common cutting and non-cutting instruments. Instruments are generally categorized into hand instruments and rotary instruments. Each procedure has special instruments to accomplish specific tasks. It is the assistant's responsibility to keep the instruments sterilized, organized, and in working condition.

CASE STUDY

Dr. Charles Thomas has been practicing dentistry for five years, and his practice has grown to the point where changes need to be made in his current tray setup system. He has three treatment rooms and one hygiene room. Dr. Thomas is willing to finance the necessary updating and would like to color code his instruments, trays, and so on.

Case Study Review

1. Before deciding on a system, what factors need to be considered?

2. Give some possible suggestions for the color-code combinations.

3. What are the benefits of having an office where a color-coding system is effectively utilized?

 To complete your study of this chapter, work the review activities that follow. Also, refer to the software that accompanies this text.

REVIEW QUESTIONS

Multiple Choice

1. The part of the dental instrument that comes straight, curved, monangle, binangle, or triple angle is called the
   a. handle.
   b. shank.
   c. working end.
   d. shaft.

2. Which of the following instruments has a four-number formula?
   a. Chisel.
   b. Angle former.
   c. Spoon excavator.
   d. Hoe.

3. The mouth mirror uses include all of the following *except*
   a. indirect vision.
   b. reflection of light.
   c. retraction.
   d. direct vision.

4. The instrument used to carve an amalgam restoration before it hardens is the
   a. Hollenback.
   b. gingival margin trimmer.
   c. Wedelstaedt chisel.
   d. T-ball burnisher.

5. The rotary instrument also known as a "Jo-dandy" is the
   a. diamond bur.
   b. sandpaper disc.
   c. carborundum disc.
   d. rubber wheel.

Critical Thinking

1. What does a bur number tell about the bur?

2. Which handpiece would the dental assistant select if the procedure included polishing the patient's teeth? Would an attachment be required?

3. List the basic hand instruments that would be necessary for an amalgam restoration procedure.

Management of Pain and Anxiety

OBJECTIVES

The student should strive to meet the following objectives and demonstrate an understanding of the facts and principles presented in this chapter:

1. Describe methods used to manage the pain and anxiety related to dental procedures.

2. Explain different types of topical anesthetics and their placements.

3. Describe types of local anesthetics.

4. List the steps for preparing for the administration of local anesthetic.

5. Identify the injection sites for the maxillary and mandibular arches.

6. Describe the equipment and materials needed to administer local anesthetic.

7. Identify supplemental techniques to administer anesthetics.

8. Discuss the role of nitrous oxide in the care of the dental patient.

9. Demonstrate the ability to assist in the administration of nitrous oxide.

KEY TERMS

carpules (p. 295)

cartridges (p. 295)

computer-controlled local anesthesia (p. 306)

field block anesthesia (p. 296)

general anesthetic (p. 294)

infiltration anesthesia (p. 296)

local anesthesia (p. 294)

nerve block anesthesia (p. 296)

nitrous oxide (p. 306)

topical anesthetic (p. 294)

vasoconstrictors (p. 295)

INTRODUCTION

One of the biggest fears for patients visiting the dentist is the injection. People have shared their "experiences with the needle" for generations. Over the years, though, many advances have been made to control patients' pain and anxiety. Improved administration techniques and equipment for management of pain and anxiety for the patient continues to be a focus of research.

Because most procedures require some form of anesthesia, the dentist may select one or a combination of methods to control pain, depending on the patient and the procedure to be completed.

ANESTHETICS AND SEDATION

General Anesthesia

When a general anesthetic is administered, the patient becomes unconscious. The anesthetic temporarily alters the central nervous system so that sensation or feeling is lost. General anesthetic is ideal for some patients for various surgeries and treatments.

The dental assistant is not involved with the administration of the general anesthetic but does assist during surgery and is responsible for dismissing and monitoring the patient during recovery.

Local Anesthesia

Local anesthesia produces a deadened or pain-free area while the dentist performs a procedure that may cause the patient uncomfortable sensations if no anesthetic were used. Sensory impulses such as pain, touch, and thermal change are temporarily blocked. Local anesthetic only works if it comes in contact with the nerve fibers that carry the impulses to the brain or the small nerve endings that pick up sensations in the tissue.

The dental assistant must be aware of the various anesthetic solutions and techniques used when administering local anesthetic. The dental assistant is responsible for preparing, safely transferring, and caring for the anesthetic syringe and accessories.

Topical Anesthesia

Before the local anesthesia is injected, the area is numbed with topical anesthetic. This material desensitizes the oral mucosa for a brief period so that the patient will not feel the "pinch" of the needle. Topical anesthetics affect the small nerve endings located in the surface of the skin and mucosa. The dental assistant must be aware of the various topical anesthetic solutions and possible patient reactions. He or she must know application sites and how to apply the anesthetic. In some states, the dental assistant can apply the topical anesthetic for the dentist before an injection.

Sedation

In some difficult cases, more frequently with children, the patient requires **sedation** or **pre-medication** prior to the administration of an anesthetic. This relaxes the patient and relieves fear and anxiety, which come with the anticipation of dental treatment. Sedation is administered in the form of pills or liquids or through gases used for **nitrous oxide sedation**. Patients who are sedated should be accompanied by responsible adults. The dental assistant follows the dentist's directions for the administration of the medication. Local anesthetic is used in conjunction with sedation to control the pain during the procedure.

TOPICAL ANESTHETICS

Topical anesthetics are placed on the surface of the oral mucosa to eliminate sensation. They also have several other uses in dental procedures, such as decreasing pain sensation for subgingival scaling, root planing, seating crowns, placing matrix bands, and performing periodontal probing. Sometimes topical anesthetic is used to depress the gag reflex that occurs when taking intraoral x-rays or impressions.

Topical anesthetics are available in gels, ointments, liquids, or metered sprays (Figure 16-1). The gels, ointments, and liquids are applied in small amounts to specific areas. The sprays are metered to control the amount of solution sprayed and to confine it to the desired area.

The **composition of topical anesthetics** is classified as either the ester or amide local anesthetics. Benzocaine is an example of an ester, and lidocaine is an example of an amide topical anesthetic. These classifications are according to chemical linkages, which define several properties of the anesthetics, including how the materi-

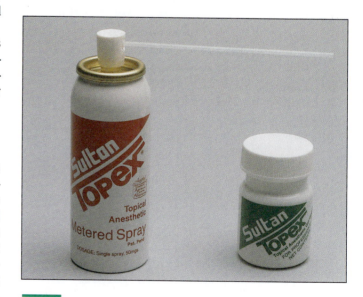

FIGURE 16-1 Examples of topical anesthetic, metered spray and gel.

als are absorbed into the system. The concentration of solution for topical anesthetics is greater than the concentration of solution used for local anesthetics. For example, lidocaine topical anesthetic is a 5 or 10 percent concentration, while the lidocaine used as a local anesthetic is a 2 percent concentration. Due to the higher concentrations of the topical anesthetics, there is a greater risk for allergic and/or toxic reactions to occur than there is with local or general anesthetics.

The **allergic reaction** is a hypersensitive reaction to the anesthetic solution. The reaction can range from mild to severe and can occur up to twenty-four hours or more after the application. Clinical manifestations include swelling, redness, ulcerations, and difficulty swallowing and breathing. Topical anesthetics also may contain flavorings that patients may be allergic to, such as banana flavor, mint, or cherry.

The **toxic reactions** are symptoms that appear due to overdose or excessive administration of the anesthetic solution. The first symptom is the stimulation of the central nervous system. The patient becomes more talkative, apprehensive, and excited, with an increased pulse rate and blood pressure. This is followed by depression of the central nervous system as the drug dissipates.

To avoid either of these reactions, review and revise the patient's medical history at each visit, taking special care to note any allergies or allergic reactions.

The ADA recommends that topical anesthetics be left on the mucosa for one minute in order for the solution to be most effective. The dentist considers the type, concentration of the anesthetic solution, treatment location, and manufacturer's directions when applying topical anesthetic. Procedure for typical placement is described later in this chapter.

LOCAL ANESTHETICS

Local anesthetics are used to manage pain for most dental procedures. The solution is injected into the soft tissues. It must come in contact with the sensory nerve fibers in order to be effective. Once the anesthetic solution anesthetizes the nerve, sensations cannot pass through to register the feeling of pain in the brain. The tissues and teeth in the affected area can be operated on without the patient experiencing any pain.

The local anesthetics used for injection are available in liquid form and supplied in premeasured **carpules** or **cartridges** (Figure 16-2).

Local Anesthetic Agents

There are two local anesthetic solutions used for injections in dental procedures. They are amide or ester chemical compounds. Some of the available agents are:

▶ The amides: lidocaine, mepivacaine, prilocaine, articaine, bupivacaine, and etidocaine

▶ The esters: propoxycaine and procaine

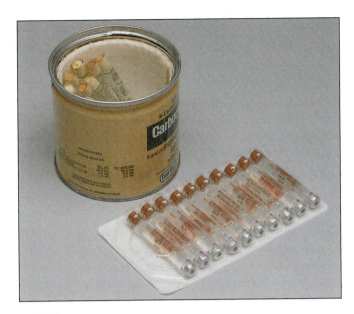

FIGURE 16-2 Variety of anesthetic cartridges (they come in can or a blister pack).

Patients may have reactions to one type of local anesthetic but not to another. Specific notations should be made on the patient's chart regarding the type of anesthetic, percent of solution, number of cartridges administered, and any reaction the patient experienced.

The Duration. Most patients want as much dental treatment completed at one time as possible. This requires an anesthetic that lasts for a long period of time. The duration of the local anesthetics can be divided into three sections:

1. **Short duration** solutions last about thirty minutes and contain no vasoconstrictor.

2. **Intermediate duration** solutions last about sixty minutes and usually contain a vasoconstrictor. Most anesthetics fall into this category.

3. **Long duration** solutions last longer than ninety minutes and contain a vasoconstrictor.

Vasoconstrictor

Vasoconstrictors are drugs that are added to the anesthetic solutions. Their function is to constrict the blood vessels around the injection site, reducing blood flow in this area. The vasoconstrictors slow the absorption of the anesthetic into the blood stream, thereby affecting the intensity and the duration of the solution in the area. Adding vasoconstrictors to the anesthetic lowers the level of local anesthetic solutions in the blood stream, which decreases the risk of a toxic reaction. Vasoconstrictors also decrease bleeding at the operating site.

The most common vasoconstrictor used in dentistry is **epinephrine**. Epinephrine is added to the local anesthetics in very small amounts. The dilution of vasoconstrictors is commonly referred to as a ratio. The most common ratios are 1 : 20,000, 1 : 50,000, 1 : 100,000, and 1 : 200,000. These ratios are listed on the cartridges and indicate one part vasoconstrictor to 20,000 or 100,000 parts anesthetic solution.

Sometimes, other drugs that patients are taking interact with the vasoconstrictor and cause reactions. Again, this information should be highlighted on the patient's medical/dental history.

Possible Complications of Local Anesthetics

A toxic reaction is a complication that also occurs with local anesthetics. Anesthetics used for dental procedures are very safe, but the possibility exists for a toxic reaction. Reactions to the anesthetic depend upon the following:

▶ The type of anesthetic solution

▶ The amount of anesthetic injected

▶ The rate at which the solution was injected and absorbed

▶ The individual patient's characteristics

Another complication of local anesthetic is **paresthesia**, the sensation of feeling numb. Paresthesia can last for hours or days beyond the temporary numbness experienced after an injection. Most patients who experience paresthesia regain sensation within eight weeks without treatment. Paresthesia may be caused by:

▶ Trauma to the nerve sheath (covering) during the actual injection

▶ Hemorrhage into or around the nerve sheath, causing pressure on the nerve

▶ Injection of local anesthetic contaminated by alcohol or disinfecting solution near a nerve

The paresthesia can be permanent if the damage to the nerve is severe enough, but this rarely occurs. If the patient calls the office following a dental procedure and complains of extended numbness, the patient should speak to the dentist and be scheduled for an examination as soon as possible. In most cases, the paresthesia is limited. The major concern brought on by the short-term numbness is that the patients may injure themselves by biting the tongue, cheeks, or lips.

Types of Injections

Three types of injections are given for dental procedures: local infiltration, field block, and nerve block. The type of injection is determined by the injection site and the innervation of the area or specific tooth.

Local Infiltration. Local **infiltration anesthesia** is an injection method that places anesthetic solution into the tissues near the small terminal nerve branches for

absorption (Figure 16-3). The local infiltration injections are used for various dental treatments, including root planing, soft tissue incision for a biopsy, gingivectomy, or frenectomy.

Field Block Anesthesia. **Field block anesthesia** is commonly referred to as local infiltration anesthesia. With the field block anesthesia, the anesthetic is deposited near larger terminal nerve branches (Figure 16-4). This prevents impulses from passing from the tooth to the central nervous system. This anesthesia is used most often for dental procedures that involve the teeth or bone on the maxillary and mandibular anterior regions. The field block anesthetic injections are given near the apex of the tooth and involve one or two teeth. Usually, the patient feels numb within two to three minutes.

Nerve Block Anesthesia. **Nerve block anesthesia** is injected near a main nerve trunk (Figure 16-5). The anes-

FIGURE 16-3 Local infiltration. Anesthetic is placed in area of treatment. *(Courtesy of Dr. Gary Shellerud)*

FIGURE 16-4 Field block anesthesia. Anesthetic is injected near larger terminal nerve ending at the apex. *(Courtesy of Dr. Gary Shellerud)*

FIGURE 16-5 Nerve block anesthesia. Anesthetic is injected close to main nerve trunk. *(Courtesy of Dr. Gary Shellerud).*

thetic prevents any pain sensation from passing from the site to the brain, including any branches of the nerve trunk. These injections eliminate sensations over a larger area than either the infiltration or the field block anesthesia. Some nerve block injections numb from the posterior region of a quadrant to the midline. The nerve block injection usually takes effect within four to five minutes.

INJECTION SITES

In order to assist effectively or place the topical anesthetic correctly, the dental assistant must know the injections sites. The sites are divided between the maxillary and the mandibular arches (Figures 16-6 and 16-7 and Tables 16-1 and 16-2).

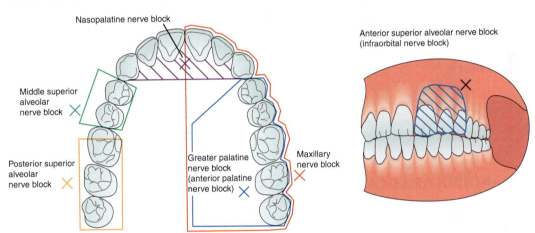

FIGURE 16-6 Maxillary arch injections and site locations.

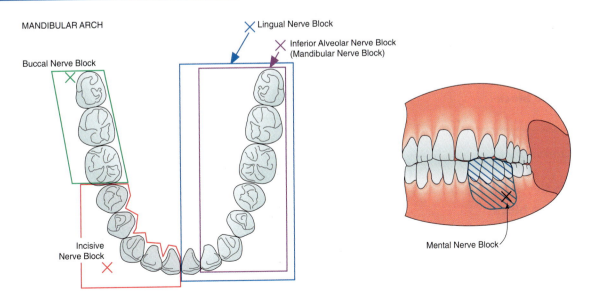

FIGURE 16-7 Mandibular arch injections and site locations.

TABLE 16-1 MAXILLARY LOCAL ANESTHESIA INJECTION SITES

Name of Injection	Affected Teeth/Tissues	Location of Injection
Infiltration (field block)	Individual teeth.	Near the apex of the tooth; most commonly used on the maxillary anteriors.
Anterior superior alveolar nerve block (also called the **infraorbital nerve block**)	Maxillary central and lateral incisors and cuspid in one quadrant.	Height of the mucobuccal fold at the maxillary first premolar.
Middle superior alveolar nerve block	Maxillary premolars in one quadrant.	Height of mucobuccal fold at the maxillary second premolar.
Posterior superior alveolar nerve block	The maxillary second and third molars, the distobuccal and palatal roots of the first molar. The buccal tissues adjacent to these teeth.	Apex of the second molar toward the distobuccal root.
Greater palatine nerve block	The hard palate and soft tissues covering the hard palate from the distal of the canine posteriorly.	Anterior to the greater palatine foramen, middle of the maxillary second molar on the palate.
Nasopalatine nerve block	The anterior one-third of the hard palate from canine to canine.	The lingual tissue adjacent to the incisive papilla.
Maxillary nerve block	The buccal, palatal, and pulpal tissues in one quadrant. Skin of the lower eyelid, side of nose, cheek, and upper lip.	Height of the mucobuccal fold above the distal of the maxillary second molar.

TABLE 16-2 MANDIBULAR LOCAL ANESTHESIA INJECTION SITES

Name of Injection	Affected Teeth/Tissues	Location of Injection
Infiltration (field block)	Individual teeth.	Near the apex of the individual tooth.
Inferior alveolar nerve block (commonly referred to as the **mandibular block**)	A mandibular quadrant including the teeth, mucous membrane, anterior two-thirds of the tongue and floor of the mouth, lingual soft tissues, and periosteum.	Inside of the mandibular ramus, posterior to the retro-molar pad, below and anterior to the mandibular foramen.
Buccal nerve block	Buccal tissue adjacent to the mandibular molars only.	Mucous membrane to the distal and toward the buccal of the last mandibular molar tooth in the arch.
Lingual nerve block	The lingual tissues and side of the tongue. Mandibular teeth to the midline.	Lingual to mandibular ramus and adjacent to maxillary tuberosity.
Mental nerve block	The mandibular premolars, canines, and facial tissues adjacent to these teeth.	Anterior to the mental foramen, between the apices of the roots of the mandibular premolars.
Incisive nerve block	Premolars, canine lateral, and central incisors. Buccal mucous membrane from the mandibular second premolar, the lips, and chin.	At the height of the mucobuccal fold in front of the mental foramen.

ANESTHETICS, SYRINGES, AND NEEDLES

The equipment necessary for the administration of local anesthetic includes a syringe, a needle, and an anesthetic carpule.

The Syringe

There are various types of syringes used for dental procedures, but the most common is the **aspirating syringe**. The aspirating syringe, recommended by the ADA, is designed to allow the operator to check the position of the needle before depositing the anesthetic solution. The aspiratory syringe has a harpoon on the end of the piston. The harpoon penetrates the rubber end of the anesthetic cartridge. Once the needle is placed in the tissues, the operator retracts the thumb ring, creating negative pressure (Figure 16-8). If the needle has penetrated a blood vessel, a thin line of blood is drawn into the cartridge. The operator then repositions the needle to avoid injecting the anesthetic into the blood vessel and retests until there is evidence that the needle is not placed in a blood vessel. The use of an aspirating syringe allows the operator to place the anesthetic for maximum benefit.

Syringes may be metal (stainless steel) or non-metal (plastic). The metal syringes are autoclavable while the non-metal syringes may be disposable or autoclavable.

Parts of the Aspirating Syringe.

▶ **Thumb ring**—Located at one end of the syringe. A ring for the operator's thumb to allow the operator to aspirate and apply force during the injection. The thumb ring does come loose and should be checked and tightened as needed before every use.

▶ **Finger grip/bar**—Supports the index and middle fingers of the operator as the anesthetic solution is administered into the oral tissues.

▶ **Syringe barrel**—Holds the cartridge. One side of the barrel is open so that the cartridge/carpule can be loaded, known as a breech-loading syringe. Opposite the open side is a "window" for the operator to view the solution left in the cartridge.

▶ **Plunger** or **piston rod**—Located inside the syringe barrel. It is a rod with the harpoon on the end. The rod is used to apply force to the rubber stopper in the anesthetic cartridge to expel the solution.

▶ **Harpoon**—A barbed tip at the end of the piston rod that engages the rubber end in the cartridge. The harpoons allows the operator to aspirate with the syringe. When the operator pulls the thumb ring back, the engaged harpoon pulls the rubber end of the cartridge.

▶ **Threaded end of the syringe**—Where the needle attaches to the syringe. This end needs to be checked to be sure it is securely on the syringe. Also, sometimes the needle attaches so tightly to the threaded end that this end loosens with the needle and can be mistakenly discarded.

Care and Handling of the Anesthetic Syringe.
Follow the manufacturers' recommendations concerning the care and handling of the autoclavable syringes. After each use, the harpoon is cleaned with a brush and the syringe is prepared for sterilization like other autoclavable instruments. Some syringes need periodic lubrication in the threaded joints and where the thumb ring meets the finger bar. The harpoon may need to be replaced if it becomes bent or dull and does not remain embedded within the rubber stopper.

The Needle

The needle is used to penetrate the tissues and to direct the local anesthetic solution from the carpule into the surrounding tissues. Most needles are made of stainless steel and are disposable.

One factor to consider when selecting a needle for a dental procedure is the length of the needle. Dental needles are available in two lengths: short (one inch) and long (one and five-eighths inch) (Figure 16-9). The selection usually depends on the operator's preference, the approximate depth of the soft tissues to be penetrated, and the aspiration potential. The short needle is used for injections that require little penetration of the soft tissues, such as the infiltration, field block injections, and the following nerve block injections: posterior superior alveolar, incisive nerve block, and mental nerve block. Periodontal ligament injections are also often administered with a short needle.

The long needle is used for injections that require the penetration of several thicknesses of soft tissue. The

FIGURE 16-8 Aspirating syringe with labeled parts.
(A) Needle adapter. (B) Piston with harpoon. (C) Finger grip. (D) Thumb ring. (E) Syringe barrel.

FIGURE 16-9 Needle parts labeled; short needle and long needle. (A) Syringe end. (B) Hub. (C) Shank of needle. (D) Bevel of needle.

long needle is used for nerve block injections, such as the infraorbital, buccal, and maxillary nerve blocks and the mandibular nerve blocks.

The other consideration when selecting a needle is the needle gauge or diameter. The needles used in dentistry are 25, 27, and 30 gauge. The smaller the gauge, the larger the diameter of the needle. Both long and short needles come in all sizes. The 25-gauge is used when there is a high risk of a positive aspiration. The internal opening of the needle, where the anesthetic solution flows through, is called the **lumen**.

Parts of the Needle.

▶ **Bevel**—The slanted tip of the needle that penetrates the soft tissues.

▶ **Shank**—The length of the needle from the hub to the tip of the bevel. It is sometimes referred to as the shaft. Along the inside of the shank runs the lumen.

▶ **Hub**—The part of the needle that attaches to the threaded end of the syringe. The hub may be a plastic or metal piece. The hub is normally pre-threaded.

▶ **Syringe end**—The end of the needle that punctures the diaphragm end of the anesthetic cartridge.

Care and Handling of the Dental Needle. The

needle is used on a patient and then disposed of in a sharps container. If the operator penetrates the tissue with the needle more than four times during a procedure, the needle should be changed, because disposable needles become dull. When opening the needle package, a seal must be broken; if the seal is already broken, do not use the needle and dispose of the needle as if it had been used. Always be aware of the location and position of the uncovered needle tip to minimize the risk of a needle stick. Keep the protective covers on the needles when they are not being used. Dispose of needles following OSHA guidelines with protective coverings and in a sharps container. (In the case of a needle stick, begin treatment and report the incident immediately to the dentist. Follow guidelines discussed in Chapter 9, Infection Control.)

The Anesthetic Cartridge

The anesthetic cartridge, also called the carpule, is a glass cylinder that contains the anesthetic solution (Figure 16-10).

Parts of the Anesthetic Cartridge.

▶ **Glass cartridge**—Contains the solution. A thin plastic label covers all glass cartridges. This provides protection to the patient, the dentist, and the assistant should the glass break. In addition, the manufacturers place pertinent information on the label (Figure 16-11).

▶ **Rubber stopper** or **plunger**—Located in the harpoon end of the cartridge. Most stoppers are treated with silicone so that they can move along the inside of the glass more smoothly. The stopper should be slightly indented from the edge of the glass cartridge.

▶ **Aluminum cap**—Located at the opposite end of the cartridge from the rubber plunger. It is a silver-colored aluminum cover that fits tightly around the neck of the glass cartridge. In the center of the end is a thin diaphragm.

▶ **Diaphragm**—Where the syringe end of the needle penetrates into the anesthetic solution. The diaphragm is made of a latex rubber.

Care and Handling of the Anesthetic Cartridges.
Carefully examine the cartridges before using them.

FIGURE 16-10 Anesthetic cartridge with labeled parts. (A) Rubber diaphragm. (B) Aluminum cap. (C) Neck. (D) Glass cylinder. (E) Rubber stopper.

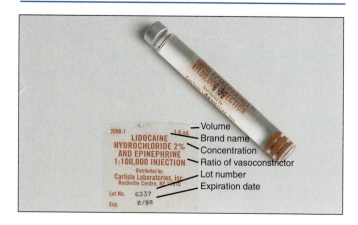

FIGURE 16-11 Anesthetic cartridge and mylar plastic label with information identified.

Things to look for include expired shelf-life dates, large bubbles, extruded plungers (caused by the solution being frozen), corrosion (caused by immersion in disinfecting solutions), or rust on the aluminum caps (caused by a broken or leaking anesthetic cartridge). If you find any of these conditions, the cartridges should be discarded.

The anesthetic cartridge is discarded after use on each patient. Be aware of the expiration date indicated by the manufacturer. The cartridges should be stored at room temperature and in a dark place. The cartridge does not need to be heated before use.

Anesthetic cartridges are stored in their original containers until they are used. The cartridges are sterilized and often come in sealed units called blister packs (refer

FIGURE 16-12 Disposable needle in a blister pack.

P R O C E D U R E

16-1 Preparing the Anesthetic Syringe

The dental assistant prepares the syringe out of the view of the patient. A topical anesthetic is applied by either the dentist or the dental assistant. The equipment and materials are on the procedure tray or stored at the dental unit.

EQUIPMENT AND SUPPLIES (Figure 16-13)

▶ Sterile syringe

▶ Selected disposable needle (Figure 6-12)

▶ Selected anesthetic cartridge

▶ 2 × 2 gauze sponge moistened with 91 percent isopropyl alcohol or 70 percent ethyl alcohol

FIGURE 16-13 Equipment and supplies needed to prepare an anesthetic syringe.

PROCEDURE STEPS (Follow aseptic procedures)

This procedure is described for a right-handed person.

1. Following aseptic procedures, select the disposable needle and the anesthetic the dentist has specified for this procedure.

2. Remove the sterilized syringe from its autoclave bag or pouch. Inspect the syringe to be sure it is ready for use.

3. Hold the syringe in the left hand and use the thumb ring to fully retract the piston rod (Figure 16-14).

4. With the piston rod retracted, place the cartridge in the barrel of the syringe. The plunger end (rubber stopper end) goes in first (Figure 16-15). To prevent contamination, do not place a finger over the diaphragm while placing the cartridge in the syringe. Once the cartridge is in place, release the piston rod.

FIGURE 16-14 Left-hand retraction of the piston rod of an aspirating anesthetic syringe.

(continued)

P R O C E D U R E   1 6 - 1 *continued*

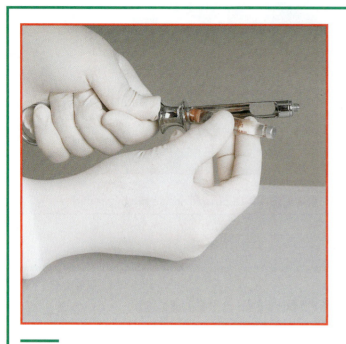

FIGURE 16-15 Technique to place a cartridge in an aspirating syringe.

FIGURE 16-16 Engage the harpoon with pressure on the finger ring (bar).

5. With moderate pressure, push the piston rod into the rubber stopper until it is fully engaged (Figure 16-16). Do not hit the piston rod to engage the harpoon, and do not hold your hand over the cartridge while engaging the harpoon.

6. Remove the protective plastic cap from the syringe end of the needle, and then screw or press the needle onto the syringe depending on the type of needle hub. Make sure the needle is secure but not too tight (Figure 16-17). A disposable needle guard is often placed on the protective cap covering the needle.

7. Carefully remove the protective cover from the needle. Holding the syringe upright, expel a few drops to ensure that the syringe is working properly. Replace the cap and place on the tray, ready for use.

FIGURE 16-17 Open the cap on the needle.

NOTE: The needle may be placed on the syringe before the cartridge. This technique also requires pressure on the thumb ring to engage the harpoon into the rubber plunger.

back to Figure 16-2). Many dentists feel the need to wipe the diaphragm with a solution before use. A 2 × 2 gauze sponge moistened with 91 percent isopropyl alcohol or 70 percent ethyl alcohol is used. A single day's supply of cartridges can be stored in a dispenser with alcohol gauze sponges in a separate container.

SUPPLEMENTAL ANESTHETIC TECHNIQUES

There are various techniques for the administration of anesthetics that supplement the infiltration and

PROCEDURE

16-2 Assisting with the Administration of Topical and Local Anesthetics

The dental assistant checks with the dentist for instructions on the type of anesthetic and needle for the procedure. The equipment and materials are either on the procedure tray or stored at the dental unit.

EQUIPMENT AND SUPPLIES *(Figure 16-18)*

▶ Patient's medical dental history and chart

▶ Basic setup: mouth mirror, explorer, and cotton pliers

▶ Air-water syringe tip and evacuator tip (HVE)

▶ Cotton rolls, cotton-tip applicator, and 2 × 2 gauze sponges

▶ Topical anesthetic

▶ Aspirating syringe

▶ Anesthetic cartridge

▶ Selection of needles

FIGURE 16-18 Equipment and supplies needed to place the topical anesthetic and pass the prepared syringe.

PROCEDURE STEPS *(Follow aseptic procedures)*

Placing Topical Anesthetic (by the dentist or the assistant)

1. After seating the patient, review and update the medical dental history.

2. Prepare the patient for the procedure and explain what you are doing and the tastes and sensations he or she may experience. (The explanations should be brief and avoid such words as "pain," "shot," and "injection.") Explain that the topical anesthetic is being applied to make him or her more comfortable during the procedure.

3. Place a small amount of topical anesthetic on a cotton-tip applicator.

4. Prepare the oral mucosa by drying with a sterile 2 × 2 gauze sponge. Keep the tissue retracted.

5. Place the topical anesthetic on the site of the injection and leave in place for one minute (Figure 16-19A-C).

Administering the Local Anesthetic

6. While waiting for the topical anesthetic to take effect, prepare the syringe if this has not been completed. Assemble the syringe, cartridge, and needle as described previously.

7. When the operator indicates, take the cotton-tip applicator and prepare to pass the syringe.

8. Check the needle bevel so it is directed toward the alveolar bone, and then loosely replace the cap on the needle. The protective cap is placed

FIGURE 16-19 (A) Dry the tissue with a gauze. *(continued)*

(continued)

P R O C E D U R E   **1 6 - 2** *continued*

FIGURE 16-19 *(continued)* (B) Placing topical anesthetic on the maxillary injection site. (C) Placing the topical anesthetic on the mandibular injection site.

on the hub of the needle so that it is secure but can be removed easily.

9. Pass the syringe below the patient's chin (or behind the patient's head), placing the thumb ring over the dentist's thumb (the dentist grasps the syringe at the finger rest and takes the syringe) (Figure 16-20). As the dentist takes the syringe, remove the protective guard. During the injection, watch the patient for any adverse signs or reactions.

NOTE: There are different methods to safely remove the cap and complete the transfer. It is important for the dentist and the assistant to establish a routine. The assistant

FIGURE 16-20 Passing the prepared anesthetic syringe.

can hold the operator's hand until they have cleared the needle.

10. The operator recaps the syringe by sliding (scooping) the needle into the protective guard or placing the needle of the syringe in a mechanical recapping device. If a second injection is given, remove the cartridge, insert a new cartridge, test the syringe by expelling a few drops, check the bevel, and position the needle for the dentist to retrieve.

NOTE: At this time, the syringe is contaminated. It is during recapping that most needle sticks occur. To prevent this from happening, the dentist should recap the needle and retrieve it after the assistant has replaced the cartridge and has repositioned the syringe on the tray or counter. There are a variety of needle holders available. These devices hold the needle cap so that the needle can be recapped while protecting the hand.

11. The recapped syringe is placed on the tray out of the way for the rest of the procedure but close in case more anesthetic is needed.

12. Rinse the patient's mouth with the air-water syringe and evacuate to remove the water, saliva, and taste of the anesthetic solution.

Unloading the Anesthetic Syringe

1. After the procedure is completed and the patient is dismissed, don utility gloves, take the syringe apart, and prepare it for sterilization.

(continued)

P R O C E D U R E   1 6 - 2 *continued*

2. Carefully remove the needle with the protective cap in place. Carefully unscrew the needle. A hemostat can be used to hold the needle while it is being removed from the syringe. Also, there are mechanical devices that cut the needle from the hub; after being cut, the needle falls into a closed container. The needle is discarded in the sharps container.

NOTE: The needle can also be removed after the cartridge.

3. Retract the piston to release the harpoon from the cartridge (Figure 16-21A).

4. Remove the cartridge from the syringe by retracting the thumb ring enough to release the cartridge. Turn the syringe until the cartridge is free (Figure 16-21B).

5. Prepare the syringe for sterilization.

(A)

(B)

FIGURE 16-21 (A) Retract the piston to release the harpoon from the cartridge and (B) Remove the cartridge from the syringe.

block injection techniques or that can be used as the only anesthetic injection technique.

Intraosseous Anesthesia

Intraosseous injection places local anesthetic directly into the cancellous bone (spongy bone). This injection is used for anesthesia in a single tooth or multiple teeth in a quadrant. The bone, soft tissue, and root of a tooth/teeth are anesthetized by the intraosseous injection. This type of anesthetic injection is useful for patients who do not like the feeling of the numb lip and tongue. It is immediate in action and is atraumatic for patients. The intraosseous injection requires a special system for administration. This technology has been modified with two parts:

1. A perforator, which is a solid needle that attaches to a slow-speed handpiece. The needle perforates the cortical plate of bone.

2. An 8-mm, 27-gauge needle that is inserted into the pre-drilled hole for administration of the anesthetic (Figure 16-22).

To ensure that this is a "painless" injection, a topical anesthetic is first placed on the tissues. Once the perforator (solid needle) is injected into the tissues, a small amount of anesthetic is administered to numb the nerve endings in this area.

Periodontal Ligament Injection

The periodontal ligament injection, or intraligamentary injection, is used for pulpal anesthesia of one or two

teeth in a quadrant and sometimes as an adjunct to another injection where the patient is only partially anesthetized. It also is used as an aid for diagnosing abscess teeth and when a patient does not want his or her lip and tongue numb.

This technique involves the insertion of the needle into the gingival sulcus along the long axis of the tooth to be treated on the mesial or distal or the root. The original pressure syringe used for the periodontal ligament injection was developed in 1905. This technique has become popular again, mainly because manufacturers have designed pressure syringes for easier administration (Figure 16-23).

FIGURE 16-22 Stabident system (Lasystem). *(Courtesy of Fairfax Dental Inc., 1-800-233-2305, e-mail: fairfax@stabident. com)*

FIGURE 16-23 Periodontal ligament injection syringe and a selection of needles.

Intrapulpal Injection

The intrapulpal injection technique deposits the anesthetic directly into the pulp chamber or root canal of the involved tooth. This injection may be used when there is difficulty in securing pain control. A 25- or 27-gauge short or long needle is used; sometimes, the needle is bent to gain access to the pulp canal.

Electronic Anesthesia

Electronic dental anesthesia has been used for a long time with low to moderate levels of success. When used with nitrous oxide inhalation sedation, the effectiveness is improved. It has been used in many dental procedures, such as placing restorations, muscle relaxation, and determining the patient's centric occlusion. Electronic dental anesthesia may be used when local anesthetics are contraindicated, such as with patients who are allergic to local anesthetics or are extremely fearful of the injection.

Computer-Controlled Local Anesthesia Delivery System

Computer-controlled local anesthesia delivery systems promise pain-free injections. These systems can be used to administer all traditional infiltration and block injections. The computer-controlled system is a microprocessor that delivers a controlled pressure and volume of anesthetic solution at a rate that is commonly below the threshold of pain. The microprocessor adjusts the pressure for low-resistant tissues to high-resistant tissues and can be used for injections on the palate and periodontal ligament.

Standard anesthetic cartridges and any size or gauge Luer Lock needle can be used with the system. On the microprocessing unit, the cartridge is twisted into place with the diaphragm end of the cartridge down and the rubber plunger up; a plastic microtubing is linked from

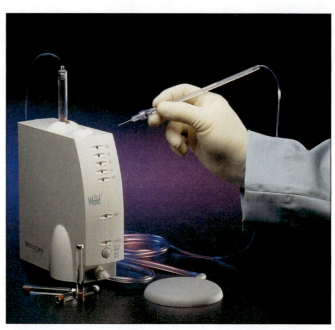

FIGURE 16-24 Computer-controlled local anesthetic delivery system (The Wand). *(Courtesy of Milestone Scientific)*

the plunger to the "handpiece," where the needle is attached. A foot control is used to activate the delivery of the anesthetic (Figure 16-24).

NITROUS OXIDE SEDATION

Nitrous oxide and oxygen gases are used together to provide relaxation and relieve apprehension for patients during dental treatment. These two gases used together allow a safe method of sedation for patients who experience great fears during dental care. This gas allows patients to maintain a conscious state while taking the "edge" off the pain so that relaxation can occur. Patients report a floating sensation, tingling fingers, and the feeling that time is passing quickly. Used safely, nitrous oxide can be a wonderful aid to allow patients to be comfortable and relaxed while receiving dental treatment.

Nitrous oxide is a stable, nonflammable gas. When used with oxygen, nitrous oxide is one of the safest anesthetic agents available. It is administered through a small nosepiece to the patient and has very little offensive odor. It raises the pain threshold without the loss of consciousness so that the patient is able to talk and follow directions.

The gas nitrous oxide was first discovered by Joseph Priestly in the early 1770s. It was thought that the gases would cure diseases. Horace Wells, a Connecticut dentist, was the first to use nitrous oxide as an anesthetic during dental surgery. He immediately recognized that it could be used to reduce pain during dental procedures.

PROCEDURE

16-3 Administration and Monitoring of Nitrous Oxide Sedation

Some states allow dental assistants to perform this task under the supervision of the dentist; in other states, the assistants will assist the dentist in administration of nitrous oxide and/or monitoring nitrous oxide.

EQUIPMENT AND SUPPLIES

▶ Nitrous oxide unit with controls and gauges

▶ Tanks of nitrous oxide and oxygen

▶ Patient nitrous nosepieces (sterile)

PROCEDURE STEPS *(Follow aseptic procedures)*

Preparation

1. Check all equipment to verify that it is working properly.

2. Check the levels of the gases to determine that the tanks are full.

Administration

1. Seat the patient and place him or her in a supine position.

2. Explain the effects, sensation, and potential hazards of nitrous oxide to the patient.

3. Have the patient give informed consent allowing the administration to continue.

4. Attach a sterile nitrous scavenger mask to the tubing (Figure 16-25).

5. Place the nosepiece mask over the nose of the patient with the tubing draped to each side.

6. Instruct the patient to breath through his or her nose slowly.

7. Begin the flow of oxygen (five plus liters per minute) and nitrous oxide. (Many offices begin with the flow of oxygen for a minute prior to the nitrous oxide. This allows the patient to become accustomed to the mask and the situation before adding the effects of the nitrous oxide.)

8. Sit with the patient and monitor for any effects as the nitrous oxide is administered. Watch for Guedel's signs, Stage I. Talk with the patient and ask him or her how he or she is feeling. (This allows

FIGURE 16-25 Nitrous oxide nasal hoods with scavenging circuit. *(Courtesy of Accutron, Inc., Phoenix, AZ)*

the baseline nitrous oxide to be identified for the patient. Adjustments are made until a comfortable level of sedation is achieved. The patient does not lose consciousness and dialogue is ongoing.)

9. Watch the patient's chest and the reservoir bag rise and fall during the breathing.

10. The local anesthetic solution is administered within a few minutes of nitrous oxide application. The patient is comfortable and the procedure can continue.

Recovery

1. When the dental procedure is nearing completion, turn off the nitrous oxide.

2. The patient will breath oxygen for a minimum of two minutes or until all signs of the nitrous oxide sedation have disappeared.

(continued)

P R O C E D U R E   **1 6 - 3** *continued*

3. Remove the nosepiece from the patient's nose.

4. Turn off the oxygen at the unit. The flow meters for the nitrous oxide and oxygen will be at zero.

5. Seat the patient upright and ask how he or she feels.

6. Ask the patient to stay seated for a minute or two until his or her head clears. (Even without having nitrous oxide, rising from the supine position may make the patient feel lightheaded.)

7. Dismiss the patient when he or she feels all right.

8. Complete all documentation on the patient's chart, including the notation about the administration of nitrous oxide.

9. The patient nosepiece is either given to the patient to save for later use or disposed of. Some offices provide plastic bags for patients to save their nitrous oxide masks for repeated use, to cut down on disposables. Patients then bring their masks back for each following appointment.

10. Disinfect the tubing.

Safety and Precautions

Safety and precautions must be practiced because of problems that are associated with nitrous oxide. Females in the first trimester of pregnancy, infertile people using in-vitro fertilization procedures, people immuno-compromised at risk of bone marrow suppression, and people with neurological complaints need special consideration. Nitrous oxide may cause fertility problems for individuals who work with and around nitrous oxide sedation on long-term bases.

Indications for Use of Nitrous Oxide Sedation.
The following patients would benefit from nitrous oxide analgesia:

▶ Patients who are fearful of dental treatment

▶ Patients who have gag reflexes that are very sensitive

▶ Patients who can breath through their noses

▶ Patients who have heart conditions (they benefit because of the oxygen and stress reduction)

▶ Patients having long appointments

Contraindications for the Use of Nitrous Oxide Sedation.

▶ Patients unable to breath through their noses

▶ Patients involved in drugs or psychiatric treatment

▶ Females in the first trimester of pregnancy

▶ Immunocompromised people at risk of bone marrow suppression

▶ Infertile people using in-vitro fertilization procedures

▶ People with neurological complaints

Equipment

Nitrous oxide is delivered to the patient through tubing connected to a nosepiece and tanks of nitrous oxide and oxygen. The gases flow through a unit that has a flow meter and adjustment on it. After the adjustments are made, the gas flows through the breathing tubes to the mask. The excess gas and air exhaled from the patient is in the reservoir bag. Nitrous oxide units can be either portable or wall mounted and distributed throughout the office (Figures 16-26 and 16-27). Cylinders of nitrous oxide gas are blue and those of oxygen are green. If a wall-mounted nitrous oxide unit is used, the gas is sent from the cylinders through pressure lines to outlets in the treatment rooms.

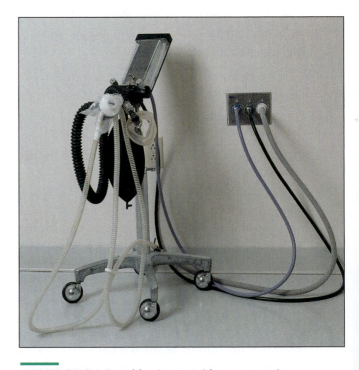

FIGURE 16-26 Portable nitrous oxide-oxygen unit.

FIGURE 16-27 Example of a wall-mounted nitrous oxide-oxygen unit with gas cylinders in remote storage area. *(Courtesy of Accutron, Inc., Phoenix, AZ)*

CHAPTER SUMMARY

Because most procedures require some form of anesthesia, the dentist may select one or a combination of methods to control pain, depending on the patient and the procedure to be completed. The dental assistant is responsible for preparing, safely transferring, and caring for the anesthetic syringe and accessories. During this time, the assistant must be aware of the various topical solutions, application sites, how to apply the topical anesthetic, and possible patient reactions. In addition, the assistant follows the dentist's directions for the administration of sedation and monitoring requirements.

CASE STUDY

Chuck Thompson, forty-five years old, was scheduled for a crown preparation. Topical anesthetic was placed, and Chuck became very talkative and excited. His pulse rate increased.

Case Study Review

1. What considerations could there be on the patient's medical history that would indicate this reaction?

2. What are the possibilities that would indicate this reaction? What kind of reaction is Chuck experiencing?

3. Are there any other symptoms to watch for?

To complete your study of this chapter, work the review activities that follow. Also, refer to the software that accompanies this text.

REVIEW QUESTIONS

Multiple Choice

1. Anesthetic that produces a deadened or pain-free area is called
   a. general anesthetic.
   b. local anesthetic.
   c. topical anesthetic.
   d. sedation anesthetic.

2. Topical anesthetics are available in all of the following forms *except*
   a. powders.
   b. gels.
   c. ointments.
   d. metered sprays.

3. An injection that deposits anesthetic near a larger terminal nerve branch and is mainly used for treatment on the maxillary or mandibular anterior regions is a(n)
   a. infiltration injection.
   b. field block injection.
   c. block injection.
   d. periodontal ligament injection.

4. All of the following are parts of the dental needle except the
   a. bevel.
   b. syringe end.
   c. plunger.
   d. hub.

5. A drug that is added to anesthetic solutions in order to reduce blood flow around the injection site is called
   a. paresthesia.
   b. vasoconstrictor.
   c. infiltration.
   d. nitrous oxide.

Critical Thinking

1. Which anesthetic solution would dentists select to administer to a patient if they wanted a stronger ratio of the vasoconstrictor?

2. What should be noted on the patient's chart in regard to the local anesthetic?

3. What types of patients would benefit most from nitrous oxide analgesia?

Dental Radiography

OBJECTIVES

The student should strive to meet the following objectives and demonstrate an understanding of the facts and principles presented in this chapter:

1. Explain the history of radiation and the use of the Hittorf-Crookes and Coolidge tubes.
2. List the properties of radiation and explain the biological effects of radiation exposure.
3. Identify the components of a dental x-ray unit and explain the function of each component.
4. Describe the safety precautions to be utilized when using radiation.
5. Explain how an x-ray is produced.
6. Describe the composition, sizes, types, and storage of dental x-ray film.
7. Explain intraoral and extraoral x-ray production.
8. Identify means of producing quality radiographs on a variety of patients.
9. Explain the bisecting and paralleling techniques.
10. List common production errors.
11. Describe the processing techniques, the composition of the solutions, and the storage of final radiographs.
12. Explain the mounting procedures.
13. Identify extraoral films and describe exposing techniques.
14. Identify normal and abnormal radiographic landmarks.
15. List standardized procedures and state policies that dental offices follow to ensure quality radiographs.
16. Identify imaging systems used for dental purposes.

KEY TERMS

ALARA (p. 316)

anode (p. 312)

automatic
   processing (p. 358)

basal cells (p. 316)

bisecting technique
   (p. 313)

bite-wing (p. 324)

blurred images
   (p. 348)

cassette (p. 363)

cathode (p. 312)

central beam (p. 320)

cephalometric
   radiographs
   (p. 365)

collimator (p. 320)

computed
   tomography
   (CT scanning)
   (p. 372)

cone cutting
   (p. 347)

cross-section
   technique (p. 337)

(continued, p. 278)

developer solution (p. 354)

digital imaging technology (p. 372)

double exposure (p. 347)

duplication technique (p. 360)

electromagnetic energy (p. 314)

elongation (p. 346)

extraoral film (p. 363)

fixer solution (p. 358)

focal spot (p. 319)

focusing cup (p. 319)

foreshortening (p. 347)

Frankfort plane (p. 365)

Gray (GY) (p. 316)

herringbone pattern (p. 349)

horizontal angulation (p. 325)

intensifying screens (p. 364)

interproximal (p. 329)

intraoral (p. 313)

kilovoltage (kV) (p. 317)

latent period (p. 317)

leakage radiation (p. 316)

long wavelengths (p. 315)

magnetic resonance imaging (MRI) (p. 372)

manual processing (p. 352)

maximum permissible dose (MPD) (p. 317)

milliamperage (mA) (p. 317)

milliroentgen (mr) (p. 317)

mitosis (p. 316)

occlusal radiographs (p. 324)

overlapping (p. 347)

panoramic technique (p. 314)

paralleling technique (p. 313)

periapical (p. 324)

primary radiation (p. 315)

radiation absorbed dose (rad) (p. 316)

radiolucent (p. 322)

radiopaque (p. 348)

radiosensitive (p. 316)

relative biological effectiveness (rbe) (p. 317)

reticulation (p. 350)

roentgens (p. 313)

roentgen equivalent man (rem) (p. 316)

scatter radiation (p. 315)

secondary radiation (p. 315)

short wavelengths (p. 315)

sievert (Sv) (p. 316)

tragus of the ear (p. 365)

thermionic emission (p. 321)

topographic technique (p. 337)

transcranial temporomandibular joint radiograph (p. 365)

tubehead (p. 319)

vertical angulation (p. 325)

x-ray tube (p. 319)

x-rays (p. 312)

INTRODUCTION

Wilhelm Conrad Roentgen (ren-ken) discovered **x-rays** in 1895 (Figure 17-1). Roentgen was a professor of physics at the University of Wurzberg in Germany. He was doing experiments with a cathode ray tube called the Hittorf-Crooks tube. This glass vacuum tube had an electrical circuit connected to each end. Roentgen, as well as a number of other physicists at this time, were interested in the stream of bluish colored light that passed from one end of the tube to the other when the electrical circuit was connected. The colored light was later discovered to be a stream of electrons that traveled from the **cathode** end to the **anode** end of the tube.

Roentgen placed an aluminum sheet with a window opening on the side of the tube in order to study the properties of the cathode ray. The room was darkened and a number of fluorescent screens were placed around the laboratory. While conducting his experiments, he noticed that a fluorescent screen on the other side of the room was glowing. Because Roentgen knew that the cathode rays (electrically negative particles) could travel only a short distance outside the cathode tube in the air, he knew he was observing a new phenomenon, an unknown ray, which he identified as an "x" ray, noting the unknown in mathematics.

Roentgen continued his experiments with the x-ray. He placed a variety of objects in front of the beam and

FIGURE 17-1 Wilhelm Conrad Roentgen (1845–1923). He discovered x-rays in 1895. *(From O. Glasser, Dr. W.C. Roentgen, 2nd edition, 1958. Courtesy of Charles C. Thomas, publisher, Springfield, Illinois)*

observed the images that were made on the fluorescent screen. For instance, when he placed metal in front of the beam, there was no visible image on the fluorescent screen. The metal blocked the beam. However, paper and wood allowed the x-ray to pass through and the glow on the fluorescent screen changed according to the density of the object. It was while placing the objects in front of the screen that he noticed he was able to see a shadow of the bones of his hand. The soft tissues of the hand allowed the x-rays to pass through, but the harder tissue of the bones stopped the x-rays.

Roentgen furthered his experiments with the x-ray and produced images on photographic plates. A couple of the first radiographs made were those of his shotgun barrel and his wife Berta's hand.

The news of the discovery of the x-ray was soon heard around the world. Roentgen was awarded the first Nobel Prize in physics in 1901 for his work. Today, units of x-ray exposure are still expressed in **roentgens** in his honor.

In Germany in 1895, Dr. Otto Walkoff was the first to take a dental radiograph, just two weeks after the discovery of the x-ray. He used a small glass plate coated with photographic emulsion and an exposure time of about twenty-five minutes to obtain his desired result.

In 1896, Dr. C. Edmond Kells, a New Orleans dentist, took the first **intraoral** radiograph using his own equipment and techniques. Later he presented a clinical demonstration of dental x-rays at a dental association meeting in North Carolina. Dr. Kells utilized a method for adjusting the x-ray beam that he called "setting the tube." In this technique, he placed his hand between the tube and the screen and adjusted the beam until he could clearly see the bones of his hand (Figure 17-2). He was unaware of the dangerous effects of radiation. Kells experienced pain and erythema (redness of the skin) on his hands from continued radiation exposure. Ongoing exposure resulted in the subsequent loss of three fingers, his hand, his arm, and eventually his life, at the age of seventy-two.

The inventor of the first dental x-ray unit was Dr. William Rollins of Boston, Massachusetts, in 1896. He reported effects of radiation exposure, noting burning of the skin on his hands. He was an early advocate of caution in the use of "x" radiation.

Dr. William D. Coolidge, a physicist, invented the hot cathode x-ray tube in 1913. This hot filament replaced the need for the residual gas of the older model and established a standard for producing x-rays that were more uniform and therefore more predictable. The first American-made x-ray machine was manufactured around this time as well.

In 1923, the Victor X-Ray Corporation, which later became known as the General Electric Corporation, developed a dental x-ray machine using the Coolidge tube in the machine head, which was cooled by oil immersion. Although the x-ray machine has been enhanced with numerous modifications to meet current application and safety requirements, this basic prototype is still used today.

FIGURE 17-2 Early radiograph. (*Courtesy of the American College of Radiology, Reston, VA*)

Around 1905, Dr. Howard Rober and A. Cieszyski, an engineer, developed the **bisecting technique**. This technique applies a geometric principle. This principle is known as the rule of isometry (discussed later in this chapter).

In 1920, Frank McCormack developed an additional technique for exposing dental x-rays called the **paralleling technique**. This technique is often called the right-angle technique. To further perfect the paralleling technique, Gordon M. Fitzgerald and William J. Updegrave developed the long cone technique and devices for positioning x-rays and refined information on how to expose the x-ray properly. Over the years, the long cone technique has become more simplified due to the change in the shape of the cone. Open-ended cylinders or rectangular tubes have replaced the pointed cone, allowing the operator to direct the x-rays more accurately. The open-ended tube, called the **position indicator device** (**PID**), is still commonly referred to as the cone.

Several doctors researched the concept of rotational panoramic machines. The desired concept was to have an x-ray of the entire dental arch on one film. To accomplish this, some machines rotated the film, others rotated the patient, and some rotated the x-ray beam. In 1959, the **panoramic technique** was developed. Dr. Paatero was credited with developing the first orthopantomograph unit that would take acceptable panoramic radiographs. Over the next ten years, a number of advances were made, and in 1980 the Panorex II was developed by Dr. Charles Morris. This machine allowed the operator to make a split or continuous image of the oral cavity.

Present radiographic technology uses the principles of tomography, where the structures in the mouth can be visualized in a chosen layer or plane while intentionally blurring out structures in other planes. This technique is not normally used in the dental offices on a routine basis.

X-ray film also has changed throughout history. At first, glass photographic plates were used. Later, film was cut to size in the darkroom and wrapped in paper and a rubber coating; this process was very time consuming. In 1913, Kodak developed the first pre-wrapped film packets. Today's x-rays come in easy-to-use sizes and a standard of quality we have come to expect. They require minimal exposure to the patient to achieve the needed results.

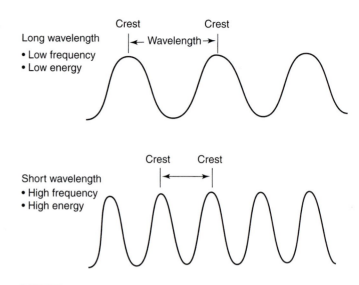

FIGURE 17-3 Wavelengths as they relate to energy, frequency, and x-ray. In dentistry, the shortest wavelength with high frequency and energy is used to expose dental film.

RADIATION PHYSICS AND BIOLOGY

Radiation is one type of **electromagnetic energy** (radiation). The most familiar forms of electromagnetic energy are radio and television waves and visible light. All electromagnetic energy has some similar properties. First, the energy travels in waves that move in straight lines at the speed of light (186,000 miles per second). Second, they consist of energy only. Therefore, energy can be sent through lines to a receiver, such as a television. No mass is involved, only the energy. Last, electromagnetic energy travels through space in the form of transverse waves. The wavelength is the distance between the peaks of adjacent waves and is called a cycle (Figure 17-3).

The length of the wavelength is the characteristic that separates the different types of electromagnetic energy into categories. Examples of electromagnetic radiation with longer wavelengths are visible light, television, and radio waves. Forms of electromagnetic radiation with shorter wavelengths are x-rays and gamma rays. The electromagnetic scale identifies the relationship between the types of energy and the length of the wave (Figure 17-4). The more cycles that pass a point in a given time, the higher the frequency. Therefore:

▶ Short wavelength with high frequency = more energy

▶ Long wavelength with low frequency = less energy

It is important that individuals working with radiation understand the behavior and nature of x-rays. Vis-

ible light is the only wavelength that is detected with your senses. Invisible x-rays, utilized for diagnosis in dentistry, carry 10,000 times more energy than does visible light. X-rays do travel in a straight line and can be deflected off an object and scatter. They are able to penetrate matter, where visible light is absorbed or reflected.

The Structure of an Atom and Ionization

Understanding the composition of an atom will aid the dental assistant in understanding the process of **ionization**, where atoms are changed into negatively or positively charged ions during radiation. Atoms make up all matter. An atom is composed of a nucleus (the inner core that is positively charged) and electrons (negatively charged particles that orbit around the nucleus). The nucleus mass is composed of subatomic particles: protons (positively charged) and neutrons (having no charge) and subatomic particles that are divided further into hadrons, leptons, and quarks.

The electrons remain stable as they rotate around the nucleus, in an orbit, unless disturbed. If they are disturbed, for example when x-ray photons collide with the atoms, electrons are lost and the remaining electrons become positive ions. These positively charged ions can then react with other atoms in tissues and other matter. This process can alter living cells and tissues and even cause permanent damage.

The patient and the operator must always be protected during exposure to ionizing radiation. Following safety guidelines, monitoring radiation, and using lead-lined protection protects individuals from the harmful effects of radiation.

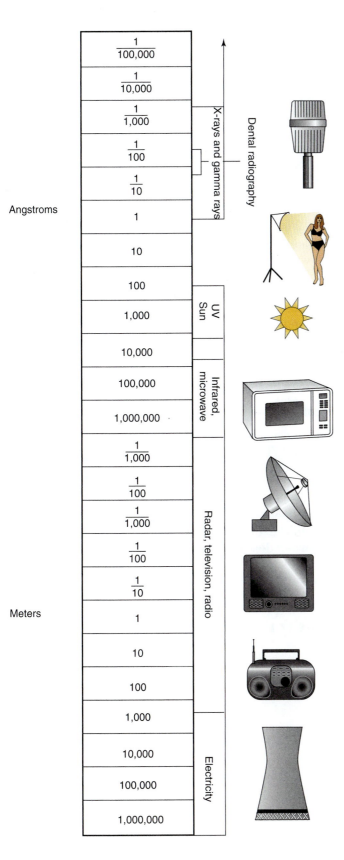

FIGURE 17-4 Electromagnetic energy spectrum. Several familiar electromagnetic energy applications in relationship to dental radiography are shown.

Types of Radiation

The wavelengths desired in dental radiographs are **short wavelengths**, or **hard radiation**. These have high frequency, high energy, and high penetrating power. **Soft radiation**, or **long wavelengths**, have low energy, low frequency, and low penetrating power. They are unsuitable for exposing dental radiographs. These soft radiation rays are often referred to as Grenz rays.

There are four types of radiation: primary, secondary, scatter, and leakage (Figure 17-5).

1. **Primary radiation** is the central beam that comes from the x-ray tube head. It consists of high energy, short wavelength x-rays traveling in a straight line. Primary radiation, often called the primary beam, is the useful x-ray that produces the diagnostic image on the x-ray film.

2. **Secondary radiation** is formed when primary x-rays strike the patient or come in contact with matter (any substance). The waves are often transformed into longer wavelengths that lose their energy.

3. **Scatter radiation** is deflected from its path as it strikes matter. Often, secondary and scatter radiation are used interchangeably. This radiation is scattered in all directions and therefore presents the most serious danger to the operator. Due to scatter radiation, the operator must stand at least six feet away from the patient while exposing x-ray film or structural shielding and out of the path of the primary beam.

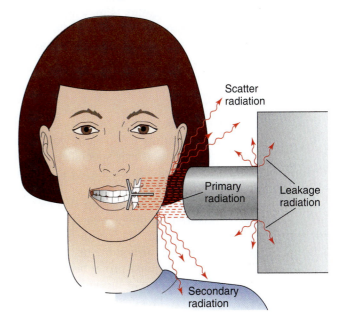

FIGURE 17-5 Primary, secondary, and leakage radiation identified on an x-ray tube and a patient's face.

4. **Leakage radiation** escapes in all directions from the tube or the tube head. The x-ray machine must be checked for leakage and should not be used until the problem is taken care of. The leakage radiation is not useful to the diagnostic process and the long wavelengths can only be harmful.

BIOLOGICAL EFFECTS OF RADIATION

X-rays can cause injury to biologic tissues. Some of these injuries heal, but some cause permanent damage. If the cell is affected by direct radiation, the cell may die immediately, change, become altered at the time of **mitosis** (cell division in the sex cells in which the number of chromosomes in each is reduced to one-half), or remain unaffected.

Somatic and Genetic Effects of Radiation

The cells in the body are divided into two groups: the somatic and the genetic. The somatic make up all the cells except the reproductive cells. The genetic cells make up all the reproductive cells, such as the ova and the sperm. The biological effects of radiation are classified according to the type of cell that is affected by the radiation. The radiation is said to be either somatic or genetic.

The somatic effects of radiation leave the individual in poor health, with cataracts, cancer, or leukemia. The effects are not passed on to the next generation; the consequence of the radiation exposure remains with the primary individual. Genetic effects may not involve the primary individual exposed to the radiation. The genetic effects cannot be repaired and they are passed on to future generations.

Radiosensitive Cells

Some cells are more **radiosensitive** than others. The more sensitive cells are immature cells, rapidly dividing cells, and cells that do not perform specialized functions. An example of rapidly dividing cells are the **basal cells** of the skin. They are sloughed off and continuously replaced. Therefore, a person may develop skin cancer due to prolonged exposure to sunlight, a high dosage of radiation, and/or frequent radiation exposures.

Today the public is more informed about the effects of radiation. Most patients request protection from radiation during pregnancy because individuals understand that the embryo is very sensitive to radiation. Radiation to an embryo may cause death, congenital malformations, or growth retardation. The effects of the radiation depend on the stage of the developing embryo and the radiation dosage that the embryo was exposed to. So, when pregnancy is suspected, every precaution is taken. All patients should receive protection with lead aprons with thyroid collars during radiation exposure.

Cells that are radioresistant or less sensitive to radiation are mature cells that rarely undergo cell divisions. Examples of radioresistant cells are nerve and muscle cells. Table 17-1 shows the levels of sensitivity of different cells.

Low-level radiation normally does not cause damage that cannot be repaired within the cells. Tissues that are radiosensitive in the dental region are the lens of the eye and the thyroid gland. Because of their location near the oral cavity, the tissues may be exposed to the primary beam (central beam) of the x-ray. Very high radiation dosages (not used in dentistry) have been known to cause cataracts in the eye and thyroid carcinoma. It is unlikely that dental x-rays would cause one of these serious effects; however, it is always necessary to utilize the least amount of radiation possible. All dental personnel use the **as low as reasonably achievable (ALARA)** concept for radiation protection. Dental offices use a thyroid shield extension on the lead apron to further protect the patients.

Radiation Units of Measurement

The terminology for measurement of radiation has changed. There are several new terms replacing the older, more familiar, terms (refer to Table 17-2).

In 1937, the International Committee for Radiological Units established the official definition of radiation quantity. A **roentgen (R)** equals the amount of radiation that will ionize one cubic centimeter of air. A **radiation absorbed dose (rad)** or **Gray (GY)** is the amount of ionizing radiation absorbed in a substance. A **roentgen equivalent man (rem)** or **sievert (Sv)** is the dose to

TABLE 17-1 TISSUE AND ORGAN RADIATION SENSITIVITY

Most sensitive	Lymphoid Reproductive cells Bone marrow Intestinal epithelium
Moderately sensitive	Skin Intestinal tract Oral mucosa
Sensitive	Connective tissue Growing bone
Less sensitive	Mature bone Salivary glands Thyroid Liver
Least sensitive	Kidney Muscle Nerves

TABLE 17-2 RADIATION MEASUREMENT TERMS

	Standard System (Traditional)	Metric Equivalent or Système Internationale (SI)
Exposure (C/kg)	Roentgen (R) 3.88×10 R =	Couloumb per kilogram 1 c/kg
Dose	Radiation absorbed dose (RAD) 100 rads =	Gray (GY) 1 Gy
Dose equivalent	Radiation equivalent man (REM) 100 rems =	Sievert (Sv) 1 Sv

which body tissues are exposed, measured in terms of its estimated biological effects in relation to an exposure dose of one R of x or gamma radiation. A **milliroentgen (mr)** is one one thousandth (1/1,000) of a roentgen (R).

Relative biological effectiveness (rbe) is the measurement unit used to compare the biological effects of different tissues irradiated by different forms of energy. Dental x-rays have arbitrarily been assigned an rbe unit of one.

Determine the rem by multiplying the rad by the rbe. Therefore, 100 rads times one equals 100 rems. The rad and the rem are considered equal for dental x-rays. The roentgen and the rad are considered equal in amount, but a rad is an absorbed dose and not the amount coming from the machine.

Occupational Exposure

Individuals who routinely use ionizing radiation in their occupations are regulated by the dose limitations defined by the National Council on Radiation Protection and Measurements. The **maximum permissible dose (MPD)** is the maximum dose of radiation that, in light of present knowledge, would not be expected to produce any significant radiation effects in a life. The MPD calls for the dose limit of occupational exposure to be at 0.05 Sv (5 rems) per year for radiation workers; non-occupational and pregnant workers are regulated at one-tenth that limit. Most resources recognize the 0.05 Sv per year maximum; however, recommendations by the International Commission on Radiological Protection call for the occupational exposure dose limits to be 20 mSv (2 rems).

Daily Radiation Exposure

The general population is exposed to two major categories of radiation daily: natural and artificial. Annually, a person encounters 3.6 mSv (360 mrem) of radiation from all sources. Natural sources make up about 55 percent of radiation exposure. It comes from the earth (radon, for instance), the sun, and the atmosphere.

About 41 percent of radiation exposure comes from artificial radiation, such as x-rays used for diagnosis, as well as from consumer products, such as television, airline travel, tobacco, and smoke alarms.

Accumulation of Radiation

The effects of radiation are accumulative. This means that the effects of the exposure increases every time the individual is exposed to radiation. This is often called the "long-term effect."

The normal aging process tends to accelerate due to the accumulation of radiation. Most adults know that the skin of individuals who have (or had) high exposure to the sun will age at an increased rate. The higher the doses, the more rapid the effects. This period of time between the direct exposure and the development of biological effects (or symptoms) is called the **latent period**.

DENTAL X-RAY UNIT/COMPONENTS

Control Panel

The **control panel** is where the circuit boards and controls are located that allow the operator to adjust the correct setting for each patient (Figures 17-6A and B). It is where the on/off switch is located along with the selection for the **milliamperage (mA)** and **kilovoltage (kV)** and the **electronic timer**.

The operator chooses the correct settings according to the individual (for example, children need less radiation), the area of the oral cavity needing diagnostic x-rays, the exposure technique used, and the film speed.

Milliamperage. Milliamperage (mA) determines the amount or quantity of electrons. The higher the milliamperage, the greater the amount of radiation. Milli (1/1,000) amperage is a measurement unit for electrical current.

Some dental x-ray machines use 10 or 15 mA. Many machines are set up with selectors for either 10 or 15 mA on the control panel. This milliamperage selector also acts as the on and off switch for the machine. Often, 10 mA is used with this type of dental x-ray machine.

(A)

(B)

FIGURE 17-6 Control panels. (A) Digital settings for milliamperage, kilovoltage, and time. (B) Manual settings for milliamperage, kilovoltage, and time.

Radiation is not produced until the electronic timer is pushed. Some of the newer units are preset at 7 mA for all x-rays. They have separate on and off switches.

Kilovoltage. Kilovoltage (kV) determines the quality or penetrating power of the central beam. The higher the kilovoltage, the greater the penetration power of the x-rays and the less exposure time that is required; therefore, there is less radiation to the patient. The quicker the radiation goes through the tissues, the greater the quality of the radiograph (showing a longer range of the gray scale). A longer range of the gray scale would show varying tissue density and provide greater diagnostic quality.

The kilovoltage meter is located on the control panel. The operator adjusts the kilovoltage selector to the desired setting. The most common settings for the kilovoltage are from 70 to 90 kV. On many of the digital machines, the kilovoltage is set automatically according to the selection of the area to be x-rayed.

Electronic Timer. The electronic timer controls the total time that rays flow from the x-ray tube. It is a rotating dial with which the dental assistant selects how many fractions of a second or impulses are needed to produce the x-ray. It takes thirty impulses to equal one-half of a second. The operator determines the number of impulses or exposure time after evaluating the technique to be used, the type of x-ray film, the target film distance, and which tissues are going to be radiographed. Again, this may be preset on the digital machines. The digital machines have touch pads and/or switches with simple drawings of adults or children on which to select patient size. By indicating the size of the patient, the amount of kilovoltage, and the area to be radiographed, the machine automatically sets the timer.

The switch to the timer is located outside the room or behind a lead barrier. The operator pushes the switch and the timer allows the electrons to flow from the x-ray tube for the indicated time. Then, it resets.

Milliamperage Seconds. Milliamperage seconds (mAs) determine the amount of radiation exposure the patient is receiving. The dental assistant calculates the milliamperage times the exposure time in order to determine the milliamperage seconds (mAs). Once set, most offices do not change the kVp and mAs, except for child and adult variations.

Arm Assembly and Tube Head

The **arm assembly** is attached firmly to the wall in the x-ray room (Figure 17-7). The flexible extension of the arm allows the operator to freely position the tube head for the various positions required for dental radiography exposures.

FIGURE 17-7 The parts of the dental arm assembly. (A) (1) Control panel. (2) Extension arm. (3) Tubehead. (4) The position indicator device (PID). (B) (1) Tubehead. (2) PID. (3) Vertical indicator scale.

The **tubehead** is where the x-ray tube and step-up and step-down transformers are located (Figure 17-7). The high voltage (step-up transformer) provides the kV needed to propel the electrons, and the low voltage (step-down transformer) adjusts the voltage down to the amount of power needed to heat the filament of the cathode and produce the milliamperage. It is where x-rays are generated. The tubehead is made of a metal casing that is lead lined or lead to limit the amount of radiation leakage. An oil bath surrounds the components in the tubehead to provide cooling as heat is given off. The heat is derived from production of the cloud of electrons and then manufacturing of the x-rays.

The **x-ray tube** is approximately six inches in length and one-half inch in diameter and is often referred to as a Coolidge tube (Figure 17-8). The tube is made from leaded glass and has a window (aperture window) of unleaded glass in the side where the x-rays exit. The tube is a vacuum tube (all air has been removed from the tube) so the electrons will be free to travel at the speed of light and not collide with air or gas molecules. On the cathode (–) side of the tube, a **focusing cup** made of molybdenum with a filament of tungsten is positioned. This is where the electrons originate. Tungsten is used because it has a high melting point, high ductility so it can be made into a fine wire, and a high atomic number so a large number of electrons develop when it is heated. The focusing cup is designed to direct the stream of electrons to the anode. The anode (+), which is located opposite the cathode, is made of a tungsten target set at an angle to direct the flow of x-rays. The small spot on the tungsten target where the electrons hit is called the **focal spot**. After the electrons hit, a great deal of heat is generated. The anode tungsten target is attached to a copper stem and then to a heat radiator to conduct the heat away from the focal spot. The heat dissipates through the copper stem and then is cooled by the heat radiator and the surrounding oil bath.

After leaving the anode, the x-rays go through the aperture or non-leaded window and encounter a solid metal **filter**, usually made of aluminum. The filter, know

FIGURE 17-8 X-ray tube.

as the inherent filter, is placed in the path of the x-rays in order to eliminate the soft x-rays (those with low penetrating power). The hard x-rays with short wavelengths, called the **central beam**, continue through the filter to the collimator (lead diaphragm). This collimator is a lead disc with an opening in the middle that restructures the beam and filters out additional weak rays. The opening limits the size of the x-ray beam that is permitted to pass through the open cone and out the position indicator device (PID). The x-ray beam size cannot exceed two and three-quarters inches in diameter. Approximately 1 percent of the kinetic energy (energy of motion) created during the x-ray process is converted into useful x-rays. The remaining 99 percent is dissipated as heat.

Bremsstrahlung radiation is the primary type of radiation in the x-ray beam going from the tubehead. Bremsstrahlung originates from a German word meaning "braking." This braking action takes place when the electrons strike the anode target. Bremsstrahlung also refers to the specific characteristics of the beam.

SAFETY AND PRECAUTIONS

It is the responsibility of the manufacturers, dental team members, and patients to follow safety and precaution measures when using radiography equipment. Steps must be used to minimize risk to the patient and all dental personnel.

Manufacturer's Responsibilities

The federal government has set up specific safety specifications that all manufacturers of dental x-ray units must meet.

- The machine must have a separate control switch to cut off the electricity to the machine. The exposure switch must have an electronic timer to stop the electricity automatically when the control switch is released.

- The cone position indicator device (PID) must be lead lined, and the x-ray tube itself must be sealed in an oil-immersed casing.

- The control panel must have indicators that display milliamperage, kilovoltage, and impulses per exposure time. Some models display the preset number for milliamperage and only two choices for kilovoltage. On a digital control panel, the timer is preset, and changes on the digital panel display according to the chosen exposure area.

- The **collimator**, fitted directly over the opening where the x-ray beam exits from the tubehead, is made of a lead plate. The opening or a hole in the middle of the lead plate of the collimator is regulated to ensure that the useful beam does not exceed 2.75 inches in diameter.

- Filtration of 2.5 mm of aluminum is required and built in the head of all x-ray machines operating at kilovoltages higher than 70.

Dentist's Responsibilities

- It is the dentist's responsibility to have all x-ray equipment installed in a safe manner and to maintain it properly. The office design must provide occupants with lead filtration protection from radiation. The location of the x-ray room and the protective lead barriers must meet specific requirements for safety that allow at least six feet in the opposite direction of the primary ray. X-ray machines must be inspected regularly, usually yearly, by the Department of Social and Health Services, state x-ray control section, to ensure proper functioning.

- The dentist must be responsible in prescribing x-rays for patients, keeping in mind that only x-rays for a proper diagnosis are necessary.

- It is the dentist's responsibility to repair x-ray equipment when necessary and to stop usage immediately when a problem is apparent.

- The dentist is responsible for having dental assistants properly credentialed and trained to expose and process radiographs. The dentist is also responsible for supervising dental assistants in these tasks.

In 1981, the Consumer Patient Radiation Health and Safety Act was enacted. This federal law requires each state to inform the Secretary of Health and Human Services how compliance with the act is accomplished.

Responsibilities of the Dental Assistant

- The dental assistant must be trained in aseptic techniques, radiation hygiene, and maintenance of quality assurance and safety.

- The dental assistant must obtain a proper education in exposure and processing techniques. He or she must have an understanding of the physics and biological effects of ionizing radiation and utilize the understanding during every radiographic exposure.

- The dental assistant must understand the ALARA principle and utilize the lead apron with cervical collar for the patient's safety each time an x-ray is taken.

- Dental assistants must label and store patient x-rays properly to prevent loss.

Responsibility of the Patient

The patient is responsible for notifying the office of any changes in health (pregnancy, for instance). The patient is responsible to present, to the best of his or her ability, a radiation history as part of the dental record.

Additional Notes Regarding Reducing Radiation Exposure

▶ Using E-type film instead of D-type film reduces the time of radiation exposure to the patient by up to 50 percent. In the past, there has been some resistance to changing from the standard D film because of quality control, but recent studies have demonstrated that E film is comparable in quality.

▶ A patient having an eighteen-film series (full mouth) using a long, round PID without a lead apron results in a genetic exposure of 0.5 mrad; with a lead apron, the genetic exposure is approximately 0.01 mrad. If a thyroid collar is used, a 50 percent reduction is noted in the thyroid area.

▶ A patient having an eighteen-film series using a rectangular PID instead of a round PID reduces the radiation exposure to the patient by approximately 60 percent (Figure 17-9). Therefore, an eighteen-film series with the lead apron is approximately 0.01 mrad.

▶ Proper filtration can reduce somatic (all tissues) exposure by 50 percent. A number of rare earth filters are being used to further reduce radiation exposure. The Radiation Health and Safety Board or the Kodak Company can be contacted for updated information on approved filters.

A dosimeter badge should be worn at all times in the dental office by any dental assistant producing radiographs (Figure 17-10). This badge is for monitoring each individual's radiation exposure in the office. It is important that the badge not be worn out of the office, because it will produce an inaccurate reading. The badges are normally read monthly, and each employee should be apprised of the outcome.

A quality assurance (QA) program should be developed for the production and processing of radiographs in the dental office.

RADIATION PRODUCTION

X-rays are produced when the operator depresses the exposure switch and starts the process of generating electricity (Figure 17-11). The electricity passes to the control panel by way of the step-down and step-up transformers, where specified instructions on the quantity and the quality of x-rays have been selected. From the setting of the milliamperage, time, and kilovoltage circuits, the electricity travels to the cathode filament. This current passes through the filament and heats it to an extremely high temperature. This process is called **thermionic emission**. When the filament reaches a certain temperature, electrons are given off. These electrons are negatively charged and therefore attracted to the positively charged anode side of the tube. The electrons travel toward the anode at a rapid speed. The focusing cup on the cathode directs the electrons to a small area (about one square millimeter in size), called the focal spot, on the anode tungsten target. The precise moment of contact is when the x-rays are produced due to the forceful collision of the electrons. At the time of the collision, the x-rays are given off the tungsten target and weaker rays go in all directions. The useful x-rays travel through the filters and collimator and out the PID (position indicator device) opening.

FIGURE 17-9 In comparison to the rectangular collimator, the round collimator exposes the patient to an increased amount of excess radiation.

FIGURE 17-10 The operator wears a film badge to detect radiation exposure.

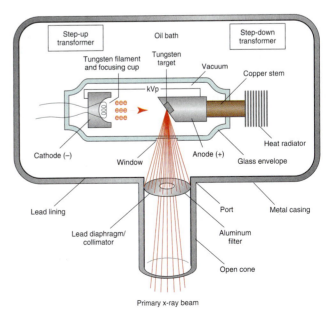

FIGURE 17-11 Production of x-rays within the tubehead.

The excess heat generated by the collision is dissipated by a heavy copper stem that takes it away from the tungsten target and cools it in oil present in the tubehead. In addition to the copper stem cooling, a bulb also takes heat into the oil bath chamber of the tubehead to increase cooling.

▌DENTAL X-RAY FILM

Composition of Dental X-Ray Film

The film used in dental radiography is composed of a flexible, thin, polyester plastic base (about 0.2 mm thick). This semi-clear base (cellulose acetate) has a slightly bluish tint in order to enhance the quality of the image. The primary function of the base is to provide support to the emulsion. It permits easy handling during the processing and makes viewing the image less difficult. The base is coated on each side by the emulsion and is attached firmly by an adhesive (Figure 17-12). The adhesive ensures that the emulsion is distributed uniformly over the base. The emulsion is made of a homogeneous mixture of silver **halide** crystals suspended in a gelatin. Halides are compounds of halogen, such as chlorine, bromine, and iodine, that combine with another element, such as silver. In dental films, silver is combined most frequently with bromine. During the process of radiation exposure, the silver halide crystals store the energy from which they have been exposed and react with the chemicals in the processing tank to form a black (**radiolucent**) region on the film. The silver halide crystals that have not been struck by the radiation are not energized and wash off the film when it processes.

This energy or latent image does not become visible until the film has been exposed to chemicals for a given time at a given temperature. If a film has been totally exposed to visible light, it appears black after the processing. If the film was not exposed to light or radiation, the film appears clear after processing. The emulsion washes off and appears as a semi-clear blue base. The emulsion is placed on both sides of the base to reduce the amount of radiation needed, and it means that the x-ray can be read from either side. On top of the emulsion is a protective coating that is used to protect the emulsion, especially from the rollers in an automatic processor.

Film Speed

The size of the crystals in the emulsion regulate the speed of the film. The larger the crystals, normally the faster the film. Dentists normally use one of two choices in dental x-ray film. The D-speed film, called Ultraspeed, is being replaced by the E-speed film, Ektraspeed. The Ektraspeed film requires approximately 40 percent less exposure time than the Ultraspeed film, therefore reducing the amount of radiation the patient is exposed to.

Film Sizes

Dental intraoral film packets come in five basic sizes (Figure 17-13). Each size is used for a specific radiographic exposure, depending on the size of the patient's oral cavity and the area to be radiographed (see Table 17-3). The film that produces the best radiographic results with the least radiation exposure for the patient is selected.

Dental Film Packet

The intraoral film packet has a sealed outer plastic wrap (Figure 17-14). Inside the wrapper, a black paper is folded around the film and a lead foil backing is placed away from the x-ray tube. The lead foil absorbs any unused radiation and the scattering of secondary radiation and film fogging. The outer plastic wrap is totally sealed to prevent any moisture from getting to the film.

FIGURE 17-13 Examples of dental x-ray film showing sizes and numbers. (Size #1, narrow anterior film size, and size #3, long bite-wing film size [not shown]).

FIGURE 17-12 The composition of the dental x-ray film.

TABLE 17-3 INTRAORAL FILM SIZES AND USES

Film Size	Description/Uses
No. 0	Child size
No. 1	Narrow anterior film size
No. 2	Adult size
No. 3	Long bite-wing film size
No. 4	Occlusal film size

The film packets also come in double packets. These film packets contain two films per packet. They take slightly more radiation for exposure but allow both the doctor and the specialist to have an original film.

Dental Film Storage

Prior to use, dental x-ray film should be stored carefully. It is sensitive to stray radiation, high temperatures, and chemicals. Ideally, the unexposed film should be stored at 50°F to 70°F (10°C to 20°C). Many dental offices store the film in the refrigerator. The dental assistants take only the needed films to the area and use disposable cups to collect and transfer the exposed radiographs.

The dental assistant should pay careful attention to the expiration date on the boxes of film. Placing the boxes of film in the storage area so that the oldest film is used first will prevent any film from expiring. Using expired film for a patient's radiographs may inhibit diagnostic quality.

After the film has been exposed and processed, it should be mounted and placed in a protective envelope. All x-rays should be handled with care so that they are not scratched and the integrity of the radiograph is not compromised. The radiographs are records of the patients' conditions at that time and may be used as legal documents.

PRODUCING QUALITY RADIOGRAPHS

Preparing for X-Ray Exposure

The dental chair should be covered with a plastic bag or at least have a barrier on the head rest and the chair controls (Figures 17-15A and B). The x-ray units should have barriers covering the dials, the exposure buttons, the cone, the tubehead, areas of the extension arm that would be touched, and any other areas that may be contaminated. If there is a door the dental assistant needs to open and close, a barrier should be placed on the door knob (plastic sandwich bags work

FIGURE 17-15 (A) Control panel. (B) Tubehead with barriers in place.

Outer package and black paper — Dental film — Black paper — Lead foil backing — Outer package

OPPOSITE SIDE TOWARD TUBE
Kodak
EKTASPEED Plus
Dental Film

FIGURE 17-14 A film packet.

well to barrier this area). An area for clean and contaminated films should be prepared.

Set up the materials needed. For example, assemble the parts of the sterile Rinn XCP instruments and select the appropriate x-ray films. Also, have a tissue available for the patient and gauze and cotton rolls for x-ray film positioning.

During the Film Exposure

The dental assistant should wear gloves, protective eyewear, and masks. After removing the exposed film from the patient's mouth, wipe the saliva from the film and place it in a paper cup or on a covered surface. Film can be purchased with a plastic barrier or separate plastic barriers can be purchased to place on the individual film packets before exposure.

Patient Exposure

Before the patient is seated, prepare the room following aseptic techniques. Review the patient's medical history and check the dental chart to confirm the number and types of x-rays the dentist has requested for diagnosis.

Establish a routine to check the x-ray machine. Check the settings for the kilovoltage, the milliamperage, and the exposure time. (Note that some x-ray machines are preset and do not require any changes.) Select the x-ray unit if the control panel operates more than one tubehead.

Escort the patient into the room, seat the patient in an upright position, and position the head rest to secure the head. Ask the patient to remove eyeglasses, partials, or any metal objects that will interfere with the x-rays (Figure 17-16). Place a lead apron with a thyroid collar on the patient, making sure it is secured and covers the patient. Explain the procedure to the patient and indicate how the patient can assist during the exposure

FIGURE 17-16 Barriers on a dental x-ray unit and a lead apron with a thyroid collar placed on a patient.

Some patients have problems with gagging. Try to get the patient to breathe through the nose and to think of something else, because psychological factors contribute to triggering the gag reflex. Talk to the patient, work quickly, and have him or her concentrate on breathing. If the patient still has problems, an anesthetic mouth rinse or a throat lozenge may be helpful. Position the tubehead in the approximate location for the film exposure before placing the film in the patient's mouth. After exposing the x-ray film, remove the film, pull the x-ray tubehead out of the way, and place the film in a cup/container or on a barrier. After all the films have been taken, remove the lead apron from the patient and place the lead apron over a bar or hang it on a hook to prevent creases or folds. If the lead apron is creased routinely, the lead may be damaged and protection from x-ray exposure would not be complete in these areas.

of the x-rays. Bring the tubehead close to the working area and proceed.

After the Films Are Exposed

After the films are exposed, the dental assistant removes his or her gloves or places overgloves on and removes the lead apron from the patient and makes a chart notation. The patient is dismissed. Following appropriate infection control procedures, remove the barriers from the dental chair, x-ray unit, and the control buttons. Dispose of barriers after each patient and disinfect the area. When handling contaminated films without barriers, wipe or spray them with a disinfectant and leave for ten minutes. If film barriers are used, remove them, along with other contaminated barriers. Films are taken to the processing area for processing.

Intraoral Techniques for Film Exposures

There are two basic techniques used for film exposures in dentistry: the **bisecting technique** and the **paralleling technique**. The bisecting technique, which is used for more specific or unique radiographs rather than the routine, is the oldest technique. The paralleling technique is widely accepted because the detail of the image is more accurate. The American Association of Dental Schools and the American Academy of Oral and Maxillofacial Radiology recommend the paralleling technique.

Bisecting Technique

The bisecting technique is used to expose **periapical**, **bite-wing**, and **occlusal radiographs** (Figures 17-17A through C). In the bisecting technique, either a film holder or the patient's finger is used to secure the film close to the tissue/tooth without bending the film. In

PROCEDURE

17-1 Radiography Infection Control

This procedure is performed by the dental assistant. The dentist designates which radiographs are needed for diagnosis. The dental assistant prepares the patient and area, takes the radiographs, and processes and mounts the films for viewing according to the infection control protocol.

EQUIPMENT AND SUPPLIES

▶ Barriers for the x-ray room

▶ X-ray film (size selected accordingly)

▶ Rinn XCP materials (assembled for use) or other paralleling technique aids

▶ Film barriers (optional)

▶ Lead apron with thyroid collar

▶ Container for exposed film

PROCEDURE STEPS *(Follow aseptic procedures)*

1. Wash and dry hands.

2. Place appropriate barriers on the dental chair, film, and x-ray equipment.

3. Prepare equipment and supplies needed for the procedure, including sterile Rinn XCP instru-ments, tissue or a paper towel, and a cup or container with the patient's name on it.

4. After the patient is seated and positioned, place on glasses and a mask and wash and dry hands. Don treatment gloves.

5. After the x-rays are exposed and removed from the patient's mouth, wipe off the x-rays and place them in a cup/container or on a covered surface.

6. When all x-ray exposures are complete, remove the lead apron from the patient. There are several ways this is done to follow aseptic protocol. The lead apron can be removed once the contaminated gloves are removed or overgloves can be placed on and the lead apron removed. If the lead apron is removed with contaminated gloves, it must be disinfected following the procedure.

7. After the patient is dismissed, remove and dispose of all barriers.

8. Any areas that were not covered with a barrier must be disinfected, including the x-ray film.

---

the bisecting technique, the central ray is directed at an imaginary line that bisects the angle created by the length (long axis) of the tooth and the film packet. The central ray must be perpendicular to this bisecting line (the Rule of Isometry). The direction of the central ray creates **vertical angulation**. An average for the vertical angulation has been pre-determined for this technique. The angulation works with most patients, but operators should determine the appropriate angle after the patient has been positioned and the film is in place (Figure 17-18) (see Table 17-4).

Principles of the Bisecting Technique. The principles of the bisecting technique include the following:

▶ The patient's head must be in the correct position for each arch. For the maxillary arch, seat the patient in an upright position and support the head so the occlusal surfaces of the maxillary teeth are parallel to the floor and the patient's nose is positioned slightly downward (Figure 17-19A). For the mandibular arch, seat the patient in an upright position and support the head slightly tilted back so the occlusal surfaces of the mandibular teeth are parallel to the floor and the patient's nose is positioned slightly upward (Figure 17-19B).

▶ The film is placed in the patient's mouth as close to the lingual surface of the tooth as possible without bending the film.

▶ Various kinds of bite-blocks and film holders can be used to hold the film. Examples include the Stabe, Snap-a-Ray, Rinn XCP, Precision, and bite-blocks. As a last resort, the patient's finger can be used to hold the film in position. Be sure the patient's finger pressure is enough to prevent film movement during exposure but not so firm as to cause the film to bend.

▶ Set the appropriate vertical angulation using the vertical angulation degree guide on the x-ray tubehead (Figure 17-20). **Horizontal angulation** is determined by directing the central ray at the teeth to be exposed, aiming the beam directly through the interproximal spaces (Figure 17-21).

FIGURE 17-17 (A) Periapical radiograph showing crowns, roots, and supporting bone. (B) Bite-wing radiograph showing crowns of teeth on both arches. (C) Occlusal radiograph showing entire dental arch.

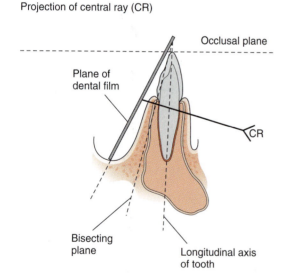

Projection of central ray (CR)

Occlusal plane

Plane of dental film

CR

Bisecting plane

Longitudinal axis of tooth

FIGURE 17-18 The principle of the bisecting technique.

▶ The film is placed in the patient's mouth so that only an edge of the film, one-eighth of an inch, can be seen beyond the occlusal surface or the incisal edge. The cone must cover the x-ray film completely. As with other techniques, the patient and the tubehead should be still during exposure.

▶ Exposure time, mA, and kVp selections are determined according to the type of film and dental x-ray machine being used.

TABLE 17-4 VERTICAL ANGULATION TABLE

Area	Maxillary	Mandibular
Incisor/lateral	+40°	–15°
Cuspids	+45°	–20°
Bicuspids (premolars)	+30°	–10°
Molars	+20°	–5°

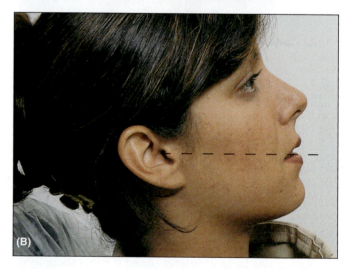

FIGURE 17-19 When exposing radiographs using the bisecting technique, the patient's head is positioned as shown for (A) the maxillary regions and (B) the mandibular regions.

Disadvantages of the Bisecting Technique. The bisecting technique disadvantages include image distortion, guesswork with the technique, patient positioning, and increased exposure to the patient's finger and hand.

The technique is still used, however, on small children, adults with small or tender mouths, some endodontic exposures, and on patients who have conditions or oral anatomies that make it difficult to use the parallel positioning instruments.

FIGURE 17-20 Example of cone positioning for vertical angulation. Numerical degree guide on the side of the tubehead is also shown.

FIGURE 17-21 Example of cone positioning for horizontal angulation.

Paralleling Technique

The paralleling technique is the technique most commonly used in exposing periapical and bite-wing radi-

FIGURE 17-22 For the paralleling technique, the following film-holding devices may be used: snap-a-ray and Rinn XCP.

ographs. It is accurate and produces excellent diagnostic-quality radiographs. There is less exposure to the patient's head and neck, and the technique is easier and requires less guess work. However, the paralleling technique is uncomfortable for small children, adults with small or sensitive mouths, or for patients with low palatal vaults. Practice helps the operator gain the skills and confidence needed to use the paralleling technique.

The paralleling technique requires the film packet and the long axis of the teeth to be parallel. The x-ray beam is directed perpendicular to this parallel line formed by the teeth and the film packet. The anatomy of the oral cavity requires the film to be placed toward the center of the mouth, with the exception of the mandibular molars, in order to keep the film packet flat and have the film parallel to the long axis of the teeth. A film holder is used for ease of technique and correct alignment.

Holders Used for the Paralleling Technique. There are a variety of film holders available for use with the paralleling technique. The function of the holder is to secure the film away from the lingual surfaces of the teeth and parallel with the long axis of the teeth. Some holders have supports to prevent the film from bending. One example is the Rinn XCP. Also, several of the holders have positioning rings that assist the operator in correct cone placement and allow the patient to be in a variety of positions for x-ray exposure. The film holders (Figure 17-22) may be simple one piece bite-blocks (snap-a-rays), hemostats with rubber bite-blocks, or they may come with several pieces, such as the Rinn XCP kit or the Precision paralleling device (Figure 17-23). It is important to be familiar with these to allow for quick and accurate assembly.

Film Positioning. When using the paralleling technique, the film should be placed in the patient's mouth with care to keep the patient relaxed and cooperative for the film and holder placement. Place the film in the film holder evenly and allow no more than one-eighth inch to extend beyond the edge of the occlusal plane

FIGURE 17-23 Rinn XCP components assembled correctly for (A) anterior exposures, (B) bite-wing exposures, and (C) posterior exposures.

Types of Film Exposures

Three types of film exposures/radiographs are used most commonly in the dental office: the periapical, bite-wing, and occlusal. The type of film used and the number of x-rays taken are determined by the dentist.

Periapical Radiographs. The **periapical radiograph** pictures the entire tooth and surrounding area (Figure 17-17A). The periapical radiographs are used to assess the health of the teeth, bone, and surrounding tissues. Tooth development and eruption stages also are seen on periapical radiographs. Abnormalities and pathological conditions are diagnosed by the dentist using these radiographs. The size of the patient's mouth usually determines the size of the x-ray film used and the number of exposures necessary.

Bite-wing Radiographs. The **bite-wing radiograph** pictures the crowns, the interproximal spaces, and the crest area of the alveolar bone of both the maxillary and the mandibular teeth (Figure 17-17B). Bite-wing radiographs usually are taken only on the posterior teeth and are used to detect caries, faulty restorations, and calculus and to examine the crestal area of the alveolar bone. The size of the patient's mouth determines the size of the film used for the bite-wing x-ray.

Occlusal Radiograph. The **occlusal radiograph** pictures large areas of the mandible or maxilla (Figure 17-17C). These radiographs can be used alone or to supplement periapical or bite-wing films. For adults, a size 4 film is used; and for children, a size 2 film may be used.

once the film/film holder is placed in the patient's mouth. The dot on the x-ray film should be positioned toward the occlusal surface. The film packet/film holder should be placed parallel to the long axis of the teeth, covering all teeth to be exposed. Keep the film packet flat and away from the lingual surface of the teeth. Vertical and horizontal angulation is obtained by keeping the cone end even with the positioning ring or following the guide of the handle with the other film holders (Figure 17-24). The positioning ring guides the cone for correct placement to ensure that the film is covered. Without the ring to act as a guide, the operator needs to visually check the film placement and direct the cone to cover the entire film.

Full-Mouth Radiographic Survey

A full-mouth radiographic survey (FMX) is composed of periapical and bite-wing radiographs. This survey includes a number of radiographs that collectively display all the teeth and surrounding structures and areas. The dentist determines what is needed for diagnosis and for the patient's records.

The number and the size of the radiographs taken depend on several factors, including what the dentist needs to view on the radiograph, the size of the patient's mouth, the number of teeth present in the oral cavity, existing conditions that may interfere with film placement, and the patient's ability to cooperate. A full-mouth survey for an adult routinely includes fourteen periapical and four bite-wing films. This number may vary depending on the factors listed and the dentist's directions.

When exposing any radiographs, an order should be followed to prevent double exposing the patient. There is no recommended sequence, so the dental assistant should decide what order he or she is comfortable with and can follow routinely. Once the films are exposed, they should be placed in a cup or on a barrier away from the unexposed film.

Bite-block

FIGURE 17-24 Correct placement of premolar bite-wing film using a film-holding device. The film is positioned so that the x-ray beams pass directly through the interproximal spaces to prevent overlapping of the teeth. The curve of the patient's arch is evaluated when placing the dental film.

Bite-Wing Series

Bite-wing radiographs are a routine part of the dental exam. They are taken as part of the full-mouth series and also at six-month intervals. These radiographs are used specifically for caries detection but also assist in the evaluation of restorations, calculus detection, assessment of the alveolar crestal bone, tooth eruption, occlusal relationships, and some pulpal pathology. Bite-wing radiographs, also known as **interproximal** radiographs, are taken of the premolar area and the molar area. The film is placed most often in a horizontal position, but in cases where the dentist wants to see more of the tooth root and alveolar bone, the film is placed vertically.

▶ Horizontal Positioning

With adults, four #2 size films are taken (one premolar and one molar on each side). Some dentists choose to use the longer #3 size film and take one on each side, but care must be used when selecting this film size because different horizontal angulations are needed on the premolars and molars to open the contacts. With children, the size of the child's mouth determines the number and the size of films to be used. Older children may need only one #2 size film on each side of the mouth, while younger children or children with small mouths may need two #1 size film on each side of the mouth.

▶ Vertical Positioning

Vertical bite-wing radiographs are requested by the periodontist as well as the general dentist. With the increase in periodontal disease, patients are requiring bite-wing radiographs that show more of the root area. Root caries, advanced periodontal pockets, and bone loss can be seen to a greater extent on bite-wing radiographs if the film is placed vertically instead of horizontally. The vertical bite-wing can be used in both the posterior and anterior areas. An adhesive tab is used to hold the film in the correct position.

PROCEDURE

17-2 Full-Mouth X-Ray Exposure with Paralleling Technique

This procedure is performed by the dental assistant. The dentist requests a full-mouth set of radiographs. The dental assistant prepares the equipment (Rinn XCP instruments), the area, and the patient; takes the radiographs; and processes and mounts the films for viewing according to infection control protocol.

This procedure explains film placement and exposure for the central incisors in each arch and one-half of the maxillary arch and one-half of the mandibular arch. The same technique would be used to expose the opposite arches.

EQUIPMENT AND SUPPLIES

▶ Barriers for the x-ray room and equipment

▶ X-ray film (appropriate size and number of films)

▶ X-ray film barriers (optional)

▶ Cotton rolls (optional)

▶ Rinn XCP materials (assembled for use) or other paralleling technique aids

▶ Lead apron with thyroid collar

▶ Container for exposed film

▶ Paper towel or tissue

PROCEDURE STEPS *(Follow aseptic procedures)*

1. Review the patient's chart.

2. Wash and dry hands.

3. Place appropriate barriers on dental chair, film, and x-ray equipment.

4. Prepare equipment and supplies needed for the procedure, including the sterile Rinn XCP instruments, tissue or paper towel, and cup or container with patient's name on it.

5. Turn the x-ray machine on and check the mA, kV, and exposure time.

6. Seat and position the patient in an upright position.

7. Have the patient remove any removable appliances, earrings, or eyeglasses that may interfere with the exposing process.

8. Place the lead apron with the thyroid collar on the patient.

9. After the patient is prepared, wash and dry the hands and don latex treatment gloves.

The film placement and vertical and horizontal angulation remain the same as with the horizontal bite-wing radiograph (Figure 17-25).

Positioning for Maxillary Arch

▶ **Maxillary Incisors** (Figure 17-26)

1. To prepare the maxillary incisors for exposure, tilt the back of the film holder slightly and insert the film vertically into the slot on the bite-block. Adjust the ring on the metal rod to cover the film. Pull positioning ring back on the metal rod, away from bite-block.

2. Bring the tubehead near the area of exposure.

3. Tilt the film/film holder downward to place in the patient's mouth. Position in the mouth away from the lingual surfaces and centered behind the incisors. Have the patient close slowly and evenly on the bite-block.

4. Holding on to the metal rod, slide the positioning ring close to the patient's face. Position the cone parallel to the metal indicating rod and place to within one-half inch of the positioning ring. The cone end should be at an equal distance from the positioning ring. This directs the central ray perpendicular to the film. The patient may help hold the metal rod to secure the film holder in position.

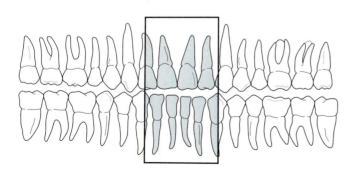

FIGURE 17-25 Anterior vertical bite-wing.

FIGURE 17-26 Maxillary incisors.

5. The incisal edges rest on the flat portion of the bite-block.

6. The diagram shows the film, tooth, positioning ring, and open end of the cone parallel to each other. The central ray will be perpendicular to the film. (No. 2 size film will show all four incisors. Teeth are centered on the radiograph, showing the apices, roots, and crowns. The bite-block may be seen as a radiopaque area near the incisal edge of the film.)

▶ **Maxillary Cuspids** (Figure 17-27)

1. For the maxillary cuspids, tilt the film/film holder, place it in the patient's mouth, and position it away from the lingual surfaces. The film is placed in the mouth, directly behind the center of the cuspid and positioned toward the midline.

2. Have the patient close slowly and center the cuspid on the bite-block. Holding the metal rod, slide the positioning ring toward the patient's face.

3. Bring the tubehead toward the ring, placing the cone end evenly around the positioning ring.

4. All planes are parallel so that the central ray will be directed perpendicular to the film plane. Because of the curvature of the maxillary arch, the distal of the cuspid is overlapping the first bicuspid on many cuspid radiographs. Note that the central ray is directed at the center of the cuspid.

▶ **Maxillary Premolars** (Figure 17-28)

1. For the maxillary premolars, tilt the film/film holder, place it in the patient's mouth, and position it away from the lingual surfaces, toward the middle of the palate.

2. Place the anterior edge of the film behind the middle of the cuspid to ensure that the film will cover the area of the two premolars.

3. While holding the film in place, have the patient close slowly on the bite-block. Hold the metal rod and slide the positioning ring toward the patient's face.

4. Bring the tubehead toward the ring, placing the open cone evenly around the ring. Note the angle of the film and the film holder, positioned so that the central ray will pass through the contact point of the first and second premolars.

5. The bite-block is centered on the premolars. On this radiograph, the distal of the cuspid is seen and the first and second bicuspids show that the contact between them is open.

▶ **Maxillary Molars** (Figure 17-29)

1. For the maxillary molars, tilt the film/film holder so that it is less vertical when entering the patient's mouth. Place the film in the patient's mouth and

FIGURE 17-27 Maxillary cuspid.

FIGURE 17-28 Maxillary bicuspids (premolars).

FIGURE 17-29 Maxillary molars.

position it away from the lingual surfaces of the molars.

2. Center the bite-block on the second molar. Have the patient close slowly on the bite-block.

3. Bring the tubehead toward the ring, placing the open end of the cone evenly around the positioning ring.

4. The diagram shows the film, tooth, and cone lined up for correct direction of the central ray. This radiograph shows the open contact between the first and second molars. The distal of the second premolar is seen. Note that the film angles are parallel to the lingual surface of the molars and placed near the middle of the palate.

Positioning for the Mandibular Arch

▶ **Mandibular Incisors** (Figure 17-30)

1. The film holder is assembled in the same way for mandibular and maxillary positions. For the mandibular incisors, tilt the film/film holder and place it in the patient's mouth, gently pressing the film on the floor of the mouth behind the incisors and away from the lingual surface.

2. Have the patient close slowly on the bite-block. Holding the metal rod, slide the positioning ring close to the patient's face.

3. Bring the tubehead close and place the cone parallel to the metal rod. The open end of the cone should be even with the ring.

4. The diagram shows how far the film needs to be placed in the mouth in order to see the entire length of the tooth. Sometimes the tongue is moved when the film is being placed. Being gentle with the placement will encourage patient cooperation.

5. The mandibular incisors are centered on the bite-block. The incisal edges of the teeth are one-eighth inch from the top of the film.

6. The central ray is directed between the two central incisors to open contact areas. The curve of the arch will cause some overlapping on the distal of the lateral incisors.

7. The drawing illustrates the film placed directly behind the incisors and as far into the mouth as the tongue attachment allows.

▶ **Mandibular Cuspids** (Figure 17-31)

1. For the mandibular cuspids, tilt the film/film holder, place it in the patient's mouth, and position it away from the lingual surface.

2. Center the bite-block on the cuspid and have the patient slowly close. Move the positioning ring close to the patient's face, bring the cone parallel to

FIGURE 17-30 Mandibular incisors.

FIGURE 17-31 Mandibular cuspid.

the metal rod, and position the open end of the cone flat with the ring.

3. Insert the film toward the floor of the mouth enough to ensure that the film covers the entire length of the cuspid.

4. The film, tooth, and the plane of the open end of the cone are all parallel. The central ray will be directed perpendicular to the film plane.

5. In the diagram, the film is angled on the center of the cuspid. As with the incisors, place it toward the base of the tongue, away from the alveolar bone.

▶ **Mandibular Premolars** (Figure 17-32)

1. For the mandibular premolars, tilt the film/film holder and place the film in the patient's mouth, gently positioning it between the lingual surface of the teeth and the tongue.

2. Place the anterior edge of the film at the middle of the cuspid to ensure that the film covers the area of the two premolars.

3. Have the patient close on the bite-block.

4. Note the position of the film as it is placed in the space between the tongue and the mandibular arch.

5. The film, teeth, and plane of the open end of the cone are all parallel. The first and second premolars are seen on this film with the contact points open.

▶ **Mandibular Molars** (Figure 17-33)

1. For the mandibular molars, tilt the film/film holder and place the film holder with the film in the patient's mouth, positioning it between the tongue and the lingual surfaces of the teeth.

2. Center the bite-block over the second molar. Hold it in the desired position, and have the patient close to secure it in place.

3. Gently place the patient's cheek over the bite-block, if this is more comfortable for the patient.

4. Align the positioning ring and cone.

5. Note how close the film is to the lingual surface. Move the tongue toward the center of the mouth to make this placement more comfortable for the patient.

6. The edge of the film is positioned only one-eighth inch above the occlusal edge.

7. The first, second, and third molars are seen on this film with the contacts open. The third molar may not be erupted into the oral cavity, but it will be seen on the film.

8. During placement, to prevent the film and film holder from moving forward, hold the bite-block in position until the patient closes firmly on it.

FIGURE 17-32 Mandibular bicuspids (premolars).

FIGURE 17-33 Mandibular molars.

▶ **Premolar Bite-Wing** (Figure 17-34)

1. To position bite-wing radiographs, a tab or positioning instrument is used. Tabs come with adhesive backs or with loops to surround the film. The positioning instrument comes with a bite-wing holder, an indicator rod, and a positioning ring.

2. Holding the film horizontally, place the tab in the center of the film or, if using a positioning instrument, make sure the film is centered on the bite-wing holder with the smooth side of the film directed toward the positioning ring.

3. The drawing/radiograph illustrates the position of the film covering the premolars with the front edge of the film to the middle of the cuspid while the back edge of the film may be to the mesial of the second molar.

4. Hold the tab and place the film near the lingual surface of the teeth in the patient's mouth, positioning the film to cover the mandibular premolars.

5. While holding the tab in place, have the patient close and slowly rotate fingers out of the way.

6. When using a positioning instrument, place the bite-wing holder in the patient's mouth, away from the lingual surface of the teeth. Position the film to cover the premolars and to be parallel to them. Have the patient close slowly on the bite-wing holder and hold it in place.

7. The cone positioning for the premolar bite-wing begins with the vertical angulation set at 0° so the cone is perpendicular to the film.

8. The horizontal angulation is positioned so that the beam is aimed directly between the contacts of the premolars and the cone is perpendicular to the film. This film placement is sometimes uncomfortable for the patient because of the alveolar ridge curvature near the cuspid. Gentleness when positioning this exposure will be rewarded with patient cooperation. When using the positioning instrument, first hold the indicator rod and then bring the positioning ring close to the patient's face.

▶ **Molar Bite-Wing** (Figure 17-35)

1. Position the film to cover the molars and the distal half of the second premolar. Place the front edge of the film at the distal of the second molar.

2. Holding the tab, place the film in the patient's mouth, away from the lingual surfaces, gently moving the tongue toward the middle of the mouth.

3. When using the positioning instrument, place it in the patient's mouth, pushing the tongue away from the lingual surfaces.

4. The vertical angulation for the molar bite-wing is set at 0° so the cone is perpendicular to the film. The horizontal angulation is directed so that the beam is between the contacts of the first and second molars. Place the cone near the patient's face, covering the film and perpendicular to the film. Look at the curve of the patient's arch rather than the patient's face to position the cone.

Occlusal Radiographs

Occlusal radiographs show a large area of the dental arch. They are used with children when periapicals are difficult to expose and with patients who have difficulty opening the mouth or controlling muscular movement. The films are placed on the occlusal surface and then the patient closes gently on the film to hold it in place.

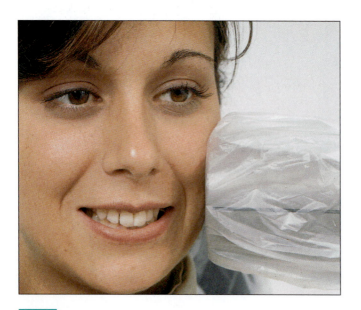

FIGURE 17-34 Premolar bite-wing using bite-wing tab.

FIGURE 17-35 Molar bite-wing using Rinn XCP.

Occlusal radiographs are used to locate or define the following: fractures, impacted teeth, foreign bodies in the bone or floor of the mouth, changes in the sizes and shapes of the arches, supernumerary teeth, cleft palate, root fragments, cysts, malignancies, tumors (odontomas), osteomyelitis, stones in the ducts of the salivary glands, and unerupted teeth.

Two techniques are used to expose occlusal radiographs: the **topographic technique** and the **cross-section technique**. Technique selection is determined by the view the dentist needs for diagnosis. With the topographic technique, the rules of bisecting are followed. The central ray is directed perpendicular to the bisecting plane. With the cross-section technique, the central ray is perpendicular to the film.

PROCEDURE

17-3 Exposing Occlusal Radiographs

This procedure is performed by the dental assistant at the direction of the dentist. The dental assistant prepares the equipment and supplies, the area, and the patient. The occlusal films are exposed using the topographic or cross-sectional technique.

EQUIPMENT AND SUPPLIES

▶ Barriers for the x-ray room

▶ Occlusal film (#2 for children and #4 for adults)

▶ Lead apron with thyroid collar

▶ Container or barrier for exposed film

PROCEDURE STEPS *(Follow aseptic procedures)*

1. Wash and dry hands.

2. Place appropriate barriers.

3. Prepare film, tissue or paper towel, and cup or container with patient's identification on it.

4. Seat the patient in an upright position and place the lead apron on the patient.

5. Wash and dry hands and don treatment gloves.

▶ **Topographic Technique**

6. For the **maxillary view**, positioning is similar to that used for the bisecting technique. The patient is positioned so that the maxillary arch is parallel to the floor.

7. The film is placed in the mouth with the smooth/plain side toward the cone.

8. Have the patient close on the film, leaving about 2 mm of an edge beyond the incisors.

9. Move the cone to a vertical angulation of +65° to +75°.

10. Direct the cone over the bridge of the nose, with the lower edge of the cone covering the incisors (Figure 17-36).

(continued)

P R O C E D U R E   **1 7 - 3** *continued*

FIGURE 17-36 Topographic occlusal radiograph of the maxillary arch. (A) Vertical film placement. (B) Horizontal film placement.

11. For the **mandibular view** using the topographic technique, the patient's head is tilted back.

12. Place the smooth side of the film on the occlusal surfaces of the teeth with the central incisors at the front edge of the film.

13. Have the patient close gently on the film.

14. The vertical angulation will vary with each patient between −40° and −55°.

15. Center the cone over the film, directing the central ray at the middle and tip of the chin (Figure 17-37).

▶ **Cross-Section Technique**

1. For the **maxillary view** using the cross-section technique, the patient should be in an upright position with the head tilted back slightly.

2. The film placement is the same as with the topographic technique. The cone is positioned over the top of the patient's head with the central ray directed perpendicular to the film.

3. Be sure the cone covers the maxillary area to be exposed (Figure 17-38).

4. For the **mandibular view**, the patient's head should be tilted backward.

(continued)

P R O C E D U R E   **1 7 - 3** *continued*

FIGURE 17-37 Topographic occlusal radiograph of the mandibular arch.

FIGURE 17-38 Cross-sectional occlusal radiograph of the maxillary arch.

(continued)

P R O C E D U R E   **1 7 - 3** *continued*

5. The film placement is the same as with the topographic technique.

6. The cone is positioned under the patient's chin with the central ray directed perpendicular to the film. The patient may have to lift the chin up in order to position the cone (Figure 17-39).

FIGURE 17-39 Cross-sectional occlusal radiograph of the mandibular arch.

Pediatric Radiographs

Radiographs play an important role in the dental health of children. They are used to detect caries, abscesses, cysts, anodontia, and fractures and to evaluate eruption stages and growth patterns. Technique suggestions associated with pediatric radiographs are:

1. Because developing tissues are sensitive to radiation, the exposure time should be reduced and the number of radiographs should be kept to a minimum.

2. The oral mucosa of young children in eruption stages is sensitive to the slightest pressure, so carefully examine the mouth for loose or erupting teeth, any parulis, pulp polyps, cold sores (herpes simplex), canker sores (aphthous ulcers), or any deviation from the normal.

3. Talk to the child and show him or her what is going to happen.

4. Evaluate the child's behavior and cooperation. Having the child help often reduces apprehension.

5. Work quickly and with confidence because children move constantly and become bored easily.

6. Evaluate the child's mouth to determine the number and size of x-ray film to be used. Select the smallest film you can to minimize discomfort and still obtain the view needed. For preschool children, 0 size film is most often used. Older children will vary from a 0 size film to sizes 1 and 2, depending on the size of the mouth, the tenderness of the tissues, and the depth of the palate and the floor of

the mouth. For occlusal views, size 2 film is used. The number of films and the size of the film used can be tailored to the individual child and the dentist's needs (Figures 17-40A through C).

7. Take anterior films first to encourage the child's cooperation.
8. The paralleling technique is most often used, with all guidelines being the same as for adults.

FIGURE 17-40 Pedodontic full-mouth survey of a child three to five years old. (A) Includes two bite-wings and two occlusals. Or (B) Includes two bite-wings, two occlusals, and four periapicals.

(continued)

FIGURE 17-40 *(continued)*
Pedodontic full-mouth survey of a child eight to twelve years old. (C) Includes two bite-wings, six anterior incisors, and four posterior periapicals.

P R O C E D U R E

17-4 Full-Mouth Pediatric X-Ray Exposure

This procedure is performed by the dental assistant. The dentist requires that a pediatric full-mouth set of radiographs be taken and identifies the eight films. The dental assistant prepares the equipment (Rinn XCP instruments), the area, and the patient; takes the radiographs; processes the films; and mounts the films for viewing according to infection control protocol.

This procedure explains film placement and exposure for the two occlusal films (maxillary and mandibular), two bite-wing x-rays, and four periapical x-rays.

EQUIPMENT AND SUPPLIES

▶ Barriers for the x-ray room and equipment

▶ X-ray film, six size #0 films and two #2 size films

▶ X-ray film barriers (optional)

▶ Cotton rolls (optional)

▶ Rinn XCP materials (assembled for use) or other paralleling technique aids

▶ Lead apron with thyroid collar

▶ Container for exposed film

▶ Paper towel or tissue

PROCEDURE STEPS *(Follow aseptic procedures)*

1. Review the patient's chart.

2. Wash and dry hands.

3. Place appropriate barriers on the dental chair, film, and x-ray equipment.

4. Assemble the sterile Rinn XCP instruments and prepare tissue or paper towel and cup or container with patient's name on it.

5. Turn on the x-ray machine and check the mA, kV, and exposure time.

6. Seat the patient in an upright position.

7. Place the lead apron with the thyroid collar on the patient.

(continued)

P R O C E D U R E   **1 7 - 4** *continued*

8. After the patient is prepared, wash and dry hands and don latex treatment gloves.

9. Explain the procedure to the patient.

Exposing Occlusal Radiographs

PROCEDURE STEPS *(Follow aseptic procedures)*

1. Wash and dry hands.

2. Place appropriate barriers.

3. Prepare film #2 for children, tissue or paper towel, and cup or container with patient's identification on it.

4. Seat the patient in an upright position and place the lead apron on the patient.

5. Wash and dry hands and don treatment gloves.

Maxillary Occlusal Film/Topographic Technique

1. For the maxillary view, positioning is similar to that used for the bisecting technique. The patient is positioned so that the maxillary arch is parallel to the floor.

2. Place the film in the mouth with the smooth/plain side toward the cone.

3. Have the patient close on the film, leaving about 2 mm of an edge beyond the incisors.

4. Move the cone to a vertical angulation of +65° to +75°.

5. Direct the cone over the bridge of the nose with the lower edge of the cone covering the incisors.

Mandibular Occlusal X-Ray/Topographic Technique
For the mandibular view using the topographic technique, the patient's head is tilted back to allow for correct placement for the bisecting technique until the mandibular arch is parallel to the floor.

1. Place the smooth side of the film on the occlusal surfaces of the teeth with the central incisors at the front edge of the film.

2. Have the patient close gently on the film.

3. The vertical angulation will vary with each patient between −40° and −55°. Center the cone over the film, directing the central ray at the middle and tip of the chin.

Deciduous Bite-Wings

1. To position bite-wing radiographs, a tab or positioning instrument is used. Tabs come with ad-hesive backs or with loops to surround the film. The positioning instrument comes with a bite-wing holder, an indicator rod, and a positioning ring.

2. Holding the film horizontally, place the tab in the center of the film or, if using a positioning instrument, make sure the film is centered on the bite-wing holder with the smooth side of the film directed toward the positioning ring.

3. Position the film covering the deciduous first and second molars with the front edge of the film to the middle of the cuspid.

4. Hold the tab and place the film near the lingual surface of the teeth in the patient's mouth, positioning the film to cover the mandibular deciduous molars.

5. While holding the tab in place, have the patient close and slowly rotate the fingers out of the way.

6. When using a positioning instrument, place the bite-wing holder in the patient's mouth, away from the lingual surface of the teeth. Position the film to cover the deciduous molars and be parallel to them. Have the patient close slowly on the bite-wing holder and hold it in place.

▶ The cone positioning for the premolar bite-wing begins with the vertical angulation set at 0°.

Positioning for Maxillary Deciduous Molars

1. For the maxillary deciduous molars, tilt the film/film holder, place it in the patient's mouth, and position it away from the lingual surfaces, toward the middle of the palate.

2. Place the anterior edge of the film behind the middle of the cuspid to ensure that the film will cover the area of the two molars.

3. While holding the film in place, have the patient close slowly on the bite-block. Hold the metal rod and slide the positioning ring toward the patient's face.

4. Bring the tubehead toward the ring, placing the open cone evenly around the ring. Note the angle of the film and the film holder, positioned so that the central ray passes through the contact point of the first and second deciduous molars.

5. Center the bite-block on the deciduous molars. On this radiograph, the distal of the cuspid is seen and the first and second deciduous molars have the contact between them open.

(continued)

Positioning for the Mandibular Deciduous Molars

1. For the mandibular deciduous molars, tilt the film/film holder, place the film in the patient's mouth, and gently position it between the lingual surface of the teeth and the tongue.

2. Place the anterior edge of the film at the middle of the cuspid to ensure that the film covers the area of the two deciduous molars.

3. Have the patient close on the bite-block.

4. Note the position of the film as it is placed in the space between the tongue and the mandibular arch. The film, teeth, and plane of the open end of the cone are all parallel. The first and second deciduous molars are seen on this film with the contact points open.

Edentulous Radiographic Survey

A series of radiographs on the edentulous (ee-**DENT**-you-lous), or toothless, or partially edentulous patient may be indicated to show cysts, impacted teeth, retained root tips or bone fragments, other pathological conditions, and normal landmarks, such as the mental foramen, mandibular canal, maxillary sinuses, and alveolar bone. As part of the routine examination, radiographs are taken before dentures and partials are made; if abnormal pathology or sensitivity is found, the patient can receive treatment before the removable prosthesis is made. Technique suggestions associated with treatment for the edentulous patient are:

1. A routine full-mouth survey consists of six anterior and eight posterior films, but these numbers can be reduced by taking fewer anterior films in smaller arches, eliminating bite-wing radiographs.

2. Either the paralleling or the bisecting technique can be used, but both will need to be modified. In the paralleling technique, cotton rolls are used with the film holder to position the film parallel to the alveolar ridge. If the patient has dentures or partials, leave the appliance in the opposing arch for better support. In the bisecting technique, the film will be almost flat. Just extend the edge of the film one-quarter inch beyond the crest of the alveolar ridge.

3. The vertical angulation will be increased. Reduce the exposure time by one-quarter the normal time in order to prevent the over-exposure of an area where teeth are missing and the bone is thinner.

4. Try using occlusal film and exposing individual quadrants and/or arches, take a panoramic film that includes both arches and surrounding area on one film, or use periapical films if areas are of a suspicious condition (Figure 17-41).

Endodontic Radiographic Technique

Radiographs are taken periodically during the endodontic procedure. The radiographs allow the dentist to check the progress of the procedure and take the neces-sary measurements. Technique suggestions associated with endodontic procedures are:

1. Use the paralleling technique to reduce distortion whenever possible.

2. Place film in a hemostat or snap-a-ray to use as a positioning device.

3. Loosen the dental dam from the frame on one side and position the film on the lingual, parallel to the tooth. If a plastic frame is not used, the metal frame may have to be removed to prevent the frame from being exposed on the radiograph and possibly distorting the image.

4. The film should cover the entire length of the tooth and the surrounding area at the apex of the root.

5. Center the tooth on the film and direct the central ray perpendicular to the tooth. The patient must keep the mouth open because of protruding endodontic instruments and materials, so work quickly (Figure 17-42).

Special Needs Patients/ Compromised Patients

Patients come to the office with a wide variety of special needs. Consideration and creativity often are required to obtain the desired radiographs. The wheelchair patient is one example where advanced preparation is needed in order to have the treatment room ready. When there is a plan in place to expose the x-ray, the procedure is much easier for everyone involved. With other special needs patients, a parent or guardian may be asked to assist in holding the patient or the x-ray steady; however, every attempt should be made to expose the x-ray by another means. Work as quickly as possible. If it is impossible to expose a periapical film, an occlusal or a panoramic film may be substituted. Technique suggestions associated with treatment for special needs patients are:

1. Before treating special needs patients, discuss how to best handle the patients with the entire office. A good time to do this is at the office meetings. The entire staff needs to work together to make the

Maxillary anterior region

Maxillary posterior region

Mandibular anterior region

Mandibular posterior region

FIGURE 17-41 Radiographs of a full-mouth series of an edentulous patient. Cone and film-holding device positioned in four areas of the mouth.

FIGURE 17-42 When a patient is positioned for an endodontic radiograph, the patient does not close on the film holder because of the reamer or file is positioned in the root canal. Radiograph shows the reamer in place.

patients' visits as simple and comprehensive as possible.

2. Prepare all areas in the office that the patient will be in before the appointment. These should include the reception room and the treatment room. For example, have extra radiation protection in the treatment room for the parent or guardian in case he or she has to hold the film in the patient's mouth (Figure 17-43).

3. Call the patient, caregiver, or guardian in advance and ask for suggestions on how to best accommodate the patient's needs.

4. Read about the patient's condition in order to better understand and communicate with him or her. For example, when working with a deaf patient, learn a few words in sign language.

Common Radiographic Errors

Errors during exposing and processing of radiographs are inevitable, especially when learning. Understanding the basic principles and practices helps to produce quality diagnostic x-rays. Practice on manikins to gain experience and work on preventing errors. Perfect x-ray technique skills to reduce the number of unnecessary retakes, which expose the patient to more radiation and require more time for everyone. However, in order to avoid common radiographic errors, it is necessary to understand what constitutes a quality x-ray.

What Is a Quality X-Ray?

▶ Desired teeth and surrounding area are on the film.
▶ Images are dimensionally accurate.
▶ The contacts between the teeth are open.
▶ The teeth are not elongated or foreshortened.
▶ The entire length of the teeth is visible, including 1 to 2 mm beyond the cusps and 4 to 6 mm beyond the apex.
▶ The film has enough contrast and density to show good detail of all anatomy.
▶ The radiograph is free of spots, stains, handling marks, and other artifacts (black lines).

Correct assembly of the film holding device will eliminate many errors. Be sure the bite-block is in the correct position for the corresponding arch. Also, be sure the film is centered in the indicating ring. Select the correct size film to cover the area to be exposed. If the film is too small, the apex may be cut off. If the film is too large, it may be difficult for the patient to hold and the x-ray may be distorted. When the film is properly placed in the mouth, a 1 to 3 mm edge of the film should show beyond the occlusal/incisal surface of the tooth. If a hemostat or snap-a-ray film holder is used, be sure to hold the film at the edge, touching just enough to hold the film secure.

Distortion. Sometimes the film will bend or curve on the palate and in the cuspid area on the mandible; when the film bends, the image will distort. During the film placement, the film may be creased. These crease marks show on the processed film as black lines (artifacts). Adjust the film position farther into the mouth, toward the midline of the palate of the maxillary, and push the tongue gently so that the film is between the tongue and the mandible (Figures 17-44 and 17-45).

Elongation. Elongation is a vertical angulation error and is caused by not having enough angulation, meaning there is not enough positive angulation on the maxillary or negative angulation on the mandibular. This error occurs more often when using the bisecting technique. In the paralleling technique, elongation is minimized if the cone end is positioned evenly against the indicating ring and the film is placed correctly.

Paralleling instruments are aids, but evaluate each cone placement. Sometimes the angulation may need to be slightly increased or decreased from the guides (Figure 17-46).

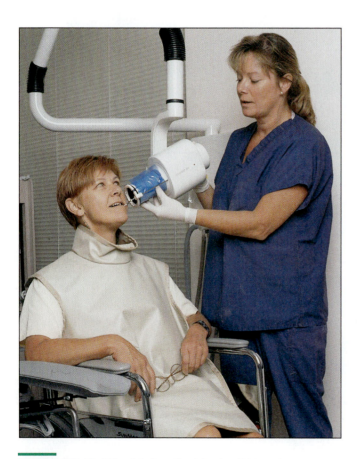

FIGURE 17-43 Wheelchair patient having intraoral radiographs taken.

FIGURE 17-44 A curved film distorts the images on the radiograph.

FIGURE 17-45 A bent film appears as a black crease or thin, dark, radiolucent line.

FIGURE 17-46 Elongation on a radiograph. Diagram shows how a film is elongated.

Foreshortening. **Foreshortening** is also a vertical angulation error. Foreshortening is the opposite of elongation and is caused by too much angulation. This error also occurs more often with the bisecting technique and

can be corrected by decreasing the vertical angulation. If the paralleling technique is used, align the cone with the film holder (Figure 17-47).

Overlapping. **Overlapping** is caused by incorrect horizontal angulation. When the cone is angled toward the mesial or the distal surfaces of the teeth instead of the interproximal areas, overlapping occurs. The cone/central ray should be directed straight at the teeth and at a 90° angle to the film in order to keep the contacts open. Remember to evaluate the film placement in regard to the curve of the arch, *not* the contour of the patient's face (cheeks) (Figure 17-48).

Cone Cutting. **Cone cutting** means that the x-ray beam missed part of the film, causing the film to be only partially exposed. Because the cone is lead lined, the shape of the cone cut on the film will match the shape of the cone (either round or rectangular). Be sure that the x-ray film is placed in the center of the cone (Figure 17-49).

Clear Film. A **clear film** indicates that the film was not exposed to any radiation. Check your machine to verify that it was turned on. If it was, then it is malfunctioning. If the exposure routine was interrupted, an unexposed film may have been placed in the cup with exposed films (Figure 17-50).

Double Exposure. Sometimes, inadvertently, film is exposed twice. A **double exposure** results in blurred images or a dark x-ray. Examine the film closely and two

FIGURE 17-47 Foreshortening on a radiograph. Diagram shows how a film is foreshortened.

FIGURE 17-48 Overlapping. Diagram shows the position of an x-ray beam to prevent overlapping.

FIGURE 17-49 Cone cut. Diagram shows correct and incorrect positions of a cone to prevent cone cutting.

FIGURE 17-50 Clear film. This film has not been exposed to x-rays.

images can be seen. Establishing a routine can help avoid double-exposed films (Figure 17-51).

Blurred Image. Blurred images result from movement of the patient's head or tubehead or from the x-ray film moving in the patient's mouth. The images are undefined and unclear. Be sure the patient can hold the film in place and hold still for the exposure. Also, make sure the tubehead is still before leaving the room (Figure 17-52).

Underexposed Film. When the film appears light and has a thin image, it may be **underexposed**. Check the mAs, kVs, and the exposure time settings for the type of film being used, the size of the patient, and the x-ray machine. Another reason for this outcome is that the cone may not have been positioned close enough to the patient's face (Figure 17-53).

Overexposed Film. When the film has a dark image, it is overexposed and too dark (dense) to see any structures clearly and accurately for a diagnosis. Use the same checks used for the light film image (Figure 17-54).

Radiopaque Film Images. Often, metal objects such as eyeglasses, earrings, and partial appliances show as **radiopaque** (not transmitting light) objects on the processed x-ray (Figure 17-55). Check for and remove objects before exposing the film.

FIGURE 17-51 Double exposure.

FIGURE 17-52 Blurred image is the result of movement during exposure. *(Reprinted courtesy of Eastman Kodak Company)*

Backward Film. Placing the film in the mouth backward or reversed causes the images on the film to be light and a **herringbone pattern** (tire track) to be seen. The white, plain side of the film is always placed facing the tubehead. If the film is reversed, the amount of x-rays that reach the film are reduced by the lead foil. The herringbone or "tire track" pattern on the foil is seen on the sides of the processed x-ray (Figure 17-56).

Film Processing Errors

Light Film Image. Light and dark film images can occur while exposing the film and during processing. A light film is said to be underprocessed. If the film is underprocessed, the developing time was too short, the developer temperature was lower than recommended, or the developing solution was "exhausted" (too weak from over-use and needs to be changed).

Another cause is the fixing process. If the film is not fixed completely, the emulsion will not be hardened sufficiently and will wash off in the water. With over-fixation, the film is left in the fixer for too long and the image bleaches out. Also, if the film was placed in the mouth backward, the result is a lighter film (Figure 17-57).

Dark Film Image. The dark film images can be caused by over-developing, the developing solution temperature being too high, the developing solution being too strong, or the film being left in the developer too long. Routinely check solutions and adjust the processing times accordingly (Figure 17-58).

Fogged Film. **Fogged films** have a gray appearance, film image detail is lost, and contrast is lessened. It is like viewing a film image through a dense fog. Fog on films can be caused by improper storage conditions,

FIGURE 17-53 On an underexposed film, the image appears light.

FIGURE 17-54 On an overexposed film, the image appears dark.

FIGURE 17-55 Example of a radiopaque image on the x-ray. Full-gold crown on lower first molar.

FIGURE 17-56 Film was placed in the patient's mouth backward. Note herringbone pattern on molars.

FIGURE 17-57 Light image due to film processing.

FIGURE 17-58 Dark image due to film processing.

outdated films, light leaks in the processing room, or light leaks from loose fittings on automatic processors and daylight loaders. Also, safelights (lights with filters under which the film can be manipulated without exposing it) may need to be adjusted or changed; for example, they may be too close to the processing area or too bright (Figure 17-59).

Partial Image. A **partial image** on the film is the result of film placement in the processing tanks when the solution levels are low. The film is not completely immersed and a partial image results. Always check the levels of the processing solutions. Daily, some evaporation takes place and the films absorb some developer, so replenish the developer regularly (Figure 17-60). To avoid the chance of a partial image, do not use the top clips on the x-ray racks.

Film Artifacts. Film artifacts are the result of not handling the films carefully or not keeping the area around the processing tanks clean. Examples of artifacts include water spots on unprocessed film, which leave clear areas on the film; fixer on unprocessed film, which leaves a white area on the film; developer, which leaves black spots. If the film is not washed/rinsed properly, a yellowish brown stain is left on the film. Black film artifacts can occur from a small charge of electricity, such as a lightening streak, when you pull the x-ray film from the packet in a dry climate. Fluoride ions on gloves that are transferred to the film during handling leave dark fingerprint smudge marks (Figure 17-61). X-rays that overlap (touch) during processing leave an artifact on the films (the artifact is in the shape of the edge or corner of the film).

Torn or Scratched Film. Rough handling of the film can lead to the emulsion on the film being torn or scratched, which leaves a white area or mark on the processed film. Films can be scratched and torn if they are not handled carefully in over-crowded tanks or during retrieval if lost off the film racks (Figure 17-62).

Air Bubbles on Film. Air bubbles are trapped on the film if it is not agitated when placed in the processing solutions. The air bubbles leave round, white spots where they were attached to the film (Figure 17-63).

Reticulation. **Reticulation** is when a film has been exposed to a high temperature followed by a low temperature. The film emulsion swells and then shrinks. The film looks like it is dried and has tiny cracks (Figure 17-64). The temperature of the solutions and the water should be monitored to ensure that they are within the recommended temperature ranges.

Streaks. Streaks on films can be caused by rollers not being clean when using automatic processors or from

FIGURE 17-61 Example of a fingerprint on an x-ray from processing solutions.

FIGURE 17-59 Film that is fogged.

FIGURE 17-60 Partial image due to low levels of processing solution.

FIGURE 17-62 A radiograph with torn or scratched emulsion.

FIGURE 17-63 Films that are not agitated well when they are placed in the processing solutions leave air-bubble artifacts on the processed film.

FIGURE 17-64 Reticulation. *(Reprinted courtesy of Eastman Kodak Company)*

FIGURE 17-65 The vertical lines on this film are a result of dirty rollers in the automatic processor. *(Reprinted courtesy of Eastman Kodak Company)*

unclean x-ray racks. Debris is picked up as the films pass though the rollers, leaving a streaked appearance on the film (Figure 17-65). Streaks from unclean x-ray racks occur during the processing procedure; debris, including processing solutions, runs from the racks onto the film.

PROCESSING QUALITY RADIOGRAPHS

Normally, the darkroom is located in the center area of the dental office or near the x-ray units for easy accessibility for the dental assistants. It is a small room where x-ray processing (develop, fix, and wash) can be accomplished. This room needs to be well ventilated and of an adequate size.

One of the main concerns of the darkroom is that it can exclude all white light. It is important that there are no light leaks from around doors, fans, and vents, because the light harms the sensitive film emulsion during processing. Safelights must be used when the film packets are opened, when attaching the film to the racks, and during processing procedures. A safelight will not affect the film emulsion because it is of a red-orange spectrum. The film is much more sensitive to the blue-green spectrum in which the wavelengths are shorter. Safelight filters need to be free of scratches and fit precisely. The safety lights need to be mounted at least four feet away from the counter surface where the films are unwrapped. It is recommended that a 15-watt incandescent bulb be used. If it must be mounted closer to the counter, a lower watt bulb, such as a 7.5 watt, needs to be used. If using indirect lighting (facing the light toward the ceiling), then a 25-watt bulb may be used with the proper filters. It was once thought that the walls of the room should be painted black, but it is currently recommended that they be in a light color to reflect the safety light. It is more important that the walls be washable because of the spills and splashes that take place during the processing procedure. If processing any films where an intensifying screen has been used, a filter that eliminates more of the light must be used (a red filter needs to be used in place of the orange). Films that have been exposed in conjunction with the intensifying screens are more sensitive to light. Therefore, orange filters for the safelight should never be used for extraoral films. A good safelight filter to use with both the intraoral films and the extraoral screen films is the GBX-2 safelight filter manufactured by Kodak.

There are no recommendations for the overhead white light. It is, however, important that it provide proper illumination for the whole room and that the switch not be placed in an area where it could be turned on accidentally.

Many offices have view boxes in their darkrooms so that x-rays can be read while still wet. This box also should be in an area where the switch cannot be turned on accidentally.

There may be a warning light outside the darkroom that indicates when x-ray processing is taking place. Also, it is advisable to have a lock on the door to prevent light exposure if the door is opened accidentally. A rotational darkroom door that allows access for individuals while maintaining darkness in the room can be utilized.

The darkroom must have a hot and cold water source, along with a drainage line. It is also necessary to have thermostatic water controls to control the intake water line and to enable adjustment of the water to maintain constant temperatures in the processing solutions. A large sink with a goose-neck faucet is recommended for use in replenishing and changing the processing solutions (Figure 17-66).

Manual Processing Equipment

The **manual processing** tanks should be made of stainless steel. The processing tank contains a large tank for the water bath and two one- or two-gallon insert tanks (Figure 17-67). The water bath has an inlet valve where the water flows in and an outlet valve or overflow pipe where the water escapes the tank. The tank comes with a tank cover that needs to be kept on at all times, except when placing or removing films, in order to prevent the solution from oxidizing or evaporating. Many of the newer insert tanks come with film retrievers that slide into the insert tanks and have bars across the top for use in placement and removal. The film retriever is used to bring the x-ray from the bottom of the tank upward so that it can be retrieved if it has mistakenly come loose

from the x-ray rack. Normally, when facing the processing tank, the developer is located on the left side of the processing tank and the fixer is on the right side. The insert tanks should never be interchanged due to the sensitivity of the processing solutions.

Other items needed in the darkroom are a thermometer, timer, processing racks, stirring rods, a dryer, and brushes or sponges with long handles (Figure 17-66). The thermometer is a special design that can be suspended in the developing solution. It is critical that the solution be checked prior to developing a set of x-rays. The dental assistant needs to know the precise temperature of the developer rather than of the water surrounding the tanks or the incoming water. It takes time for the developer and the surrounding water temperature to equalize; therefore, it is important to check the developer solution each time.

No darkroom is complete without a timer. The correct monitoring of the processing time is critical in producing quality x-rays. An accurate timer that can be set easily and has a loud alarm must be utilized.

Processing racks, sometimes called intraoral film hangers, come in a number of sizes, ranging from one to twenty clips. They are made of stainless steel and, except for the single film hanger, have equal numbers of clips on each side. If the film hanger has defective clips, it should be discarded. It causes films to be lost or it may scratch films on other racks.

Stirring rods or paddles are utilized first thing in the morning and first thing in the afternoon to stir the developer and fixer solution. They should be marked according to the solution and not used interchangeably.

FIGURE 17-66 A manual processing room with equipment.
(A) Thermostatic water gauge.
(B) Thermostatic water control.
(C) Disinfectant solution.
(D) Timer.
(E) Silver recovery unit.
(F) Manual tank.
(G) Floating thermometer.
(H) X-rays on rack.
(I) Dryer.
(J) Storage for stirring rod, solutions, view box, and cleaning supplies.
(K) Safelight is above manual tanks.

FIGURE 17-67 (A) Typical manual processing tank showing developer and fixer insert tanks in the water bath. (B) Line drawing of manual processing tank.

Dental x-ray dryers are used after the processing is complete. The x-rays are left on the racks and placed in the dryer, suspended from a rod over a fan and heat element to dry. This process takes between fifteen and twenty minutes. An alternative to this procedure is to hang the x-rays from a towel rack or rod and to let them air dry. It is important that the x-rays not touch and that the drying is out of the way in a clean area to prevent dust and other debris from collecting on the x-ray.

Long-handle brushes or sponges are used to clean the inside of the processing tanks. There should be one brush for the developing tank and one for the fixing tank. These brushes should be marked and never be interchanged. After use, they should be rinsed and stored separately.

Preparation for Processing

The developing and fixing solutions are normally prepared from liquid concentrates, following the manufacturer's instructions. They come in two-packs with color-coded lids and labels (Figure 17-68). Verify that the correct solution is placed in the proper tank to prevent cross-contamination of the chemicals. After checking the date on the solution, carefully open the top and pour the developer into the developing tank. Add water, about 68° or slightly cool to the touch, to the indicator line at the top of the tank. The fixer is prepared in the same manner. After the insert tanks are in the processing tank, start the water coming through the inlet valve. The water can run in fairly quickly during this time. When it is up to the point where it is flowing out the outlet or overflow pipe, adjust the water to a slow, steady flow. Each insert tank is then stirred with the appropriate stirring paddle to mix the chemicals completely. Check the temperature of the developing solution; if it is around 68°, it is ready to process x-rays. A time/temperature chart is located on each of the developer/fixer solution packages. Have the chart available in the darkroom for review. Charts may vary slightly from manufacturer to manufacturer.

Temperature	Duration in the Developer
80°F	2½ minutes
75°F	3 minutes
70°F	4 minutes
68°F	4½ minutes
60°F	6 minutes

FIGURE 17-68 Manual processing developer and fixer solution. *(Reprinted courtesy of Eastman Kodak Company)*

The optimum temperature is from 68° to 70°. If the temperature goes 20 degrees either way from the optimum, the chemicals in the solutions may be destroyed and will have to be discarded. It is necessary to change the solutions every three to four weeks in order to maintain optimum processing, under normal use. If there is heavy use, change solutions more often.

Each day, a test film should be processed to compare to the film that was processed the first day the solutions were changed. If a change is seen in the processed films, then the solutions may not be effective. It is important to keep a log of the date you last changed the solution. Also, check the solution visually to ensure that it is not cloudy or dark. This also may indicate that the solution needs to be changed.

Replenishing the Processing Solutions. The processing solutions may need to be replenished periodically. The solutions may be low prior to the time of changing the solutions. If this happens, open a pack of the concentrated developer solution and add a fifty/fifty consistency of developer and water. In other words, add the same amount of developer as water to the developer insert tank. The fixer is different because water comes from the water bath of the processing tank on the x-rays into the fixer during each processing sequence. Therefore, add straight fixer to the fixer insert tank to replenish it.

Manual Film Processing Technique

After the solutions are stirred with the appropriate stirrers and the temperature in the developer is checked, it is ready to process x-rays. The work area must be clean and dry. Obtain the correct processing rack and write the patient's name, date, and number of x-rays on the identification tab at the top with a pencil. The x-rays themselves may be in a cup. If they have come directly from the patient's mouth, wear gloves while the x-rays are carefully unwrapped and placed on the racks. Do not touch any portion of the film directly. Other ways to handle the aseptic technique are to disinfect the x-rays prior to bringing them into the darkroom or use preplaced protective coverings on the films themselves, which are removed, and place the uncontaminated films in a cup ready for processing. It is not important which technique is used, but a standard policy needs to be followed so that cross-contamination does not take place (Figure 17-69).

The overhead light is turned off and the safety light is turned on. The door is locked if it is possible. When the eyes are accustomed to the safety light, unwrap the film; pull back the plastic coating, the black paper, and the lead foil; and attach the film to the hanger. Hold the film by the edges to confirm that it is securely on the hanger. Place each film on the x-ray rack in the same manner. When this process is completed, lift the lid off the processor and place the rack in the developer solution. Be sure to agitate the films in the solution by quickly raising and lowering the films several times into

the solution before attaching the rack to the side of the tank. This ensures that the films are bathed totally in the solution and that no bubbles are on the surface of the film. Place the lid on the processing tank and wait four and one-half minutes if the temperature is at 68°. The timer should be set immediately after the lid is on. When the time is up, open the lid cover (safety lights only) and lift the rack from the developer. Carefully shake off excess solution and then place the rack in the water bath solution. The x-ray films need to be rinsed for at least thirty seconds in the running water (middle portion of the tank). The rinsing stops the process of the developing solution. After thirty seconds, raise the rack and let the excess water drain off. Place the film in the fixer insert tank. The tank cover is then replaced over the tank and the timer is set again. The time for processing in the fixer is twice that of the developer; therefore, process for nine minutes at 68°. After the fixing time is complete, the films are removed from the fixer solution and placed in the wash bath in the center of the tank for the final rinse. The films are rinsed by clear running water for about twenty minutes. When this is complete, the films are removed and hung from a towel rack or placed in an electric dryer for fifteen to twenty minutes. The films are then ready for mounting.

Composition of the Processing Solutions

The Developer. The **developer solution** has a pH above 7 and chemically reduces the exposed area of the emulsion, making it visible to the naked eye. The pH scale is from 0 to 14, with 7 as neutral. Anything above 7 is considered to be acid and anything below 7 is considered to be alkaline.

The following components make up the developing solution: hydroquinone, elon, sodium carbonate, sodium sulfite, potassium bromide, and water. **Hydroquinone** is extremely sensitive to changes in temperature and is inactive when the temperature is below 60°. Hydroquinone is a reducing agent, or a chemical that blackens the exposed silver halide crystals. Even though this chemical acts slowly, the image gains density steadily during the developing process. Hydroquinone is responsible primarily for the film contrast. **Elon** is a reducer that also blackens the exposed silver halide crystals. Elon is not affected greatly by the temperature changes. It acts quickly and is responsible for giving detail to the film. The reducers cannot develop unless they are in an alkali medium. **Sodium carbonate** is often used as an alkaline medium in the developer. It softens and swells the emulsion so that the reducers can reach the silver crystals. If the solution has too much alkaline medium, over-swelling of the emulsion takes place, causing blisters on the film.

The reducers and the alkaline medium are affected by oxygen. The oxygen in the air and solution can spoil the developer. Therefore, a preservative is used to slow

MANUAL PROCESSING KODAK INTRAORAL DENTAL X-RAY FILM

Correct manual processing makes a definite contribution to the quality of a radiograph. It is also a fact that properly processed film requires only the minimum of exposure. The importance of correct processing cannot be over-emphasized. The three fundamentals for good processing are fresh solutions, adequate equipment, and a standardized method.

This chart describes and pictures the basic steps in correct time/temperature processing.

GENERAL RULES

Timer and Thermometer. Both must be accurate and in good working order. It is essential to use them routinely.

Chemicals. In preparing solutions, follow directions on the packages exactly. Maintain levels of the solutions in the tanks with proper amounts of replenishment solutions. The solutions must cover the top films on the hanger.

KODAK Dental X-Ray Developer is recommended for the times in the chart below. KODAK Liquid X-Ray Developer and Replenisher or KODAK Rapid X-Ray Developer can also be used, but under controlled processing conditions there may be some differences in speed, contrast, and gross fog.

Film Handling. Handle film carefully when attaching it to a hanger to avoid finger marks or abrasions. Be sure films do not touch tank walls, films, or another hanger.

1 STIR SOLUTIONS

Dilute developer and fixer solutions as directed on the container. Stir to equalize both the temperature and the distribution of the chemicals in the solution. Use a separate paddle for each solution. Note: Stir gently. Do not whip.

2 CHECK TEMPERATURE

Check temperature of developer with an accurate thermometer.

3 SET TIMER

Set the timer for recommended development time based on temperature of the developer. Do not start the timer until after Step 5.

DEVELOPMENT TIMES	
65° F (18.5°C)	6
68° F (20.0°C)	5
70° F (21.0°C)	$\frac{1}{2}$
72° F (22.0°C)	4
75° F (24.0°C)	3
80° F (26.5°C)	$2\frac{1}{2}$

4 LOAD FILM HANGER (under safelight conditions)

Remove films from packets and attach carefully to a multiple-clip hanger, such as the KODAK Dental Processing Hanger No. 45. Avoid finger marks, scratching, or bending.

FIGURE 17-69 Kodak manual processing step-by-step chart. *(continued) (Reprinted courtesy of Eastman Kodak Company)*

5 IMMERSE FILM IN DEVELOPER

Completely immerse the film in the developer. Do it smoothly and without pause to prevent streaking. Start timer.

6 AGITATE FILM

Immediately raise and lower hanger (agitate it) several times so that the film surfaces are thoroughly bathed to remove air bubbles.

7 RINSE THOROUGHLY

When the timer bell rings, remove hanger from the developer. Place film in rinsing section for thirty seconds with clean running 60° to 80° water. Lift from rinse and drain into wash tank. Do not drain back into developer tank.

8 FIX ADEQUATELY

Place film in the fixer solution. Agitate the hanger vigorously. Generally, film should remain in fixer for twice the time required to "clear" it. See specific instructions for fixing times. Do not view film before it is cleared.

9 WASH COMPLETELY

Place film in the washing compartment. Wash for at least twenty minutes in running water. Eight volume changes per hour are recommended.

10 DRY

The films are removed from the water, hung from a towel rack, or placed into an electric dryer for fifteen to twenty minutes.

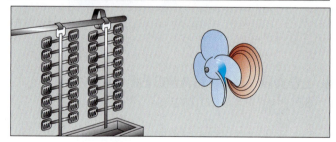

FIGURE 17-69 Kodak manual processing step-by-step chart. *(continued)*

PROCEDURE

17-5 Processing Radiographs Using a Manual Tank

This procedure is performed by the dental assistant. The assistant prepares the equipment, supplies, and the area. The exposed radiographs are taken to the darkroom by the dental assistant to process.

EQUIPMENT AND SUPPLIES

▶ Barriers for the darkroom counter

▶ Exposed radiographs

▶ X-ray rack

▶ Processing tank

▶ Safety light

▶ Timer

▶ Thermometer

▶ Pencil

▶ Electric film dryer

PROCEDURE STEPS *(Follow aseptic procedures)*

1. Wash and dry hands (gloves must be worn if the x-rays are contaminated).

2. Make sure the area is clean and free of splashes. Place barriers on the counter in the darkroom.

3. Check the temperature of the developer with the thermometer. Also, check the processing chart for the corresponding temperature and time information.

4. Check the volumes of the processing solutions to ensure that they do not need replenishing. (Replenish if necessary.)

5. Stir the developer and fixer if it is the first processing being completed that morning or afternoon. Stir the solutions with the corresponding stirring rods. Do not interchange.

6. Check the x-ray rack to ensure that the clips are in working order.

7. Label the x-ray rack in pencil with the patient's name, date of exposure, and the number of x-rays taken.

8. Turn on the safelights and turn off the white lights.

9. Remove the films from their wrappers and place on the x-ray racks. (Use gloves if the x-rays are contaminated.)

10. Check each film to make sure it is attached securely and placed in a parallel manner so that it is not touching the adjacent film.

11. Place in the developer tank and agitate the rack slightly in the developing solution to eliminate bubbles on the surface of the emulsion.

12. Place the tank cover on the processing tank. Set the timer for four and one-half minutes if the temperature of the developer is at 68°. The area can be cleaned up and the barrier and x-ray wrappers are disposed of.

13. When the timer goes off, remove the x-ray rack from the developer, letting the excess solution drip into the developer prior to placing the rack in the running water (the middle area in the processing tank). Let it rinse for thirty seconds.

14. Remove the x-ray rack from the rinsing, let the excess water drip off, and then immerse the rack in the fixing solution for ten minutes. If the dentist needs to view the patient's x-rays, they can be removed after three minutes and then returned to the fixer for the remaining time.

15. Replace the processing lid and set the timer for ten minutes.

16. After the ten minutes, remove the x-ray rack from the fixer and place it in the running water at the center of the processing tank. The final wash takes twenty minutes to complete.

17. The rack of x-rays can be removed from the water after twenty minutes and placed in an x-ray dryer for an additional fifteen to twenty minutes or until drying is completed.

18. When the x-rays are dry, remove them from the rack and place them in a labeled x-ray mount.

this process. **Sodium sulfite** prevents oxidation and increases the life span of the developing solution by two to four weeks.

If the chemicals work too fast, a film fog appears and the x-rays are unclear. A restrainer such as **potassium bromide** is used to slow the developing process to a practical speed and prevent film fog.

The last ingredient used to mix all these chemicals together is water. It is recommended that distilled water be used so that no additional chemicals are brought into the developing solution.

The Fixer Solution. The fixer solution removes the unexposed and undeveloped crystals from the film emulsion as well as stops the developing process. The following components make up the fixer solution: sodium thiosulfate, acetic acid, potassium alum, and water. **Sodium thiosulfate**, or hyposulfite, is known as the "hyp" agent. It is responsible for removing the unexposed and undeveloped crystals from the film. The chemical that stops the developing action and provides the required acidity for sodium thiosulfate to work is **acetic acid**. The third chemical in the fixer is sodium sulfite, and it works much as it does in the developer, by preserving the solution and preventing oxidation. **Potassium alum** is the chemical that shrinks the emulsion gelatin and hardens it. This hardening process protects the film from abrasion and helps the films dry more quickly. The final ingredient is water. It is used as a medium to incorporate the chemicals. It is not as critical to have distilled water in the fixer as it is in the developer.

Used fixer solution stains clothing; the silver salts accumulate in it and form spots that may not show up until after the garment is laundered. If the fixer solution has spotted the clothing before being washed, rinse it first in unused fixer solution and then thoroughly with water before laundering. There are several products on the market for treating stains on dental uniforms.

Disposing of the Fixer and Developer (OSHA Guidelines). Disposal of the fixer and developer solution must follow OSHA hazardous waste guidelines. Silver is present in the fixer solution and must be disposed of properly. It cannot be washed down the sink. Both the used developer and fixer solution should be put in a leak-proof container and disposed of by a company specializing in biohazard waste. The solutions also can be treated in dental offices that have silver recovery units, which take the silver from the solutions. The treated solutions can then be disposed of.

The lead in the film packet is also a hazardous material. The lead can be saved in a container and sold along with the recovered silver to a metal recycling company.

Automatic Processor

Automatic processors are used in most dental offices (Figure 17-70). Automatic processors are easy to use and reduce processing time. The x-rays are consistently

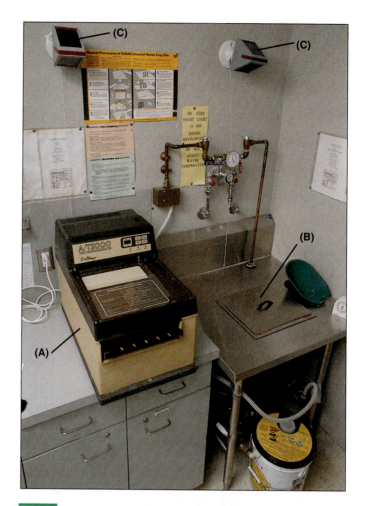

FIGURE 17-70 (A) Automatic film processor. (B) Manual processing tank in darkroom. (C) Safelights.

of a good quality. Most processors are compact and require minimum space in the darkroom. If space in the darkroom is a problem, some processors have daylight loading units that can be added. With the daylight loading units, the processors can be placed wherever they are convenient to use. One important factor to consider when using automatic processors is that maintenance of the units and daily chemical control is essential.

Although automatic processing follows the same basic steps as manual processing, the order in which the film is soaked in solutions is different. With automatic processors, a series of rollers move the x-ray film through the developing compartment, the fixing compartment, the water compartment, and, last, through the drying compartment before depositing it onto a tray (Figure 17-71).

The rollers are moved by gears, belts, or chains that must be lubricated and maintained according to manufacturer's instructions. The x-ray film is processed in four to seven minutes depending on the temperature of the developing solution. The temperature also determines the speed at which the rollers are set. Automatic processing is done at temperatures between 85°F and

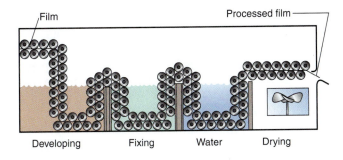

Film   Processed film

Developing   Fixing   Water   Drying

FIGURE 17-71 The inside of a typical automatic film processor.

95°F. This increase in temperature greatly reduces the total processing time. The rollers move the film through each compartment and also "squeeze" off the excess solution between compartments. This prevents processing chemicals from being carried into the next stage of processing.

Automatic Processing Solutions. The **automatic processing solutions** are designed specifically for automatic processors and are not interchangeable with solutions used for manual processing. In automatic processing solutions, the developer has chemicals added to prevent the emulsion from becoming soft and sticking to the rollers. The solution also has an agent that reduces the swelling of the emulsion so the films will not absorb too much developing solution. Automatic processing solutions are used to replenish solutions daily. Some machines have the ability to replenish the solutions automatically each time a film is fed into the unit.

Care of the Automatic Processor. Proper care of automatic processors is critical. To ensure quality x-ray film processing, daily and weekly maintenance must be followed. Read the manufacturer's instructions and set a schedule for maintenance. Designate a staff member to be the "quality assurance controller" for x-ray processing. Here are a few general guidelines:

▶ Every morning, check the solution levels and add solutions where needed. Turn the water on so that fresh water is running continuously, or place fresh water in the units without water hookup. Place on the lid securely and run a film through the processor to remove any debris.

P R O C E D U R E

17-6 Processing Radiographs Using an Automatic Processor

This procedure is performed by the dental assistant. The dental assistant prepares the equipment, the supplies, and the area. The exposed radiographs are taken to the automatic processor by the dental assistant to process.

EQUIPMENT AND SUPPLIES

▶ Exposed radiographs

▶ Automatic x-ray processor with daylight loader

PROCEDURE STEPS *(Follow aseptic procedures)*

1. Turn on the automatic x-ray processor at the beginning of each day. This ensures that it is warmed up and ready to process after the x-rays are exposed. (The chemicals must be heated to the correct temperatures or the x-rays will appear light and the diagnostic quality will be diminished.)

2. Wash and dry hands.

3. Place exposed radiographs in the daylight loader with two additional containers.

4. Place on gloves and position gloved hands through the sleeves of the daylight loader.

5. Remove each radiograph from its packet and place the film in the container that is not contaminated. Be careful not to touch and contaminate the film as the packet is removed.

6. Place the empty packets in a contaminated cup.

7. After all x-rays are unwrapped, remove the gloves and place them in a contaminated container.

8. With clean hands, feed the unwrapped films into the machine *slowly*. Start on one side of the processor and rotate to the other side. Repeat. If using a film holder, place all films in the holder and release for processing. Continue until all films are placed in the processor.

9. Remove processed films from the outlet area and place in a labeled x-ray mount.

▶ Every night, turn off the water. Lift off the lid and place it slightly ajar to prevent fumes from accumulating and condensing (which can cause films to fog) and processor motor problems.

▶ Weekly, rinse the rollers with warm water and then soak them as recommended by the manufacturer.

▶ Solutions should be changed between two and six weeks depending on use and how much the solutions were replenished. Cleaning solutions recommended by the manufacturer should be used routinely.

▶ Rinse the rollers completely before replacing them in the compartments. Each compartment has a plug that needs to be securely in place before the tanks are filled.

Duplicating Radiographs

Dental x-rays can be duplicated so that the originals never have to leave the office. The need for duplication is increasing because more patients have dental insurance, patients request that x-rays be sent to specialists, and requests are made to forward x-rays when patients move to new areas. Also, malpractice suits have increased, which require radiographs for defense support. Copies of x-rays can be made by a duplication process in the darkroom. These copies offer protection for the dentist as well as reference sources for the patient.

The **duplication technique** requires the purchase of duplicating film and a duplication machine. The film comes in a variety of sizes and can be processed either manually or with an automatic processor. Duplicating film has emulsion on one side only and is coded with a notch in the upper right corner, when the emulsion side is facing you. Duplicating film is a direct positive film; thus, if an increase in film darkness (density) is desired, the exposure time is reduced.

Duplicating machines have light sources with glass over them. The lid closes with a latch to prevent light leaks. There is a setting for viewing the x-rays and a timing selector. These machines are not large and fit conveniently on a counter top.

P R O C E D U R E

17-7 Processing Duplicating Technique

This procedure is performed by the dental assistant. The dental assistant prepares the equipment, the supplies, and the area. The radiographs to be duplicated are taken to the darkroom by the dental assistant to duplicate.

EQUIPMENT AND SUPPLIES

▶ Duplicating film and radiographs to be duplicated

▶ X-ray duplicating machine

▶ Automatic x-ray processor with daylight loader

PROCEDURE STEPS *(Follow aseptic procedures)*

1. Place the x-rays in the desired position on the duplicator (Figure 17-72). Make sure the dot on the film is upward (convex).

2. If the machine has a viewing light, turn it on to assist during placement of the x-rays.

3. Turn off the viewing light and under safelight conditions, place the duplicating film over the x-rays with the emulsion side facing downward so that it is contacting the x-rays (the notch will be in the upper left corner).

4. Cover with the lid and latch tightly. Set the timer to four to five seconds (this may vary with machines).

FIGURE 17-72 Example of a radiographic duplicator and film.

5. Activate the machine to expose the film.

6. When completed, remove the duplicating film under safelight conditions and process the film.

MOUNTING RADIOGRAPHS

Each radiograph has a raised dot on it to help with the mounting process. The film pack is placed in the patient's mouth so that the raised dot, or convex side, is toward the x-ray cone. Mounting the radiographs so that the dot is toward the operator means that the operator is looking at the film as if the operator were facing the patient. The patient's left side would be on the operator's right side facing the film mount. This type of mounting is called labial mounting. The ADA recommends that dental offices use the labial mounting. An x-ray viewbox may be used to mount dental radiographs. A viewbox is a lighted box that has a white, frosted surface so that x-rays can be viewed easily for diagnostic purposes.

The other type of mounting is called lingual mounting. This is where the depressed dot (concave side) is toward the operator and therefore the operator is viewing the films from the inside out, or from a position inside the oral cavity looking outward. This type of mounting has the patient's left side on the operator's left side. Both systems of mounting are used in the dental offices today; however, the labial system is used more widely.

There are a number of different mounts available (Figure 17-73). They range in sizes from 1, 2, 4, 7, 14, 16, 18, 20, and 28 windows. Bite-wing x-ray mounts normally come in either 2 or 4 windows. The 14 or 16 window mounts are used most commonly for periapical mounts. The 18 or 20 windows are used most often for full-mouth (both periapical and bite-wing) mounting.

Mounts can be purchased in a number of different materials. They should be stiff enough to keep the films rigid and hold them securely in place. The most commonly used mounts are made from plastic or cardboard. The plastic mounts come in clear, frosted, or dark coloring. The advantage of plastic mounts is that they are water repellent and can be reused. Disadvantages are that the plastic mounts can crack or split and, if the operator uses the clear mounts, they can give off a glare around the films and inhibit diagnosis (the frosted and dark mounts cut out the glare).

The cardboard mount is normally less expensive than the plastic mounts and blocks out any glare around the film. It can be reused if pencil is used to write in the patient's name. The cardboard mounts have an area for each film to slide into place. Some operators prefer one type of mount over another. The disadvantages of a cardboard mount are that it is not water resistant and it bends and breaks easily.

After selecting the correct mount, place the x-rays on a clean counter in front of a viewbox. If mounting a full mouth set of x-rays, divide the x-rays into three groups: bite-wings, anterior periapicals, and posterior periapicals. It is easy to identify the bite-wing x-rays because they have both the crowns of the mandibular and the maxillary teeth on them. Individuals may find it easier to mount the bite-wings x-rays first to reference them for the placement of the periapicals. However, there is no set pattern for which x-rays should be mounted.

The four bite-wing x-rays are mounted so that the molar x-rays are on the outside and the corresponding bicuspid x-rays are on the inside, just as if looking directly at the patient (Figure 17-74). Notice the curve of spee (or formation of a smile pattern), which comes from the curvature of the mandible on correctly mounted x-rays. Check carefully that the dots are convex, the molars are on the outside, the bicuspids are on the inside, and the occlusal plane is curved in a smile pattern.

Now mount the anterior periapical x-rays. The maxillary anterior teeth are always larger and wider than the mandibular anterior teeth. The maxillary central teeth are normally the easiest to identify. Locate them and place them in the full-mouth mount in the center upper portion. They should be placed as they are in the mouth, with the incisal edge in the middle of the mount and the roots toward the outside of the mount. Find the mandibular central x-rays (they will appear to have the smallest teeth on them). Place them directly below the maxillary teeth with the incisal edges toward each other. There are four cuspid x-rays (two maxillary and two mandibular) left to mount. Look for the maxillary

FIGURE 17-73 Various full-mouth, bite-wing, and single-film mounts.

FIGURE 17-74 Full-mouth mount with bite-wing x-rays in place.

cuspids first. They will appear larger and may show the maxillary sinuses near the distal side of the apex of the roots. Remember that the roots always tend to curve distally. Mount both the maxillary and the mandibular cuspid x-rays in the correct position with the lateral sides toward the centrals and the bicuspid sides outward. Make sure that all the incisal edges come together in the middle, just like the mouth does.

The mandibular and maxillary posterior films are differentiated from each other on the basis of root and crown shape, along with anatomic landmarks. The maxillary posterior x-rays may show the nasal cavity or sinuses. The maxillary premolars usually have two roots and the molars have three roots. The roots of the maxillary molars may look unclear because of the lingual root showing through the mesial and distal roots. Mount the maxillary molars on the upper part of the mount toward the outside. The bicuspids will be placed between the molars and the anterior cuspids. The bicuspid and molar x-rays that have been placed in the mount must match each other as well as the corresponding crowns of the bite-wing x-rays. Identify the same restoration in several x-rays (it may be from different angles but still

FIGURE 17-75 Full-mouth x-rays mounted with correct placement references.

should appear similar). The mandibular periapical x-rays should be mounted in much the same manner as the maxillary. The molars will have two roots that are more clearly defined than the maxillary; the bicuspids will have one root. After all the x-rays are in the mount, do a quick check to see whether all the x-rays are mounted similar to the position of the teeth in the mouth (Figure 17-75). It may take several practices to be able to quickly identify any incorrectly mounted x-rays and to replace them correctly.

PROCEDURE

17-8 Mounting Radiographs

This procedure is performed by the dental assistant. A viewbox may be utilized when mounting the radiographs.

EQUIPMENT AND SUPPLIES

▶ Radiographs

▶ Lighted viewbox

▶ X-ray mount (using full-mouth, 18 x-ray mount)

▶ Clean, dry surface

PROCEDURE STEPS *(Follow aseptic procedures)*

1. Wash and dry hands.

2. Label the x-ray mount with the patient's name and the date of the exposure (in pencil).

3. Turn on the viewbox (optional).

4. Place the radiographs on a clean surface so that all dots are convex or outward to viewing.

5. Categorize all x-rays into three groups: bite-wings (four in number), anterior (six in number), and posterior (eight in number).

6. Place the bite-wing x-rays in the mount, making sure the dots remain convex, the molars are toward the outside, and the bicuspids (premolars) are toward the inside. Make sure that the x-rays are mounted according to the curve of the spee.

7. Place the anterior x-rays in place, with the maxillary on the upper and the mandibular on the lower. The incisal edges should be closest to each other in the mount and the roots positioned as they grow. The centrals are placed in the middle with the cuspids on the outer sides. (The maxillary centrals are much larger than the mandibular centrals.)

8. Place the remaining posterior x-rays. The molars should be toward the outside and the bicuspids (premolars) toward the inside. The maxillary molars have three roots and the mandibular molars have two roots. Both should be placed according to how they are in the mouth, with the roots opposite each other and the biting surfaces more closely positioned.

9. Review the mounted x-rays to verify that they have been placed properly.

STORAGE OF PATIENT RADIOGRAPHS

Patients' radiographs are stored in the treatment record. If they are removed from the mount, they are placed in a small envelope with the patient's name, date, and number of x-rays enclosed labeled on the outside. Each state has regulations on the length of time radiographs must be saved (because they are considered legal records). Dental assistants should inquire about the statutes of limitations in their states.

LEGAL IMPLICATIONS OF RADIOGRAPHS

 As stated above, x-rays are legal records and should not be destroyed. They belong to the dentist and should not be given to the patients. If a patient switches to another dentist, send a duplicate of the x-rays to the new dentist; keep the original for the office files.

EXTRAORAL RADIOGRAPHS

Extraoral radiographs are used by the dentist to identify large areas of the skull on one radiograph. These radiographs give the dentist an overall view and are used most often in conjunction with periapical, bite-wing, and occlusal radiographs. Orthodontists and oral maxillofacial surgeons routinely use extraoral radiographs, especially panoramic and cephalometric exposures.

Panoramic Radiography

Many dental offices have panoramic radiography machines (Figure 17-76). Panoramic machines take a radiograph that shows the entire maxilla and mandible on one film (Figure 17-77). Panoramic radiography is commonly known and named after the brand name of the panoramic x-ray machine. There are many types of panoramic machines, but most use the same principles of technique. The film holder (**cassette**) and the x-ray head rotate opposite each other around the patient's head. Because they are connected by bars extending from the top of the machines, they rotate at the same speed. The result is an x-ray that extends from the condyle on one side of the patient's head to the condyle on the other side. There is some overlapping and loss of detail, but panoramic radiographs are valuable when an overall assessment of the patient is needed. Panoramic x-rays can be taken on adults, children, edentulous patients, patients who have trismus (lack the ability to open the mouth very wide), and patients in wheelchairs.

Panoramic x-rays give the dentist a general view of the following:

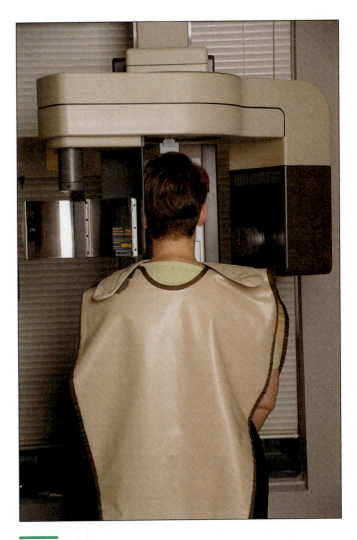

FIGURE 17-76 Patient positioned in a panoramic x-ray machine.

- The entire dentition
- Nasal and orbital areas
- Alveolar bone
- Carious lesions
- Fractures, cysts, tumors
- Malocclusion
- Maxilla and mandible
- Sinuses
- Unerupted teeth
- Dental appliances and restorations
- Periodontal disease
- Temporomandibular joint

Extraoral Film. The **extraoral film** comes in a variety of large sizes, ranging from 5×12 for the panoramic to 8×10 for the cephalometric exposure. The film is not

FIGURE 17-77 A panoramic radiograph.

FIGURE 17-78 (A1) Hard cassette for panoramic x-ray. (A2) Intensifying screen. (B) Soft cassette.

wrapped individually; it comes in a box of fifty or more. Therefore, the film must be loaded into the cassettes in the darkroom *under safelight conditions.* The box must be closed carefully to prevent light exposure to the remaining film in the box.

Extraoral film is screen film, requiring the use of screens for exposure. The film is placed between two intensifying screens in the cassette holder. Screen film is sensitive to the light emitted from the intensifying screens rather than to radiation. The film must be sensitive to the type of light emitted by the screen particles. It is important to have extraoral film that is designed specifically for the type of intensifying screens being used.

Cassettes. **Cassettes** are used to hold the film during exposure. They are either flat, hard containers that open on the back or flexible, thin sleeves that open on one end (Figures 17-78A and B). Both prevent light from coming through but allow x-rays to pass through. The cassettes must be marked to distinguish left or right because there is no raised dot on the film. Also, care must be given not to scratch the screens and to keep them clean and free of stains and debris. Cassettes usually are lined with **intensifying screens**. The action of the x-rays on the film is increased or "intensified"; therefore, the exposure to the patient is decreased. A substance called phosphor is used on the screens. The phosphor emits light when struck by x-rays. Some phosphors emit blue light and others emit green light. It is important to use film that is sensitive to the kind of light the phosphor emits. The green-light phosphors are known as "rare earth" phosphors and are faster; thus, the patient receives fewer x-rays during exposure.

Film-Holding Devices

The panoramic machines have cassette holders attached to them. With other extraoral exposures, the cassette holder may be attached to a wall or the patient may hold the cassette. With some extraoral exposures, the cassette is placed on a flat surface and the patient's face is laid against it.

Panoramic Exposure Technique Suggestions

There are many types of panoramic machines. Each machine has specific instructions for successful exposures on a variety of patient. Be sure to read and follow these specific instructions. There are a few points to follow with all panoramic exposures:

▶ The patient always should wear a lead apron *without* a thyroid collar. The collar interferes with the image and, because the x-ray beam is directed upward, the x-ray exposure to the thyroid gland is minimal.

▶ The patient needs to be still during the entire exposure. Each machine has some type of chin rest, biteblock, and head positioners to prevent movement.

▶ Explain the procedure to the patient, including the rotation of the machine and what to do during the exposure. Remove bulky sweaters, coats, hair clips, or anything that may interfere with the rotation of the x-ray tubehead. Also remove earrings, necklaces, and dental appliances.

▶ Place the cassette in the machine, prepare your patient, carefully take the readings, set the machine, and take the exposure. Release the patient and remove the cassette for processing and reloading.

FIGURE 17-79 Patient positioned for a lateral cephalometric radiograph.

FIGURE 17-80 A lateral cephalometric radiograph.

Cephalometric Radiographs

Cephalometric radiographs (*cephalo* means head and *metric* means measurement) are used to assess the patient's skeletal structure and profile (Figure 17-79 and 80). The cephalometric radiographs are used mainly by orthodontists in treatment planning for their patients, but some oral maxillofacial surgeons and general practitioners include these radiographs for patient assessment. The patient's bony structure as well as soft tissues are recorded on the cephalometric radiograph. Lateral or posterior anterior views are used for orthodontic measurements, examination of the sinuses, implant evaluation, and TMJ assessment. Use of a cephalometric unit is the accurate way to ensure that the patient is positioned in a manner that can be duplicated as the patient grows and as repeated radiographs are needed for comparison. The unit consists of a cephalostat, or head-holding device; a cassette holder for an 8 × 10 inch cassette; and an x-ray tubehead.

For lateral views, position the patient by placing the left side of his or her head against the cassette, positioned so the midsagittal plane is parallel to the cassette. The **Frankfort plane**, or line from the **tragus of the ear** to the floor of the orbit, of the patient is parallel to the floor. The x-ray beam is directed perpendicular to the cassette.

For posterior anterior radiograph views, the patient faces the cassette with the Frankfort plane parallel to the floor and the x-ray beam directed at the occipital bone and perpendicular to the cassette (Figures 17-81A and B).

Lateral Jaw Radiograph. The **lateral jaw radiograph** can be used if the dental office does not have a panoramic x-ray machine. Large areas of the jaw can be radiographed by using a 5 × 7 inch or an 8 × 10 inch film cassette and having the seated patient hold the cassette next to his or her face and resting on his or her shoulder. The x-ray tubehead is positioned on the opposite side and directed so that the central ray is perpendicular to the patient's head and the cassette. The x-ray exposure time is increased because of the layers of tissue and bone. The patient's head is positioned differently depending on the area the dentist needs to view.

The Transcranial Temporomandibular Joint Radiograph. The **transcranial temporomandibular joint radiograph** is taken with the patient holding a cassette against the side of the head and the cone/central x-ray positioned on the opposite side of the patient's head, slightly above and behind the external auditory meatus. Positioning devices assist in the correct alignment for the x-ray (Figures 17-82 and 17-83). The radiograph can be taken with the patient's mouth open or closed.

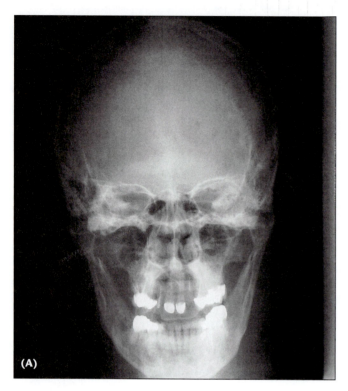

(A)

Film

Central ray

(B)

FIGURE 17-81 (A) Posterior anterior radiograph. (B) Line drawing of posterior anterior radiograph, labeled.

FIGURE 17-82 Patient positioned for a transcranial lateral position TMJ radiograph with mouth closed.

FIGURE 17-83 Transcranial TMJ radiograph with mouth closed, showing the relationship of the condyle to the glenoid fossa.

RADIOGRAPHIC INTERPRETATION

Being familiar with the terminology used in radiographic interpretation will make the dental assistant better prepared to perform radiograph procedures (refer to Table 17-5).

Learning landmarks make radiographic interpretation much easier and more meaningful. The following structures are defined and identified on radiographs and/or in diagrams, showing both normal and abnormal landmarks. The dental assistant interprets radiographs in order to be prepared for the dentist and the procedure.

The terms begin with the tooth and the surrounding tissues, then cover the maxilla and the mandible. Periapical, occlusal, and panoramic radiographs are used to show each term, but the landmark may be seen on more than one type of radiograph.

TABLE 17-5 TERMINOLOGY USED IN RADIOGRAPHIC INTERPRETATION

Terminology	Explanation
Anatomical landmarks	Anatomical areas that assist in identification for mounting x-rays and communicating with the dentist and the patient. (The dental assistant does not diagnose x-rays but can interpret the images on the x-ray and recognize what is normal and what is abnormal.)
Radiopaque	Structures that are dense and do not allow rays to pass through them. The x-rays are blocked or absorbed to varying degrees depending on the density of the structure. The structures show up in light gray to white shades on the x-ray, depending on the density.
Radiolucent	Show up on x-rays in shades of dark gray to black. The structure is not dense, x-rays penetrate in varying degrees.
Diagnosis	To know; the art or act of identifying disease.
Interpretation	To explain the meaning of something.
Superimposition	One structure is lying over another.

Note: Radiopaque and radiolucent are comparative terms. They are used to compare one structure or substance to another.

The Tooth and the Surrounding Tissues
(Figure 17-84)

Enamel: A radiopaque area on the crown of the teeth.

Dentin: The area just inferior to the enamel; it is less radiopaque than enamel.

Cementum: Radiopaque like dentin; look for the thin covering on the root(s).

Pulp chamber: A radiolucent area surrounded by dentin. The pulp horns can be seen; these projections usually correspond with the cusps of the tooth, as seen on the x-ray.

Pulp canals or root canals: The radiolucent areas in the root. They extend from the pulp chamber to the apex of the tooth.

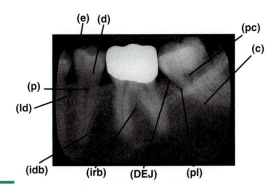

FIGURE 17-84 X-ray identifying teeth and surrounding structures: (d) Dentin. (e) Enamel. (p) Pulp canal. (DEJ) Dentinoenamel junction. (pc) Pulp chamber. (c) Cementum. (pl) Periodontal ligament (black line). (ld) Lamina dura (white area of cortical bone). (irb) Interradicular bone. (idb) Interdental bone.

Periodontal ligament/space: The radiolucent area that surrounds the root(s) of the tooth.

Lamina dura: The radiopaque line of cortical bone that surrounds the root(s) of the tooth and the periodontal ligament.

Cortical plate: The dense compact bone that forms the tooth socket.

Interradicular bone: The alveolar bone found between the roots of a tooth; it shows radiopaque on the x-ray.

Interdental bone: Alveolar bone found between two teeth; it shows radiopaque.

The Mandibular Landmarks (Figure 17-85)

Mental foramen: A radiolucent area located between the roots of the premolar.

Mandibular canal: This canal is radiolucent but it is outlined by radiopaque lines that extend from the mandibular foramen to the mental foramen.

External oblique ridge: A ridge on the external surface of the mandible extending from the middle of the rami to beyond the molar area. This ridge runs in an oblique line but curves more to the middle third of the molars than the internal oblique ridge.

Trabecular patterns: The spongy/cancellous bone that surrounds the teeth and forms the mandible. The spongy bone pattern is shown as radiopaque with radiolucent spaces.

Alveolar crest: The compact edge of the cortical bone that shows as radiopaque between the teeth.

FIGURE 17-85 X-ray identifying mandibular landmarks on panoramic film; (mf) Mental foramen. (mc) Mandibular canal. (eor) External oblique ridge. (ac) Aveolar crest. (c) Condyle. (cor) Coronoid. (bom) Border of mandible. (s) Symphysis. *(Courtesy of Dr. Rodney Braun and Dr. Chris Chaffin)*

Mandibular retromolar area: The area behind the last mandibular molar; it shows varying tissues in this triangular space.

Lingual foramen: The radiolucent area located on the lingual surface of the mandible at the midline/symphysis.

Genial tubercle: The raised areas of bone that surround the lingual foramen.

Internal oblique ridge: A ridge of bone on the mylohyoid ridge internal surface of the mandible that runs from the middle of the rami to the third molar region. Sometimes it continues past the molars up to the cuspid area; this extension is known as the mylohyoid ridge and shows superimposed over the root area.

Mandibular foramen: The radiolucent area in the middle of the ramus of the mandible on the interior surface.

Condyle: The back projection on the top of the ramus; it shows radiopaque and is articulated in the glenoid fossa.

Coronoid process: The front projection of the tip of the ramus; it shows radiopaque.

Medial sigmoid notch: The indented area between the condyle and coronoid processes on the ramus; also known as the coronoid notch or the mandibular notch.

Ramus: The section of each side of the mandible that runs vertical.

Body of the mandible: The section of the mandible that runs horizontally.

Border of the mandible: The lower edge of the body of the mandible that is made of compact bone.

Symphysis: The "chin" area, or the anterior portion of the mandible.

Hyoid bone: A "U"-shaped bone suspended by ligaments below the mandible but anterior to the larynx; it is occasionally seen on dental x-rays

Nutrient canals: The radiolucent paths that extend toward the alveolar crest.

The Maxillary Landmarks (Figure 17-86)

Hard palate: The radiopaque structure that forms the roof of the mouth.

Incisive foramen: A radiolucent area located at the midline of the palate behind the central incisors.

Maxillary suture: Also known as the median palatine suture, it is a radiolucent line that joins the right and left halves of the maxillary bone and palatine bones.

Zygomatic process: The process on the external surface, which begins around the first molar region.

Malar: Forms the cheek and is also known as the zygomatic bone.

Nasal septum: A radiopaque line that divides the nasal fossae.

Nasal cavities: The two side-by-side openings of the nose.

Nasal conchae: The bony, scroll-shaped plates in the lateral walls of the nasal cavity.

Maxillary sinuses: The left and right cavities located above the apices of the teeth, which can extend from the canines to the molar area.

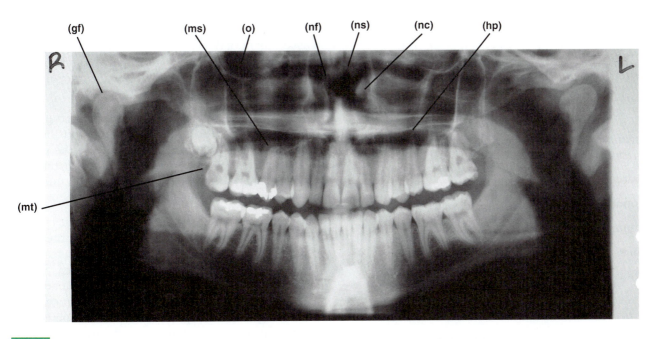

FIGURE 17-86 X-ray identifying maxillary landmarks. (gf) Glenoid fossa. (hp) Hard palate. (ns) Nasal septum. (nc) Nasal conchae. (ms) Maxillary sinuses. (o) Orbit. (mt) Maxillary tuberosity. *(Courtesy of Dr. Rodney Braun and Dr. Chris Chaffin)*

Infraorbital foramen: The radiolucent area located below the inferior border of the orbit (eye socket).

Orbit: The bone that circles the eyeball.

Maxillary tuberosity: A radiopaque area behind the most posterior molar on the maxilla.

Glenoid fossa: A depression on the lower border of the temporal bone where the condyloid process of the mandible articulates as the temporomandibular joint.

Mastoid process: A process of the temporal bone that lies in the lower, anterior section just behind the ear (auditory canal).

External auditory meatus: The radiolucent area in the temporal bone for the auditory canal.

Hamular process: A slender projection of bone that lies behind/posterior and medial to the maxillary tuberosity.

Styloid process: The projection of bone, larger than the hamular process, which comes from the temporal bone and lies behind the glenoid fossa.

Conditions or Artifacts on X-Rays. The following are conditions or artifacts that may appear on x-rays (Figure 17-87):

FIGURE 17-87 X-ray showing artifacts that may appear, such as calculus, caries, and an abscess. *(Courtesy of Dr. Rodney Braun and Dr. Chris Chaffin)*

- Dental caries
- Implants
- Impacted tooth
- Recently extracted tooth
- Root canal with reamer
- Periodontal pocket
- Orthodontic bands
- Overhang
- Calculus
- Attrition
- Abscesses
- Cysts
- Vertical bone loss
- Eyeglasses

- Vertebra
- Metallic restoration
- Bridge
- Fracture
- Mixed dentition
- Abrasion
- Drifting
- Supernumerary tooth
- Horizontal bone loss
- Earrings
- Edentulous patient
- Cement base/lining
- Root canal restoration
- Pins/posts
- Cervical burnout

QUALITY ASSURANCE

A quality assurance program refers to routine procedures that have been developed to ensure the highest quality and minimal risk to the patients in radiation exposure. It is a program that tests the equipment, solutions, and procedures to ensure that consistent high quality is maintained.

Several aspects of the equipment should be checked each year by the state regulatory agencies:

- Kilovoltage output
- Milliamperage output
- Exposure timer working properly
- Half value layer (HVL)
- Focal spot size
- Beam alignment and beam size
- X-ray output and reproducibility of exposure
- Stability of tubehead

These recommendations were published in the *Recommendations for Quality Assurance in Dental Radiography* by the American Academy of Dental Radiology. It is important that the date of the test, the type of the test performed, the individual name of the person performing the test, and the results be kept in a service log. Include documents of any service work in the log. Radiographic units are like any equipment and must be calibrated occasionally in order to work at the optimum level.

Implementation of a quality assurance (QA) program and assessment of the variables that affect x-ray quality greatly benefit the patients and operators. The tests used for routine assessment give the accuracy needed to provide good diagnostic x-rays.

- One of the most important aspects of a QA program is monitoring film processing. Make sure your lighting conditions in the darkroom are safe. Use the proper filters for the films currently in use. If the faster films are used, then the red filter is correct. If in question, check with a state regulatory representative.

- Another area of concern are the white light leaks in the darkroom. A simple way to evaluate the darkroom for possible light leaks is to do a "coin test." On the counter in the immediate processing area, place a coin on an unwrapped, unexposed x-ray film under the safelight for two to three minutes. Then, process the film using standard procedures. If the outline of the coin is evident on the film after processing, then the safelight illumination is inadequate or a white light leak is possible (Figure 17-88). Document the results in a log and date it. Correct any problems and do the test again. This test should be done monthly.

A technique for monitoring the quality of the processing solutions is to use a step wedge. Use a commercial step wedge or make a step wedge by placing several lead foil pieces, from x-ray film packets, together in a stair-step manner and soldering them (Figures 17-89A and B). Expose twenty x-rays the first day that the processing solution is changed. Make sure it is stirred, and check the temperature. Then, process one of the x-rays. This processed film will become a standard to evaluate the other films. Choose a density in the middle of the film to be used for comparison. Store the other nineteen exposed x-rays in a cool, dry place. Every day or two process another of the x-rays and compare it to the first

FIGURE 17-88 Unexposed film with a coin on it for the safelight test.

FIGURE 17-89 (A) Manufactured step wedge. (B) Step wedge made from lead foil from x-ray film packets.

(B)

FIGURE 17-90 (A) Spin top used in checking time accuracy and exposed x-ray showing results of the spin top test. (B) Impulses indicated by markings on the x-ray.

one. The same middle density on these later films should be comparable to the first one. If the later film differs from the standard by two or more steps, check the processing solution.

Other areas to be checked include the last time the solution was changed or replenished, the water temperature, the processing time, and whether the solutions have been contaminated. After checking all possibilities and correcting the problem, process an additional test x-ray to compare to the standard film.

▶ Monthly, the x-ray machine can be checked by using several additional equipment items. To test the timer, a spin top is needed (Figure 17-90A). Place the film (normally size #4) on the sitting area of the x-ray chair. Select the mA and kVp values and the number of impulses to be tested. Place the spin top on the film, place the PID over the top and film, set it to spin, make the exposure, and process the film. Count the number of dots visible on the film to interpret the results (Figure 17-90B). The number should correspond to the number of impulses selected on the machine.

▶ To evaluate the effectiveness of the milliamperage, use the step wedge and place it on a size #2 film and position the PID so that it covers the film. Then, expose the film. Do this each month; if the appearance of the corresponding shade varies more than two steps, the mA should be checked and adjusted by a qualified service person (Figure 17-91).

▶ To measure the kVp, a dosimeter and charger are needed (Figure 17-92). Make sure the dosimeter is charged and at the 0 reading. Place the dosimeter on a surface, place the PID over it, and expose the dosimeter. It should show a reading of the appropriate kVp. If it does not, have it checked by a qualified service person.

FIGURE 17-91 Comparison made of two x-rays exposed using the step wedge. (A) Standard processed when the solution was first prepared. (B) Standard processed after replenishment of the solution had taken place.

FIGURE 17-92 A dosimeter used in evaluation of the kilovoltage. (A) Dosimeter charger. (B) Dosimeter.

If a problem is apparent, it is important that no radiographs be taken until the problem is fixed. Quality control cannot be overlooked. Each step of the procedure must be followed carefully, including the storage of the unexposed films, use of a lead apron with a thyroid collar, proper placement of the film and cone in order to reduce retakes, and correct, final labeling of the film mount from which the diagnosis is to be made. All the steps in between are important to minimize radiation to the patient. It is important that each dental assistant has the proper training to take x-rays. Every patient deserves competent, quality service.

1. Set high standards for quality assurance.
2. Follow a consistent procedure to maintain control.
3. Check equipment, solutions, and procedures often.
4. Keep a log of daily, monthly, and yearly procedures used to maintain quality radiographs.

IMAGING SYSTEMS

Imaging systems are used frequently by dental professionals. The systems most commonly used are the **computed tomography (CT scanning)** and the **magnetic resonance imaging (MRI)**. The image systems are found in hospitals or specialized clinics.

Advances also are being made in **digital imaging technology**. These computerized systems are the future in dental radiology and will be in every dental office. Dental assistants continually need to be up-to-date concerning these systems as they are integrated into the dental office.

Computed Tomography (CT Scanning)

CT scanning is used to plan implant surgery and to locate and define lesions associated with the oral cavity.

Computed tomography has eliminated the use of x-ray film but still uses ionizing radiation as the source of energy. The patient is placed in a CT unit, where the radiation and image detector rotate around him or her. The information is transmitted to a computer, which calculates an image and displays it on a monitor. The image can be transferred to a film for later study. The computer is able to produce images in all dimensions or planes, although the original image is taken in one plane, the **axial plane**. This is where the original CAT scan (computed axial tomography) came from. CT scanning is the accepted term for computed tomography (Figure 17-93).

Magnetic Resonance Imaging (MRI)

The MRI techniques are used mainly in diagnoses of temporomandibular joint (TMJ) disease. They enable the dentist and radiologists to look at the soft tissues of the TMJ with very little risk to the patient. These techniques use low energy electromagnetic radiation instead of ionizing radiation. The patient is placed in a unit that contains powerful primary and secondary coils. The primary coils produce the magnetic field, while the secondary coils maintain the magnetic field and alter the primary magnetic field to receive information from different planes of the body. The secondary coils also transmit and receive radio frequency pulses or magnetic signals.

Digital Imaging (Computed Dental Radiography)

Digital imaging is a computerized system that reduces x-rays received by the patient by over 90 percent. This computer technology allows the dentist to take an x-ray of

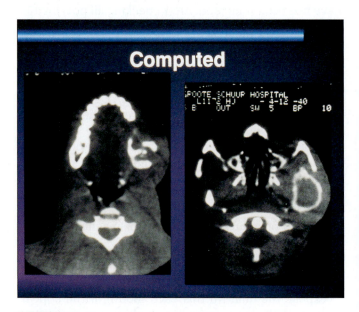

FIGURE 17-93 CT scan of the skull in the coronal plane. *(Courtesy of Dr. Gary Maxwell)*

an area in the patient's mouth and show the image on a computer screen. The image can be stored, printed, or sent to another dental office by means of a fax or modem. The equipment needed includes a computer, digital imaging software, sensors, a fax/modem, and a printer.

Digital imaging eliminates the processing step involved in producing traditional dental x-rays. A sensor is selected and placed in the patient's mouth. Then, a receptor is positioned and the exposure is made. The sensors come in sizes that correspond to film sizes: 0.1 and 2. Adult and pediatric periapicals and bite-wings can be taken with this system. The dentist can change the contrast, density, or color of the digital radiograph without exposing the patient to additional x-rays. However, the ability to correctly position the sensor and the receptor is still needed to produce a detailed, quality radiograph. Positioning technique errors are the same as with traditional x-ray exposure; therefore, placing the sensors takes the same time and skill.

The dentist has instant results and the ability to enhance, contrast, zoom, take exact measurements, make notes on the radiograph, and alter the color. Patients have visual images to view when the dentist is discussing areas of concern.

 The main disadvantage is the initial expense of the equipment and the time required to become efficient in the use of the digital system technology. Computers and computer technology are constantly improving and changing dentistry. Digital x-ray technology is part of this change (Figure 17-94).

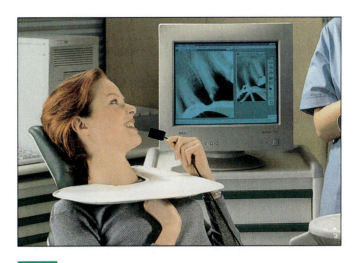

FIGURE 17-94 Intraoral digitizing unit. *(Courtesy of Dentsply/Gendex)*

CHAPTER SUMMARY

It is the responsibility of the manufacturers, dental team members, and patients to follow safety precaution measures when using radiography equipment. Steps must be used to minimize risk to the patient and all dental personnel.

The dentist is responsible for having dental assistants properly credentialed and trained to expose and process radiographs. The dentist is also responsible for supervising dental assistants in these tasks. In 1981, the Consumer Patient Radiation Health and Safety Act was enacted. This federal law requires each state to inform the Secretary of Health and Human Services how compliance with the act is accomplished.

The dental assistant must be trained in aseptic techniques, radiation hygiene, and maintenance of quality assurance and safety and must obtain a proper education in exposure and processing techniques. He or she must have an understanding of the physics and biological effects of ionizing radiation and utilize the understanding during every radiographic exposure and must understand the ALARA principle and utilize the lead apron with cervical collar for the patient's safety each time an x-ray is taken. The assistant must label and store patient x-rays properly to prevent loss and thus the need for x-rays being retaken.

CASE STUDY

Dr. David Candell has requested that Coral Nicolus have a full-mouth series of x-rays. Coral is a new patient and has not had x-rays taken for over five years. Dr. Candell wants radiographs to see the condition of the teeth and supporting bone. Coral is in good health except for having difficulty opening her mouth very wide. It would be uncomfortable for a periapical size #2 film to be placed in her mouth for exposure.

Case Study Review

1. What alternatives does the dental assistant have to periapical exposures?

2. Would the information the dentist requested be visible on the panoramic exposure?

3. Does the patient have any limitations that would alter this procedure?

4. Does the dentist have to be informed of changes before the radiographs are exposed?

To complete your study of this chapter, work the review activities that follow. Also, refer to the software that accompanies this text.

REVIEW QUESTIONS

Multiple Choice

1. This professor of physics discovered x-rays in 1895:
   a. Dr. C. Edmond Kells
   b. Dr. Otto Walkoff
   c. Dr. William Rollins
   d. Wilhelm Conrad Roentgen

2. When the interproximal spaces on a radiograph are overlapped, what is the error the result of?
   a. Vertical angulation.
   b. Horizontal angulation.
   c. Improper film placement.
   d. improper film processing.

3. When processing films in an automatic processor, what is the sequence of the solutions?
   a. Developer, fixer, water.
   b. Developer, water, fixer.
   c. Water, developer, fixer.
   d. Fixer, developer, water.

4. What is the optimal temperature for processing x-rays in the automatic processor?
   a. 85° to 95°F.
   b. 68°F.
   c. 100°C.
   d. 75°F.

5. When viewing properly mounted x-rays, where is the dot on the film mounted?
   a. So that it is raised or convex.
   b. So that it is depressed or concave.
   c. So that it is placed in the middle of the film.
   d. In any position.

Critical Thinking

1. The patient appears to have a fractured mandible. The dentist requests that an x-ray be taken. What type of x-ray would be the most beneficial for diagnosing a fractured mandible? Would the dental assistant be able to obtain this x-ray clinically?

2. If the radiographs were dark after processing, what areas would the dental assistant want to check to correct the problem?

3. List three primary errors that may be apparent on routine bite-wing x-rays, and explain how they can be corrected.

Dental Specialties

Endodontics

OBJECTIVES

The student should strive to meet the following objectives and demonstrate an understanding of the facts and principles presented in this chapter:

1. Define endodontics and endodontist.

2. Describe pulpal and periapical disease.

3. Identify diagnostic procedures.

4. Identify instruments used in endodontic procedures and describe their functions.

5. Identify materials used in endodontics and describe their functions.

6. Describe endodontic procedures and the responsibilities of the dental assistant.

7. Explain surgical endodontic procedures and the instruments used.

KEY TERMS

abscess (p. 378)

apical periodontitis (p. 378)

apicoectomy (p. 391)

barbed broaches (p. 382)

cellulitis (p. 378)

electronic pulp tester (p. 380)

endodontics (p. 378)

exudate (p. 378)

files (p. 382)

fistula (p. 378)

Glick #1 (p. 386)

gutta percha (p. 380)

hemisection (p. 393)

intracanal instruments (p. 382)

irreversible pulpitis (p. 378)

master cone (p. 389)

non-vital pulp (p. 378)

obturating (p. 385)

osteomyelitis (p. 378)

percussion (p. 379)

periapical abscess (p. 378)

pulpal necrosis (p. 378)

pulpectomy (p. 390)

pulpotomy (p. 390)

radiographs (p. 379)

reamers (p. 383)

retrograde filling (p. 392)

reversible pulpitis (p. 378)

root amputation (p. 391)

root canal sealer (p. 384)

rubber stops (p. 383)

spreaders (p. 385)

transillumination test (p. 382)

vital pulp (p. 378)

INTRODUCTION

Endodontics is the branch of dentistry that deals with the diagnosis and treatment of diseases of the pulp and the periapical tissues. Endodontic procedures include diagnosis, root canal treatment, and periapical surgery.

The endodontist has advanced education and training in the field of endodontics. General dentists, who can also treat the pulp and periapical tissues, render the same standard of care within their education and experience, but then refer the patient to an endodontist for those cases requiring advanced knowledge and training.

The general dentist sends written instructions and radiographs to the endodontist to avoid miscommunication. The endodontist also often communicates with the referring dentist concerning the patient's treatment and prognosis.

The Endodontic Team

The staff in the endodontist's office shares similar responsibilities as the general dental office staff, except there is an increase in communication with other dental offices because most of the patients are referrals.

The endodontist is assisted by dental assistants who perform traditional assisting responsibilities in addition to expanded duties specific to endodontics as allowed by the state Dental Practice Act.

PROGRESS OF PULPAL AND PERIAPICAL DISEASES

The healthy pulp is said to be a **vital pulp**. When the pulp or periapical tissues are irritated or injured, the result is inflammation. Advanced dental decay is one of the main sources of irritation. Other irritations or injuries include impact trauma, fractures, invasive restorative procedures, and adverse reactions to dental materials. The degree of pulpal inflammation depends on the severity and duration of the irritation or injury and the ability of the tissues to respond. The patient may or may not have symptoms that indicate the degree of the inflammation of the **non-vital pulp**.

Pulpal Diseases

Pulpal diseases include reversible pulpitis, irreversible pulpitis, and pulpal necrosis.

▶ **Reversible pulpitis**—The pulp is inflamed but able to heal when the irritant is removed. Causes include incipient caries, enamel fractures, and occlusal attrition. Symptoms include sensitivity to hot and cold. Treatment involves removing the irritant and placing sedative materials to soothe and heal the pulp.

▶ **Irreversible pulpitis**—The inflammation continues until the pulpal tissue cannot recover. Symptoms include pain to the patient that may be short and sharp or dull and continual. The treatment for irreversible pulpitis is root canal therapy or extraction.

▶ **Pulpal necrosis**—The death of the pulpal cells, often the result of irreversible pulpitis. The symptoms and treatment for pulpal necrosis are similar to those for irreversible pulpitis. As the pulp inflammation progresses, **exudate** (**ECKS**-you-dayt), or pus, and gas form in the pulp chamber. If the tooth is sealed and the exudate cannot escape, pulpal necrosis is rapid. If the exudate drains through caries or exposure to the oral cavity, the process is slowed. A fistula is a tubelike passage that forms sometimes to drain an abscess from the apex of a tooth to the oral cavity.

Periapical Diseases

When the infection in the pulp reaches the apex of the tooth, it continues into the periapical area. The intensities of the inflammation and the host response determine the extent of the infection. Periapical disease includes apical periodontitis and periapical abscess.

▶ **Apical periodontitis**—Pulpal inflammation extends into the periapical tissues. This acute condition subsides if the irritation is removed. If the process continues and the irritant is not removed, the apical periodontitis becomes a chronic inflammation. A radiograph of the area shows an interruption of the lamina dura and destruction of the periapical tissues (Figure 18-1). The immediate area of chronic apical periodontitis is usually classified as a **granuloma** or a **cyst**. A granuloma consists of numerous cells of the inflammatory process. If a granuloma is left untreated and the irritation continues, a cyst forms. A cyst is filled with liquid and semi-solid materials and is partially lined with stratified squamous epithelium (**SKWAY**-mus ep-ih-**THEE**-lee-um) and surrounded by connective tissue.

▶ **Periapical abscess**—A localized destruction of tissue and accumulation of exudate in the periapical region. The patient's reaction can range from moderate to severe discomfort and/or swelling. The treatment includes releasing the pressure by creating an opening into the pulp chamber, removal of the necrotic pulp, and root canal therapy.

Related Terms

▶ **Fistula** (**FIS**-tyou-lah)—A path to the external surface, created to drain the **abscess** (Figure 18-2).
▶ **Cellulitis** (sell-you-**LYE**-tis)—When the abscess spreads into the facial tissues, causing swelling and discomfort.
▶ **Osteomyelitis** (**oss**-tee-oh-**my**-eh-**LYE**-tis)—an advanced stage of periapical infection that spreads into and through the bone.

FIGURE 18-1 Radiograph of tooth with apical abscess (Dark shadow at the apex). *(Courtesy of Clifton A. Caldwell, DDS, FICD, FACD)*

FIGURE 18-2 Patient with gingival abscess. Red area above tooth #8 near frenum. *(Courtesy of Dr. Gary Shellerud)*

ENDODONTIC DIAGNOSIS

Endodontic diagnosis includes patient medical and dental history; clinical examination, including pulp testing; and review of communication from the referring dentist about the case. Each office has a routine procedure that is carefully followed to ensure that all pertinent information is gathered.

Medical History

The first step is for the patient to fill out a medical history. Once completed, the history is reviewed and clarified to ensure that accurate and complete information is gathered. The medical history may reveal information that relates to previous treatment of the tooth pulp that would be used in diagnosis.

Dental History

The dental history provides the endodontist with past dental experiences and also the signs and symptoms of the current concern. The dental history opens the way for the *subjective examination* (the problem explained in the patient's words). The patient should be allowed to describe the type of pain, sensitivity to heat and cold, the duration, and any other symptoms.

The Clinical Examination

The clinical examination, or the *objective examination,* includes evaluation of the extraoral tissues. Facial asymmetry, swelling, redness, and external fistulas are some of the indications to the problem the patient may be experiencing.

During the intraoral examination, the soft tissues are thoroughly evaluated and palpated, looking for any abnormalities or signs of inflammation. A visual examination of the teeth may reveal caries, discoloration, or fractures, but clinical tests are usually performed for a complete diagnosis. Clinical tests are performed by the dentist to diagnose the patient's situation correctly. Following are some of the testing procedures.

Radiographs. **Radiographs** are often the most useful of the diagnostic tools. Radiographs are taken and processed immediately so that the dentist can refer to them. If the inflammation has extended beyond the apex of the tooth and has bone involvement, a radiolucent area will be apparent. Detailed periapical x-rays with accurate positioning and good contrasting qualities are necessary to view the area around the end of the root of the tooth.

Palpation. **Palpation** of the soft tissues is performed by the endodontist. Pressure is applied to the mucosal tissue near the apex of root of the suspicious tooth. Normally, one or more additional teeth are palpated for comparison. Around the indicated tooth, the area may be soft and raised (pus filled).

Percussion. **Percussion** is performed by tapping on the occlusal or incisal surface of the tooth. The handle of a mouth mirror is often used (Figure 18-3). The tapping is first done on a control tooth and then on the symptomatic tooth. The control tooth should be the same tooth in the opposite arch. The patient may experience mild to moderate pain if there is periodontal inflammation and sharp pain if there is periapical inflammation.

FIGURE 18-3 Percussion test with handle of instrument.

FIGURE 18-4 Mobility test.

Mobility. Mobility is evaluated to determine the condition and involvement of the supporting structures of the tooth. Teeth that move 2 to 3 mm should not have root canal therapy because they lack sufficient support. Mobility is tested by placing the handle of an instrument or a finger on the lingual surface and the handle of another instrument on the facial surface of the tooth and applying pressure (Figure 18-4).

Cold Test. Cold testing is accomplished by using either dry ice, ethyl chloride, or a piece of ice (ice is the most common and easiest to use). The tooth is isolated and dried; then, the ice (usually the water that is frozen is a sterilized, anesthetic carpule) is applied to the facial surface of the tooth (Figure 18-5). The ice test is more effective on the anterior teeth than the more insulated posterior teeth. A normal tooth will respond within a few seconds. If the response to the cold is intense and long-lasting, irreversible pulpitis is indicated. Teeth with necrotic pulps will not respond to the cold test.

Heat Test. Heat testing uses several heat sources. Examples include a small ball of **gutta percha** heated by a flame, the heated end of a ball burnisher, or frictional

heat from running a rubber cup on the tooth surface. Heat is applied to the tooth and, if the pain increases and lasts, there is a distinct chance of irreversible pulpitis (Figure 18-6).

> Gutta percha is a thermoplastic material used to fill the canal.

Electric Pulp Testing/Digital Pulp Testing. Electric pulp testing does not measure the degree of tooth vitality but indicates whether the tooth is vital or nonvital. Like other pulp tests, the **electronic pulp tester** can produce a false reading (Figure 18-7A). Therefore, other tests should be completed for comparison and determination of the pulp vitality. Electronic pulp testing units are usually battery operated and deliver high-frequency currents that can be varied. The current creates an electrical stimulus to the tooth.

Most pulp testers operate in a similar manner. The main difference in the **digital pulp tester** is that it gives a digital readout, which most dentists prefer (Figure 18-7B).

FIGURE 18-5 Cold test on patient with ice stick.

FIGURE 18-6 Heat test on patient with gutta percha ball.

(A)

(B)

FIGURE 18-7 (A) Electronic pulp tester. (B) Digital pulp testing probes. *(Courtesy of Analytic Endodontics)*

P R O C E D U R E

18-1 Electronic Pulp Testing

EQUIPMENT AND SUPPLIES

▶ Basic setup: mouth mirror, explorer, and cotton pliers

▶ Electronic pulp tester

▶ Conducting medium, such as toothpaste

PROCEDURE STEPS

Follow these steps to electronically test the pulp (test control tooth first):

1. Place a small amount of toothpaste on the tip of the electrode (the toothpaste acts a conduct-ing medium). Dry the tooth before using the electrode.

2. Ask the patient to signal when he or she notices a sensation, which is usually a tingling or hot feeling.

3. Place the tip on the facial surface of the tooth and gradually increase the power. **CAUTION**: Do not place the electrode on a metal restoration.

4. If the patient feels any sensation, some degree of tooth vitality is indicated. If no sensation is felt, the pulp may be necrotic.

Transillumination Test. The transillumination test involves the use of a strong fiberoptic light that transmits light through the crown of the tooth. The light produces shadows that may indicate vertical fractures.

Selective Anesthesia. Sometimes the patient is unable to identify which tooth or which arch is causing the problem. In these cases, after talking with the patient and completing the clinical examination, **selective anesthesia** is used. One area of the patient's mouth is selected and an injection is given. If anesthetic in this area alleviates the discomfort, the problematic quadrant has been determined. Usually, selective anesthetic is utilized on the maxillary teeth beginning in the most suspicious anterior area and then progressing to the posterior area.

Removal of Caries. The removal of dental caries is necessary in some patients to determine the condition of the pulp. If the patient has no symptoms but the radiograph shows deep caries and the tooth responds positively to other tests, caries removal will further determine the status of the pulp. The dentist uses the dental handpiece to remove the decay and determine whether there is reversible or irreversible pulpitis. Depending on the prognosis of the tooth, the endodontist would place a temporary sedative restoration or a permanent restoration.

Treatment Plan

Once all the information has been gathered and the dentist has made a diagnosis for root canal therapy, the patient is informed of the necessary treatment. The patient needs to sign a consent form and make appointments and financial arrangements before treatment begins. To minimize anxiety and answer questions, the office may give endodontic pamphlets or show videos to inform the patient about the upcoming procedure.

ENDODONTIC INSTRUMENTS

Characteristics of Intracanal Instruments

Endodontic **intracanal instruments** are made of stainless steel and nickel titanium alloy wire. They are flexible, fracture resistant, smooth, able to maintain sharp cutting edges, and corrosion resistant. The wire is twisted and tapered into instruments called files and reamers. To ensure consistency in the sizes and lengths of the intracanal instruments, the ADA and manufacturers have standardized a number and color-code system (Figure 18-8). The intracanal instruments have precise diameters and lengths that are consistent from manufacturer to manufacturer. Intracanal instruments range in size from 08 to 140 and in length from 21 to 25 mm.

FIGURE 18-8 Reamers showing standardized numbers.

Barbed Broaches

Barbed broaches are made of fine metal wire with tiny, sharp projections or barbs along the instrument shaft. The barbs are angled to allow a smooth entry but catch tissue when retracted. Broaches are used for removal of soft tissue from the pulp canal. The dentist selects a broach that is large enough to remove pulpal tissue but small enough so that it will not bind in the canal.

Barbed broaches are supplied in various diameters, ranging from xxx-fine to coarse. The handles are either metal or plastic and are color coded (Figure 18-9).

Files

Endodontic **files** are used to enlarge and smooth the canal. They are long, tapered, twisted instruments that

FIGURE 18-9 Barbed broach.

are moved in an up-and-down motion inside the canal. They are available in a variety of diameters and types. The handles of the endodontic files are color coded according to standardized measurements. For example, a size 15 file is color coded white, and a 20 is yellow.

The standard files are known as **K-type files**. These tightly twisted files are used to scrape the walls of the canal, widen them, and remove necrotic tissue. The K-type file is rotated in the canal and then removed from the canal (Figure 18-10A).

The **Hedström files** are manufactured by a different process than the K-type files (Figure 18-10B). They are shaped like pine trees or appear to look like stacks of cones. The edges of the Hedström files are very sharp and cut more aggressively. These files are only used in a push-and-pull motion; they are not rotated like the K-type files because they will bind in the canal due to their design.

Reamers

Reamers are used with a "reaming" or twisting motion. They have long twisted shanks like the files, but the blades are spaced much farther apart (Figure 18-11). The cutting action is completed as the reamer is re-volved out of the canal. They are color coded and num-bered according to size, similar to the files. Reamers are not used as frequently as the files are.

Different methods are available to store and organize reamers and files). Some of the storage containers can be sterilized and are designed to hold a range of the intracanal instruments. The larger organizers often have measuring gauges for setting stops, as parts of the units. Finger rings are much smaller, holding only a few

FIGURE 18-11 Close-up view of a reamer.

FIGURE 18-12 Various intracanal instrument organizers for storage and sterilization and a sponge holder/ring for use at the chair. (*Courtesy of Premier Dental Products Company*)

instruments at one time (Figure 18-12). They come with disposable styrofoam pads.

Rubber Stops

Rubber stops (also called file stops, endo stops, or markers) are placed on reamers and files to mark the length of the root canal (Figure 18-13). These small, cir-cular, silicone disks have pre-punched holes in the cen-ter for easy application. The length is determined by holding a file with a rubber stop against a radiograph and adjusting the stop to match the incisal or cusp edge (Figure 18-13). The marked file is then measured on a small millimeter gauge. This number is recorded for future reference and for marking other intracanal instru-ments.

Gates-Glidden Drills

The Gates-Glidden drills are used with latch attachments on slow-speed handpieces. The drills are long-shanked and elliptically shaped with blunt, football-shaped ends. They run in a clockwise direction. They are supplied

FIGURE 18-10 (A) K-type file. (B) Hedström file.

FIGURE 18-13 Examples of rubber stops and how they are positioned on a file.

FIGURE 18-14 A Gates-Glidden drill. The tip of the drill is elliptically shaped and has a non-cutting end.

FIGURE 18-15 A Peeso reamer. The blades are long and parallel with non-cutting ends. *(Courtesy of Premier Dental Products Company)*

in six sizes and are marked near the notch portion of the shank. The marks indicate the size; for example, #1 drill has one stripe and #6 has six stripes. The #1 is equal to a size 50 K-type file, with each consecutive size increasing in diameter (Figure 18-14). Gates-Glidden drills are used in the upper portion of the canal to prepare the opening access by removing the obstructing dentin.

Peeso Reamers

The Peeso reamers have parallel cutting sides rather than the elliptical shape of the Gates-Glidden drills (Figure 18-15). They are used with latch attachments on slow-speed handpieces. Peeso reamers are supplied in a variety of sizes, beginning at 0.70 mm for #1 and increasing 0.20 mm for every subsequent size, ending at #6. The handles are striped to indicate the corresponding sizes. These instruments are supplied with or without safe tips. The Peeso reamers are used to prepare the canal for a post and to reduce the curvature of the canal orifice for straight-line access.

Lentulo Spirals

The Lentulo spiral is a long, twisted, wire instrument used to spin **root canal sealer**, or cement, into the canal (Figure 18-16). The spirals are used with slow-speed handpieces and latch attachments.

Endodontic Spoon Excavator

The spoon excavator has a very long shank that allows the instrument to reach into the coronal portion of the tooth. The spoon-ended excavator removes deep caries, pulp tissue, and temporary cement. The doubled-ended instrument has a right and a left end (Figure 18-17A).

FIGURE 18-16 A Lentulo spiral used to place root canal sealer in the canal.

Endodontic Explorer

The endodontic explorer is designed to aid in locating the orifices (opening) of the canals. It is a double-ended instrument with long, tapered ends that have sharp points. This stiff-ended explorer is designed specifically for endodontic procedures (Figure 18-17B).

Endodontic Spreaders, Pluggers, and the Glick #1

Spreaders and pluggers (condensors) are instruments used to laterally condense materials when obturating (sealing/filling) the canal. Both of these instruments have long, tapered working ends. The spreaders are pointed on the ends, while the pluggers are flat. Both of these instruments are supplied with either instrument metal handles or "finger-type" plastic handles (Figures 18-18A and B). The spreaders are used to adapt the gutta percha into the canal (lateral condensation), and the pluggers are used to condense the filling material to provide space for additional gutta percha cones (Figure 18-18C).

FIGURE 18-18 Endodontic spreaders. (A) Finger spreader. (B) Handled spreader. (C) 1. Endodontic condensors. 2. Glick #1.

FIGURE 18-17 (A) An endodontic spoon excavator. (B) An endodontic explorer. *(Courtesy of Hu-Friedy Mfg. Co., Inc.)*

The **Glick #1** instrument is used to remove the excess gutta percha from the coronal portion of the canal and condense the remaining gutta percha in the canal opening (Figure 18-18C).

ENDODONTIC MATERIALS

Absorbent Paper Points

Paper points are used to dry canals, place medications, and take cultures of the canal (Figure 18-19). Paper points are absorbent and are supplied in various sizes, from x-fine to coarse. They come conveniently packaged and are supplied either sterile or non-sterile. Locking cotton pliers are used to transport paper points to and from the tooth being endodontically treated.

Gutta Percha

Gutta percha is used to obturate the canal. It is a thermoplastic material that is flexible at room temperature yet stiff enough to be placed into the root canal. Gutta percha cones are supplied in graduated sizes, from x-fine to large (Figure 18-20).

Gutta percha endodontic obturation systems are also available. These systems include metal cores coated with gutta percha. The gutta percha and cores are heated with units specific to the system or with an open

FIGURE 18-19 Examples of various sizes of paper points.

FIGURE 18-20 Thermafil obturators and Gutta percha points.

flame and then inserted by hand or with low-speed handpieces into the root canal (Figure 18-20).

Silver points are rarely used any more to obturate the canal. They are used much like the gutta percha but are not as flexible. However, the silver points may be removed and replaced with gutta percha.

Irrigation Solutions

During the root canal treatment, the root canal is frequently irrigated to remove debris. Sterile water can be used for irrigating, but the most common biomechanical cleaner is **sodium hypochlorite**, which is household bleach. This solution is mixed with water (50/50) and loaded into a Luer-Lock syringe. The canal is irrigated with the sodium hypochlorite/water solution, which disinfects and dissolves necrotic tissue. The dental assistant places the evacuator close to the tooth to remove the debris and solution.

Root Canal Sealers and Cements

Root canal sealers used with obturating materials prevent microleakage in the canal. A variety of materials are used as sealers, including zinc oxide-eugenol, calcium hydroxide, and glass ionomer. They are supplied in powders/liquids, pastes, and capsule forms (Figures 18-21A through C). Sealers are mixed to a smooth, even consistency and then inserted into the canal using paper points, the Lentulo spiral, or files or by placing the sealer directly on the gutta percha.

Equipment Assisting Endodontic Procedures

 As technology advances, new equipment is being developed to assist in endodontic procedures.

▶ The **apex finder** measures the distance to the apex of the tooth and displays the information on a digital readout.

▶ The **vitality scanner** allows the dentist to scan each tooth in minutes (Figure 18-22). The scanner indicates endodontic problems in the early stages. The probe on the scanner records a reading and then automatically resets for the next tooth.

▶ The **heating unit** can be controlled or continuous. It has many applications, including heat for vitality testing, warming the gutta percha for obturation, and providing heat for bleaching procedures.

▶ The **endodontic handpiece** is an attachment to a low-speed handpiece. The handpiece supplies quarter-turn motion consistently and evenly. It duplicates the manual motion needed during the cleaning and enlarging of the root canal. The endodontic handpiece can be used with all hand instruments.

FIGURE 18-21 Root canal sealer. (A) Powder/liquid. (B) Two-paste system. (C) Capsules.

FIGURE 18-22 A vitality scanner can scan the entire mouth and test in minutes. *(Courtesy of Analytic Endodontics)*

ENDODONTIC PROCEDURES

Root Canal Treatment

Root canal treatment is usually completed in two appointments, but this does vary depending upon the degree of infection and the dentist's judgment. Many times, the dentist decides to postpone filling the canal to allow more time to treat the infection. When this occurs, the canal is irrigated, sometimes medicated, and a temporary filling is placed in the coronal portion of the tooth. The patient is rescheduled for a continuation of the procedure.

The procedure begins with the dentist opening the coronal portion of the tooth with a dental high-speed handpiece and burs. This is followed by cleaning and enlarging the canal. Restoring of the canal is also known as obturation. During this phase of treatment, the pulp canal is permanently filled and sealed.

General Steps in Root Canal Therapy

The following general steps in root canal therapy can be divided into two or more appointments depending on the preference of the dentist and the extent of the infection process. Steps 1 through 8 would take place on the first appointment. Steps 6, 7, and 9 would be done at the second appointment. Once completed, the patient would follow Step 10.

1. Administer the anesthetic.
2. Isolate the area.
3. Gain access to the pulp.
4. Locate the canals.
5. Remove the pulpal tissues.
6. Enlarge and smooth the root canal.
7. Irrigate the root canal.
8. Place temporary filling.
9. Obturate (seal) the root canal.
10. Refer patient to a general dentist for final restoration.

Sterilization Procedures

Endodontic instruments must be sterilized before they are used and/or during the course of cleaning and shaping the canal. Sometimes instruments are sterilized at chairside, using a small glass bead or salt sterilizing unit (refer to Chapter 9, Infection Control).

The reamers and files are fragile and should be examined closely before use. If there is any concern about the ability of the instrument to function correctly, it should be discarded. Some manufacturers recommend one procedure use for reamers and files.

P R O C E D U R E

18-2 Root Canal Treatment

This procedure is performed by the dentist, who is assisted by the dental assistant. The following sequence will indicate steps involved in a root canal treatment that requires two appointments.

EQUIPMENT AND SUPPLIES

▶ Basic setup: mouth mirror, explorer, and cotton pliers

▶ Endodontic explorer and spoon excavator

▶ Locking cotton pliers

▶ Saliva ejector, evacuator tip (HVE), air-water syringe tip

▶ Cotton rolls, cotton pellets, and gauze sponges

▶ Anesthetic setup

▶ Dental dam setup

▶ High-speed handpiece and assortment of burs

▶ Low-speed handpiece

▶ Irrigating syringe and solution (sodium hypochlorite or hydrogen peroxide)

▶ Barbed broach, assorted reamers and files, and rubber stops

▶ Paper points (assortment)

▶ Temporization materials

▶ Permanent obturating materials (gutta percha or silver points and root canal sealer)

▶ Heat source

▶ Endodontic spreaders, pluggers, and the Glick #1

▶ Articulating forceps and paper

PROCEDURE STEPS *(Follow aseptic procedures)*

Administer Anesthetic

1. Administer topical and local anesthetic for endodontic treatment just as with restorative procedures in general dentistry.

2. Usually the dentist will anesthetize the patient at every appointment, but it is up to the dentist's discretion. After the first appointment, when the pulp chamber has been opened and the canals have been cleaned, the dentist may determine that anesthetic is unnecessary.

3. Prepare the syringe and assist during the administration of the anesthetic.

Isolate the Area

1. Place the dental dam, isolating the tooth being endodonically treated. Besides isolating the tooth, the dam improves visibility and protects the tooth from saliva and solutions used in endodontic treatment.

2. Once the dental dam is placed, wipe the area with a disinfectant to remove bacterial contaminants.

Gain Access to the Pulp

1. The dentist uses the high-speed handpiece and a round or fissure bur to gain access to the pulp. The opening is made through the crown of the tooth and should be sufficient to expose the pulp chamber and permit access for intracanal instruments.

2. Evacuate and maintain good visibility for the dentist.

3. Once access to the pulp has been gained, the endodontic explorer is used to locate the main and accessory canals.

Remove the Pulpal Tissues

1. The dentist inserts a barbed broach into the canal and withdraws the pulpal tissue to remove pulpal tissues.

2. Receive the barber broach in a gauze sponge.

Enlarge and Smooth the Root Canal

1. Using the periapical radiograph, the dentist estimates the length of the root of the tooth (Figure 18-23). An apex finder may also be used. Rubber stops are used to mark the length of the tooth on files and reamers. A series of small files are used to remove debris and enlarge the canals. Canals must be at least a #25 file before Gates-Glidden burs can be used. As the files enlarge, the diameter of the canal, the size of the files, and/or the Gates-Glidden burs increase, respectively.

(continued)

P R O C E D U R E   **18 - 2** *continued*

FIGURE 18-23 Measuring the length of the root using a radiograph and reamer.

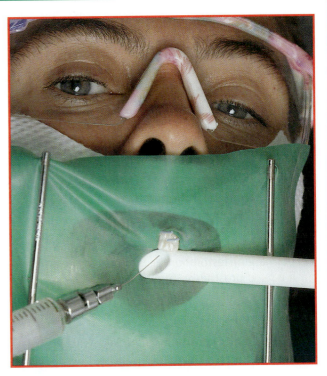

FIGURE 18-24 Irrigating the root canal.

2. Prepare the stops on the files and reamers according to the dentist's instructions. This measurement must be precise for each hand instrument. (The duties of the assistant may vary greatly depending on the preferences of the dentist. For example, some dentists may want the assistant to sterilize the reamers and files at chairside, or they may want radiographs taken periodically.)

3. Keep the files and reamers in order and free from debris.

Irrigate the Root Canal

1. Periodically, the canal is irrigated to remove debris (Figure 18-24). After the canal is flushed, it is dried with paper points.

2. Prepare the solution in the disposable syringe and transfer it to the operator. As the operator flushes the solution into the canal, evacuate the area. Then, transfer paper points in locking pliers to the operator and receive the used saturated points in a gauze sponge.

NOTE: At this time, the dentist may decide to place a temporary restoration and reappoint the patient in several days to two weeks.

3. Prepare the temporary restorative materials and either place the temporary or assist the dentist in placement.

4. Remove the dental dam and dismiss the patient.

Obturate the Root Canal

1. Obturation of the root canal is routinely performed at the second appointment. After the patient is seated, the temporary is removed and the canal is flushed to remove debris.

2. Radiographs are taken periodically throughout the procedure for the dentist to evaluate the progress. Once the canal is adequately enlarged and free of disease, it is permanently filled to prevent debris, fluids, and bacteria from entering the canal. There are many materials and techniques available to fill the canal, but gutta percha materials are most common.

3. The dentist selects a gutta percha point as the **master cone**. The cone should be no more than 1 mm short of the prepared length. The dentist inserts the cone into the canal to check the fit. If the master cone is the correct length and fits snugly near the apex, the cone is removed and the root canal sealer is prepared.

4. The root canal sealer is mixed and then placed in the canal with a Lentulo spiral and/or a master cone dipped in the sealer and placed in the canal.

5. A spreader is used to create space for additional accessory gutta percha cone. Dip each accessory

(continued)

gutta percha cone into the root canal sealer and transfer it to the dentist for placement. Transfer the spreader to create space for the subsequent cones. Repeat this procedure until the canal is filled (Figure 18-25).

6. Once the canal is filled, the excess gutta percha in the crown of the tooth is removed with a hot Glick #1 or a heated plugger. The warm gutta percha is vertically condensed into the cervical portion.

7. Hold a 2 × 2 gauze to remove any excess gutta percha from the instruments.

8. A final radiograph is taken.

9. The coronal portion of the tooth is sealed with a permanent restoration or a temporary restoration if a fixed prosthesis is the treatment choice.

10. The dental dam is removed and the patient's mouth is rinsed.

11. The patient's occlusion is checked with articulating paper.

12. Give the patient postoperative instructions and dismiss him or her.

NOTE: The patient returns to the general dentist for the final restoration of the tooth. Follow-up radiographs may be taken at six months and at one-year intervals.

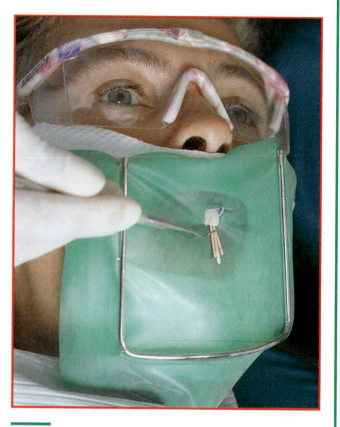

FIGURE 18-25 Root canal filled with gutta percha cones and sealer.

Pulpectomy

A **pulpectomy** is the removal of all pulpal tissues beginning in the coronal portion of the tooth and terminating 1 to 3 mm short of the apex in the root canal of a tooth. This procedure is used in the treatment of deep caries in permanent teeth. The pulpectomy procedure is the first stage of root canal treatment; cleaning and enlarging the canal usually follows.

Pulpotomy

A **pulpotomy** involves removal of the pulp in the coronal portion of the tooth, leaving the pulp in the root canal intact and vital.

A pulpotomy is indicated for:

▶ Primary teeth with pulp exposures

▶ Treatment in emergency situations where there is pulpal exposure

▶ Teeth with deep carious lesions

▶ Apexogenesis (ay-**PECKS**-oh-jen-ah-sis) (treatment of vital tooth where the root is not completely developed)

▶ Fractured anterior teeth (Figure 18-26)

FIGURE 18-26 A fractured central incisor with pulp exposure indicates the need for a pulpotomy. *(Courtesy of George J. Velis, DDS)*

SURGICAL ENDODONTICS

Endodontic treatment has a high rate of success; however, situations arise where surgical endodontic treatment is necessary in order to save the involved tooth from extraction. Surgery is performed in the area surrounding the roots of the teeth. These surgeries involve a facial surface incision through the tissue to expose the underlying bone. An opening through the alveolar bone is made to expose the root area where surgical endodontic treatment is performed.

Surgical techniques include apicoectomy, root amputation, and hemisection.

Apicoectomy

One of the most common endodontic surgical procedures is an **apicoectomy** (a-pee-koh-**ECK**-toh-me). In this procedure, the apex of the root and infection surrounding the area are surgically removed. The indications for this treatment include:

▶ Extreme curvature of the root, preventing root canal instruments from reaching the apex

▶ The root canal is hypercalcified, obstructing root canal therapy

▶ A previous endodontic treatment did not adequately seal the canal due to additional canals, fractures, or other causes of endodontic failure

▶ Gaining access to the apex of the root canal for examination and treatment

Root Amputation

Root amputation is a surgical procedure to remove one or more roots of a multi-rooted tooth. The root is

PROCEDURE

18-3 Apicoectomy

This procedure is performed by the dentist, who is assisted by the dental assistant.

EQUIPMENT AND SUPPLIES

▶ Basic setup: mouth mirror, explorer, and cotton pliers

▶ Endodontic explorer and spoon excavator

▶ Locking cotton pliers

▶ Saliva ejector, surgical evacuator tip, and air-water syringe tip

▶ Cotton rolls and gauze sponges

▶ Anesthetic setup

▶ Scalpel and blades

▶ Periosteal elevator and tissue retractors

▶ High-speed handpiece and assortment of burs (handpiece is specifically designed with a very small head)

▶ Surgical curettes

▶ Irrigating syringe and a sterile saline solution

▶ Hemostat and surgical scissors

▶ Amalgam setup

▶ Suture setup

PROCEDURE STEPS (*Follow aseptic procedures*)

1. Anesthetic is administered to prepare the patient.

2. The dentist makes a flap incision with the scalpel and lifts the tissue away from the bone with a periosteal elevator (Figure 18-27). Retract the tissue for the dentist throughout the procedure.

FIGURE 18-27 Apicoectomy procedure begins with a flap incision.

(continued)

P R O C E D U R E   **18 - 3** *continued*

3. Transfer instruments and keep the site clear and clean using the surgical evacuator and tissue retractors.

4. The high-speed handpiece is used by the dentist to gain access to the root apex through the bone (Figure 18-28).

FIGURE 18-28 A dental handpiece is used to remove the bone and expose the root tip.

5. The dentist removes debris and infection around the apex of the root with a surgical curette (apical curettage) (Figure 18-29).

FIGURE 18-29 Apical curettage. Removing infection and debris with a surgical curette.

6. Evacuate and remove debris from instruments with a gauze sponge.

7. Prepare the handpiece and the sterile saline irrigation syringe.

8. The high-speed handpiece and burs are used to remove a section of the exposed root tip (Figure 18-30). The root tip is beveled for better access. The area is rinsed with the sterile saline to prepare the root to receive the **retrograde filling** material.

FIGURE 18-30 Opening the root apex in preparation for the retrofill.

9. Retrograde filling material is placed in the prepared cavity (Figure 18-31). Amalgam is commonly used, but gutta percha, zinc oxide eugenol, and composites are also used.

Amalgam restoration

FIGURE 18-31 Retrofill being placed in root canal at the apex of the tooth.

(continued)

P R O C E D U R E 18 - 3 *continued*

10. Flap replacement and suturing are the final steps of this procedure. The flap is returned to position and held in place for a few minutes. The dentist then sutures the flap into place.

11. Prepare the sutures and assist during placement. Once the suturing procedure is completed, give the patient postoperative instructions, a prescription for pain medication, and dismiss him or her.

amputated at the point where the root meets the crown. The most common indication for the root amputation procedure is extensive bone loss around the root or furcation of the tooth (Figure 18-32).

Hemisection

Hemisection is the surgical removal of one root and the overlying crown. The tooth is separated buccolingually though the bifurcation, and the affected or diseased portion of the tooth is removed. Surgical burs, chisels, elevators, and forceps are used for this procedure. The indications for a hemisection are the same as for the root amputation (Figure 18-33).

Once the hemisection is complete, the remaining tooth and root are restored with a fixed prosthesis. The tooth may only need a crown, or it may become part of a bridge.

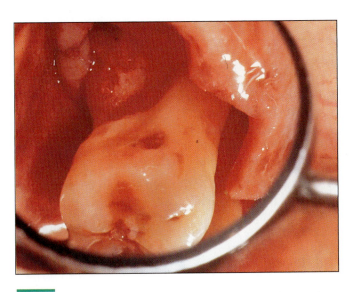

FIGURE 18-32 Root amputation on a mandibular first molar. The crown is saved; however, the diseased root is surgically removed. *(Courtesy of Dr. Gary Shellerud)*

FIGURE 18-33 Hemisection on a mandibular first molar. One root and one-half of the crown over the root are removed. *(Courtesy of Dr. Gary Shellerud)*

CHAPTER SUMMARY

Endodontics is the branch of dentistry that deals with the diagnosis and treatment of diseases of the pulp and periapical tissues. Procedures include diagnosis, root canal treatment, and periapical surgery.

The endodontist is assisted by the dental assistants who perform traditional assisting responsibilities in addition to expanded duties specific to endodontics as allowed by the state Dental Practice Act.

Endodontic diagnosis includes patient medical and dental hsitory; clinical examination, including pulp testing; and review of communication if the patient is sent from a referring dentist.

CASE STUDY

Gerold Frank, sixty-seven years old, came into Dr. Lamb's office for an examination of his mandibular right side. He has been experiencing pain and inflammation in this area. Upon examination, Dr. Lamb suspects that the mandibular first molar is causing Mr. Frank's problem.

Case Study Review

1. What are the key indications for treatment?
2. What clinical tests should be prepared?
3. What is a possible treatment?
4. What information should be given to Mr. Frank concerning his treatment?

To complete your study of this chapter, work the review activities that follow. Also, refer to the software that accompanies this text.

REVIEW QUESTIONS

Multiple Choice

1. Which of the follow diseases is a localized destruction of tissue and accumulation of exudate in the periapical region?
   a. Periodontitis.
   b. Apical periodontitis.
   c. Osteomyelitis.
   d. Periapical abscess.

2. The clinical examination for endodontic diagnosis includes all of the following *except*
   a, radiographs.
   b. sweet test.
   c. mobility.
   d. cold test.

3. What instrument is used to enlarge and smooth the root canals?
   a. Barbed broach
   b. Endodontic file.
   c. Endodontic reamer.
   d. Peeso reamer.

4. Root canal treatment is most often completed in
   a. two appointments.
   b. three appointments.
   c. four appointments.
   d. five appointments.

5. What procedure is performed to gain access to the apex of the root canal?
   a. Pulpotomy.
   b. Root canal treatment.
   c. Apicoectomy.
   d. Root amputation.

Critical Thinking

1. Describe the difference between a pulpectomy, a pulpotomy, and a root canal treatment.

2. Is anesthetic always administered for root canal treatment? Explain.

3. What is the difference between the K-type files and the Hedström files?

Oral and Maxillofacial Surgery

OBJECTIVES

The student should strive to meet the following objectives and demonstrate an understanding of the facts and principles presented in this chapter:

1. Describe the scope of oral and maxillofacial surgery.

2. Identify the various surgical instruments used in this type of surgery and describe their functions.

3. Explain aseptic procedures followed in the oral surgeon's office.

4. Describe the evaluation procedures for new patients.

5. Describe how to prepare the patient for surgical treatment.

6. Explain surgical procedures, including tray setups and assisting responsibilities.

7. List postoperative instructions given to patients.

8. List and describe the types of dental implants and explain the procedures they are used with.

9. Explain the oral surgeon's relationship with the hospital.

KEY TERMS

alveolitis (p. 413)

alveoplasty (p. 405)

biopsy (p. 411)

dental implants (p. 414)

elevators (p. 401)

endosteal implants (p. 417)

excisional biopsy (p. 411)

exfoliative cytology (p. 411)

extraction forceps (p. 401)

hemostats (p. 398)

incisional biopsy (p. 411)

informed consent (p. 405)

luxates (p. 406)

maxillofacial (p. 396)

mouth props (p. 397)

mucoperiosteum (p. 400)

needle holders (p. 398)

orthognathic surgery (p. 417)

osseointegration (p. 414)

periosteal elevator (p. 400)

retractors (p. 397)

rongeurs (p. 400)

root tip picks (p. 401)

subperiosteal implant (p. 414)

surgical aspirating tips (p. 399)

surgical bone files (p. 400)

surgical chisels (p. 400)

surgical curettes (p. 399)

surgical mallet (p. 400)

surgical scalpels (p. 397)

surgical scissors (p. 399)

tissue forceps (p. 397)

INTRODUCTION

Oral and **maxillofacial** surgery is the branch of dentistry that focuses on the diagnosis and treatment of diseases, injuries, and malformations. It involves surgery for both functional and esthetic aspects of the face, jaws, mouth, neck, and head. This specialty is sometimes referred to as oral surgery.

The general dentist refers surgical cases that go beyond his or her scope of training to the oral surgeon. Although the general dentist studies surgical procedures, the number of surgical procedures performed in the general dentist's office depends on individual preference and training. Upon graduating from dental school, a surgeon receives a minimum of four more years of advanced training in anatomy, anesthesia, pain control, and surgical procedures in and out of the hospital setting before receiving a degree in oral and maxillofacial surgery.

The Oral and Maxillofacial Surgeon's Office

There are a variety of settings for the oral surgeons' offices, just as there are for other dental offices. Some surgeons prefer to be close to a hospital if they routinely perform surgeries in a hospital setting.

The oral surgeon's office includes areas similar to the general office, with the addition of a recovery area. Some offices have separate areas for patients recovering from general anesthesia. Often, there is a large reclining chair or bed in this area so that the patient can lie down. Postoperative instructions and prescriptions are given to the patient or the patient's support person in the recovery area.

The Oral and Maxillofacial Surgery Team

The oral surgery office team varies according to the goals of the surgeon concerning the practice. In addition to the oral and maxillofacial surgeon, the team usually consists of the receptionist, the business office staff, the dental assistants, and, in some offices, a nurse or an anesthesiologist.

Oral and Maxillofacial Surgeon. The oral and maxillofacial surgeon performs the following: patient examination; diagnosis; teeth extraction; cyst and tumor removal; temporomandibular joint treatment; biopsies; and emergency, reconstructive, and implant surgeries. The oral surgeon works mainly in the office setting but also goes into the hospital to perform complicated surgeries and to treatment emergencies. Like all professionals, the oral surgeon continually attends seminars and courses to advance knowledge and skills.

Receptionist and Business Staff. The receptionist and the business staff perform many of the same duties in the oral surgery office as they would in the general dental office. Because the majority of the oral surgeon's patients are referred by other dental and medical offices, communication and recordkeeping responsibilities increase. The patient's x-rays and written information must be received in the surgeon's office before the patient's appointment. When the patient first arrives at the office, he or she is given forms to fill out. Appointments for treatment are scheduled and insurance claims and financial arrangements are completed before the day of the surgery.

Surgical Dental Assistant. The surgical dental assistant's responsibilities often vary depending on the size of the practice. For example, a dental assistant may be responsible for sterilization and room preparation, the seating and dismissing of patients, pre- and postoperative care, and assisting the oral surgeon during all procedures.

Typical responsibilities of a surgical dental assistant are:

▶ Perform traditional duties, such as instrument transfer and maintaining the operating field during the procedure

▶ Assist with the administration of intravenous sedation and analgesics

▶ Take and record vital signs

▶ Prepare the treatment rooms

▶ Sterilize instruments

▶ Ensure that all presurgery steps are completed and any materials or prosthetics required are ready

▶ Prepare the patient for treatment

▶ Maintain asepsis throughout the procedure

▶ Stabilize the patient's head and mandible during surgery, if necessary

▶ Provide postoperative care of the patient

▶ Clean the treatment room

▶ Remove sutures (if this is a legal expanded function)

> The option to become a Certified Dental Assistant in Oral and Maxillofacial Surgery (COMSA) is available upon successful completion of an examination administered by the Dental Assistant National Board.

ORAL SURGERY INSTRUMENTS

Surgical instruments are designed to apply adequate pressure in specific areas in order to remove bone tissue or teeth. Surgical instruments are made of stainless steel (so they can be sterilized after each use) or disposable plastics.

Scalpel

Surgical scalpels are surgical knives used to *incise* or *excise* the soft tissue in a precise manner with the least amount of trauma.

Scalpels are designed in two sections: the handle and the blade (Figure 19-1). The metal handle is slim and straight and is designed to accommodate detachable, disposable blades. A common handle is the Bard Parker style. This handle is flat and has a metric ruler. The blades are very sharp and are supplied in a variety of lengths and designs. The blades are used once and then disposed of in the sharps container. Blades are made of surgical carbon steel and are numbered according to shape. Common blades used are #15 for surgical procedures and #11 and #12 to incise and drain.

Disposable scalpels are also available. They have plastic handles with metal blades. Disposable scalpels are supplied in sterile packages and are disposed of after one use.

> When removing or replacing blades on the scalpel handle, use cotton pliers, a hemostat, or a blade protector to avoid injury. Practice placing and removing the blades to familiarize yourself with the mechanics of this skill. Disposable surgical blade removers are available. The scalpel blade is placed in a plastic cap of the removers and removed from the handle. The blade is left in the cap and discarded.

Retractors

Retractors are used to deflect tissue away from the surgical site so that the view is unobstructed. Careful handling of retractors is necessary in order to avoid traumatizing the tissue. There are several types of retractors: tissue retractors, cheek and lip retractors, and tongue retractors.

Tissue retractors are supplied in either forceps (hinged) type (**tissue forceps**) or cotton-plier style. The working end of both types of retractors has small teeth to assist in grasping the tissue securely (Figure 19-2).

Cheek and **lip retractors** are used to hold the patient's cheeks away from the operating site. They increase visibility by retracting the cheeks and expanding the viewing area. Cheek retractors are made of metal or plastic (Figure 19-3 and 4).

Tongue retractors are placed between the border of the tongue and the lingual surfaces of the teeth. The dental assistant gently but firmly retracts the tongue from the operating site. Tongue retractors are spoon shaped or have long blades (Figure 19-3 and 4). Tongue retractors also are used to retract the cheeks. They are placed on the buccal mucosa and then the tissue is retracted for a clear view.

Mouth Props

Mouth props are used to prevent the patient from closing during the procedure. Sometimes, the long appointment, the type of anesthesia administered, or the physical condition of the patient requires the use of props. Mouth props are made of hard rubber, silicone, plastic, or stainless steel. They are supplied in child and adult sizes. The prop is inserted into the patient's mouth with the tapered end toward the posterior teeth. This allows the muscles to relax while keeping the mouth open.

Another type of mouth prop is the Molt mouth gag, which is hinged and has handles, a ratchet release, and

FIGURE 19-1 Metal scalpels, variety of blades, and blade removal cap.

FIGURE 19-2 Tissue retractors. *(Courtesy of Miltex Instrument Co., Inc., Lake Success, NY)*

FIGURE 19-3 (A) Tongue and cheek retractors. (B) Lip, tongue, and cheek retractors.

FIGURE 19-4 (A) Tongue retractor. (B) Cheek retractor in patient's mouth.

FIGURE 19-5 Mouth prop positioned in patient's mouth.

beaks. Molt mouth gags are supplied in pediatric, child, and adult sizes. The beaks are closed when inserted into the patient's mouth, and the handle is gently squeezed, which opens the beaks and the patient's mouth. The forceps are locked in this position until the release is engaged (Figure 19-5).

Hemostats

Hemostats have multiple uses during surgical procedures. They are used to retract tissue, remove small root tips, clamp off blood vessels, and grasp loose objects. A hemostat is a forceps with working ends that are not sharp but long, serrated, or grooved beaks. They have locking handles that can be manipulated with one hand (Figure 19-6).

Hemostats are supplied in a variety of sizes to accommodate the uses of the instrument. Tissue, bone, and tooth fragments are easily grasped and removed with the hemostat. There are various types, including the Kelly and the Halstead-Mosquito. Hemostats come with straight and curved beaks.

Needle Holders

Needle holders are similar to hemostats and function in much the same manner. They are forceps with straight beaks, but needle-holder beaks are shorter than hemo-

FIGURE 19-6 (A) Hemostats. (B) Needle holder. *(Courtesy Miltex Instrument Co., Inc., Lake Success, NY)*

stat beaks. The needle holder has fine serrations with a groove down the center of each beak to hold the suture needle. They are supplied in a variety of sizes (Figure 19-6).

Surgical Scissors

Surgical scissors are used to cut sutures and to trim soft tissue. They are supplied in a variety of sizes and shapes (Figure 19-7). They are made of stainless steel and should be used only for surgical procedures in order to maintain their sharp edges. The surgical scissors have pointed beaks with either straight or angled blades.

Surgical Aspirating Tips

Surgical aspirating tips are made of either metal or plastic. The metal tips are sterilizable, while the plastic tips are discarded after one use. The surgical aspirating tips are long tubes that are either very slender or taper to small openings. The tips are used to aspirate blood and debris from the surgical site (Figure 19-8). A stylet is used to clear blood and tissue from the surgical tips.

Surgical Curettes

Surgical curettes are used for curettage and debridement of the tooth socket or the diseased tissue. They

FIGURE 19-7 Surgical scissors.

FIGURE 19-8 Surgical aspirating tips.

are double ended and have either straight or curved shanks; the working end of the instrument is spoon shaped. Surgical curettes are available in a variety of sizes (Figure 19-9).

Surgical Chisels and Mallets

Surgical chisels are used to remove or shape the bone. They can be used alone if the bone is soft, but if the bone is dense, a **surgical mallet** is used with the chisel. The chisel is positioned on the bone, and mallets are used to gently tap the end of the chisel. Chisels and mallets also are used to split teeth into smaller portions for easier removal.

Chisels are available in either beveled on one surface or bi-beveled (beveled on both sides). The bi-beveled chisels are used to split a tooth, while the single-beveled chisel is used to remove and shape the bone (Figure 19-10).

Surgical Bone Files

Surgical bone files are usually double-ended instruments. They are supplied in a variety of sizes and shapes. Bone files are used in a back-and-forth motion to smooth the edges of alveolar bone. They trim and smooth the bone after the teeth have been extracted

and the rongeurs have contoured the bone (Figure 19-11).

Rongeurs

Rongeurs (**RON**-jeers) are hinged forceps that have springs in the handle. They are used to trim and shape the alveolar bone after extractions. The beaks are sharp and have cutting edges, similar to fingernail trimmers. There are several sizes and shapes of rongeurs. When multiple teeth are removed and a denture is to be seated, rongeurs are necessary to contour the ridges of the alveolar bone and eliminate sharp edges (Figure 19-12).

Periosteal Elevator

The **periosteal elevator** is an instrument of many uses and is included on most surgical tray setups. It is often used to detach the **periosteum** (bone covering) and gingival tissues from around the tooth prior to the use of extraction forceps. The periosteal elevator is also used to reflect and lift the **mucoperiosteum** (mucosa and periosteum) from the bone.

FIGURE 19-9 Surgical curettes.

FIGURE 19-10 Surgical chisel and mallet.

FIGURE 19-11 Surgical bone file.

FIGURE 19-12 Rongeurs.

Periosteal elevators are double-ended instruments with a variety of working-end combinations. Often, one end is pointed and the other is rounded (Figure 19-13).

Elevators

Elevators are used by the surgeon to loosen and remove teeth, retained roots, and root fragments. Elevators are designed in different shapes and sizes to accommodate the variety of tasks, operating techniques, and tooth morphology. They are single-ended instruments with large, bulbous, or T-shaped handles to allow for a firm grip. Being able to firmly grip the elevator allows the surgeon to exert the necessary force. The working ends of elevators may be straight or angular and are often paired left and right. Elevators are referred to by manufacturer's number or by designer names. Two common designer elevators are Potts and Cryers (Figure 19-14B and C).

Apical elevators are similar to the elevators with the large handle but have smaller working ends. They are either straight or angular and have longer, narrower blades to loosen and remove roots or root or bone fragments (Figure 19-14A).

(A)   (B)

(C)

FIGURE 19-14 Extraction elevators. (A) Apical. (B) Potts or T-handled. (C) Cryers. *(Courtesy of Miltex Instrument Co., Inc., Lake Success, NY)*

FIGURE 19-13 Periosteal elevators.

Root tip picks or elevators are even thinner and longer than the apical elevators. They are paired left and right and are also either straight or angled. The root tip picks are designed to tease the root tips or fragments out of the bone socket. They are delicate instruments that break if too much force is applied (Figure 19-15).

Forceps

Extraction forceps are used to remove teeth from the alveolar bone. They are hinged instruments with a variety of handles and beak styles. Specific forceps are used on certain teeth or in certain areas of the mouth. The dental assistant should be able to identify which forceps his or her dentist routinely uses. One way to learn

FIGURE 19-15 Root tip picks.

the forceps is by the manufacturer's number. Each instrument has a number imprinted on the handle and is labeled with an "L" or "R" for left or right. For example, a #88R is used on the maxillary right first and second molars.

Another way to identify the forceps is to learn how the design of the forceps is applicable to tooth morphology. Careful study of the various shapes of the beaks will allow determination of forceps for:

▶ The maxillary or mandibular teeth

▶ The right or left quadrant

▶ Anterior or posterior teeth

▶ Accommodating the anatomy of the teeth

For example, on #53R for the maxillary molars, there is one beak that is pointed for placement in the bifurcated buccal root. For the maxillary molars (88L), there is a pointed single beak on the buccal to be placed between the two buccal roots and a split beak on the lingual to engage the single lingual root.

The curve of the shank of the forceps indicates whether the forceps should be used on the maxillary or mandibular. Mandibular forceps are often at more of a right angle, and the maxillary are straight, slightly curved, or have two angles (like bayonets). For example, #17 forceps are used on the mandibular first and second molars; the beaks form an angle with the handle. The for-

FIGURE 19-16 Maxillary extraction forceps. (A) Incisors and root tips. (B) Incisors and cuspids. (C) #150 incisors, cuspids, bicuspids and roots—universal. (D) #88R and #88L first and second molars. (E) #53R and #53L first and second molars. (F) #210 third molars—universal. *(Courtesy Miltex Instrument Co., Inc., Lake Success, NY)*

ceps for the maxillary first and second molars has two angles in the working end of the forceps.

Some forceps are **universal forceps** and can be used on any of the four quadrants. For example, #101 forceps can be used for bicuspids and deciduous teeth in either arch. Other forceps can be used on either side in the same arch. For example, #150 forceps can be used for maxillary incisors, bicuspids, and roots on the left or right quadrant.

Forceps that are used on the anterior or the posterior teeth can be distinguished by the width of the beaks. For example, on mandibular forceps #151, the beaks are smaller in order to fit the incisors, bicuspids, and roots, while mandibular molar forceps #17 are wider to accommodate the width of the molars.

The shapes of the forceps beaks are designed to accommodate the anatomy of the specific teeth. For example, mandibular first and second molar forceps have narrow, pointed beaks to engage the bifurcated roots of these molars. These forceps are often called the "cow horns" because of their shape.

Extraction forceps are held in a palm grasp by the operator. Some handles are straight, while others have "finger rings" or hooks on the handles. The selection is the preference of the dentist.

To better visualize and learn the forceps, divide them into the arches and teeth they are used on (Figures 19-16 and 19-17).

ASEPSIS IN ORAL SURGERY

Like all dental offices, the oral and maxillofacial surgery office follows a plan for infection control. It is critical to prevent cross-contamination. The oral surgery office is at a higher risk because of the increased possibility of contact with blood.

Extraordinary care of surgical equipment and supplies is necessary in order to prevent accidental exposure. In the sterilizing room, an area should be designated for "unclean" trays, where the contaminated tray is taken apart and disposable sharps are placed in a marked sharps container. Expendable items such as gauze, cotton rolls, and so on are placed in marked hazardous waste containers. The instruments are cleaned and bagged or wrapped for sterilization. The bags are carefully marked with the procedure and date. The instruments are sterilized according to various methods, such as steam autoclaving, dry heat, or chemical vapor. Current OSHA guidelines should be followed (see Chapter 9, Infection Control).

Storage of Contaminated Instruments

If contaminated instruments cannot be processed immediately, they should be presoaked to prevent blood and debris from drying on them.

FIGURE 19-17 Mandibular extraction forceps. (A) Incisors, bicuspid, cuspids, and roots. (B) #151 incisors, cuspids, and roots—universal: (C) #23 first and second molars—universal "cow horns"; (D) #15 first and second molars—universal with finger ring; (E) #222 third molars—universal. *(Courtesy Miltex Instrument Co., Inc., Lake Success, NY)*

The Dentist and the Dental Assistant

The dentist and the dental assistant must follow the routine requirements of personal protective equipment (PPE) for all surgical procedures. One change is in the handwashing procedure. For oral surgery, the surgical hand scrub is completed before donning sterile gloves.

PATIENT CONSIDERATIONS

On the first visit, a medical history is completed by the patient. If surgery is anticipated, the surgeon may consult with the patient's physician about the patient's medications and physical conditions that may impact the surgical procedure.

Radiographs are sent from the general dental office to the oral surgeon's office before the patient is scheduled.

PROCEDURE

19-1 Surgical Scrub

This procedure is performed by the oral surgeon and the dental assistant before donning sterile gloves for a surgical procedure.

EQUIPMENT AND SUPPLIES

▶ Antimicrobial soap

▶ Sterile scrub brush or foam sponge

▶ Disposable sterile towels

PROCEDURE STEPS *(Follow aseptic procedure)*

1. Remove watch and rings before the scrub.

2. Use an antimicrobial soap, such as chlorhexidine gluconate.

3. Wet hands and forearms up to the elbows with warm water.

4. Dispense about 5 ml of soap into cupped hands and work into a lather.

5. Beginning with the fingernails, scrub the fingers, hands, and forearms with a surgical scrub brush.

6. Rinse thoroughly with warm water.

7. Repeat the procedure with soap but without the scrub brush.

8. Rinse with warm water, beginning at the fingertips and moving hands and forearms through the water and up so that the water drains off the forearms last (Figure 19-18). This prevents the hands from being recontaminated.

9. Dry hands and arms thoroughly with disposable sterile towels.

10. Don sterile surgical gloves.

NOTE: The surgical scrub was commonly referred to as the "five-minute scrub," but studies have indicated that scrub times of three to four minutes are as effec-

FIGURE 19-18 (A) Completion of surgical scrub. (B) Materials for surgical scrub.

tive as five-minute scrubs. The recommendation is to follow scrub product manufacturer's instructions and OSHA guidelines. Do not use a brush so stiff that it creates microscopic abrasions on the skin.

Periapical radiographs are commonly used for extractions, but extraoral radiographs such as panoramic, occlusal, lateral skull, cephalometric, and computerized tomography also may be required. (Specific extraoral exposures are explained in Chapter 17, Dental Radiography.)

 The oral surgeon completes a thorough examination. Once the diagnosis is made, the treatment options are explained to the patient. The patient must carefully read and sign an **informed consent** form prior to the procedure. The informed consent identifies and explains the surgery the patient is to receive and acknowledges any risks involved in the treatment.

PATIENT PREPARATION

Whether a general anesthetic is administered will determine the preoperative instructions given to the patient. It is important for the patient to follow the instructions carefully, prior to his or her appointment.

Typical Preoperative Instructions for the Patient

1. Wear loose-fitting clothing and low-heeled shoes. Your shirt should be short sleeved or easy to roll up.
2. Remove contact lenses before surgery.
3. Notify the dentist if a cold, a sore throat, a fever, or another illness develops prior to surgery.
4. Do not consume alcoholic beverages twenty-four hours before surgery.
5. Arrange transportation to and from the office on the day of the surgery.
6. When a physical examination is requested by the oral surgeon, have the physician send written approval prior to surgery.
7. Some medical conditions, such as rheumatic heart disease or artificial heart valves, require prophylactic antibiotics to be taken prior to surgery.
8. If the surgery is in the morning, do not eat anything after midnight. This includes medicines, food, and all fluids.*
9. If the surgery is in the afternoon, drink only water, juice, tea, or coffee prior to six a.m. After six a.m., take absolutely nothing by mouth.*

 * Food, liquids, or medications in the stomach when general anesthesia is administered may cause vomiting. The vomit may then be aspirated into the lungs.

Patient Preparation

1. The patient is escorted to the treatment room. The dental assistant checks the following: any changes in the medical history, whether the patient followed the preoperative instructions, and whether prescribed medication was taken as directed.

2. The patient is given an antimicrobial rinse.
3. The patient is seated and a full-length drape is placed on him or her. The patient is then reclined to a routine position for the dentist.
4. A sterile towel is placed over the patient's chest.
5. Vital signs are taken and recorded. The patient is prepared for administration of the intravenous sedation.

ORAL SURGERY PROCEDURES

 Common procedures performed in the oral surgeon's office are routine extractions, multiple extractions and alveoplasty, surgical removal of impacted third molars, biopsy procedures, and dental implant surgery.

Routine or Uncomplicated Extractions

Routine or uncomplicated extractions include the removal of permanent or primary teeth that are erupted into the oral cavity. These surgeries are usually less involved than other surgeries. The dental assistant prepares the tray setup and selects forceps and elevators for the specific tooth to be extracted.

Multiple Extractions and Alveoplasty

Multiple extractions are needed when the patient is going to have a full or partial denture. The extraction process is similar for one tooth or for several teeth, but after several teeth have been removed, the bone and soft tissue must be contoured and smoothed. The contouring process is called an **alveoplasty**. The alveolar ridge must be free of any sharp edges or points to achieve the best comfort and function for the patient. If both the maxillary and the mandibular teeth are to be extracted at one appointment, the maxillary teeth are extracted first. This prevents hemorrhage and debris from contaminating the mandibular extraction site during surgery. Routinely, the dentist starts at the most posterior tooth and moves anteriorly.

Impacted Teeth Extractions

Extracting impacted teeth is one of the most common procedures the oral surgeon performs, especially third molar extractions (Figure 19-23). There are many factors that determine the difficulty of the impacted tooth extraction, including the depth, position, or angulation of the tooth in the bone. The teeth may be impacted in soft tissue or in the bone. If the teeth are impacted in bone, dental handpieces and surgical burs are required in order to gain access. Additional surgical instruments are utilized to facilitate the removal of the tooth from the bone. Often, all third molars are removed at one appointment.

PROCEDURE

19-2 Routine or Uncomplicated Extraction

The dental assistant assists the oral surgeon throughout this procedure. The dental assistant must be prepared and thinking ahead to anticipate the surgeon's needs.

EQUIPMENT AND SUPPLIES (Figure 19-19)

FIGURE 19-19 Tray setup for uncomplicated extraction.

- Mouth mirror
- Gauze sponges
- Surgical HVE tip
- Retractor for the tongue and the cheek
- Local anesthetic setup
- Nitrous oxide setup (optional)
- Periosteal elevator
- Straight elevator
- Extraction forceps
- Hemostat/needle holder
- Surgical curette
- Suture setup

PROCEDURE STEPS (*Follow aseptic procedures*)

1. The surgeon examines the site of extraction. *The dental assistant transfers the mouth mirror and explorer to the surgeon. The patient's x-rays are mounted on the viewbox for the dentist to review.*

2. Topical anesthetic is placed on the mucosa and local anesthetic is administered. *The dental assistant prepares the topical anesthetic and transfers it to the surgeon (if allowed by the state Practice Act,*

the dental assistant can place the topical anesthetic). The syringe is prepared and transferred to the surgeon. The dental assistant then observes the patient.

3. Either the periosteal or a straight elevator is used by the oral surgeon to determine whether the patient is adequately numb, to separate epithelial attachment from around the tooth, and to initiate alveolar bone expansion around the neck of the tooth (to accommodate forceps placement). *The dental assistant transfers and receives elevators and has gauze ready to remove blood or debris from the instruments. The dental assistant maintains the operating field, adjusts the light, and retracts tissues as needed.*

4. Once the tooth is loosened in the alveolus, forceps are placed securely on the tooth and, with a firm grasp, the surgeon **luxates** (moves or dislocates) the tooth and then removes it from the socket. This may be easy, or the tooth may have to be subluxated (rocked back and forth), rotated, and lifted several times before the bone around the tooth is spread enough to lift the tooth out of the socket. *During this time, the dental assistant transfers forceps and elevators as needed by the surgeon, keeps the instruments clean of debris, and retracts the cheek or tongue. The dental assistant should observe the patient for signs of anxiety or syncope. Once the tooth is extracted, the forceps beaks and tooth are received in the palm of the dental assistant's hand while transferring gauze to the surgeon (Figure 19-20). Once the forceps*

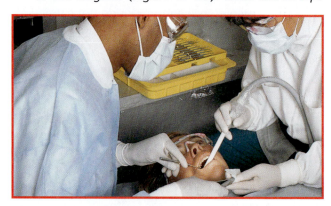

FIGURE 19-20 Dental assistant receiving extraction forceps with tooth in beaks.

(continued)

and tooth are placed on the tray, the tooth is examined for fractured roots.

5. The alveolus (socket) is examined for fractured root tips and debris. A surgical curette is used to remove bone chips, granulation tissue, and abscesses/cysts. *The dental assistant evacuates the alveolus using the surgical HVE tip, then transfers the surgical curette. A gauze is held close to the patient's chin to remove debris from the curette.*

6. Once the tooth and any fragments are removed, the area is debrided and the wound is covered with a folded, moistened gauze as a pressure pack. The patient is instructed to bite down on the gauze to apply pressure. This aids in controlling the bleeding and the formation of the blood clot.

7. The dentist may place sutures at this point in the procedure. *The dental assistant prepares the sutures and assists during placement (see Chapter 28, Advanced Chairside Techniques). The dental assistant debrides the site with the HVE and has the moistened gauze folded and ready to place.*

8. *The dental assistant checks and cleans the patient's face, returns the patient to a sitting position, and allows a few minutes before giving postoperative instructions. The patient is then dismissed.*

P R O C E D U R E

19-3 Multiple Extractions and Alveoplasty

The procedure is performed by the oral surgeon, who is assisted by the dental assistant. This sterile procedure involves the removal of several teeth and contouring the bone. Responsibilities of the dental assistant include evacuation and instrument transfer.

EQUIPMENT AND SUPPLIES (Figure 19-21)

FIGURE 19-21 Tray setup for multiple extractions and alveoplasty.

▶ Mouth mirror

▶ Gauze sponges

▶ Surgical HVE tip

▶ Luer lok syringe and sterile saline solution

▶ Retractor for the tongue and cheeks

▶ Local anesthetic setup

▶ Nitrous oxide setup (optional)

▶ Scalpel and blades

▶ Hemostat and tissue retractors

▶ Periosteal elevator

▶ Straight elevator

▶ Extraction forceps (selected for the teeth being extracted)

▶ Surgical curette

▶ Root tip picks

▶ Rongeurs

▶ Bone file

▶ Low-speed handpiece and surgical burs

▶ Suture setup

PROCEDURE STEPS (*Follow aseptic procedures*)

1. The surgeon examines the teeth to be extracted.

2. When several teeth are going to be extracted, the

(continued)

P R O C E D U R E   **19-3** *continued*

patient may request general anesthesia. The patient will be prepared for intravenous sedation, which is followed by local anesthetic. The local anesthetic reduces bleeding at the extraction site and postoperative pain. *The dental assistant prepares the materials necessary for the local and intravenous anesthetic and then assists in the administration.*

3. The teeth are removed by the same techniques described for the routine extraction.

4. After the teeth have been extracted and any root tips or debris removed, the alveoplasty procedure begins. The alveoplasty usually is accomplished one quadrant at a time. The surgeon makes an incision on the buccal and lingual surface, to remove the interdental papillae and to expose the crest of the alveolar bone. The flap of tissue is reflected for clear vision. *The dental assistant transfers the scalpel and evacuates the area as necessary, receives the scalpel, and transfers the periosteal elevator to reflect the soft tissue. The dental assistant uses tissue forceps to retract the tissue and maintain the operating area.*

5. Rongeurs and/or surgical burs are used for the initial trimming and contouring of the alveolar bone. *The dental assistant transfers the rongeurs and/or the low-speed handpiece with surgical burs and keeps them free of debris. The dental assistant intermittently uses the HVE and the irrigation syringe with sterile saline solution to maintain the operating field.*

6. Final contouring and smoothing are done with the bone file. The area is rinsed with sterile saline

solution. At this point, a **plastic stint** (clear denture base material, molded to the same shape and size as the denture) is placed in the patient's mouth. Areas that are impinging on the stint can be seen by the surgeon. The surgeon continues to contour the bone until all interferences are removed. *The dental assistant transfers instruments and continues to maintain the surgical site. The stint needs to be kept clean, so the dental assistant removes blood and debris from the stint between placements.*

7. The buccal and lingual flaps are repositioned and sutured into position. *The dental assistant prepares the suture materials and, once the tissue is in position, the suture is transferred for placement. The dental assistant assists during the suture procedure and holds the tissue as the surgeon places the sutures (see Chapter 28, Advanced Chairside Functions.).*

8. A folded, moist gauze pack is placed over the surgical site or the immediate denture is seated. *The dental assistant prepares the gauze pack and transfers it to the surgeon. If the patient receives an immediate denture, the dental assistant readies the denture and transfers it to the surgeon for placement.*

9. The patient is allowed to recover and then postoperative instructions are given both verbally and written.

10. The patient is scheduled for a postoperative examination and suture removal.

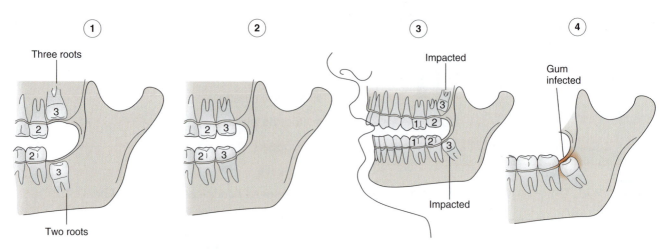

Wisdom teeth (No. 3 above) develop *inside* the bone. Crowns form first, then the roots.

If the jaw grows long enough, the wisdom teeth can erupt and be used.

If the jaws are not long enough by age 16, wisdom teeth stay trapped *(impacted)* inside the bone.

Impacted wisdom teeth can cause:

(A) Infection of the gums over or around them.

FIGURE 19-22 Problem caused by impacted wisdom teeth.

(continued)

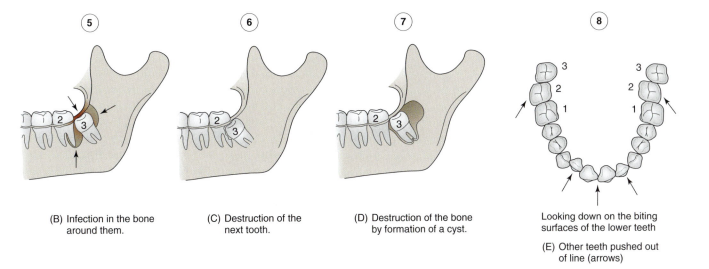

(B) Infection in the bone around them.

(C) Destruction of the next tooth.

(D) Destruction of the bone by formation of a cyst.

Looking down on the biting surfaces of the lower teeth

(E) Other teeth pushed out of line (arrows)

FIGURE 19-22

P R O C E D U R E

19-4 Removal of Impacted Third Molars

This procedure, bony impaction, is performed by the oral surgeon, who is assisted by the dental assistant. This is a sterile procedure. Because the teeth are impacted, the surgeon will first have to expose the teeth by incising the tissue and removing the bone (Figure 19-22). The dental assistant transfers instruments and maintains the operating site.

EQUIPMENT AND SUPPLIES

▶ Basic setup: mouth mirror, explorer, and cotton pliers

▶ Gauze sponges

▶ Surgical HVE tip

▶ Irrigating syringe and sterile saline solution

▶ Retractor for the tongue and the cheek

▶ Local anesthetic setup

▶ Nitrous oxide setup (optional)

▶ Scalpel and blades

▶ Hemostat and tissue retractors

▶ Periosteal elevator

▶ Straight elevator

▶ Extraction forceps (if needed)

▶ Root tip picks

▶ Surgical curette

▶ Rongeurs

▶ Bone file

▶ Low-speed handpiece and surgical burs

▶ Suture setup

PROCEDURE STEPS *(Follow aseptic procedures)*

1. The anesthetic is administered. Oral sedation may be used with local anesthetic, but the most common is intravenous (IV) anesthesia. *The dental assistant prepares and transfers the anesthetic and/or assists with the IV.*

2. When the patient is adequately anesthetized, an incision is made along the ridge, distal to the second molar. The scalpel incises the mucoperiosteum to the underlying bone. Depending on where the impacted tooth lies, a flap incision may be made to ensure adequate vision for the surgeon. *The dental assistant transfers the scalpel and maintains the operating field with the surgical HVE (Figure 19-23A).*

3. The periosteal elevator is used to retract the tissue from the alveolar bone. *Once the tissue is incised, it must be reflected from the bone. The dental assistant transfers the periosteal elevator and evacuates. When the flap is completed, the dental assistant retracts the tissue (Figure 19-23B).*

(continued)

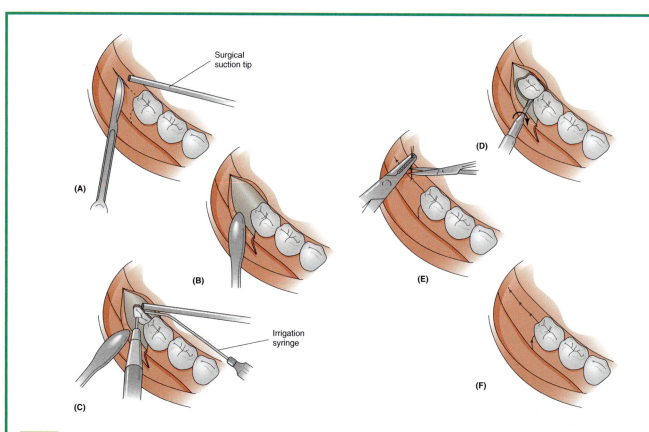

FIGURE 19-23 Steps to remove impacted third molars. (A) Flap incision is made, assistant evacuates the area. (B) Periosteal elevator is used to retract the tissue. (C) Surgical bur is used to remove the bone over the tooth. The dental assistant evacuates and irrigates the area. (D) Elevator luxates and removes the tooth. (E) Sutures are placed. (F) Completion of surgery.

4. The surgeon uses a surgical bur and handpiece or a chisel and mallet to remove the bone over the tooth. *The dental assistant receives the periosteal elevator and transfers the handpiece and bur or the chisel. The dental assistant continues to evacuate as needed* (Figure 19-23C).

5. Once the tooth is exposed, it can often be luxated and lifted from the socket with elevators or forceps. If this is not possible, the tooth may be sectioned or divided for removal. This involves dividing the tooth into two or more parts. Burs and/or the chisel are used to separate the tooth in half to remove part or all of the crown of the tooth from the root portion. *The dental assistant passes elevators and forceps. The dental assistant keeps the area clear with the HVE and periodically transfers the surgeon new gauze* (Figure 19-23D).

6. When the tooth is removed, it is placed on a flat surface and examined to ensure that all of the tooth has been removed.

7. Curettes are used to remove the follicle (sac of thickened membrane) and debride the socket. The rongeurs, bone files, or burs may be used to contour the bone margins. The area is then irrigated with sterile water and evacuated. *The dental assistant transfers instruments and removes debris from the working ends with gauze. The dental assistant prepares the irrigating syringe with sterile water and evacuates the area thoroughly.*

8. The tissue flap is replaced to its normal position over the wound, and the operator sutures the area. *The dental assistant prepares the suture and places it in the needle holder and transfers it to the oral surgeon. The cheeks are then retracted so that the surgeon can place the sutures* (Figures 19-23E and F). *The dental assistant has a folded, moist gauze ready to place when suturing is completed.*

9. The patient is allowed to recover and is given postoperative instructions, an ice pack, and a prescription for pain before being dismissed. The patient will need to schedule an appointment for suture removal in five to seven days. *The dental assistant stays with the patient during recovery. When the patient is ready to leave, the dental assistant notifies the patient's escort and verifies that the patient has the necessary prescription(s) and postoperative instructions.*

Biopsy Procedures

With every patient, the dentist and staff must be aware of any abnormal tissue. Through the clinical examination, x-rays, or patient complaints, the presence of pathology may be discovered. Early detection of premalignant and/or malignant conditions can save lives. Once the suspicious lesion or area is recognized, the dentist will want a **biopsy**. The biopsy procedure, performed by an oral surgeon, involves removal of tissue from a suspicious area, either totally or partially, for microscopic examination and diagnosis. There are three types of biopsy techniques: excisional, incisional, and exfoliative.

The Incisional Biopsy. The **incisional biopsy** involves removal of a small section of the lesion, which includes a small border of normal tissue (Figure 19-24A). This technique is often performed on lesions larger than 1 cm in all dimensions, where total removal is more difficult and patient appearance and function are impaired.

The Excisional Biopsy. The **excisional biopsy** involves removal of the lesion completely, including a border of the normal tissue surrounding it (Figure 19-24B). The excisional biopsy is performed for smaller lesions such as fibromas. The total removal of the lesions does not interfere with the patient's appearance or functioning.

The Exfoliative Cytology. The **exfoliative cytology**, or "smear biopsy," involves removal of a layer of cells from the surface of the lesion. This is a non-surgical procedure in which the gathered cells are spread on a glass slab. This technique is used as an adjunct to the surgical biopsy techniques and is also performed by an oral surgeon.

Postoperative Care of the Patient

Following oral surgery, the patient is given postoperative home-care instructions. The instructions are given routinely by a dental assistant at the direction of the surgeon. The dental assistant gives the instructions verbally to the patient and the patient's escort. In addition, a written copy of the instructions with the office phone number is given to the patient, along with necessary prescriptions.

Postoperative Home-Care Instructions

It is important to carefully read and follow these instructions in order to prevent needless worry. Have someone with you for twenty-four hours following the surgery. Treatment continues until the healing process is completed.

What to expect:

1. **Discomfort** reaches a peak when the anesthetic wears off and sensation returns.
2. **Swelling** is normal following a surgical procedure. The swelling will continue up to twenty-four hours after surgery and can persist for four to five days. Facial discoloration may appear but will disappear in a day or so.

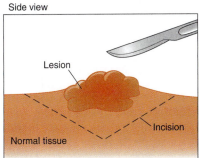

(A) (B)

FIGURE 19-24 Biopsy techniques.

P R O C E D U R E

19-5 Biopsy

This procedure is performed by the oral surgeon, who is assisted by the dental assistant. The dental assistant readies all materials that are sent to the laboratory as well as the tray setup.

EQUIPMENT AND SUPPLIES

▶ Mouth mirror

▶ Local anesthetic setup

▶ Retractors (tongue, cheek, and tissue)

▶ Gauze sponges

▶ Surgical HVE tip

▶ Scalpel and blades

▶ Tissue scissors and hemostat

▶ Small container with a preservative solution, such as formalin

▶ Suture setup

PROCEDURE STEPS (*Follow aseptic procedures*)

1. The patient is anesthetized with local anesthetic.

2. A scalpel blade is used to incise or excise the lesion and a border of normal tissue. *The dental assistant transfers the scalpel with the specific blade the surgeon prefers and has the HVE ready for use, if necessary. The dental assistant uses caution to remove only blood and saliva and not the tissue being removed for biopsy.*

3. Tissue forceps are used to lift the biopsy specimen once freed from the underlying tissue and to place it in a small, covered container. *The dental assistant retracts the cheeks and tongue, if needed, and uses gauze to control hemorrhage. The dental assistant has the specimen container ready for the surgeon. Care is taken not to touch the outside of the specimen container in order to prevent contamination. Once the tissue biopsy in placed in the container, the dental assistant replaces the cap tightly.*

4. The biopsy site is closed with sutures. The surgeon then prepares the biopsy and the necessary information to be sent to the pathology laboratory. *The dental assistant assists during the placement of sutures by transferring the suture needle and thread on needle forceps, retracting tissues, and transferring the suture scissors.*

5. The patient is dismissed and scheduled for an appointment in one week for the results of the biopsy and suture removal. *The dental assistant gives the patient postoperative instructions. The dental assistant gathers the pertinent information and prepares the biopsy container for pickup by the pathology laboratory.*

---

3. **Bleeding** or oozing may occur for the first twelve to twenty-four hours after surgery. The surgeon will place a sterile gauze in your mouth to bite on immediately following surgery. Remove the gauze when the oozing has stopped.

4. **Difficulty opening mouth, a sore throat,** and **earaches** are not uncommon, especially if third molars were removed.

What to do:

1. Begin taking pain medication before the discomfort begins and the anesthetic wears off. Over-the-counter analgesics are suggested for minor discomfort, and the surgeon will prescribe a stronger medication for pain control, if necessary. Take medications as directed to avoid nausea and vomiting.

2. Use an ice pack to reduce the swelling as soon as possible. Apply the pack to the face over the extraction site for twenty minutes and then remove for twenty minutes (twenty minutes on, twenty minutes off). Continue this cycle intermittently throughout the first twelve to twenty-four hours. After forty-eight hours if the swelling has not subsided, use moist heat.

3. The best means to control bleeding is pressure. To accomplish the pressure needed, place a folded gauze over the surgical site and bite down. Change the sterile gauze pads as needed. If the bleeding persists, insert a wet tea bag over the surgical site and bite down for about twenty minutes. Tea contains tannic acid, which assists in the clotting process.

4. A soft diet should be followed for twenty-four hours. Eat a well-balanced diet with soups, fruit juices, milk shakes, and other foods, as tolerated. Drink fluids to prevent dehydration and temperature elevation.

5. Take medications to prevent infection as directed.
6. Continue brushing and flossing areas not involved in surgery.
7. Sleep with your head elevated to reduce swelling.
8. Avoid vigorous physical exercise.
9. Rest as much as possible for the first couple of days following surgery to promote healing.

Things to avoid:

1. Avoid strenuous physical activity for forty-eight hours.
2. Do not suck through a straw and avoid spitting.
3. Do not smoke or chew gum.
4. Do not drive, drink alcohol, or operate machinery while taking pain medication.
5. If immediate dentures have been inserted, do not remove until your next appointment, usually within twenty-four hours of surgery.

6. Do not rinse vigorously for forty-eight hours after surgery. After this time, rinse gently with warm salt-water solution.

IF YOU HAVE ANY QUESTIONS OR PROBLEMS, PLEASE CALL THE OFFICE.

DR. _____ TELEPHONE # _____

Postsurgical Complications

Alveolitis (alveolar osteitis), or **dry socket**, is the most common complication following an extraction. The loss of the blood clot leaves a dry socket, which is very painful. Alveolitis usually develops between the third and the fifth day after surgery. In the normal process after an extraction, blood oozes into the socket and begins clotting. The clot is later replaced by connective tissue and eventually bone tissue. In some extractions, this process does not happen and the blood clot either

P R O C E D U R E

19-6 Treatment for Alveolitis

This procedure is performed by the oral surgeon who is assisted by the dental assistant.

EQUIPMENT AND SUPPLIES (Figure 19-25)

▶ Mouth mirror

▶ Surgical HVE tip

▶ Local anesthetic setup (may be required)

▶ Surgical scissors

▶ Surgical curettes

▶ Irrigating syringe and warm, sterile, saline solution

▶ Iodoform gauze or sponge

PROCEDURE STEPS (*Follow aseptic procedures*)

1. Anesthetic may be administered. The sutures are removed.

2. The surgeon may gently curettage the area inside the socket to stimulate the formation of a new blood clot.

FIGURE 19-25 Tray setup for alveolitis treatment.

3. The alveolus (socket) is gently irrigated with the warm saline solution. *The dental assistant prepares the syringe and maintains the area by retraction and evacuation.*

(continued)

4. The alveolus is gently packed with a medicated dressing. Narrow strips of iodoform gauze or iodoform sponge are used for packing the socket. *The dental assistant prepares and transfers the materials to the surgeon for placement* (Figure 19-26).

5. The surgeon prescribes medication for pain control, and the patient is scheduled to return in one to two days to repeat this process.

FIGURE 19-26 Examples of iodoform gauze and sponge packing materials. Dental assistant prepares to pass the gauze packing.

does not form or forms and is lost. The exact etiology for this phenomenon is not clear, but insufficient blood supply to the area, infection, or trauma seem to play a role. The mandibular third molars seem to be the most frequent sites for dry socket to occur.

The signs are extreme pain, foul breath and taste, exposed bone, and an empty socket.

DENTAL IMPLANTS

Dental implants are becoming an increasingly popular procedure to replace missing teeth. The implant is a metal screw or metal framework that is placed in the bone (Figure 19-27). Titanium is used because it is compatible with human tissue. The implant becomes fused with the bone tissue. This process is called **osseointegration**. Once the implant is integrated and stable in the bone, a fixed or removable prosthesis is fabricated. The prosthesis may be a single crown, bridge, partial, or denture.

Dental implants give the option for a fixed or permanent restoration that is both functional and esthetic. For patients with little bone to support a denture or partial, dental implants restore confidence, comfort, and function. Implants also allow for missing teeth to be replaced without involvement of the adjacent teeth.

The patient who is interested in dental implants should be in reasonably good health with adequate alveolar bone, have a positive and cooperative attitude toward the implant treatment, and be dedicated to the care of the implants once they are placed.

It can take up to nine months to complete all phases of the dental implant process, and the treatment is more expensive than traditional treatment. Patients must be advised that it is a surgical procedure and that there is a chance for infection and other complications.

Types of Implants

The two most common types of dental implants include the subperiosteal and the endosteal.

Subperiosteal Implants. The **subperiosteal implant** is often used on patients whose dentures have failed because the alveolar bone has atrophied (wasted away). Subperiosteal implants are most commonly placed on the mandible. The titanium implant rests on top of the alveolar bone with abutment posts or bars above the mucoperiosteum in the cuspid and first molar area. The

(A)   (B)

FIGURE 19-27 Dental implant. (A) Actual size of implant. (B) Model of the implant used for patient education.

denture connects to this structure for support and retention (Figure 19-28).

The subperisoteal implant requires one or two surgeries, depending on the technique.

Single-Surgery Technique This technique involves fabricating the impression for the implant on a model. The model is constructed by using computed tomography (CT) scans. After the implant is fabricated on the model, surgery is performed to incise the tissue and expose the alveolar bone. The implant is seated on the bone and the tissue is sutured back into place.

Two-Surgery Technique During the first surgery, the tissue is incised and the alveolar bone is exposed. Then, an impression is taken. The impression is sent to the laboratory for the subperisoteal implant to be fabricated. Within a week, the patient returns to the office for the

FIGURE 19-28 Example of subperiosteal implant.

P R O C E D U R E

19-7 **Dental Implant Surgery**

 The following procedure is for the placement of an endosteal implant for a single tooth replacement. This is a two-stage procedure in which the appointments are scheduled three to four months apart. During the presurgery appointment, the treatment is explained in detail and the patient signs a written consent for the implant surgery. Radiographs are taken, impressions for diagnostic casts are made, surgical templates (guides) are fabricated, and financial arrangements are completed. The patient is given intravenous sedation for this procedure.

EQUIPMENT AND SUPPLIES (Figure 19-29)

For first surgical procedure:

▶ Intravenous sedation and local anesthetic setup
▶ Mouth mirror
▶ Surgical HVE tip

(A)

(B)

FIGURE 19-29 (A) Tray setup for implant surgery. (B) Surgical barrier kit.

P R O C E D U R E   **1 9 - 7** *continued*

▶ Sterile gauze and cotton pellets

▶ Irrigation syringe and sterile saline solution

▶ Low-speed handpiece

▶ Sterile template

▶ Sterile surgical drilling unit

▶ Scalpel and blades

▶ Periosteal elevator

▶ Rongeurs

▶ Surgical currette

▶ Tissue forceps and scissors

▶ Cheek and tongue retractors

▶ Hemostat

▶ Bite-block

▶ Oral rinse

▶ Betadine

▶ Implant instrument kit

▶ Implant kit

▶ Suture setup

For second surgical procedure:

▶ First seven items from first procedure

▶ Electrosurgical (cautery) unit and tips (Figure 19-30)

▶ Hydrogen peroxide

PROCEDURE STEPS

First Surgery for Endosteal Implants

1. The patient is prepared and IV sedation is administered. Local anesthetic is administered. *The dental assistant prepares and assists during the administration of sedation and anesthetic.*

FIGURE 19-30 Electrosurge cauterizing unit.

2. The surgical template is seated in the patient's mouth. The target is marked through the template into the soft tissues.

3. The template is removed and the surgeon incises the tissue to expose the ridge of bone. *The dental assistant prepares and transfers the scalpel and blade while maintaining the operating site.*

4. A periosteal elevator is used to reflect the overlying tissues. Special spiral burs are used to prepare for the implant. *The dental assistant changes burs as size increases and irrigates with the sterile saline solution.*

5. The implant is partially placed and then tapped or threaded into position. *The dental assistant opens the sterile implant and transfers it to the surgeon. A special inserting mallet or ratchet wrench is transferred, and the dental assistant readies the healing cap and contra-angle screwdriver.*

6. A healing cap is screwed into the implant. *The dental assistant passes the healing cap and the contra-angle screwdriver (Figure 19-31A).*

7. Once the implant and healing cap are positioned, the flap is repositioned and sutured.

8. The patient is allowed to recover and given postoperative instructions.

Second Surgical Procedure

1. Local anesthetic is administered.

2. The template is positioned over the osseointegrated implant and a sharp-pointed instrument is

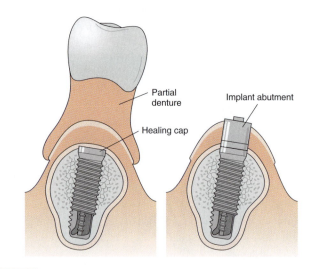

Partial denture

Healing cap

Implant abutment

FIGURE 19-31 Implant placement procedure for the (A) first-stage and (B) second-stage surgery for an endosteal implant.

used to mark the site. *The dental assistant transfers the sterile template and a sharp-pointed instrument.*

3. The template is removed and the soft tissue is excised with an electrosurgical loop. Once the healing screw is exposed, it is removed. *The dental assistant receives the template and evacuates as the electrosurgical loop is used. Once the tissue is excised, the dental assistant receives the healing screw in a gauze sponge.*

4. The inside of the implant is cleaned with hydrogen peroxide on a sterile cotton pellet. *The dental assistant prepares the cotton pellet and transfers it to the surgeon.*

5. The implant abutment is placed so that it extends slightly beyond the mucosa. The mucosa is then sutured around the abutment. *The abutment is transferred to the surgeon and then the dental assistant prepares the suture material and assists during the suturing* (Figure 19-31B).

6. The patient is given postoperative instructions and is dismissed.

second surgery. The tissue is opened and the implant is seated. A transitional appliance is used while a final denture is made, which usually takes four to six weeks.

Endosteal Implants. The **endosteal implants** are placed in the bone surgically. These implants are used to replace a single tooth and for patients who are partially edentulous. The endosteal implants are placed when there is sufficient ridge width and at least 2 mm between the implant and the mandibular canal.

These implants are, in themselves, expensive, as is the equipment required to place them. There are two basic designs of the endosteal implants: the *blade* and the *screw* (Figure 19-32).

The technique for the endosteal implants is a two-stage insertion system. (Procedure 19-7) The implant is placed in the alveolar bone and then allowed to heal for three to four months. The second surgery follows osseointegration of the implant. An incision is made over the implant and a healing cap is placed. After the tissues have healed, the patient returns for the crown, bridge, or partial denture.

HOSPITAL DENTISTRY

Most procedures are performed in the oral maxillofacial surgeon's office, but some cases require a hospital setting. The surgeon follows the protocol of the hospital to meet scheduling, staffing, and credentialing standards. Some hospitals allow dental assistants to assist the oral surgeons, after the dental assistants meet the hospital standards on asepsis and operating room protocol.

Patients who require hospitalization for dental treatment include:

▶ Trauma victims with facial and jaw fractures.

▶ Patients with high-risk conditions or diseases (e.g., heart disease or diabetes)

▶ This also includes patients with mental or physical disabilities who could not tolerate surgery in an office setting.

▶ Patients who require extensive surgical procedures such as temporomandibular joint surgery or **orthognathic surgery**.

(A)

(B)

FIGURE 19-32 Example of endosteal implants. (A) The blade. (B) The screw.

CHAPTER SUMMARY

The dental surgery team may vary according to the goals of the surgeon concerning the practice. In addition to the oral and maxillofacial surgeon, the team usually consists of the receptionist, the business office staff, the dental assistants, and, in some offices, a nurse or an anesthesiologist.

The surgical dental assistant's responsibilities often vary depending on the size of the practice. The option to become a Certified Dental Assistant in Oral and Maxillofacial Surgery (COMSA) is available upon successful completion of an examination administered by the Dental Assisting National Board.

CASE STUDY

Josiah Scott, forty-five years old, had his maxillary first molar removed a few years ago. The patient is not experiencing any pain but has noticed that his teeth seem to be shifting. The adjacent teeth are rotating into the space left by the first molar, and the opposing first molar is super-erupting. Mr. Scott is scheduled for an examination by Dr. Manwell, who is an oral surgeon.

Case Study Review

1. Why would Mr. Scott make an appointment with an oral surgeon?

2. What procedure would correct Mr. Scott's problem?

3. What would the dental assistant need to prepare for the examination appointment?

4. What other dental professionals would be involved in Mr. Scott's treatment?

To complete your study of this chapter, work the review activities that follow. Also, refer to the software that accompanies this text.

REVIEW QUESTIONS

Multiple Choice

1. Which of the following instruments is used to retract tissue, remove small root tips, and clamp off blood vessels?
   a. Needle holder.
   b. Hemostat.
   c. Tissue retractor.
   d. Surgical curette.

2. Which teeth are "cow-horn" forceps used to extract?
   a. Maxillary bicuspids.
   b. Maxillary molars.
   c. Mandibular bicuspids.
   d. Mandibular molars.

3. During surgical handwashing, the dental assistant scrubs with a scrub brush and then repeats the process with soap but without the scrub brush. How long does it take to complete this process?
   a. Fifteen seconds.
   b. Thirty seconds.
   c. One minute.
   d. Five minutes.

4. Before the surgery is scheduled but after the patient's records and examination are completed, the patient must
   a. sign an informed consent.
   b. sign a waiver from the patient's general dentist.
   c. register with the oral surgeon's office.
   d. bring proof of identification to the oral surgeon's office.

5. Which of the following biopsy techniques is non-surgical and is used as an adjunct to the other surgical techniques?
   a. The incisional biopsy.
   b. The excisional biopsy.
   c. The exfoliative cytology.

Critical Thinking

1. Why are the maxillary forceps designed for the left or the right quadrant and the mandibular forceps are not?

2. If a patient is having multiple extractions in preparation for a full denture, identify and explain the procedure that immediately follows the extractions.

3. List the dental assistant's responsibilities during surgical procedures.

Oral Pathology

OBJECTIVES

The student should strive to meet the following objectives and demonstrate an understanding of the facts and principles presented in this chapter:

1. Define oral pathology and identify the dental assistant's role in this specialty.

2. Characterize the process of inflammation.

3. Identify oral lesions according to their placement.

4. Identify the oral diseases and the lesions related to biological agents.

5. Describe the oral diseases and the lesions related to physical agents.

6. Identify the oral diseases and the lesions related to chemical agents.

7. Identify the oral conditions related to hormonal disturbances.

8. Identify the oral conditions related to developmental disturbances.

9. Distinguish the oral conditions related to nutritional disturbances.

10. Identify the conditions and the lesions of oral neoplasms.

11. Identify the oral lesions related to HIV and AIDS.

12. Describe the conditions related to miscellaneous disorders affecting the oral cavity.

KEY TERMS

abscess (p. 423)

actinomycosis (p. 423)

angular cheilitis (p. 432)

ankylosis (p. 429)

anodontia (p. 429)

aphthous ulcers (p. 424)

biopsy (p. 422)

blister (p. 423)

bulla (p. 423)

candida albicans (p. 432)

canker sores (p. 424)

cleft lip (p. 429)

cleft palate (p. 429)

cyst (p. 423)

dysplasic cells (p. 433)

ecchymosis (p. 423)

etiology (p. 422)

fissured tongue (p. 431)

Fordyce's spots (p. 431)

granuloma (p. 423)

hematoma (p. 423)

herpes labialis (p. 424)

herpes zoster (p. 424)

herpetic gingivostomatitis (p. 424)

herpetic whitlow (p. 424)

histamine (p. 422)

human immunodeficiency virus (HIV) (p. 435)

(continued)

INTRODUCTION

Oral pathology is defined as the study of oral diseases, their causes (if known), and their effects on the body. A dental assistant does not diagnose oral pathological diseases but may alert the dentist to abnormal conditions in the mouth. The dental assistant must recognize abnormal conditions and know how to prevent disease transmission, how the identified pathological condition may interfere with planned treatment, and what effect the condition will have on the overall health of the patient.

Oral pathology can originate from a number of different agents or disturbances. Biological, physical, and chemical agents may bring on a disease condition that exhibits signs within the oral cavity. Hormonal, developmental, and nutritional disturbances will also show disease signs within the mouth. Other disorders and reactions to stress and **antigenic** (capable of causing the production of an antibody) substances, as well as neoplasms and cysts, develop within the oral cavity. The dental assistant has a different viewpoint of the patient's oral cavity sitting on the opposite side of the patient. Anything that appears to be atypical should be brought to the attention of the dentist for further investigation, without alarming the patient. Any unusual oral **lesions**, an all-encompassing term for abnormal structures in the oral cavity, must be more closely observed by the dentist. The dentist may **palpate** (feel with fingers) or perform a procedure called a biopsy on the suspicious lesion. A **biopsy** (the removal of a small amount of the tissue surgically) is an accurate method of diagnosing many illnesses. After the diagnosis is made, further study is done to identify the **etiology** (cause of the disease). This biopsy normally is sent to a pathologist for examination under the microscope and further diagnosis. The dentist includes any information that he or she observes clinically or through palpation, such as size, location, color, and texture. Other information about the lesion may include how long the lesion has been present, if it is painful to touch, whether the area seems hot, and what the patient identifies as starting the situation. All of this information, as obtained from the patient, should be documented. Any additional information that the doctor thinks is pertinent should be sent to the laboratory along with the biopsy.

INFLAMMATION

The body responds to disease and injury with a process known as **inflammation**. Specialized cells in the area give off a number of chemicals, one of which is called a **histamine**. Histamine is said to bring about the inflammation process. It increases blood flow to the involved area and causes redness and heat. It also makes the blood capillaries more hyperemic (increased amount of blood) and fluid oozes from them into the tissues, causing swelling. When the nerve endings in the area are stimulated by these chemicals, the pain occurs. Four conditions are an essential part of the body's response to injury or disease: redness (erythema), heat, swelling (edema), and pain.

Inflammatory Process

▶ Redness
▶ Heat
▶ Swelling
▶ Pain

White blood vessels are attracted to the chemicals of inflammation. White blood vessels seek out the area to help destroy the invading microorganisms and aid in the healing process. The area is encircled by a fibrous connective tissue to prevent the spread of the condition to any other area.

ORAL LESIONS

The abnormal tissues in the oral cavity, called lesions, are further classified according to their placement in the surface of the mucosa. They can be classified as above the surface, below the surface, or even or flat with the surface of the oral mucosa.

Lesions Classified Above the Surface of the Oral Mucosa

▶ A **blister** is a raised area, usually oval or circular in shape, that is fluid filled. This fluid leaks from the blood vessels to underlying layers of skin following some type of trauma, such as burn, friction, or disease. This fluid protects the damaged tissue.

▶ A **bulla** (**BULL**-ah) is a large (greater than one-half inch in diameter) fluid-filled blister.

▶ A **hematoma** is a lesion caused by bleeding from a ruptured blood vessel, which appears as a raised bruised area due to the collection of localized, clotted blood. Dental assistants should watch for a hematoma after oral anesthetic. Even the best clinicians may nick a blood vessel during an injection, resulting in hematoma. The dental assistant alerts the dentist about the condition and then applies pressure to the area to disperse the blood in the tissue, which alleviates the pressure in the area.

▶ A **papule** is a small (less than one-half inch in diameter), solid, raised area of skin. The surface of the papule may be pigmented in color and either smooth or bumpy in texture.

▶ **Plaque** is any raised or flat patch in the oral mucosa. This term is not to be confused with dental plaque, which causes dental caries (see Chapter 2, Oral Health and Nutrition).

▶ A **pustule** is a small, pus-containing blister. A person may see a pustule during non-infective acne. A pustule at the end of an eyelash follicle is a **stye**.

▶ **Vesicles** are small, fluid-filled blisters.

Lesions Classified Below the Surface of the Oral Mucosa

▶ An **abscess** is a concentrated area of pus formed as a result of infection by microorganisms. Dental abscesses are periapical (at the apex of the tooth) or periodontal, caused by microorganisms invading the periodontal membrane of the tooth (see Chapter 23, Periodontics).

▶ A **cyst** is a fluid or semi-solid fluid-filled sac. The causes of cysts are numerous. In dentistry, cysts normally occur as a result of a duct leading from a fluid-forming gland becoming blocked. Cysts can develop around the crown of an undeveloped tooth prior to eruption.

▶ **Erosion** is the defect left from a trauma or an injury. It may arise from a person biting the cheek. The margins of the cheek erosion are red and painful.

▶ An **ulcer** is due to destruction of the mucous membrane and appears as an open sore on the tissue. The ulcer may appear shallow or crated deeply and is normally inflamed and painful.

Lesions Classified Even or Flat with the Surface of the Oral Mucosa

▶ **Ecchymosis** (**eck**-ih-**MOH**-sis) is a medical term for bruising of the tissue.

▶ A **macule** (**MACK**-youl) is a spot of different texture or color on the skin.

▶ A **patch** is an area of skin that appears differently either in color and/or texture.

▶ **Petechiae** (pee-**TEE**-kee-ee) are small spots, red or purple in color, that occur in the skin or mucosa tissue. They are caused by localized hemorrhage.

▶ **Purpura** (**PUR**-pew-rah) is caused by bleeding within underlying tissues. These purplish or reddish brown areas or spots of discoloration can range in size from the diameter of a pin head up to one inch. Small purpura normally are referred to as petechiae, and the larger are called ecchymoses or bruises.

Lesions Classified Flat or Above the Surface of the Oral Mucosa

▶ A **granuloma**, associated with chronic inflammation, appears as a neoplasm or tumor that is filled with granulation tissue. The suffix "oma" refers to neoplasms or tumors.

▶ A **neoplasm** is the medical term for tumor. This new, abnormal growth that serves no usefulness can be either malignant (life threatening) or benign (non-life threatening).

▶ A **nodule** is a small lump of tissue, either hard or soft, that is usually more than one-quarter inch in diameter. A nodule may either protrude from the tissue or form beneath the surface of the tissue.

BIOLOGICAL AGENTS

A number of microorganisms cause oral diseases that are manifested through lesions in the head and neck.

Actinomycosis

Actinomycosis is an infection caused by a bacterium. First, a painful swelling appears, and later pus and yellow granules discharge from the area. Poor oral hygiene or microorganisms obtaining access to the bone through the dental socket after a tooth removal are thought to be contributing factors.

Herpes Simplex

Herpes simplex can occur in Type I, which appears above the waist (normally around the mouth), or Type II, which may appear in the oral cavity but normally appears below the waist, commonly called genital herpes. The Type I infection has occurred in about three-fourths of middle-aged adults. Forms of the virus are responsible for cold sores (painful blisters around the mouth). These blisters, commonly called fever blisters, can appear solitary or in a cluster of small blisters on the lips, called **herpes labialis** (Figure 20-1). Normal inflammation encompasses the area.

The virus responsible for the disease is transmitted through physical contact and is seen normally in children around the age of six as **herpetic gingivostomatitis** (the initial infection). Adults often unknowingly pass the virus, which is infectious both during the onset of the vesicular stage and throughout the crusted stage, to children during kissing. It exhibits symptoms much like the flu. Fever, along with body aches, is apparent, followed by scattered ulcers in the oral mucosa or on the lips. The lesions appear as nicks in the tissue and are extremely sore. These vesicle ulcerations vary in size from a pin head to one-quarter inch in size. The symptoms reappear throughout life and usually last from seven to fourteen days. If the condition is caught early, medication is available to alleviate the discomfort (see Chapter 8, Microbiology).

Dental assistants must exert extreme care while working with patients who have herpes. Stretching and pulling of the lesion causes the patient significant discomfort. The dentist may choose to reschedule the patient after he or she has recovered from the herpes outbreak. The dental assistant must pay special attention to eliminating cross-contamination and maintain asepsis. The herpetic virus lasts on a counter top or work surface for up to four hours. Health-care workers are known to develop the infection if barriers are not used. If the exposure is significant, gloves are not worn, and a break in the skin is accessible to the virus, **herpetic whitlow** may occur. This is a crusting ulceration on the fingers or hands that is extremely painful.

Any patient with apparent ulcers from the herpes virus that last longer than a month should be tested for immunodeficient diseases, such as HIV.

Aphthous Ulcers

Common ulcerations that recur in the oral cavity are **aphthous** (**AF**-thus) **ulcers**. These painful ulcers appear circular with yellow centers and erythematous (red) halos surrounding the lesions (Figure 20-2). The yellow necrotic center is due to the dead or dying epithelium cells. The cause of this ulcer is unknown, but the bacteria microorganism in streptococci has been apparent in numerous cases. Aphthous ulcers are referred to by patients as **canker sores**, and they are not contagious. A patient may have as few as one or as many as six sores at one time. Heredity, trauma, stress, food allergens, and hormonal changes are associated with the recurrence of this ulceration.

Aphthous ulcers last from ten to fourteen days, and topical anesthetics are used to treat the painful symptoms. Patients may have to be rescheduled for dental treatment, because these sores cause significant discomfort if they are touched or stretched.

Herpes Zoster

Herpes zoster (shingles) appears as unilateral, painful lesions that can last up to five weeks. This virus, which causes varicella in children, may lay latent and then activate at a time when the person is immunodeficient. Patients with human immunodeficiency virus (HIV) or advanced cancers are predisposed to herpes zoster. Acyclovir™ has been used successfully to treat the symptoms of these painful ulcers in some cases.

Syphilis

Syphilis, the venereal disease caused by bacteria that may be treated with antibiotics, has three primary

FIGURE 20-1 Herpes lesions on the lips, called herpes labialis. (*Courtesy of Joseph L. Konzelman, Jr., DDS*)

FIGURE 20-2 Aphthous ulcer on the buccal mucosa. (*Courtesy of Joseph L. Konzelman, Jr., DDS*)

stages. The first stage shows with a primary lesion about one-half inch in diameter that is hard and raised (Figure 20-3). This lesion, called a *chancre,* appears normally on the lip. The chancre first ulcerates and then becomes crusted over. It appears much like a herpetic lesion. The chancre disappears within five weeks, and no clinical manifestations of the disease appear in the oral cavity until two months to one year later.

The second stage begins with flu-like symptoms, followed by one of two types of lesions. These lesions, a mucous patch or a split papule, are both extremely infectious. In the tertiary or third and final stage of syphilis, a **gumma** or localized lesion appears. The final stage of syphilis may occur many years after non-treatment of secondary syphilis. This lesion destroys bone and cartilage.

Children born to mothers with syphilis may have teeth with enamel hypoplasia or teeth that have been altered, because of the infection, during the **morphodifferation** and **dentinogenesis** cycles of tooth development. The anterior dentition appears to be dented on the incisal edges, called **Hutchinson's incisors** (Figure 20-4). The permanent molars may appear more rounded with the occlusal surface, resembling a mulberry. Due to their appearance, they are called **mulberry molars** (Figure 20-5).

Thrush

Thrush is the common name for the fungal infection of *candidiasis* in children. It appears as a white, thick covering over the oral mucous membranes. The white covering can be removed by wiping it with a 2×2 gauze. This fungal infection often originates as the newborn

FIGURE 20-4 Hutchinson's incisors from prenatal syphilis. *(Courtesy of Dale Ruemping, DDS, MSD)*

FIGURE 20-5 Mulberry molars from prenatal syphilis. *(Courtesy of Dale Ruemping, DDS, MSD)*

travels through the birth canal. The fungal microorganism can grow in increasing numbers in this warm, moist environment and causes very little discomfort to the child. Treatment is to wipe the involved area and apply topical antifungal drugs to the area.

PHYSICAL AGENTS

Several physical agents can cause oral clinical manifestations. These trauma-induced ulcerations are most often self-induced. The patient may bite the inside of

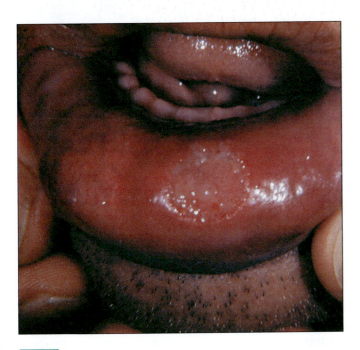

FIGURE 20-3 Lip chancre from primary syphilis.

the cheek; have an accident, such as fall on a blunt object, or wear an ill-fitting dental appliance, such as a denture. The dental team must use great care not to induce other traumas during dental care. The edge of the high-volume evacuator (HVE) has a rough edge that can cut or lacerate the patient's tissue if not handled properly. Other physical agents, such as instruments, can cause trauma by tearing or bruising the tissue if not utilized carefully. The dental assistant must constantly watch as instruments and materials are transferred to and from the mouth.

SAFETY Cotton rolls that are placed in an area that becomes overly dry and that are removed quickly can cause a gingival ulcer. The tissue adheres to the cotton roll so that when it is removed, the top layer of gingival tissue is also removed. To avoid this, the dental assistant can moisten the cotton roll prior to removing it.

Denture Irritation Causing Hyperplasia

An ill-fitting denture can cause small ulcers that, after continued irritation, become folds of excess tissue called **hyperplasia** (Figure 20-6). In the palatal area, the ruga(e) palatine become inflamed and swollen nodules. These nodules reduce in size and the redness disappears if the patient does not wear the denture for several days. Soft tissue lining material can be placed in the denture by the dentist to allow the palate to heal prior to relining or remaking the denture.

Amalgam Tattoo

An **amalgam tattoo** can occur when amalgam particles become trapped in the tissue, either during oral surgery or during an amalgam procedure (Figure 20-7). The gingival tissue in the immediate area appears blue to gray in color. No treatment is necessary, because the tattoo is asymptomatic and harmless. To prevent this condition from occurring, the dental assistant should flush the area with water to remove any amalgam particles after treatment, especially when the tissue is severely abraded. Use of a dental dam also aids in preventing amalgam tattoos.

FIGURE 20-7 Amalgam tattoo. (A) In the oral cavity. (B) On a periapical x-ray. *(Courtesy of Joseph L. Konzelman, Jr., DDS)*

FIGURE 20-6 Hyperplasia from denture irritation. *(Courtesy of Joseph L. Konzelman, Jr., DDS)*

Radiation Injury

Patients receiving excess radiation due to cancer treatment around the oral cavity may experience a number of side effects. Excess radiation may cause the developing teeth to be malformed, dwarfed, or without roots. This deformity depends on the stage of tooth development. The soft tissue may show reddening, with apparent ulcers due to excess radiation. After the area has healed, the tissue within the area may appear pigmented. Spider-like vessels may appear in skin that appears to be atrophied.

CHEMICAL AGENTS

A number of chemical agents can cause oral lesions. Some of the materials used in dentistry are caustic and may cause chemical burns. These agents include phenol, sodium hyperchlorate, zinc chloride, and aspirin. The chemicals in tobacco also cause oral lesions. Certain drugs will also induce oral lesions that the dental assistant will see from time to time. The most common chemical agents seen in patient's oral cavities in the dental office are aspirin burns, nicotine stomatitus, and chewing-tobacco lesions.

Aspirin Burn

Some people place aspirin over the root area of the tooth to alleviate discomfort prior to seeking dental treatment. The placement of the aspirin causes a lesion that is white in color and rough in texture (Figure 20-8). Soreness is apparent after the aspirin is removed and prior to complete healing.

Nicotine Stomatitis

Nicotine stomatitis is another condition that the dental assistant is likely to see in the dental office (Figure 20-9). Pipe smokers are more likely to develop nicotine stomatitis than cigarette smokers. It is caused by the heat and the irritating effect of the chemicals in tobacco. The reason that it is seen more in pipe smokers is that they normally place the pipe, in the same area, repeatedly. The end of the pipe then gives off a great deal of heat and tobacco in a concentrated area.

The affected area of tissue first turns red in response to the irritation. If the irritation continues, the tissue shows as whitened and red **hyperkeratinized** nodules. Hyperkeratinized tissue is where the epithelium tissue builds up a layer of keratin as a protective coating. The **orifices**, or openings of the salivary glands, appear red and inflamed. The patient should be made aware of this condition and encouraged to stop smoking. Normally, the condition clears up totally if the patient ceases to smoke.

Chewing Tobacco (Snuff) Lesion

Another lesion caused by tobacco is due to chewing tobacco (snuff). It appears in the oral vestibule, normally the lower anterior area between the lip and the teeth. It appears as wrinkled, white, thickened tissue. Like nicotine stomatitis lesions, the severity of a snuff lesion depends on how often the smokeless tobacco is used and how sensitive the individual is to this product (Figure 20-10). Individuals smoking other drugs, such as

FIGURE 20-8 Aspirin burn. *(Courtesy of Joseph L. Konzelman, Jr., DDS)*

FIGURE 20-9 Nicotine stomatitis. *(Courtesy of Joseph L. Konzelman, Jr., DDS)*

marijuana, may exhibit the clinical signs of tobacco irritation. Marijuana irritations normally are apparent in the middle anterior section of the lips, both maxillary and mandibular. This tissue appears red in the early stages and white with thick, wrinkled tissue in the later stages. This occurs primarily because a device such as a "roach clip" is used to hold the drug as it is smoked down to a very small piece; therefore, the heat and the drug create the condition on the lips.

Hairy Tongue

A condition in which the filiform papillae of the tongue become elongated and appear like hairs is called **hairy tongue** (also referred to as the black hairy tongue) (Figure 20-11). This "hair" normally becomes stained by tobacco, food, or other microorganisms, making it appear dark in color. A hairy tongue may appear without known cause, but it is normally associated with chemotherapeutic agents such as drugs, hydrogen peroxide mouth rinses, and antibiotics. Treatment of this condition is to stop the known cause, if applicable, and use good oral hygiene, including brushing the tongue. In extreme cases, the filiform papillae grows so long that it causes the person to gag. If this happens, the papillae can be trimmed to alleviate the gagging.

Gingival Hyperplasia

A condition known as **gingival hyperplasia** occurs when the connective tissue grows over the teeth (Figure 20-12). This fibrous mass is not uncomfortable to the patient but can inhibit eating and alter the patient's appearance. A number of substances can cause this condition: plaque, orthodontic braces, and various drugs. Phenytoin (Dilantin™) causes this symptom in about one-half of the patients being treated with this medication. The condition is then referred to as **Dilantin hyperplasia**.

The condition normally is reduced after the irritant is removed or the patient stops taking the drugs, but that

FIGURE 20-11 Hairy tongue.

FIGURE 20-10 Snuff lesion. *(Courtesy of Joseph L. Konzelman, Jr., DDS)*

FIGURE 20-12 Gingival hyperplasia. *(Courtesy of Joseph L. Konzelman, Jr., DDS)*

solution is not always preferable. If ongoing drug therapy is necessary, the tissue can be removed surgically and recurrence is probable.

HORMONAL DISTURBANCES

Oral conditions can be caused by a change in the individual's hormonal balance. Going through puberty or pregnancy causes hormonal changes that affect the oral tissues. An individual who notices a soreness in the gingival tissue must pay close attention to oral hygiene so that the condition does not progress.

Pregnancy Gingivitis

Pregnancy gingivitis occurs in about 5 percent of pregnant women. The gingival tissues appear enlarged and inflamed. A few pregnant women with this condition also develop pregnancy tumors. Both of these conditions clear up once the hormonal balance returns to normal, but good oral hygiene practices must be followed to control gingivitis and bleeding.

Pyogenic Granuloma

Often called pregnancy tumor, **pyogenic** (**pie**-oh-**JEN**-ick) **granuloma** is also found in males and non-pregnant females (Figure 20-13). This overgrowth of granulation tissue occurs as a result of local irritation. This red, vascular mass ranging in size from a few millimeters to several centimeters grows rapidly. It normally is not painful and can be excised. The cause is hormonal disturbances, and the lesion may grow back if the situation continues. Therefore, it is not prudent to remove the lesion during the pregnancy unless it is uncomfortable for the patient.

FIGURE 20-13 Pyogenic granuloma. *(Courtesy of Joseph L. Konzelman, Jr., DDS)*

Other factors, such as calculus on the teeth, should be removed to eliminate irritation to the area.

Puberty Gingival Enlargement

Adolescents going through puberty can experience gingival enlargement due to hormonal changes. The condition appears much like pregnancy gingivitis as the gingival tissue is enlarged, bleeds easily, and appears soft and swollen. This condition is more common in girls than in boys. It corrects itself after the hormonal balance is stabilized again and good oral hygiene practices are maintained.

DEVELOPMENTAL DISTURBANCES

A wide range of anomalies can take place if any stage of embryo development is disturbed. In the oral cavity, anomalies occur in about one in every 800 children born. These **congenital** (present at birth) conditions are genetic (inherited). Other anomalies are caused by outside agents, such as alcohol, drugs, or the mother having had a disease during pregnancy, such as syphilis (refer to biologic agents).

One such developmental disturbance is clefting in the oral cavity. The most common clefting resulting from developmental disturbances are the **cleft lip** and the **cleft palate** (see Chapter 5, Embryology and Histology). The majority of these conditions are **innocuous** (harmless); however, some conditions cause eating, speaking, and esthetic difficulties. The construction of an opturator (an appliance to aid in swallowing) for the cleft palate may be necessary to treat the condition.

Disturbances in Tooth Development

As the teeth are developing, a number of disturbances can take place.

Amelogenesis Imperfecta. **Amelogenesis imperfecta** is a genetic (inherited) condition of the teeth in which the enamel is discolored, partially missing, or extremely thin. These teeth may be more susceptible to dental caries. Treatment may consist of composite restorations that cover the entire surface of the teeth.

Ankylosis. **Ankylosis** is a condition in which the tooth, cementum, or dentin fuses with the alveolar bone, restricting movement of the tooth as well as eruption. An ankylosed tooth appears below the normal occlusal plane of the adjacent teeth. If, during the removal of third molars, this condition becomes apparent, it is much more difficult to remove the tooth. The tooth will not come from the socket in a normal manner and may have to be separated from the bone by the dentist.

Anodontia. **Anodontia** occurs when teeth are congenitally missing. This condition can affect primary or permanent teeth or both. It is most often seen in permanent third molars. Many individuals only develop one or two of their third molars, or "wisdom teeth." Some individuals never develop any third molars.

Dentinogenesis Imperfecta. **Dentinogenesis imperfecta** is a condition in which the enamel appears to be opalescent and chips away from the dentin soon after eruption of the tooth. This hereditary condition normally appears in both the deciduous and permanent teeth. The pulp chambers are obliterated, as are the root canals. Normally, these patients present with attrition (wearing away) due to a lack of enamel.

Fusion. **Fusion** is a condition in which the enamel and dentin of two or more individual teeth join together. The incisal or occlusal surface may show an indentation between the two teeth, and they normally are much broader in appearance. This condition most often is seen in mandibular anterior deciduous teeth.

Gemination. **Gemination** may appear much like a fusion, but in this case a single tooth bud attempts to divide. The indentation on the incisal or occlusal surface is apparent.

Macrodontia. **Macrodontia** teeth are abnormally large. The entire dentition may manifest itself in macrodontia teeth, or only two teeth may develop in this manner.

Microdontia. **Microdontia** teeth are the opposite of macrodontia: They are abnormally small. This condition often is seen in individuals with Down syndrome or in individuals born with congenital heart disease. These small teeth can be apparent in the entire dentition or only show in one or two teeth. Commonly, the maxillary laterals show as microdontia teeth. In this area, their shape is often peg shaped and small.

Neonatal Teeth. **Neonatal teeth** (natal teeth) are present at the time of birth or within the first month after birth. Normally, the baby sheds these teeth very quickly, because the roots are not formed yet.

Supernumerary Teeth. **Supernumerary teeth** are extra teeth. They appear dwarfed in size and shape but normal in all other aspects. Supernumerary teeth are seen most frequently in the maxillary anterior or in the third molar area, both maxillary and mandibular.

Twinning. **Twinning** is a condition in which the germination process has been successful and two separate teeth are made from one tooth bud. The tooth appears as a clone of the original tooth in both shape and size.

Oral Tori

Boney outgrowths of tissue in the oral cavity that are benign (non-malignant) in nature are called **tori**. If they are located in the maxillary hard palate, they are termed *torus palatinus*. If they are located in the mandibular canine or premolar region, they are termed *torus mandibularis*.

Torus palatinus are normally seen close to the midline but can occur on the lateral borders (Figure 20-14). Approximately one in every five adults has a maxillary tori, and about one in every twenty has a mandibular tori. Tori mandibularis are more annoying, because food debris can collect beneath them (Figure 20-15). Both conditions of tori present with surfaces of hard bone covered with thin coverings of tissue. A dental assistant must be careful while taking oral radiographs. He or she should examine the oral cavity carefully before placing the radiograph into position. The radiographs can abrade the tissue and cause the patient discomfort if placed directly on the tissue covering the boney growths.

These growths are not removed unless the patient needs a prosthetic appliance, such as a denture or a

FIGURE 20-14 Torus palatinus. *(Courtesy of Joseph L. Konzelman, Jr., DDS)*

FIGURE 20-15 Torus mandibularis. *(Courtesy of Joseph L. Konzelman, Jr., DDS)*

lower partial. The growths are then surgically removed to allow room for the dental appliance.

Exostoses

An enlargement or a nodular outgrowth of dense lamella (thin structure extending from the facial surface) bone that appears on the facial surfaces of the mandibular and the maxillary palates is called **exostosis**. These enlargements, which appear much like toris, may be variations of the same developmental disturbance. There is no treatment, unless a dental appliance is necessary or the enlargements hamper the mastication (chewing) function for the patient.

Fordyce Spots (Granules)

In about 80 percent of the population, numerous light-yellow spots in the oral cavity are present. These round lesions, called Fordyce's spots, are sebaceous oil glands near the surface of the epithelium (Figure 20-16). They can be found anywhere in the oral cavity but most often are on the buccal mucosa. No identified causes are known, and no treatment is necessary.

Fissured Tongue

A fissured tongue occurs in about 5 percent of the population (Figure 20-17). It appears as a wrinkled, deeply grooved surface on the tongue. Fissured tongue may be symmetrical or irregular in pattern. The patient may experience discomfort due to retention of debris in the deep fissures. No treatment is necessary, although the patient may use a home irrigating device to clean the fissures occasionally.

FIGURE 20-17 Fissured tongue. *(Courtesy of Joseph L. Konzelman, Jr., .DDS)*

Bifid Tongue

If the two lateral halves of the anterior two-thirds of the tongue fail to fuse completely, a condition known as **bifid tongue** occurs. It appears as an extra tag of muscle at the end of the tongue. No treatment is necessary, unless the extra tag of tongue is annoying; then, it is surgically removed.

Ankyloglossia

The term commonly used for **ankyloglossia** is "tongue tied" (Figure 20-18). This is a condition in which the

FIGURE 20-16 Fordyce's spots. *(Courtesy of Joseph L. Konzelman, Jr., DDS)*

FIGURE 20-18 Ankyloglossia. *(Courtesy of Joseph L. Konzelman, Jr., DDS)*

lingual frenum is attached near the tip of the tongue. This limits movement of the tongue and may interfere with the enunciation of specific sounds. This condition can be corrected with a simple surgical procedure, which enables the individual to overcome any related speech problems. A dental assistant should watch for this condition in children. Under the direction of the dentist, while waiting for the anesthetic to begin, ask the child to stick the tongue out and move across the upper lip from side to side. Note if a restriction is present, and bring this information to the attention of the dentist for further evaluation.

NUTRITIONAL DISTURBANCES

The oral cavity can reveal a number of conditions due to poor or improper diet. It is important to consult with all patients about eating a well-balanced diet (see Chapter 2, Oral Health and Nutrition).

Angular Cheilitis

Vitamin B complex deficiency results in a condition known as **angular cheilitis**. A lesion forms in the corner of the mouth, involving both the mucous membrane and the skin (Figure 20-19). This condition may also occur if the patient constantly licks the corners of the mouth (commissures) or if the patient loses vertical dimension of the face. A loss of vertical dimension occurs when a person overcloses the mouth because the occlusal plane is worn down or the bone structure beneath a denture is deteriorated. The end of the chin is

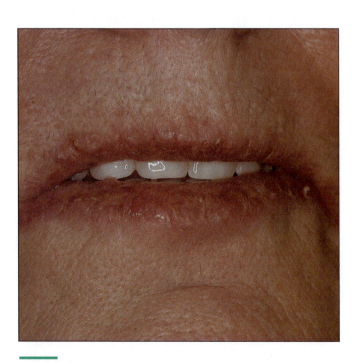

FIGURE 20-19 Angular cheilitis. *(Courtesy of Joseph L. Konzelman, Jr., DDS)*

closer to the tip of the nose and the corners of the mouth cave in, which allows saliva to pool in them. This condition permits microorganisms to grow; as a result, fungal **opportunistic infections** such as *candida albicans* are often found in this area.

The treatment for this condition is correction of vitamin B deficiency or the use of antifungal drugs to treat the infection. The dentures can be remade or the teeth crowned and extended in length to correct the loss of vertical dimension.

Glossitis (Bald Tongue)

Another condition reportedly caused by the lack of the vitamin B complex is **glossitis**. Glossitis literally means "inflammation of the tongue." The filiform papillae on the tongue are absent, and the tongue appears to be smooth, hence the name "bald tongue." The tongue may be sore and the patient may experience difficulty in eating. A well-balanced diet aids in the correction of this condition.

NEOPLASMS

As stated earlier, a neoplasm is a medical term for tumor. This group of lesions has great potential for becoming **malignant** (cancerous). The dental assistant should be knowledgeable about the causes of these diseases and perform careful clinical examinations for any premalignant lesions. Even if it is known that a tumor is benign (harmless), it is important that all lesions are brought to the attention of the dentist, without alarming the patient. It could save someone's life if the tumor is recognized early.

Oral Cancer Warning Signs

▶ Sore in the oral cavity that does not heal within one month

▶ Lumps and swelling in the oral cavity, on the lips, or on the neck

▶ White lesions or rough lesions in the mouth or on the lips

▶ Dryness in the mouth over a period of time for no apparent reason

▶ Numbness in or around the oral cavity

▶ Soreness or burning sensation in or around the oral cavity

▶ Difficulty speaking, chewing, or swallowing

▶ Repeated bleeding in a specific area of the mouth for no apparent reason

---

Leukoplakia

A white, leathery patch that cannot be identified as any other white lesion is termed **leukoplakia (loo-koh-PLAY-**

FIGURE 20-20 Leukoplakia. *(Courtesy of Joseph L. Konzelman, Jr., DDS)*

FIGURE 20-21 Lichen planus. *(Courtesy of Joseph L. Konzelman, Jr., DDS)*

kee-ah) (Figure 20-20). A biopsy is required to identify the lesion further. The dentist normally views these lesions with concern, because they can be precipitating factors to cancer. They are found throughout the oral mucosa and can be very dense or very diffuse. The operator is not able to wipe the lesion off with a 2 × 2 gauze as he or she could with thrush. Often, leukoplakia is seen in the lower lip of a person who uses chewing tobacco. Excessive alcohol and tobacco usage, vitamin A deficiency or trauma normally are associated with the lesion.

If a biopsy is performed, the results normally show **hyperkeratinization**, a thickening of the outer layer of the skin due to an increased amount of keratin. This condition is similar to developing corns on the feet due to constant irritation. Biopsies also could reveal **dysplasic cells**, abnormal cell features such as size, shape, and rate of multiplication. Often, dysplasic cells become malignant.

Lichen Planus

The initial skin lesion of **lichen planus** appears normally on the lower leg or ankle. This lesion is a flat-topped papule, dark red or violet in color. The oral lesions (reticular lichen planus) begin as small, white papules that group and form interlacing white lines known as **Wickham's striae** (Figure 20-21). In most cases, they are on the buccal mucosa. An erosive form of the lesion (erosive lichen planus) causes the loss of oral epithelium in the areas of infection. Both are fairly common, with reticular lichen planus being asymptomatic and erosive lichen planus usually being more tender and painful. A patient may exhibit pain while eating, and some foods may aggravate the condition. The treatment is topical steroid therapy.

Controversy over whether lichen planus is a premalignant condition exists in all texts. Patients should be examined periodically for any changes in this condition.

Erythroplakia

Any red patch of tissue in the oral cavity that cannot be associated with inflammation is termed **erythroplakia** (eh-**rith**-roh-**PLAY**-kee-ah). Most commonly, this condition appears in the soft palate, retromolar pad area, or the floor of the mouth. Usually, it is seen in patients over sixty years of age who have chronically used tobacco and alcoholic beverages.

This lesion is of great concern, because almost 100 percent of the biopsies show up premalignant or malignant. Treatment depends on the extension of the lesion. In early stages, it can be removed surgically; however, in later stages, it is necessary to treat the lesion with radiation and chemotherapy.

Squamous Cell Carcinoma

A carcinoma is a malignant neoplasm (tumor) that can spread, or **metastasize**, into the surrounding tissue and nodes in the body. Normally, it first appears as an ulcerated area in the soft tissues of the mouth. A **squamous cell carcinoma** is a cancer of the squamous epithelium (Figure 20-22). Nine out of ten oral cancers are squamous cell carcinoma.

The factors associated with causing carcinomas are sunlight exposure and extended use of tobacco and/or alcohol. Normally, squamous cell carcinomas are seen in adults forty years or older but also have been found in younger patients. More cases have been documented in males than females. Squamous cell carcinoma is found primarily on the floor of the oral cavity under the tongue, on the sides or borders of the tongue, and on the soft palate tonsil area.

FIGURE 20-22 Squamous cell carcinoma. *(Courtesy of Joseph L. Konzelman, Jr., DDS)*

The lesion may first appear as a thickened, white plaque that develops into an ulcer. As it grows, this ulcer seems to encompass other tissues. Soon, a rolled border appears with the center tissue. The mass continues to grow, rising above the normal tissue level.

Treatment for squamous cell carcinoma depends on the size, site, and spread of the tumor. Early detection is essential, because if the carcinoma metastasizes into the lymph nodes, the survival rate diminishes greatly.

Basal Cell Carcinoma

The most common form of skin cancer is **basal cell carcinoma**. The lesions normally appear on the neck, ear, face, lip, and head. Because it is the area primarily exposed to sun rays, the face is the main area on which the lesions appear. Fair-skinned individuals are more susceptible to basal cell carcinoma. Males over forty have more occurrences of basal cell cancer than females (Figure 20-23).

These cells, unlike squamous cells, stay contained and normally do not metastasize. They invade the area around them as they grow. The lesion first appears as a nodule and then ulcerates, the borders rise, and the center develops into a crater.

Treatment is to surgically remove the lesion. Patients commonly develop more than one lesion. Careful clinical examinations of the head and neck can be done during six-month recall appointments to identify any other lesions at a early stage.

Papilloma

A lesion of squamous epithelium tissue that is benign in nature is called a **papilloma**. A papilloma resembles a

FIGURE 20-23 Basal cell carcinoma.

cauliflower in appearance because it seems to have a number of projections coming from one origin (Figure 20-24). It is not caused by continued irritation, as are many of the neoplasms, but occurs after the individual has been infected by a virus. A number of viruses have resulted in a similar type of lesion. This lesion ranges in color from white to red and is normally 1 to 3 cm in size.

Treatment of the papilloma is to surgically remove it and a small amount of normal epithelium cells at the base of the lesion.

Fibroma

A **fibroma** is a benign tumor of connective tissue cells (the cells that surround and support structures) (Figure 20-25). A fibroma is a reactive hyperplasia rather than a true neoplasm. It presents in the oral cavity as a dome-shaped, pink-colored, smooth-surfaced lesion less than 2 cm in diameter. Normally, it is found on the buccal (cheek) surface, proximal to where the teeth occlude. The fibroma occurs because of continued irritation of

FIGURE 20-24 Papilloma. *(Courtesy of Joseph L. Konzelman, Jr., DDS)*

FIGURE 20-25 Fibroma. *(Courtesy of Joseph L. Konzelman, Jr., DDS)*

the teeth biting together. The continued trauma causes the connective tissue to grow. This benign tumor may be surgical excised or left without treatment. Recurrence of a fibroma is rare.

ORAL LESIONS RELATED TO ACQUIRED IMMUNODEFICIENCY SYNDROME (AIDS) AND HUMAN IMMUNODEFICIENCY VIRUS (HIV)

Acquired Immune Deficiency Syndrome (AIDS) is a deficiency of the immune system due to the infection of **human immunodeficiency virus (HIV)**. Healthy individuals can combat most microorganisms that cause dis-

ease, but individuals who suffer from **HIV** and have suppressed immune systems do not fare as well. With a depressed immune system, opportunistic infections such as herpes virus, hepatitis, tuberculosis, candidosis, and pneumonia can overcome the individual's system. Individuals with full-blown AIDS may get cancers and lymphoma of the brain and eventually die. There is no cure for AIDS, and treatment is for complications associated with it. Patients who are infected with HIV, the cause of AIDS, have specific oral manifestations related to the disease.

Patients with AIDS are much more susceptible to periodontal lesions than healthy individuals. The gingival tissue becomes inflamed, red, and bulbous, and bone loss occurs. Bacteria and yeast microorganisms are found in the infected area. This condition is extremely painful and bleeds readily when touched. Normal oral hygiene techniques fail to be as effective as they would be for a healthy individual.

Treatment consists of extremely good oral hygiene, root planning and curettage, rinses, and antibiotic therapy.

Hairy Leukoplakia

In the early 1980s, a raised, white-patch lesions called **hairy leukoplakia** was identified in patients known to be infected with HIV (Figure 20-26). It appears much like the lesion candidosis but cannot be removed by wiping with gauze. Hairy leukoplakia is a white, patterned lesion normally found on the borders of the tongue. This lesion is not painful, and no treatment is available. If the patient has not been tested for HIV, the dentist may suggest testing.

Candida Albicans

AIDS patients and patients who have had cancer treatment such as chemotherapy and are immunodepressed

FIGURE 20-26 Hairy leukoplakia. *(Courtesy of Joseph L. Konzelman, Jr., DDS)*

are likely to develop an infection called **candida albicans**. Patients undergoing antibiotic therapy for a long time also may show with the lesions. Candida albicans, a fungus infection much like thrush or moniliasis, is the first oral lesion manifesting from HIV infection. The membrane presents as a white, thick, plaque-like covering in linear patterns on top of a red, inflamed surface. It can be present on numerous oral membranes but normally appears on the tongue and buccal mucosa. Patients often report a burning sensation in the area of the infection. Treatment consists of antifungal medications such as Nystatin™ (see Chapter 12, Pharmacology).

Kaposi's Sarcoma

A number of AIDS patients present with an unusual malignant vascular tumor called **Kaposi's sarcoma** (Figure 20-27). AIDS patients are susceptible to other malignant tumors, such as squamous cell carcinoma and lymphoma, but, until the 1980s and the development of AIDS, Kaposi's sarcoma rarely was seen in the world. In patients with AIDS, Kaposi's sarcoma is aggressive and spreads rapidly.

The lesions, a diffuse blue-purple in color, appear all over the body, especially on the face, arms, and the palate. They are either flat or nodular and, as the tumor enlarges, it becomes a hemorrhagic neoplasm. Bleeding and pain are present in the more advanced stages.

Treatment is low-dose radiation and/or chemotherapeutic drugs. The prognosis (outcome) is poor at this stage, and a number of people die from the lymphoreticular neoplasms related to this disease.

MISCELLANEOUS DISORDERS

The dental assistant may see other disorders in the oral cavity. Any lesion appearing abnormal should be brought to the attention of the dentist.

Acute Necrotizing Ulcerative Gingivitis (ANUG)

The tissues present with bleeding, infection, pain, and a foul odor in a condition known as acute necrotizing ulcerative gingivitis (ANUG) (Figure 20-28). This infectious disease is seen primarily in young adults and adolescents. Poor hygiene, lack of sleep, poor nutrition, and stress are precipitating factors to this disease. It was referred to as "trench mouth" years ago due to the fact that many soldiers developed ANUG as they were fighting in the trenches. It is also seen on college campuses around the time of finals, due to the precipitating factors of the disease being present.

ANUG is very painful and must be treated with a thorough debridement and cleaning of the area. Antibiotics may be prescribed along with oral rinses of hot water. Immaculate oral hygiene also is necessary to treat ANUG. After the condition resolves, the tips of the papilla will, from that time forward, appear to be blunted or flat.

Mucocele

When a trauma happens to a minor salivary gland, a **mucocele** (**MYOO**-ko-seal) can result (Figure 20-29). This normally takes place on the mandibular anterior lip where a patient accidentally bites into the tissue. If this is at the place of a minor salivary gland, a duct may

FIGURE 20-27 Kaposi's sarcoma. *(Courtesy of Joseph L. Konzelman, Jr., DDS)*

FIGURE 20-28 Acute necrotizing ulcerative gingivitis. *(Courtesy of Joseph L. Konzelman, Jr., DDS)*

FIGURE 20-29 Mucocele. *(Courtesy of Joseph L. Konzelman, Jr., DDS)*

FIGURE 20-30 Geographic tongue. *(Courtesy of Joseph L. Konzelman, Jr., DDS)*

be closed off. The mucocele may appear like a bubble on the inside of the lip.

Occasionally, a stone-like particle may block the saliva duct opening. If this happens, the gland fills with fluid and enlarges. The gland may be opened and the fluid expressed from the area. Recurrence may necessitate total removal of the duct and gland.

Varix

Varix is a condition primarily seen in the elderly. The blood vessels become weakened and extended. Normally, this condition occurs in the oral cavity beneath the tongue or on the buccal mucosa. These dark-purple, extended vessels in the oral cavity are related to the **varicose veins** in other parts of the body. They should be noted on the patient's chart, but no treatment is necessary.

Geographic Tongue

Less than 2 percent of the population has an inflammatory condition that affects the tongue, called geographic tongue (Figure 20-30). It affects the dorsal and lateral surfaces of the tongue and shows as red, smooth patches absent of filliform papillae. Geographic tongue presents with patches that are normally surrounded by an elevated white or yellow border. The area of the patches make up an ever-changing pattern on the tongue that resembles a map of the world. The condition may have periods of remission. The condition is not painful, and treatment is unnecessary.

Anorexia Nervosa and Bulmia

The diseases anorexia nervosa (loss of 15 percent of body weight and an intense fear of fat) and bulmia (episodes of out-of-control eating followed by purging) have several implications in oral pathology. Anorexia nervosa is a disease in which extreme aversion to food is present, and accompanying symptoms of induced vomiting (bulmia) have a direct impact on oral health.

Due to the constant vomiting, the lingual surfaces of the anterior teeth become decalcified and the enamel is eroded. The occlusal surfaces of the posterior teeth become eroded, causing existing restorations to deteriorate. Rampant caries and enlargement of the parotid glands are also problems, along with the other disease symptoms that are life-threatening.

Treatment is for symptoms and maintaining comfort until this personality disorder can be reversed. The patient is encouraged to practice immaculate oral hygiene and to rinse the mouth after purging to decrease the number of microorganisms and the acidity. The teeth may be sensitive where the enamel has eroded. Toothpaste for sensitive teeth is suggested as treatment.

Bell's Palsy

Bell's palsy (named for the Scottish surgeon Sir Charles Bell) is a temporary paralysis of the muscles on one side of the face. The cause is unknown but thought to be related to herpes zoster (shingles). One side of the face droops down, and the patient cannot close the eye or smile. Some individuals have pain in the ear on the affected side. Taste is diminished, and sounds seem unnaturally loud. Most cases clear up without treatment, but analgesics can be given for symptoms of discomfort and corticosteroid drugs can be given to reduce inflammation in the nerve.

CHAPTER SUMMARY

The dental assistant, who sits opposite the dentist, has a different view of the patient's oral cavity. Anything that appears to be atypical should be brought to the dentist's attention, without alarming the patient.

The dental assistant does not diagnose oral pathological diseases but identifies abnormal conditions in the mouth. Further, the dental assistant must know how to prevent disease transmission, how the identified pathological condition may interfere with planned treatment, and what effect it will have on the overall health of the patient.

CASE STUDY

Toby Edward, twenty years old, was just given an injection by Dr. Smile. The dental assistant notices that the area where the injection was given is swelling and appears like a raised, bruised area. The patient feels no discomfort because the anesthetic has taken effect.

Case Study Review

1. What pathologic condition may be present in Toby Edward's mouth?

2. What should the dental assistant do to treat this condition?

3. What is the prognosis of this condition?

To complete your study of this chapter, work the review activities that follow. Also, refer to the software that accompanies this text.

REVIEW QUESTIONS

Multiple Choice

1. The first stage of syphilis manifests in a lesion called a
   a. gumma.
   b. chancre.
   c. mucous patch.
   d. split papule.

2. An oral condition that is common in children and appears as a white, thick covering over the oral mucous membranes is called
   a. a papule.
   b. a bulla.
   c. a hematoma.
   d. thrush.

3. All of the following are caused by chemical agents except
   a. aspirin burn.
   b. hairy tongue.
   c. nicotine stomatitis.
   d. pustule.

4. A condition in which the tooth, cementum, or dentin fuses with the alveolar bone is called
   a. amelogenesis imperfecta.
   b. ankylosis.
   c. anodontia.
   d. fusion.

5. A vitamin B complex deficiency results in a condition known as
   a. candida albicans.
   b. Fordyce's spots.
   c. glossitis.
   d. angular cheilitis.

Critical Thinking

1. If a dental assistant is taking radiographs on a patient who presents with a torus mandibularis, what should be done?

2. A patient presents with a "bald tongue." What are the conditions that may cause this condition? Is it uncomfortable for the patient? What will aid in the correction of this condition?

3. What are the warning signs of oral cancer?

Orthodontics

OBJECTIVES

The student should strive to meet the following objectives and demonstrate an understanding of the facts and principles presented in this chapter:

1. Define orthodontics and describe the orthodontic setting.

2. Define the role of the dental assistant in an orthodontic setting.

3. Define and describe occlusion and malocclusion.

4. Identify the causes of malocclusion.

5. Describe preventive, interceptive, and corrective orthodontics.

6. Explain the process of tooth movement.

7. Describe the preorthodontic appointment for the diagnostic records.

8. Describe the consultation appointment and the roles of the patient and the orthodontist.

9. Differentiate between fixed and removable appliances.

10. Identify and give the function of the basic orthodontic instruments.

11. Describe the stages of orthodontic treatment.

12. Explain the procedure for removing the orthodontic appliances and how the teeth are retained in position after removal of the appliances.

KEY TERMS

activator (p. 451)

Angle's classification (p. 443)

arch wires (p. 448)

brackets (p. 448)

buccal tubes (p. 449)

buccoversion (p. 443)

corrective orthodontics (p. 445)

distoversion (p. 443)

elastics (p. 449)

fixed appliances (p. 445)

headgear (p. 451)

interceptive (p. 444)

ligature wire (p. 449)

linguoversion (p. 443)

malocclusion (p. 442)

normal occlusion (p. 442)

orthodontic bands (p. 448)

overbite (p. 451)

removable appliances (p. 445)

resorption (p. 445)

separators (p. 453)

space maintainer (p. 451)

springs (p. 449)

INTRODUCTION

Orthodontics is a specialty of dentistry that deals with the recognition, prevention, and treatment of malalignment and irregularities of the teeth, jaws, and face. Patients seek orthodontic treatment for esthetic and functional reasons.

Ortho means straight; *odont* means tooth.

The general dentist completes two additional years of study after finishing dental school to become an orthodontist. Although the general dentist may perform limited orthodontic treatment, most patients requiring tooth alignment are referred to an orthodontist. The general dentist and the orthodontist work together to provide the best treatment for patients. Treatment may extend several years as the child patient grows and develops.

Although the orthodontic practice treats mainly children and young adults, the number of adult patients who see an orthodontist is increasing. Adults seek orthodontic treatment for both cosmetic and functional reasons.

THE ORTHODONTIC PRACTICE

Orthodontic Office

The orthodontic office is designed to facilitate a number of patients at different stages of treatment. Specific rooms or areas are used for examination, diagnostic records, and treatment consultations before treatment begins. The treatment area contains several dental chairs and units. This area is an "open bay," meaning there are no walls separating the dental units (Figure 21-1). The laboratory in the orthodontic office is where appliances and models are fabricated. This area contains equipment and materials necessary to pour impressions, trim study models, and construct orthodontic appliances.

Orthodontic Team

The orthodontic team consists of the orthodontist, reception and business office staff, office coordinator, the orthodontic/dental assistants, and laboratory technician(s).

The Orthodontist. The orthodontist examines the patient, makes the diagnosis for treatment, and performs the orthodontic procedures. He or she checks and evaluates the progress of the patient throughout treatment.

The Reception and Business Office Staff. The receptionist greets patients and schedules appointments. The business staff takes care of financial arrange-

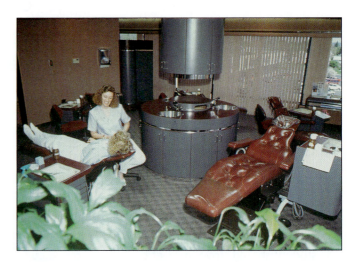

FIGURE 21-1 (A) Treatment area in an orthodontic office. The chairs are arranged in an "open bay." *(continued next page)*

ments and manages the business administration of the office. They maintain communication with the patients, parents, and the general dentist during the course of treatment.

The Office Coordinator. The office coordinator makes sure the office is run smoothly and efficiently. The coordinator provides information to families considering orthodontic treatment and coordinates the orthodontic assistant's responsibilities during the various phases of patient treatment.

The Laboratory Technician. The laboratory technician may pour and trim diagnostic models and working casts. The technician constructs orthodontic appliances and retainers to the specifications of the orthodontist.

The Orthodontic Assistant. The orthodontic assistant has a variety of responsibilities depending on the size of the practice and the number of assistants. The functions also vary with each state's Dental Practice Act. Generally, the orthodontic assistant has the following responsibilities:

▸ Seats and dismisses the patient

▸ Takes study model impressions

▸ Takes and processes intraoral radiographs (if not provided by the general dentist)

▸ Takes and processes extraoral radiographs (panoramic and cephalometric)

▸ Does the tracing on cephalometric radiographs

▸ Performs general chairside assisting responsibilities during the treatment appointments

▸ Cleans the patient's teeth at various stages of treatment

▸ Maintains and sterilizes instruments

▸ Maintains inventory and supplies

FIGURE 21-1 *(continued)* (B) Blueprint of an orthodontic office. *(Courtesy of Burkhart Dental Supply)*

▶ Performs routine maintenance of equipment

▶ Gives oral hygiene instructions

▶ Gives instructions on appliance wear and care

▶ Prefits bands before cementation*

▶ Removes excess cement from bands and brackets*

▶ Applies sealants to teeth to be bonded*

▶ Checks for loose and broken appliances at each appointment*

▶ Places and removes arch wires and ligatures*

▶ Removes bands and brackets*

*(Allowed by the state Dental Practice Act)

To become a credential orthodontic assistant, a specialty examination must be passed. The examinations are administered by the Dental Assisting National Board (DANB) and/or the individual state Board of Dentistry. DANB administers an examination and, upon successful completion, the candidate is awarded the title of Certified Orthodontic Assistant (COA).

OCCLUSION AND MALOCCLUSION

The dental assistant must understand the terminology related to occlusion in order to effectively assist the dentist during orthodontic treatment.

Normal Occlusion

Normal (or ideal) occlusion describes the contact relationship of the mandibular arch with the maxillary arch. This usually focuses on occlusal contacts, alignment of teeth, and arrangement and relationship of the teeth within and between the arches.

In normal occlusion:

▶ The mandibular teeth are in maximum contact with the maxillary teeth and the teeth are not rotated or abnormally spaced.

▶ The maxillary anterior teeth overlap the incisal edge of the mandibular anterior teeth by 2 mm.

▶ The maxillary posterior teeth are one cusp distal to the mandibular posterior teeth.

▶ The mesial buccal cusp of the maxillary first permanent molar occludes in the buccal groove of the mandibular first molar (Figure 21-2).

Malocclusion

Malocclusion is any deviation from normal occlusion, including misalignment of a single tooth, a group of teeth, or an entire arch. There are many variations of malocclusion. Table 21-1 shows the most common

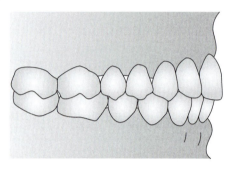

FIGURE 21-2 Example of normal occlusion.

TABLE 21-1 ANGLE'S CLASSIFICATIONS OF MALOCCLUSION AND FACIAL PROFILES

Class Name	Molar Relationship	Description	Illustration	Facial Profile
Neutrocclusion	Mesiobuccal cusp of maxillary first permanent molar occludes with the buccal groove of the mandibular first permanent molar.	Similar to normal occlusion with individual teeth or groups of teeth out of position.	Class I	Mesognathic
Distocclusion	Buccal groove of the mandibular first permanent molar is distal to the mesiobuccal cusp of the maxillary first permanent molar.	Division 1— Maxillary teeth in labioversion	Class II, Division 1	Retrognathic
		Division 2— Linguoversion of mandibular teeth	Class II, Division 2	Retrognathic
Mesioclusion	Buccal groove of the mandibular first permanent molar is mesial to the mesiobuccal cusp of the maxillary first permanent molar.	Mandibular teeth mesial to normal position	Class III	Prognathic

method of classification, called **Angle's classification**. Also included in the table is the matching facial profile.

> In 1899, Edward Angle established a system to classify malocclusion. It is still commonly used today.

Malposition of Individual Teeth and Groups of Teeth

There are numerous variations in the position of the *individual teeth* in the alveolar bone. The following terms describe these deviations:

▶ **Torsoversion**—Tooth is rotated or turned.

▶ **Mesioversion**—Tooth is mesial to normal position.

▶ **Distoversion**—Tooth is distal to normal position.

▶ **Linguoversion**—Tooth is lingual to normal position.

▶ **Labioversion** or **buccoversion**—Tooth is tipped toward the lip or cheek.

▶ **Supraversion**—Tooth extends above the normal line of occlusion.

▶ **Infraversion**—Tooth is positioned below the normal line of occlusion.

▶ **Transversion** or **transposition**—Tooth is in the wrong order in the arch.

Groups of teeth sometimes deviate from the normal tooth positions. Table 21-2 lists the term, gives a description of the variation, and shows an illustration.

TABLE 21-2 MALPOSITIONS OF GROUPS OF TEETH

Term	Description	Illustration
Anterior cross-bite	Abnormal relationship of a tooth or a group of teeth in one arch to the opposing teeth in the other arch. In anterior cross-bite, the maxillary incisors are positioned lingually to the opposing mandibular incisors.	
Posterior cross-bite	Abnormal relationship of teeth in one arch to the opposing teeth in the other arch. In posterior cross-bite, the primary or permanent maxillary posterior teeth are positioned lingually to the mandibular teeth.	
Edge-to-edge bite	Incisal surfaces of the maxillary anterior teeth meet the incisal surfaces of mandibular anterior teeth.	
End-to-end bite	Maxillary posterior teeth meet the mandibular posterior teeth cusp-to-cusp instead of in the normal fashion.	
Open bite	Failure of the maxillary and mandibular to occlude (meet).	

TABLE 21-2 *(continued)*

Overjet (horizontal overlap)	An abnormal horizontal distance between the labial surface of the mandibular anterior teeth and the labial surface of the maxillary anterior teeth.	
Overbite (vertical overlap)	Normally, the maxillary teeth extend vertically over the incisal one-third of the mandibular anterior teeth. When the vertical overlap is greater than this, the person is said to have an overbite.	
Underjet	Maxillary anteriors positioned lingually to the mandibular anteriors with excessive space between the labial of the maxillary anteriors and the lingual of the mandibular anteriors.	

ETIOLOGY OF MALOCCLUSION

The etiology or cause of malocclusion falls into one of three categories: genetic, systemic, or local.

1. **Genetic** or **heredity** factors may be responsible for deviations such as supernumerary teeth, facial and palatal clefts, abnormal jaw relationships, abnormal teeth-to-jaw relationships, and congenitally missing teeth.

2. **Systemic** factors include systemic diseases and nutritional disturbances that upset the normal schedule of dentition development during infancy and early childhood.

3. **Local** factors include trauma and habits such as thumb sucking, tongue sucking, mouth breathing, bruxism (involuntary grinding or clenching of teeth), and nail biting.

TYPES OF ORTHODONTIC TREATMENT

Orthodontic treatment involves much more than straightening teeth. The scope of treatments in orthodontics includes:

▶ Maintaining or establishing a normal or functional occlusion

▶ Improving the esthetic appearance of the face

▶ Eliminating problems that may disrupt normal development of the teeth and facial structures

▶ Correcting several facial and oral deformities through cooperative work with the oral and maxillofacial surgeon

Orthodontic treatments are divided into cases where malocclusion may be prevented or intercepted and cases where malocclusion already exists and correction is needed.

Preventive or Interceptive Orthodontics

Orthodontic treatment may be **preventive** or **interceptive**. Often, the general dentist and the pediatric dentist provide treatment. In complex cases, the general dentist works with the orthodontist on a treatment plan for the patient.

Common treatments that are considered preventive or interceptive include:

▶ Placing restorations to prevent premature loss of teeth

▶ Placing space maintainers to hold space for a missing tooth

▶ Recognizing any deviation from the normal

▶ Observing growth patterns and development of teeth and bones

- Correcting bad habits affecting the oral cavity as early as possible

- Extracting teeth to prevent overcrowding

- Removing deciduous teeth to provide space for permanent teeth

Corrective Orthodontics

Corrective orthodontics involves improving existing problems. This type of orthodontics is primarily accomplished on children in the last stage of mixed dentition entering full permanent dentition. Treatment of adults may also fall into corrective orthodontics.

Common treatments that are considered corrective orthodontics include:

- Placement of fixed or removable appliances. **Fixed appliances**, which are attached to the teeth and cannot be removed by the patient, include "braces," bands, brackets, arch wires, and ties. **Removable appliances**, which are inserted into the mouth and removed by the patient, include functional retainers.

- Orthognathic surgery for severe cases.

PROCESS OF TOOTH MOVEMENT

Orthodontic appliances are devices that move teeth by applying force. They also hold teeth in position. The appliances are carefully designed to achieve the desired movement and position of the teeth. The teeth are allowed to be moved through the process of **resorption**, which eliminates tissues no longer needed by the body. The teeth are retained in position through the process of **deposition**, which creates and deposits new cells.

The force of the orthodontic appliance compresses the periodontal ligament and reduces the blood supply to one side of the tooth. Specialized bone cells called **osteoclasts** cause the bone to resorb, or break down. As the tooth moves into the new space, the periodontal ligaments on the other side of the tooth are stretched, causing tension. As the tension increases, bone cells called **osteoblasts** deposit new bone to hold the tooth in its new position.

The principles of tooth movement are the same for all patients regardless of age; however, the rate of movement may be slower in the adult patient. Redeposited bone tissue takes six to twelve months for osteogenesis to take place. Thus, appliances such as retainers are required to hold the teeth in position. Overall, tooth movement depends on:

- Magnitude of force

- Duration of the application of force

- Direction of the force

- Distribution of the force

PREORTHODONTIC TREATMENT

Often, the patient's first visit to the orthodontist is for a preliminary examination. This enables the orthodontist to make an initial recommendation as to whether treatment is advisable at that time or should be delayed until there is further dental development. If treatment is delayed, follow-up appointments may be scheduled periodically to evaluate the patient's growth patterns. If treatment is advised, an appointment is scheduled for diagnostic records.

To ensure successful treatment, the orthodontist must have the cooperation of the patient and the support of the patient's family. This is an important aspect, because orthodontic treatment may take several years to complete. The patient must be willing to follow the directions of the orthodontist concerning appliances and also maintain good oral hygiene.

Diagnostic Records

Diagnostic records for orthodontic treatment include a medical and dental history, clinical examination, panoramic x-rays, cephalometric (**SEF**-ah-loh-meh-trick) x-rays, intraoral and facial photographs, and plaster study models of the teeth.

Medical–Dental History

Treatment begins with a complete medical history to evaluate the general health of the patient. Some conditions and medications have an effect on the patient's response to treatment or may require that the process proceed at a slower pace. Treatment may last for several years, so the medical history must be reviewed periodically.

The dental history provides information about the patient's past exposure to dental treatment. For example, caries incidence, missing teeth, and whether or not the patient has received routine dental care or only emergency dental care impacts the outcome of the orthodontic treatment. The dental history gives the orthodontist a guideline when designing the overall treatment plan to facilitate specific needs of the patient.

Clinical Examination

The dentist evaluates the results of an extensive examination of the face, jaws, and teeth, looking for symmetry between them. The teeth are evaluated for size, shape, color, and position. The jaws are examined for size, shape, and relationship to one another. The Angle classification of occlusion is often used to determine what classification the patient is in on both sides of the mouth.

The oral cavity is also examined for abnormal functional and neuromuscular patterns, such as tongue sucking, tongue thrusting, mouth breathing, and bruxism.

Radiographs

The orthodontist takes radiographs as part of the diagnostic procedure. The most common type of radiographs for orthodontics are the panoramic and the cephalometric. Some intraoral films are also taken for more detail of a particular area.

Panoramic x-rays are taken for an overall view of the dentition and surrounding area. Impacted teeth, abscesses, supernumerary teeth, or disorders of the temporomandibular joint can be determined from the panoramic film (Figure 21-3).

Cephalometric films are taken to evaluate the growth patterns and to determine the course of treatment. The cephalometric radiograph is a lateral view of the patient's head that shows the jaw and the teeth. The cephalometric radiograph tracings are done to determine the relationship of certain landmarks. These cephalometric tracings are either done manually using tracing paper and a special pen or by computer (Figures 21-4A and B). Cephalometric radiographs are taken periodically during treatment to monitor the patient's oral facial growth.

Photographs

Intraoral and extraoral photographs are taken as part of the patient's records before and after treatment. Facial photographs include a full frontal view and a profile view (Figure 21-5A). These are used to evaluate the symmetry and balance of the face.

Cheek retractors and mirrors are used when exposing intraoral photographs (Figure 21-5B and C). Intraoral photos are a visual record of the teeth and are used for planning treatment.

Study Models

Study models or diagnostic casts are used as part of the patient's record. They show how the teeth, mouth, and arches relate to one another. The study casts allow the study of the sizes and positions of the teeth along with the widths and lengths of the arches.

(A)

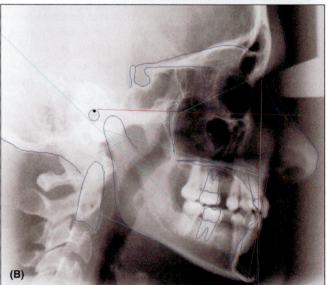

(B)

FIGURE 21-4 (A) Cephalometric radiograph. (B) Cephalometric tracing on radiograph. *(Courtesy of Dr. Steven Gregg)*

The first step is to take an alginate impression of the patient's teeth. The impression is then poured in stone or orthodontic plaster, trimmed, and finished. Orthodontic models are very detailed and symmetrical (Figure 21-6). The finished study models are used in the case presentation as visual aids and are kept as a reference throughout the patient's treatment.

▮ THE CONSULTATION APPOINTMENT

After the diagnostic appointment, the patient (and a parent if the patient is under the age of 18) is scheduled for a consultation appointment. The orthodontist studies the information gathered, makes a diagnosis, and prepares a treatment plan before the patient's appointment. Sufficient time must be allowed to present all the

FIGURE 21-3 Panoramic radiograph needed for diagnosis. *(Courtesy of Dr. Steven Gregg)*

FIGURE 21-5 (A) A full frontal view and profile view. (B) Intraoral photographs of the dentition from various angles and (C) Dentition from various angles using mirrors and cheek retractors.

FIGURE 21-6 Orthodontic study models symmetrically trimmed.

information to the patient (and parents). Radiographs, photographs, study models, and other visual aids are used in the presentation. During the consultation, the treatment, duration of treatment, involvement, and costs are explained. The responsibility of the patient is reviewed at this time so it is understood what he or she must do to facilitate treatment progress as planned. If the patient accepts the treatment plan, consent papers are signed and financial arrangements are made.

Sometimes, the age and development of the individual patient indicate that treatment be divided into several phases. The first phase may involve the patient wearing removable appliances and/or headgear. The patient is often in mixed dentition, and the treatment may last several months to two years. The next phase is the fixed appliance phase, which is started when the patient is in full permanent dentition.

ORTHODONTIC APPLIANCES

Orthodontic appliances are classified into two categories: fixed appliances and removable appliances.

Fixed Appliances

Fixed appliances are attached to the teeth and cannot be removed by the patient. The appliances are directly bonded onto the tooth or cemented into place with dental cement. The treatment is more controlled with fixed appliances, because the patient cannot remove them. Fixed appliances are commonly known as **braces** (Figure 21-7).

Orthodontic Bands. **Orthodontic bands** are thin bands of stainless steel that are carefully fitted around each tooth. Bands are supplied in a variety of sizes and are presized on the patient's model before cementation. Glass ionomer, polycarboxylate, or zinc phosphate cement is commonly used for cementing orthodontic bands. Bands are used on the posterior teeth because they provide the means to hold and control tooth movement. Depending on the individual case, various attachments such as brackets or buccal tubes are placed on the bands (Figure 21-8A).

Brackets. **Brackets** are attachments that are either welded to the bands or bonded directly to the teeth. Brackets for the posterior teeth are made of stainless steel and are welded directly to the band. Brackets for the anterior teeth are made of stainless steel, ceramic, or acrylic and are cemented or directly bonded to the teeth. The ceramic and acrylic brackets are popular because they are barely noticeable on the anterior teeth (Figure 21-8B).

FIGURE 21-8 (A) Orthodontic band with brackets and buccal tubes. (B) Metal brackets. (C) Tooth-colored brackets. *(Courtesy of Rita Johnson, RDH and Dr. Vincent DeAngelis)*

FIGURE 21-7 Patient in full braces. Posterior teeth are banded and the anterior teeth have brackets only. *(Courtesy of Rita Johnson, RDH and Dr. Vincent DeAngelis)*

The functions of the bracket is to hold the arch wire in place and to transmit the force of the arch wire to move the tooth.

Arch Wires. **Arch wires** fit into brackets and are secured by ligature ties or elastics. The arch wire is placed in the bracket and through a buccal tube on a posterior molar and then at each bracket; ligature wire or elastics are wrapped around the bracket. Arch wires are supplied in different shapes (square, round, and rectangular), diameters, and compositions, which alter the effect of the treatment (Figure 21-9A).

The function of the arch wire is to apply force to either move the teeth in or hold the desired positions. The position of the arch wire is changed throughout treatment as the teeth move.

Ligature Wire and Plastic Rings. **Ligature wire** and **plastic rings** are used to hold the arch wire to the brackets. Ligature wire is a very thin, flexible wire that usually

(A)

(B)

(C)

FIGURE 21-9 (A) 1. Various arch wires. (B) Ligature wire used to secure the arch wire to the brackets. (C) Elastic bands, "o," and chain elastics also used to secure the arch wire to the brackets.

comes in precut lengths or on spools (Figure 21-9B). The wire wraps around the bracket and then is tightened by twisting the wire, which ties or "ligates" the arch wire to the bracket. Plastic rings, also called elastic ties, are small bands that are supplied in a variety of colors. The elastic bands slip over the bracket to secure the arch wire. Also commonly used are elastic chains. The chain is a continuous chain of "Os." The elastic chain attaches several adjacent teeth together. This continuous pressure brings the teeth together (Figure 21-9C).

Buccal Tubes. **Buccal tubes** are small cylinders of metal welded to the molar bands, usually on the buccal surface. Their function is to provide a means of attachment for the arch wire to the band in the posterior area (Figures 21-8 and 21-10).

Springs. **Springs** are specially bent or shaped wires that are attached to the main arch wire. There are two main kinds of springs: the *finger spring* and the *coil spring*. The finger spring provides gentle pressure to individual teeth (Figure 21-11A). The coil springs exert a pressure to expand and compress spaces without losing the working force (Figure 21-11B).

Elastics. **Elastics** are rubber bands or elastic threads that are available in a variety of sizes. Elastics provide force for movement. They are often used between the upper and lower arches. Elastics are attached to hooks or buttons that are secured on the band or brackets.

TECH · A new advancement in ligature ties are the fluoride-releasing ties that aid in reducing decalcification of the tooth (Figure 21-12).

Special Fixed Appliances

There are several fixed orthodontic appliances that are not part of routine "braces." These appliances are cemented in place and have a specific function for a specific treatment or phases of treatment. They include the lingual braces, lingual arch wire, space maintainer, and palatal expansion appliance.

FIGURE 21-10 Diagram of full braces: bands with buccal tubes, brackets, arch wire, ligature wire, elastics, and finger springs. *(Courtesy of Rita Johnson, RDH and Dr. Vincent DeAngelis)*

FIGURE 21-11 (A) Finger spring on palate. (B) Coil spring.

FIGURE 21-12 Patient in full braces with rubber elastic from one arch to another. The rubber bands provide the force for movement. (*Courtesy of Rita Johnson, RDH, and Dr. Vincent DeAngelis*)

Lingual Braces. Lingual braces, sometimes called invisible braces, are attached to the lingual surface of the teeth. These braces have allowed patients who were apprehensive about their appearances during treatment an option to conventional braces. When the braces are placed on the lingual surfaces they are much less noticeable. The disadvantages to the lingual braces include placement and maintenance. It is difficult to

keep the areas dry during cementation, and they are troublesome for the patient to maintain.

Lingual Arch Wire. The lingual arch wire is placed on the lingual surface instead of the facial. Orthodontic bands are placed on the first permanent molars, and the arch wire is closely adapted to the lingual surfaces of the teeth. The function of the lingual arch wire is to maintain the arch by holding the teeth in position until the permanent teeth erupt (Figure 21-13A).

FIGURE 21-13 (A) Patient with a lingual arch wire. (B) Space maintainer to hold the space when a tooth is lost prematurely. (C) Palatal separating appliance. (*Courtesy of Rita Johnson, RDH, and Dr. Vincent DeAngelis*)

Space Maintainer. The space maintainer is composed of a band and a wire loop soldered together (Figure 21-13B). Its function is to maintain a space for the permanent tooth to erupt after the premature loss of the primary tooth. There are several varieties of space maintainers that can be adapted to the patient's teeth.

Palatal Separating Appliance. The palatal separating appliance is composed of an acrylic palatal portion that is split along the midline. The acrylic palatal portion is attached to bands, and the bands are cemented to the posterior teeth for stability. In the middle of the acrylic is a screw-like device that can be adjusted to expand the arch. The function of the palatal separating appliance is to spread the mid-palatal suture. This process takes about two to three weeks. Bone tissue fills in the opening and closes the space (Figure 21-13C).

Removable Appliances

Removable appliances are designed to be inserted into the mouth and removed by the patient. There are numerous varieties of removable appliances and many ways to categorize them. The more commonly used removable appliances include headgear, functional appliances, retainers, and positioners.

Headgear. Headgear consists of a strap that goes behind the patient's head or neck and a facebow that attaches to buccal tubes on molar bands. There are many designs to meet the individual patient's needs. Headgear is used to apply force to move teeth, to restrain or alter cranial-facial bone growth, and to reinforce stability of intraoral appliances. Usually, patients wear headgear for a specific number of hours each day (Figure 21-14).

Functional Appliances. Functional appliances are removable appliances that are routinely used before fixed appliances are placed. Functional appliances are used while the teeth and cranial-facial skeleton are still developing. There is a wide variety of functional appliances. Some guide newly erupting teeth into position, some change the direction of cranial-facial skeletal growth, and some inhibit the growth rate of one arch. The activator is the original functional jaw orthopedic appliance, and it has been modified many times. The activator is used to expand the width of the maxillary arch, for minor tooth movement, to make changes in skeletal growth patterns, and to reduce overbite (projection of upper teeth over the lower). The most common activators are the Bionator, the Herbst, and the Frankel (Figures 21-15A, B, and C).

FIGURE 21-14 Headgear is used to apply force to move teeth. The straps are adjustable. *(Courtesy of Rita Johnson, RDH and Dr. Vincent DeAngelis)*

FIGURE 21-15 (A) Patient with Bionator appliance. (B) Bionator appliance. (C) Herbst appliance. *(continued next page)*

FIGURE 21-15 *(continued)*
(D) Patient with Frankel appliance. (E) Frankel appliance.
(Courtesy of Dr. Steven Gregg)

Retainers. Retainers are custom-made appliances fitted to the patient's arch. They are made of acrylic or metal wire and acrylic and are secured in the patient's mouth by wires braced against and/or around the teeth. They are used to retain the teeth in position after the fixed appliances have been removed. The Hawley is an example of a retainer (Figure 21-16).

Tooth Positioner. The **tooth positioner** is a flexible rubber or soft-plastic appliance that surrounds the crowns of all teeth, in both arches, when positioned in the patient's mouth. Positioners are custom made for the patient after the removal of fixed appliances. Their function is to maintain the ideal position of the teeth upon completion of fixed treatment (Figure 21-17).

ORTHODONTIC INSTRUMENTS

There is a wide variety of orthodontic dental instruments. Following are commonly used instruments and their functions (Figures 21-18, 21-19, and 21-20):

FIGURE 21-16 Hawley appliance.

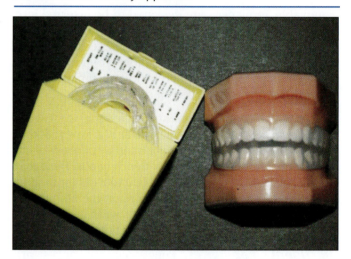

FIGURE 21-17 Tooth positioner.

▶ Coons ligature tying pliers—Manipulate ligature wire

▶ Mathieu needle holder—Tie ligature wire and place elastic ligatures

▶ Ligature director—Tucks twisted ligature wire ends into the interproximal spaces (a small condenser may also be used)

▶ Pin and ligature cutter or light wire cutter—Cut thin ligature wire

▶ Howe pliers—Utility pliers to manipulate ligature wire

▶ Band seater—Seats posterior metal bands

▶ Bite stick band seater—Uses force of occlusion to seat the band

▶ Band driver—Pushes the band into place

▶ Posterior band removing pliers—Removes posterior bands

FIGURE 21-18 Orthodontic instruments. (A) Mathieu needle holder. (B) Ligature director. (C) Pin and ligature cutter. (D) Howe pliers.

FIGURE 21-20 Orthodontic instruments. (A) Bird beak pliers. (B) Three prong pliers. (C) Weingart utility pliers. (D) Tweed loop pliers. (E) Distal-end cutting pliers.

ORTHODONTIC TREATMENTS

CDA Orthodontic treatment begins after the patient has finished the consultation appointment, the general dentist has restored all areas of decay, and the patient has been given a prophylaxis and fluoride treatment.

The orthodontic treatment sequence is as follows:

1. Application of separators
2. Placement of the posterior bands
3. Placement of the anterior brackets
4. Placement of the arch wire
5. Interval checkups
6. Completion appointment

Separators

A few days before the bands are placed on the posterior teeth, the patient is scheduled for placement of **separators**. Separators are placed in the contact areas between the teeth, forcing the teeth to spread apart to accommodate the orthodontic bands. There are several types of separators: elastics, steel spring, or brass wire.

Elastic Separators. Elastic separators are used because they provide a constant force as the teeth move, are easy to apply, and are more comfortable for the patient. The elastic separators are small circles that are stretched for placement. They fit around the contact area and, when released, apply a constant pressure until the teeth move apart, usually within a couple of days. The dental assistant may be permitted, in some states, to place and remove these separators.

FIGURE 21-19 Orthodontic instruments. (A) Band biter. (B) Band driver (pusher). (C) Posterior band removing pliers. (D) Band contouring pliers. (E) Bracket forceps.

▶ Band contouring pliers—Stretches and shapes the posterior bands to adapt to the tooth

▶ Bracket forceps—Holds brackets for placement and positioning

▶ "Bird beak" pliers—Contours wire and forms springs

▶ Three-prong pliers—Adjusts and bends wire and clasps

▶ Weingart utility pliers—Places the arch wire

▶ Tweed-loop pliers—Forms loops and springs in wire

▶ Distal-end cutting pliers—Cuts the distal ends of the arch wire

PROCEDURE

21-1 Placement and Removal of Elastic Separators

After the diagnosis, the first treatment appointment is to place separators to prepare the teeth for the orthodontic bands. Following the dentist's directions, the dental assistant places the separators. The patient has the separators removed and the bands placed several days following this procedure.

EQUIPMENT AND SUPPLIES (Figure 21-21A)

▶ Basic setup: mouth mirror, explorer, and cotton pliers

▶ Separation pliers

▶ Separators (wire or elastic)

▶ Dental floss or tape (optional technique)

▶ Scaler

PROCEDURE STEPS (*Follow aseptic procedures*)

Placement of Elastic Separators with Separating Pliers

FIGURE 21-21A Separating pliers, Howe pliers, and elastics.

1. First, examine the patient's mouth using the mouth mirror.

2. Place the elastic separator over the beaks of the separating pliers. Squeeze the pliers to secure the elastic on the pliers.

3. Further squeeze the pliers to stretch the elastic separator and place it between two teeth in a back-and-forth motion similar to the motion used when flossing. Insert one side of the elastic band below the contact in the interproximal space.

4. Release the tension on the separating pliers and remove the pliers. Repeat this process on all interproximal spaces around the teeth that are going to receive metal bands.

Placement of Separators with Dental Floss (Figure 21-21B)

FIGURE 21-21B Placement of separators. Dental floss to stretch the elastic separator for placement.

1. Place two lengths of dental floss through an elastic separator.

2. Fold over each floss length until the ends meet. Pull each piece of floss by the ends to stretch the elastic.

3. Using the back-and-forth motion, insert the separator into place.

(continued)

P R O C E D U R E   **2 1 - 1** *continued*

4. Once the separator is in place, release the floss and pull free.

Removal of Elastic Separators
(Figure 21-21C)

1. Using a scaler or an explorer, insert one end into the ring of the elastic separator.

2. Place a finger over the top of the separator to prevent the separator from snapping and injuring the patient.

3. Pull gently on the instrument toward the occlusal until the elastic is free of the contact.

FIGURE 21-21C Removal of elastic separators. *(Courtesy of Rita Johnson, RDH, and Dr. Vincent DeAngelis)*

P R O C E D U R E

21-2 Placement and Removal of Steel Spring Separators

This technique involves the placement and removal of the steel spring separators.

EQUIPMENT AND SUPPLIES

▶ Basic setup: mouth mirror, explorer, and cotton pliers

▶ Dental floss

▶ Bird beak or #139 pliers

▶ Steel spring separators

FIGURE 21-22 Steel spring separator.

PROCEDURE STEPS *(Follow aseptic procedures)*

Placement of Steel Spring Separators
(Figure 21-22)

1. Using the selected pliers, grasp the shortest side or leg of the spring separator.

2. Place the curve-hook of the spring separator under the contact from the lingual side.

3. Release the short side of the spring separator and slide it under the contact.

4. The coil is on the facial side; test the placement by gently pressing on the spring.

Removal of Steel Spring Separators

1. Place the finger of one hand over the spring to prevent injury to the patient.

2. Place one end of a scaler in the coil and lift upward.

3. Once the longest side of the spring is free of the lingual embrasure, pull the coil toward the facial aspect.

P R O C E D U R E

21-3 Placement and Removal of Brass Wire

This procedure involves the placement and removal of brass wire separators.

EQUIPMENT AND SUPPLIES

▶ Basic setup: mouth mirror, explorer, and cotton pliers

▶ Spool of brass wire (Figure 21-23)

▶ Hemostat

▶ Ligature wire cutter

▶ Condenser

Placement of Brass Wire Separators

1. Bend brass wire into C-shape, leaving a "tail" portion.

2. Starting from the lingual surface, place one part of the wire under the contact using a hemostat.

3. Fold the other part of the wire over the contact and pull toward the facial. Bring the ends of the wire together and twist.

4. Cut the twisted ends with the ligature cutting pliers and tuck them into the gingival embrasure.

FIGURE 21-23 Spool of brass wire used to separate the teeth.

Removal of Brass Wire Separators

1. Lift the brass wire carefully near the occlusal surface on the lingual side. Cut the wire using ligature cutting pliers.

2. Use the hemostat to remove both sections of the wire from under the contact on the facial side.

Selection of Orthodontic Bands

The patient returns to the office in a few days to have the separators removed and the orthodontic bands placed. The bands may be selected and sized on the patient's study model before the appointment, or the selection may take place directly on the patient, during the appointment. The bands are supplied in a wide variety of sizes for each tooth in the arch. They often have identifying code, printed on one surface. The code is helpful when selecting the bands and replacing the unused, sterilized bands.

Once the bands have been selected, they are tried on the teeth in the following way:

1. Place the band over the occlusal and apply pressure with a finger. The band should move toward the cervical third of the tooth.

2. The band pusher is used to push the band onto the tooth so that the margins of the band are beyond

FIGURE 21-24 Band pusher is used to seat the band on the tooth. *(Courtesy of Rita Johnson, RDH and Dr. Vincent DeAngelis)*

the occlusion (Figure 21-24). The band is adjusted until it fits closely to the contours of the tooth.

3. After all the bands have been sized, they are removed and placed on a model or band block.

4. The orthodontist or lab technician then prepares the bands for final cementation by smoothing the margins of the bands with a handpiece and bur. If the bands have brackets or buccal tubes, the bands are fitted with pins or wax in the openings to prevent cement from filling the bracket holes and the buccal tubes.

Band Cementation

Orthodontic bands are cemented using a variety of cements, including glass ionomer, polycarboxylate, and zinc phosphate. Although zinc phosphate cement has been used for many years, glass ionomer cement is becoming the preferred cement because it releases fluoride, which helps prevent decay under the bands during treatment.

Generally, the cement is thick for orthodontic band cementation and has a long setting time to permit final seating and adaptation. Follow manufacturer's instructions and technique suggestions.

P R O C E D U R E

21-4 Cementation of Orthodontic Bands

The orthodontic bands are prepared specifically for the patient. The orthodontist places the bands on the teeth to accomplish the task needed to correct the patient's malocclusion. The dental assistant mixes the cement and prepares the band for seating.

EQUIPMENT AND SUPPLIES (Figure 21-25)

▸ Basic setup: mouth mirror, explorer, and cotton pliers
▸ Cotton rolls and gauze
▸ Saliva ejector and HVE
▸ Slow-speed handpiece with rubber cup and prophy paste
▸ Selected and prepared bands
▸ Band pusher
▸ Bite stick
▸ Scaler
▸ Cement of choice
▸ Paper pad or glass slab
▸ Cement spatula
▸ Plastic filling instrument (PFI)

PROCEDURE STEPS (*Follow aseptic procedures*)

1. Once the separators are removed, the teeth are given a rubber cup polish.

2. The patient's mouth is rinsed thoroughly. The teeth are dried and cotton rolls are placed for isolation in the areas where the bands are to be placed.

FIGURE 21-25 Selection of bands and armamentarium for cementation.

3. Mix the cement according to the manufacturer's directions and load the first band. Place cement from the gingival edge, covering the inside of the band. Once the band is ready, transfer it to the

(continued)

P R O C E D U R E   **21-4** *continued*

dentist. There are many methods to transfer the bands. Some orthodontists prefer placement on the mixing slab or pad in order. Others like the bands passed on the end of the spatula or on a piece of wax or masking tape. Transferring the band needs to be made as easy as possible. Position the bands so that the orthodontist can pick them up in the order of sequence of placement (Figure 21-26A).

4. The orthodontist seats the band on the tooth. Transfer the band driver and any other instrument the orthodontist might request until the band is properly seated.

5. The banding procedure is repeated. Continue to fill the bands and transfer them to the operator until all bands have been cemented or until the cement becomes too thick and a new mix is required. If a new mix is required, clean the instruments with a wet gauze or an alcohol wipe and mix additional cement.

6. Once all bands are in place, the cement is allowed to set. During this time, clean the cement off all used instruments.

7. After the cement is set, remove the excess cement with a scaler. When all the cement has been removed, the protective pins or wax is (are) removed from the brackets and the patient's mouth is rinsed (Figure 21-26B).

FIGURE 21-26 (A) Assistant passes the band filled with cement to the operator. (B) Excess cement is removed from the tooth around the band. *(Courtesy of Rita Johnson, RDH and Dr. Vincent DeAngelis)*

Direct Bonding Brackets

The placement of brackets directly on the anterior teeth is a popular choice of treatment. Patients like the brackets because they are more esthetic than the full bands and it is easier to maintain good oral hygiene. The brackets are often purchased in kits or sets. The kit includes brackets from the left second bicuspid to right second bicuspid on both arches.

The brackets are bonded to the tooth surface with a similar material and technique used to restore anterior teeth composite resin.

Placement of the Arch Wire

The orthodontist selects and shapes the arch wire, so once the bands and brackets are placed, the arch wire can be positioned and secured in place. The arch wire is commonly secured into the brackets with elastic or stainless steel ligatures (ties). There is also a bracket that does not require ligature ties; instead, the bracket has a slot that opens for placement and removal of the arch wire. It is called the "Damon SL" (Figure 21-27).

FIGURE 21-27 Damon SL bracket. *(Courtesy of Dwight H. Damon, DDS, MSD)*

PROCEDURE

21-5 Direct Bonding of Brackets

This procedure involves bonding the brackets to the teeth.

EQUIPMENT AND SUPPLIES

▶ Basic setup: mouth mirror, explorer, and cotton pliers

▶ Cotton rolls and gauze

▶ Saliva ejector and HVE

▶ Slow-speed handpiece with rubber cup and pumice

▶ Bracket kit

▶ Retractors for the cheeks and lips

▶ Bracket forceps

▶ Acid etchant

▶ Bonding agent

▶ Scaler

PROCEDURE STEPS (*Follow aseptic procedures*)

1. The first step is to polish the teeth that are to receive brackets with a rubber cup and pumice (Figure 21-28A). (Polishing paste with fluoride is not used because some of the ingredients will interfere with the bonding process.)

2. The patient's mouth is rinsed and dried. Cotton rolls are placed in the area where brackets are to be bonded and retractors are positioned.

3. The acid etchant is placed on the enamel surface. The etchant remains on the tooth for a specific amount of time, following the manufacturer's directions. Prepare the etchant and transfer it to the operator. Maintain the operating field to be sure it stays dry.

4. Rinse the patient's mouth long enough to ensure that all the etchant is removed from the tooth surface (approximately thirty seconds) and then dry the tooth/teeth. The teeth will have a chalky appearance.

5. Prepare the bonding agent according to the manufacturer's directions and apply it to the back of the bracket (Figure 21-28B). Transfer the agent to the dentist for placement on the tooth. Then, pass the bracket. The orthodontist positions it on the tooth. Any excess bonding agent is removed with a scaler or similar instrument from around the bracket.

FIGURE 21-28 Steps in the placement of direct bonded brackets. (A) Clean the tooth surface. (B) Apply the bonding agent to the back of the bracket, and (C) place the bracket and light cure. (*Courtesy of Rita Johnson, RDH, and Dr. Vincent DeAngelis*)

6. The brackets are then held in position on the tooth until the bonding material is set chemically or with a curing light (Figure 21-28C).

7. Remove the cotton rolls and the retractors from the patient's mouth.

P R O C E D U R E

21-6 Placement of the Arch Wire and Ligature Ties

This procedure involves the placement of the arch wire and ligature ties.

EQUIPMENT AND SUPPLIES

▶ Basic setup: mouth mirror, explorer, and cotton pliers

▶ Cotton rolls and gauze

▶ Saliva ejector and HVE

▶ Selected arch wire

▶ Weingart pliers

▶ Bird beak pliers

▶ Elastics or ligature wire

▶ Ligature cutting pliers

▶ Ligature tying pliers

▶ Distal-end cutting pliers

▶ Condenser

PROCEDURE STEPS

1. Insert the arch wire into the buccal tubes on the molar bands using the Weingart pliers. If the wire is too long, cut off the ends with the distal-end cutting pliers.

2. The arch wire is placed in the brackets' horizontal slots along the arch (Figure 21-29). This may be accomplished with plastic rings/elastic ties, ligature wire, or the Damon SL bracket.

Elastic Ties Placement

3. The elastic ties are slipped over the brackets using ligature tying pliers or a hemostat. The ring ties are spread and placed on the gingival extensions of the brackets, pulled over the arch wire, and then wrapped around the occlusal extensions of the brackets (Figure 21-30).

Ligature Wire Ties Placement

4. Hold the ligature wire between the thumb and the index finger. Wrap the wire around the occlusal and gingival wings of the bracket in a distal-mesial direction. Cross the ends of the wire together. Using a hemostat or ligature tying pliers, twist the ends of

FIGURE 21-29 (A) Arch wire is cut to size with distal end cutting pliers and (B) placed into buccal tubes. *(Courtesy of Rita Johnson, RDH and Dr. Vincent DeAngelis)*

FIGURE 21-30 Elastic rings being placed on anterior bracket. *(Courtesy of Rita Johnson, RDH and Dr. Vincent DeAngelis)*

(continued)

P R O C E D U R E   2 1 - 6 *continued*

the wire together for several rotations. Repeat the process to secure the arch wire (Figure 21-31A).

5. The twisted ends of the ligature wire, called the "pigtail," are cut with ligature wire cutting pliers to 3 to 4 mm (Figure 21-31B and C).

6. The pigtail is bent into the embrasure space with a condenser (Figure 21-31D).

7. After all the pigtail ends have been tucked into place, run a finger over the area to check for sharp ends.

8. Check the distal ends of the arch wire. Cut any excess with distal-end cutting pliers.

9. If the patient's treatment requires rubber elastics bands, they are placed at this appointment. The patient is shown how to place and remove them. The rubber bands stretch with time, so the orthodontist will give instructions on how often to change the rubber bands. The patient is given a sufficient number of elastics with instructions to call the office for more, if needed.

FIGURE 21-31 (A) Ligature wire being looped around the brackets. (B) Ligature wire is twisted. (C) Ligature wire is cut with cutting pliers, (D) and tucked into the embrasure space. *(Courtesy of Rita Johnson, RDH, and Dr. Vincent DeAngelis)*

Oral Hygiene Instructions

Oral hygiene instructions are given to the patient once the braces are in place. With fixed braces, food and debris have many places to hide and attach to, making the patient more caries susceptible. Good oral hygiene is necessary to prevent plaque buildup in these areas. The dental assistant educates and motivates the patient. This process is continued throughout the treatment.

(A)

(B)

FIGURE 21-32 Toothbrushing with fixed appliances in place. Toothbrush properly positioned on the (A) maxillary teeth and (B) mandibular teeth.

Keeping some patients motivated can be a challenge, and numerous approaches must be used.

The instructions include:

▶ **Brushing**—The patient is given an orthodontic toothbrush and shown how to brush around the fixed appliances in order to remove plaque. The toothbrush is contoured to fit around the brackets and into the space between the band and the gingival margin. The patient will need to spend more time after meals and at bedtime to keep the teeth clean (Figures 21-32A and B).

▶ **Flossing**—Supply the patient with a floss threader to thread the floss under the arch wire and through the

FIGURE 21-33 Floss being threaded under the arch wire.

interproximal area. Motivating the patient to take the time to floss routinely may be a challenge (Figure 21-33).

▶ **Diet**—The patient should avoid certain foods that may damage the bands, arch wire, or brackets. Foods that are sticky, crunchy, and hard should be avoided. Examples include caramels, chewing gum, popcorn, and raw vegetables (unless they are cut into small pieces).

▶ **Fluoride rinses**—These may be prescribed for the patient's home use during orthodontic treatment.

Periodic Office Visits for Adjustments

As time passes and the teeth begin to move, the patient will need to see the orthodontist for adjustments. These appointments are usually short, unless the arch wire needs to be changed. The orthodontist reviews the patients' progress, checks the appliances, and makes any adjustments. The dental assistant performs some of these responsibilities under the direct supervision of the dentist.

These appointments also are used for oral hygiene checks. If the patient is not doing an adequate job, the dental assistant reviews brushing and flossing with the patient and talks with the patient to motivate and encourage.

COMPLETION APPOINTMENT

Once the teeth have moved into position and the orthodontist is satisfied with the treatment, the braces are removed. The patient receives a coronal polish and an impression is taken for construction of a retainer or positioner in order to hold the teeth in position for the alveolar bone to stabilize the new positions of the teeth.

PROCEDURE

21-7 Completion Appointment

When the orthodontist determines that the patient's teeth have moved to the desired positions, the appliances are removed.

EQUIPMENT AND SUPPLIES

▶ Basic setup: mouth mirror, explorer, and cotton pliers
▶ Cotton rolls and gauze
▶ Scaler
▶ Ligature wire cutting pliers
▶ Hemostat
▶ Bracket and adhesive removing pliers
▶ Posterior band remover
▶ Ultrasonic scaler (optional)
▶ Prophy angle, cups, and prophy paste
▶ Alginate impression material and selected tray

PROCEDURE STEPS *(Follow aseptic procedures)*

1. The ligature ties are removed first. They are loosened with a scaler or an explorer and then cut with the ligature wire cutting pliers.

Elastic Bands

2. Elastic ties are removed with a scaler.

3. The tip of the scaler explorer is placed under the elastic and rolled over the bracket wings until the elastic is released (Figure 21-34).

FIGURE 21-34 Removal of the elastic rings. Insert the end of a scaler explorer under the elastic and roll the elastic rings over the wings of the bracket. *(Courtesy of Rita Johnson, RDH, and Dr. Vincent DeAngelis)*

Ligature Wire Ties

4. Place the beaks of the ligature wire cutting pliers where the wire is exposed and cut the wire.

5. Carefully remove the wire from the wings of the bracket. Repeat on each tooth until all the ligature wires are removed.

6. Using a hemostat, remove the arch wire from the brackets (Fiure 21-35). Pull the arch wire from the buccal tube on one side. Then, hold it securely to prevent injury to the patient while removing the opposite end.

7. To remove the anterior brackets, use a bracket and adhesive-removing pliers. The lower beak of the pliers, with a very sharp edge, is placed from

FIGURE 21-35 Removal of ligature wire. Pull twisted "pigtail" wire from the embrasure. Cut the wire. Unwind from the wings of the bracket in an occlusal direction. *(Courtesy of Rita Johnson, RDH, and Dr. Vincent DeAngelis)*

(continued)

FIGURE 21-36 Removal of brackets.

the gingival edge of the bracket; the upper beak, with a nylon tip, is placed on the occlusal edge of the bracket. When the pliers are squeezed together, the sharp lower beak breaks the bond and removes some cement (Figure 21-36).

8. To remove the posterior bands, band-removing pliers are placed with the cushioned end on the buccal cusp. The end with the blade is placed against the gingival edge of the band. The band is gently lifted toward the occlusal surface (Figure 21-37).

9. This process is repeated on the lingual surfaces until the band is free.

10. Cement and direct bonding materials are removed from the tooth surface with a hand scaler, an ultrasonic scaler, and/or a finishing bur.

FIGURE 21-37 Removal of band with the band removal pliers.

11. A rubber cup polish is completed. Photographs may be taken.

12. An alginate impression is taken of both arches. The impressions are sent to the lab to be used in the construction of the retainer.

13. The patient is reappointed for later that day or for the next day. The retainer or positioner is then placed.

14. The patient is given instructions on placement and removal of the removable appliance and the wearing schedule.

CHAPTER SUMMARY

The orthodontic team consists of the orthodontist, reception and business office staff, office coordinator, the orthodontic assistants, and laboratory technicians. The orthodontic assistant has a variety of responsibilities, depending on the size of the practice and the number of auxiliaries. The functions also vary with each state's Denal Practice Act.

To become a certified orthodontic assistant, a specialty examination must be passed.

CASE STUDY

Chaz Danton, twelve years old, had an appointment with the orthodontist, Dr. Snyder. Chaz has an overbite and a receded mandible. When eating crunchy foods, such as toast and pizza crust, the palate becomes inflamed and irritated. Chaz is missing his permanent bicuspids.

Case Study Review

1. What should the dental assistant prepare for Chaz's appointment?

2. Is Chaz's age a factor in the orthodontist's diagnosis?

3. What stage of tooth eruption should the dental assistant expect Chaz to be in? What primary teeth are normally present?

To complete your study of this chapter, work the review activities that follow. Also, refer to the software that accompanies this text.

REVIEW QUESTIONS

Multiple Choice

1. When individual teeth are turned or rotated in the socket, they are said to be
a. infraversion.
b. linguoversion.
c. transposition.
d. torsoversion.

2. Which of the following types of orthodontic treatment involves placement of fixed appliances?
a. Preventive treatment.
b. Interceptive treatment.
c. Corrective treatment.

3. Orthodontic tracings are made using which of the following types of radiographs?
a. Bite-wing radiographs.
b. Periapical radiographs.
c. Cephalometric radiographs.
d. Panoramic radiographs.

4. To secure the arch wire in position on the posterior bands, use
a. buccal tubes.
b. brackets.
c. springs.
d. plastic rings.

5. All of the following are true statements about orthodontic brackets *except*
a. brackets are welded onto orthodontic bands or bonded directly to the teeth.
b. brackets are made of stainless steel, ceramic, or acrylic.
c. brackets hold the bands in place on the teeth.
d. brackets hold the arch wire in place.

CRITICAL THINKING

1. Do you have any individual teeth that are out of alignment? Using orthodontic terms, describe the deviations and identify the malpositioned teeth.

2. Which foods should the orthodontic patient avoid? What are some alternative suggestions?

3. Name the three categories of causes of malocclusion. Give three examples in each category. Have you or anyone in your family had an orthodontic condition? Trace the etiology to one of the categories.

Pediatric Dentistry

OBJECTIVES

The student should strive to meet the following objectives and demonstrate an understanding of the facts and principles presented in this chapter:

1. Define pediatric dentistry as a specialty.

2. Describe the pediatric office and team members.

3. Explain common behavior characteristics of children of various ages.

4. Describe child behavior management techniques.

5. Explain the role of the parent or guardian in pediatric dentistry.

6. Identify common procedures in pediatric dentistry.

7. Identify the equipment unique to pediatric dentistry.

8. Explain common emergencies in pediatric dentistry and the treatment for these emergencies.

9. Identify the signs of child abuse and the procedure for reporting suspected child abuse cases.

KEY TERMS

apexogenesis (p. 475)

avulsed tooth (p. 479)

behavior management (p. 470)

direct pulp capping (DPC) (p. 474)

fluoride applications (p. 472)

hand-over-mouth (HOM) technique (p. 471)

indirect pulp treatment (IPT) (p. 474)

maturation (p. 469)

modeling technique (p. 470)

mouth guards (p. 472)

objective fears (p. 470)

open bay (p. 468)

pedodontics (p. 468)

pit and fissure sealants (p. 472)

pulpectomy (p. 476)

pulpotomy (p. 474)

space maintainers (p. 472)

spot-welded matrix bands (p. 473)

stainless steel crowns (p. 476)

subjective fears (p. 470)

T-band matrix (p. 473)

tell, show, and do technique (p. 470)

tongue thrust (p. 472)

traumatic intrusion (p. 479)

INTRODUCTION

The pediatric dental practice provides dental care for children and is often referred to as **pedodontics**. The pediatric specialist treats children from birth through the eruption of their second permanent molars. The pediatric practice sometimes treats medically, mentally, or emotionally compromised adults. The scope of the pediatric treatment for child patients includes restoring and maintaining the primary, mixed, and permanent dentition and applying preventive measures for dental caries, periodontal disease, and malocclusion. Although there has been a decrease in the number of dental caries found in children, the restorative aspect is still a comprehensive part of the practice. The primary focus of the pediatric dental practice is preventive treatment and dealing with the compromised adult patient.

The pediatric specialist is concerned with the basic needs and special requirements for treatment of the young patient. The pediatric dentist has special training in child growth, development, and behavior management. This training enables the pediatric dentist to successfully treat the emotionally and physically developing child and the special needs patient.

The general dentist, other specialists, and physicians refer patients to the pediatric specialist for treatment. The general dentist, orthodontist, and pediatric dentist work closely to ensure the best overall dental care and education for the child patient.

The Pediatric Dental Office

The pediatric office is open and friendly to make the child patient feel comfortable and secure. Pediatric offices are creative and imaginative in the office setting. The decor is often bright and designed with things children are attracted to. The waiting room usually has an area for coloring or reading, a cage or tank holding small animals or fish, toys for various age groups, and a display area with pictures of patients (Figure 22-1).

In some pediatric offices, the treatment areas are designed with several dental chairs arranged in one open area. This **open bay** concept allows the children to see each other. It is reassuring for the child patient to know that other children are there and receiving treatment. Many offices have headphones with a variety of programs or music available or televisions with either movies or patient education programs running.

Often the pediatric office will include a "quiet room" for patients who are difficult to manage. This room is separate and closed off from the others so that if there are patient management problems, they will not upset the other children in the office.

The Pediatric Dental Team

The composition of the pediatric dental team is the same as the general dental office team. The difference may be

FIGURE 22-1 Reception area in a pediatric practice including various toys, an activity area, books, and television with video.

the personalities of team members and the true desire to work with children. The whole staff needs to enjoy children and be sincere and honest in their actions and feelings. To be effective in the management of children, the dental team must be upbeat, motivated, and aware.

The pediatric staff usually do not wear white uniforms but often wear bright colors and designs. Safety glasses and gloves are routinely worn, but masks may not be. If it is necessary to wear a mask, explain to the child why a mask is being worn. To make the mask look less threatening, some masks can be purchased that have designs printed on them, or the child or dental assistant can draw a happy face or a cartoon character on the mask.

The Dental Assistant's Role in Pediatric Dentistry

The role of the dental assistant in the pediatric practice varies depending on the areas of responsibility. One aspect is the management of the child. Another is the work at chairside. Skills the assistant performs at chairside vary in every office and from state to state depending on the state Dental Practice Act. When the assistant works independently, he or she assumes the authority role and must maintain control of the child.

In many offices, the assistant plays the dominant role in greeting the child, escorting him or her to the treatment area, and preparing him or her for treatment. When the dentist comes into the room, the assistant transfers the attention and control to the dentist. The assistant's role during treatment is to support the dentist in a manner that the assistant and the dentist have discussed. Usually, this is office policy and a good topic for staff meeting discussions.

The dental assistant is also an educator, both for the child and the parents. The assistant answers questions or refers them to the pediatric dentist. Topics that might be discussed include oral hygiene techniques, dental nutrition, tooth eruption, and application of fluoride.

BEHAVIOR CHARACTERISTICS OF CHILDREN AT VARIOUS AGES

Each child develops on his or her own special time schedule, but there are some common levels of psychological and physical growth. **Maturation** is growth to a certain level and then learning on that level. The child may be seven years old but not mature enough to learn on this level. Development takes longer for some than for others, and environment, age, experiences, and other people all influence psychological growth. Table 22-1 gives some general characteristics of behavior in children at various ages. These are generalizations and not meant to be limiting.

Understanding the behavior of children at different ages will give the dental assistant a better way to establish a relationship with children. Having some idea of their learning levels, communication abilities, and interests enables the assistant to understand the patient and effectively manage the child to make his or her experience with dentistry a positive one. The age from two to six years is the best age to introduce dental care in the dental office.

PATIENT MANAGEMENT

Patient management is a team effort. Successful treatment is the result of how well the patient is managed. The dental team must work together and know each other's responsibilities and roles. A positive, trusting relationship with some children takes time and effort. The dental team must have consistent management policies and procedure sequences and consistently use the same terminology when speaking with patients.

Longevity with staff members provides the opportunity to better respond as a unit. Over time, the team will

TABLE 22-1 GENERAL BEHAVIOR CHARACTERISTICS OF CHILDREN AT VARIOUS AGES

Ages	Behavior
Two to six years overall	Likes to be with parents and siblings. Likes to play (e.g., having a "ride" in the dental chair, seeing the "squirt gun," and so on). Can respond to the dentist's instructions and understands simple explanations. Transitional time from infantile behavior patterns to the more independent pre-school child.
Two to four years	Short attention span. Wide variety of interests. Parallel play without bothering other children. Responds to fantasy.
Four to six years	Shows feelings with facial expression. Parents are very influential. Greatest number of management problems. Needs constant reassurance. Moves to integrated play. Shows some tolerance with dislikes.
Six to twelve years overall	Period of socializing. Asserts independence. Difference in boys and girls more noticeable.
Six to nine years	Learning to get along with people and regulations of society. Friendships are important. Usually prefers to come in for treatment without parent. Likes to collect things. Aware of place in society and likes to belong to a group. Likes to be spoken to directly.
Nine to twelve years	Usually not difficult to manage. May be passive in responses. Girls are more mature. Will respond if things are explained. Boys sometimes act like they know it all. Like to be treated as adults.

encounter different management problems; once the problems have occurred, discuss them and decide how they will be handled in the future.

Fear is a large factor in behavior problems with children. Some of the fears are based on feelings, attitudes, and concerns that have developed from suggestions of others, including parents, siblings, and friends. These are called subjective fears. Other fears, which are based on the child's own experiences, are known as objective fears.

When a child has questions, the dental team should give honest, brief, and simple answers. Try to relate the answer to something the child already knows about or has experienced. For example, relate the pinch of an injection to the pinch of a mosquito.

Behavior Management Techniques

There are many behavior management techniques. A few are covered here to give the dental assistant some ideas. The following are taken from the American Academy of Pediatric Dentistry's published *Standards of Care for Behavior Management*.

Tell, Show, and Do. With the tell, show, and do technique, the assistant names a dental instrument and demonstrates the use of the instrument, often using either his or her hand or fingers or the child's hand. Once the child is comfortable, the instrument is utilized (Figure 22-2).

Voice Control. Speaking calmly but firmly lets the child know the dentist is in control and is serious about the treatment and the child's behavior.

Distraction. Distract the child's attention from perceived unpleasant procedures. Watching videos, listening to tapes, or getting the child to think of something pleasant are methods of distraction (Figure 22-3).

Nonverbal Communication. Nonverbal communication gains the attention of the child and guides his or her behavior. The dental team's facial expressions, postures, and contact with the child reinforces positive behavior.

Modeling. The modeling technique pairs a timid child in dental care with a cooperative child of a similar age. The open bay treatment areas provide the opportunity for the modeling process.

Positive Reinforcement. Give the patient positive reinforcement at the appropriate time. Every child does something right during the dental visit. Praise him or her in order to reinforce the positive behavior. Be sure the praise or positive reinforcement is honest, sincere, and for worthy behavior.

Gentle Restraints. Sometimes a child's behavior during treatment requires management for his or her own protection from possible injury. Some children need gentle restraint of the arms and legs to reduce or eliminate movement. This is for the safety of the patient and the operator.

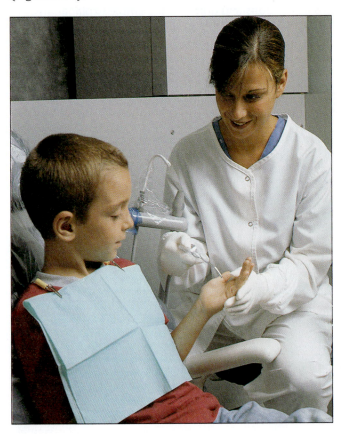

FIGURE 22-2 Dental assistant showing a child how the air-water syringe operates.

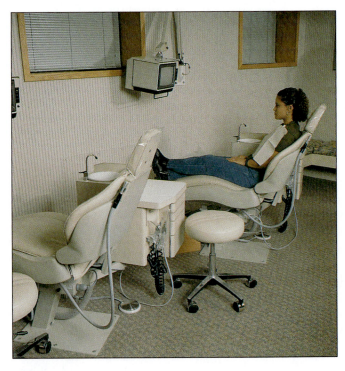

FIGURE 22-3 Child watching a television and listening with earphones.

Hand-over-Mouth (HOM). The **hand-over-mouth (HOM) technique** works to gain the child's attention for establishing communication, eliminate inappropriate avoidance responses, enhance the child's self-confidence in coping during treatment, and ensure safety during delivery of care. The dentist places his or her hand over the patient's mouth and, in a very calm voice, explains behavior expectations. The hand is removed when behavior is appropriate. The process is reapplied, if neces-

sary. HOM requires informed consent and, although effective, this technique is not used often.

Mild Sedation. An anxious child may benefit from sedation. Conscious sedation and nitrous oxide inhalation are two forms used in the pediatric office. They both require informed consent before being administered. Conscious sedation and nitrous oxide inhalation are preoperative or intraoperative. Both reduce anxiety and movement by the patient, increase tolerance for longer periods, and enhance communication. Sedation aids in the treatment of mentally, physically, or medically compromised patients.

General Anesthesia. If a child is extremely fearful or uncooperative or if the patient has certain physical, mental, or medical conditions, general anesthesia is administered for treatment. This provides a safe, efficient, and effective means for dental care. General anesthesia requires informed consent from the child's parent or guardian.

ROLE OF THE PARENT OR GUARDIAN

Parents or guardians often require assistance to best prepare the child for dental care. Sometimes, their past experiences influence how they feel about dental treatment, and this is transmitted to the child. Then, the child becomes apprehensive and hesitant.

Many offices have suggestions for parents to help prepare the child for treatment. There are pamphlets, books, and videos to instruct the parents on how to explain what the child is going to experience in the dental office. It is important that the child's questions be answered truthfully but in terms they understand and with minimal explanation. If the parents are not sure of the treatment or how to answer the questions, they should tell the child to ask the dentist.

When the first appointment is made, the parent should be informed of what to expect. This usually means examining the child's teeth and taking x-rays. A treatment plan may include restorations and preventive treatment. The parents are encouraged to discuss concerns they might have with the dentist, away from the child.

Each office has a policy on parents coming into the treatment room with the child during the appointment. The dental assistants need to know how the dentist feels about having the parents with the child during

treatment. Some dentists feel that they can manage the child better if the parents are not in the treatment room. Others feel that as long as the parents do not interfere, they can remain. The parents usually are eager to cooperate with the office policies. If the child insists that the parent comes into the treatment area, offer him or her a chair near the foot of the patient's chair so he or she is are not in the direct view of the child when the child is reclined and the dentist and dental assistant are seated. The dental team remains focused on establishing a relationship with the *child.* On occasion, the dentist may use the presence of the parents to control behavior. For example, the dentist might say that if the child cooperates, the parent can stay in the treatment area, but if the child does not cooperate, the parents will be asked to leave. Some dentists feel that if the child does not behave, it is the parent's responsibility to manage the child in order for dental care to be completed.

Parents generally are very supportive if they are informed, know what is happening, and know what is expected of them.

PROCEDURES IN PEDIATRIC DENTISTRY

The first appointment with the pediatric dentist may be for a routine examination followed by treatment, or it may be an emergency appointment due to an injury. Dental care for children involves both the primary and permanent dentition. Sometimes the parents may question the need to restore primary teeth, because they are not permanent and will be replaced. The primary dentition is restored for the following reasons:

▶ The primary teeth are needed to hold space for the permanent teeth.

▶ They maintain the functions of the teeth in chewing, speech, and esthetics.

▶ They act as guides for the permanent dentition during eruption.

Educating the parents to understand the importance of the primary teeth is necessary with all types of pediatric dental treatment (see Appendix B, Development of Human Dentition).

The Examination

The examination of a child patient is similar to that of an adult. The gingiva, supporting tissues, and oral mucosa are checked. The surfaces of the teeth are examined with a mouth mirror and an explorer. Radiographs are exposed to show the conditions of the primary teeth and the positions and development of the permanent teeth (refer to Chapter 17, Dental Radiography, for suggestions and types of pediatric x-ray exposures).

The patient's medical/dental history is recorded by the parent or guardian. The medical history provides information about past dental experiences, any allergies, facial habits, illnesses, and general development of the child.

Preventive Procedures

Preventive procedures in pediatric dentistry include educating both the child and parent regarding diet suggestions, oral hygiene techniques, the use of fluorides, pit and fissure sealants, use of mouth guards for sport activities, and preventive orthodontic treatment.

Oral Hygiene Techniques. Oral hygiene techniques are coordinated with the child's age and physical ability (see Chapter 2, Oral Health and Nutrition, for oral hygiene techniques for children). The parent is given information on toothbrushing and flossing techniques in order to assist the child.

Coronal Polishes. Coronal polishes followed by **fluoride applications** and **pit and fissure sealants** are routine procedures the child receives during examination appointments. If the water is not fluoridated in the area, fluoride is prescribed by the dentist. The dental assistant should review the fluoride therapy plan with the parents periodically.

Mouth Guards. Children who are actively involved in contact sports should be fitted for **mouth guards**. The guards offer protection from premature loss of the teeth or from fractures. There are various types of mouth guards. Some are made in the dental office, such as the custom-fit mouth guard. This mouth guard is made in the office using a study model and vacuum-formed material (Figure 22-4). There are also commercial "do-it-yourself kits" available, where the material comes in various sizes. It is heated under warm water and then molded to the individual arch.

Preventive and Interceptive Orthodontic Treatment. Preventive and interceptive orthodontic treatment includes a variety of orthodontic treatments. Two common procedures are the placing space maintainers and correcting oral habits.

Space Maintainers. **Space maintainers** are designed to maintain a space until the permanent tooth erupts. The space is the result of the premature loss of a primary tooth. A space maintainer may be a *fixed* or *removable appliance*. The appliance is designed to meet the needs of the child patient. Fixed space maintainers are more commonly used because they are cemented permanently in place so that the patients cannot take them in and out (refer to the Chapter 21, Orthodontics, for more information on space maintainers).

Oral Habits. **Oral habits** such as thumb sucking and tongue thrusting may need intervention because they can lead to abnormal muscle function, distorted growth of the jaw, malocclusion, changed facial contour, and problems with speech.

Thumb sucking is a controversial subject with many opinions on whether the habit should be "treated." Most orthodontists leave the thumb sucking of a child alone until the child's maxillary anterior teeth erupt; hopefully, by then, the habit will be gone. Most dentists begin some form of treatment if the child continues to suck his or her thumb at age five. Treatment includes counseling with the child and the parents, "gentle persuasion," and behavior modification techniques. Fixed appliances, such as cribs and rakes, are also used if the habit continues (Figure 22-5).

Tongue thrusting is a habit in which the child's tongue pushes against the anterior teeth during swallowing, causing an anterior open bite. Treatment for this habit includes myofunctional exercises (therapy) or the use of appliances.

FIGURE 22-4 Examples of mouth guard material and formed mouth guard.

FIGURE 22-5 Crib appliance to stop the child from sucking his thumb. *(Courtesy of Steven Gregg, DDS)*

Restorative Procedures

Restorative procedures are similar to those performed on adult patients. The materials used in pediatric dentistry are the same materials used in the restoration of permanent teeth. Amalgam is used most frequently for posterior teeth, while composite resins are used on anterior teeth and some posterior teeth. Badly decayed teeth are protected with stainless steel crowns that are permanently cemented in place. In very rare cases, partials and dentures are made for pediatric patients.

The difference between pediatric and adult restorative procedures is the size of the instruments. Examples of instruments and materials that are reduced in size include the dental high-speed handpiece and burs, dental dam material, and dental dam clamps. The dental dam material is smaller in size and the width of the jaws of the clamps is smaller to accommodate the primary teeth. The high-speed handpiece has a compact head to allow for better access in the child's mouth. The burs have shorter shanks.

Pedodontic Matrices. The **dental matrices** used in restorative procedures are adapted to the sizes and shapes of the teeth. The tofflemire matrix is used in pediatrics, but custom matrices are more common (see Chapter 28, Advanced Chairside Techniques). Two cus-

FIGURE 22-6 T-bands, straight and curved.

tom matrices are the **T-band matrix** and the **spot-welded matrix bands**.

The T-bands are designed for and used on primary teeth. They are often made of brass strips that are "crossed" at one end. They come in various designs and sizes. The T-bands do not require retainers, are adjustable, and can be secured on the tooth (Figure 22-6).

Spot-welded matrix bands also are used for primary teeth. The custom-made bands are used for Class II

P R O C E D U R E

22-1 T-Band Placement

For this procedure, the tooth has been prepared and a matrix is assembled and placed on the tooth. The dentist places the T-band unless the state Dental Practice Act allows the dental assistant to perform this skill.

EQUIPMENT AND SUPPLIES

▶ T-band assortment

▶ Burnisher

▶ Cotton pliers or hemostat

▶ Crown and collar scissors

PROCEDURE STEPS *(Follow aseptic procedures)*

1. Prepare the T-band ahead of time by selecting the appropriate band size.

2. Loop the band to shape the approximate diameter of the tooth.

3. Fold the "T" ends over the band loop, leaving a circle with long tail or end.

4. The band is placed on the tooth, into the interproximal space covering the margins of the preparation.

5. The portion of the band where the "T" is folded is placed on the buccal surface, away from the margins of the preparation.

6. The band is tightened by pulling on the free end (tail) until the band is tight around the tooth.

7. The free end is bent back toward the "T" to secure the band. The excess band is removed with scissors.

8. The band is burnished and a wedge is placed as needed.

9. To remove the T-band, fold back the overlapping section of band to loosen the band. Use cotton pliers to remove the band from the tooth.

P R O C E D U R E

22-2 Spot-Welded Matrix Band Placement

For this procedure, the tooth has been prepared for a restoration and the spot-welded matrix band is prepared by the dental assistant at chairside.

EQUIPMENT AND SUPPLIES

▶ Spot-welded matrix band material

▶ Crown and collar scissors

▶ Cotton pliers, hemostat, or Howe pliers

▶ Burnisher

▶ Spot-welding unit

PROCEDURE STEPS *(Follow aseptic procedures)*

1. Cut an approximate length of matrix band material. Turn on the spot-welding unit to warm it up.

2. Loop the matrix material around the tooth, bringing the ends of the material together on the buccal surface.

3. Pinch the band tightly together with a hemostat, cotton pliers, or Howe pliers.

4. Bend the excess material to one side.

5. Take the band to the spot-welding unit and spot weld the band together to form a circle the diameter of the tooth (Figure 22-7).

6. Trim off the excess and sharp edges of the band.

7. Replace the band on the tooth with the welded area on the buccal surface. Place wedges in the interproximal and contour.

FIGURE 22-7 Spot-welding the matrix band.

8. To remove the band after the amalgam has been placed, cut the lingual aspect of the band and pull the band in an occlusal/buccal direction with cotton pliers.

---

restorations. The matrix material comes in rolls of one-quarter to three-sixteenths-inch widths and 0.002 gauge thickness. This custom matrix does not require a retainer to be secure on the tooth, but a spot-welding machine is required. This band is made quickly at chairside.

Pulp Therapy in Primary and Young Permanent Teeth

Caries or traumatic injuries can damage both primary and permanent teeth. The teeth are assessed to determine the status of the pulp. The duration, frequency, and location of pain is recorded. The clinical assessment includes a visual examination and radiographs. The extent of the lesion is determined by the following:

if there is a fistula (pathway from an abscess to the mucosa), if the tooth is mobile, if there is any swelling, and/or if there is sensitivity to heat or percussion.

Vital Pulp Therapy. Vital pulp therapy involves the removal of tissue that is potentially infected (this procedure will maintain the tooth in a healthy state so that the tooth is not lost) and focuses on the reparative ability of the pulp. There are three choices in treatment depending on the status of the pulp: **indirect pulp treatment (IPT)**, **direct pulp capping (DPC)**, or a **pulpotomy**.

If the pulp is not yet exposed, indirect pulp treatment (IPT), also known as indirect pulp capping, is indicated. In this case, the pulp has not yet been exposed, but there is a chance that the pulp will be exposed while removing the caries. The technique involves:

1. Leaving a thin layer of sound or carious dentin with no evidence of pulp exposure (Figure 22-8A)

2. Placing a medicament and a temporary restoration that seals completely (Figure 22-8B)

3. Leaving the medicament and restoration for six to eight weeks

4. Opening the tooth and removing the remaining caries

5. Placing a restoration

If the pulp has been exposed through mechanical or traumatic means but there is a chance for a favorable response, a direct pulp capping (DPC) procedure is indicated. The patient should be informed of the possible outcomes with the direct pulp capping treatment. It may be successful and the pulp will heal, or the infection may continue and the tooth will abscess. In the case of an abscess, root canal treatment may be required. The DPC procedure involves placing a medicament, often calcium hydroxide, directly over the

FIGURE 22-8 Indirect pulp treatment.

exposed pulp. The tooth is then restored or a temporary restoration is placed.

If the pulp of a primary or young permanent tooth has been exposed, a pulpotomy procedure may be indicated to remove a portion of the pulp. For primary teeth, a pulpotomy keeps the pulp vital with no prolonged adverse signs, no internal resorption, and no harm to succedaneous teeth. For the young permanent teeth, a pulpotomy maintains the pulp vitality and allows enough time for the root end to develop and close (in these cases, the treatment is referred to as **apexogenesis**).

P R O C E D U R E

22-3 Pulpotomy

This procedure is performed by the dentist with the help of a dental assistant. The dental assistant prepares the treatment room, patient, equipment, and supplies. The tooth is opened and treated before a temporary restoration is placed.

EQUIPMENT AND SUPPLIES

▶ Amalgam setup

▶ Formocresol

▶ Sterile round burs

▶ Zinc oxide-eugenol cement (ZOE or IRM)

PROCEDURE STEPS (*Follow aseptic procedures*)

1. Anesthetic is administered.

2. Place the dental dam.

3. Using the high-speed handpiece, a large opening is made in the occlusal surface of the tooth, exposing the coronal portion of the pulp (Figure 22-9A).

FIGURE 22-9 Pulpotomy procedure.

4. The coronal portion of the pulp is then removed with a spoon excavator or round bur (Figure 22-9B).

5. Prepare a sterile cotton pellet by wetting it in a Formocresol solution. The dentist places the pellet in the chamber for five minutes. (Formocresol is

(continued)

bactericidal—It preserves a thin layer of the remaining pulp tissue to control hemorrhage) (Figure 22-9C).

6. After the hemorrhage is controlled, the cotton pellet is removed and the pulp chamber is rinsed and dried.

7. Mix zinc oxide-eugenol to a base consistency and transfer it to the dentist. A layer of zinc oxide base

is placed in the chamber over the remaining pulp (Figure 22-9D).

8. Place the restoration, such as amalgam, remove the dental dam, and check the occlusion. Stainless steel crowns also are used if there is little tooth structure remaining. Sometimes, the dentist will choose to place a temporary restoration instead of a final restoration. This delays the final treatment until the outcome of the injured pulp is known.

Non-Vital Pulp Therapy. Non-vital pulp therapy may be indicated for both primary and newly erupted permanent teeth. The tooth is extracted or a **pulpectomy** is indicated. This procedure involves the complete removal of the dental pulp (see Chapter 18, Endodontics).

Stainless Steel Crowns

Stainless steel crowns are used on both primary and permanent teeth. On primary teeth, stainless steel crowns are placed until the permanent dentition erupts. On permanent teeth, stainless steel crowns are placed until an individual can have them replaced with cast

gold or porcelain fused to metal crowns. Indications for use of a stainless steel crown include:

▶ Extensive carious lesions

▶ Hypoplastic or hypocalcified teeth

▶ Treatment following a pulpotomy or pulpectomy procedure

▶ Primary tooth is used as an abutment tooth for space maintainer

▶ Temporary restoration of fractured teeth

Stainless steel crowns come in a variety of sizes and can be purchased individually or in complete kits (Figure 22-10).

FIGURE 22-10 Stainless steel crown kit. *(Courtesy of 3M Dental Products Division)*

PROCEDURE

22-4 Stainless Steel Crown Placement

This procedure is performed by the dentist with the help of the dental assistant. The assistant maintains the operating field, mixes materials, and assists in the preparation of the stainless steel crown.

EQUIPMENT AND SUPPLIES

▶ Basic setup: mouth mirror, explorer, and cotton pliers

▶ Cotton rolls and gauze

▶ HVE and saliva ejector

▶ High-speed handpiece with selected burs

▶ Low-speed handpiece with green stone and rubber abrasive wheel

▶ Spoon excavator

▶ Selection of stainless steel crowns

▶ Crown and collar scissors

▶ Contouring and crimping pliers

▶ Mixing spatula, paper pad, and permanent cement

▶ Articulating forceps and paper

▶ Dental floss

PROCEDURE STEPS *(Follow aseptic procedures)*

1. Local anesthetic is administered and the tooth is prepared similar to the preparation for a cast gold crown. The high-speed handpiece with tapered diamonds is commonly used. Transfer instruments and evacuate during the preparation of the tooth.

2. The circumference and height of the tooth are reduced.

3. Decay is removed in the conventional methods and cavity medications are placed.

4. A stainless steel crown is selected from the kit, and it is tried on the tooth. The crown must fit around the circumference of the prepared tooth and contact the adjacent teeth, mesially and distally. Assist the dentist in the selection of the crown. (Some states do not allow dental assistants to perform the function of fitting the crown.)

5. Once the crown is selected, the crown and collar scissors are used to adjust the occlusal-gingival height (Figure 22-11A). The gingival margin of the crown should extend one millimeter beyond the margin of the tooth preparation.

6. A green stone is used to smooth the rough edges of the crown. This area is polished with a rubber abrasive wheel (Figure 22-11B).

7. Place the crown on the tooth and check the patient's occlusion with articulating paper. Make

(A)

(B)

FIGURE 22-11 (A) Stainless steel crown selected and trimmed with crown and collar scissors. (B) Crown margins smoothed with green stone. *(continued next page)*

(continued)

adjustments, if necessary. Use dental floss to check the contacts. Prepare the articulating paper, dry the tooth, and transfer the paper. Receive the articulating forceps and paper and prepare the handpiece, if necessary.

8. Using contouring and crimping pliers, contour the crown, and then crimp the cervical margins of the crown in toward the tooth (Figure 22-11C).

9. The crown is removed and the tooth is dried thoroughly.

10. The cement is mixed and placed in the crown and on the tooth (Figure 22-11D). Mix the cement and place it in the crown. Transfer the crown to the dentist for placement.

11. Remove the excess cement from around the crown.

12. Rinse the patient's mouth and then dismiss the patient.

FIGURE 22-11 *(continued)* (C) Crown contoured with contouring pliers; the margins are then crimped with crimping pliers. (D) Crown placed on tooth.

EMERGENCY TREATMENT FOR TRAUMATIC INJURIES

Fractured Teeth

Fractured teeth are a common emergency in the pediatric practice (Figure 22-12). The anterior teeth are most often involved. The child should be seen by the dentist as soon as possible after the accident. The dentist examines the teeth, documents the history of the accident, performs vitality tests, and takes radiographs. Treatment is determined by the extent of the injury and the vitality of the pulp (see Table 22-2 for classifications of fractures and suggested treatment).

At this initial appointment, the pulp is treated and a temporary restoration is placed if needed for protection. Generally, the dentist will wait three to six months for further treatment. This gives the pulp a chance to recover without additional injury. If the tooth recovers in six months, a permanent restoration is placed.

FIGURE 22-12 Fractures of anterior teeth. *(Courtesy of Dale Ruemping, DDS, MSD)*

TABLE 22-2 CLASSIFICATIONS OF TOOTH FRACTURES AND TREATMENT

Classifications	Treatment
Enamel	Smooth the rough edges.
Enamel and dentin are involved in the fracture	Exposed dentin is protected with glass ionomer, calcium hydroxide, and a bonding agent with composite restoration.
Enamel, dentin, and the pulp are involved	Depending on the clinical examination, a direct pulp capping, pulpotomy, or pulpectomy may be indicated.
Crown is fractured with pulp exposure	Root canal treatment, if indicated. Post and cast crown are completed to stabilize and protect the tooth.

Traumatic Intrusion

Traumatic intrusion occurs when the teeth are forcibly driven into the alveolus so that only a portion of the crown is visible. The treatment for intrusion is to allow the teeth to re-erupt on their own, or the dentist will reposition the teeth and splint adjacent teeth to hold position. These teeth may become non-vital and later require endodontic treatment.

Traumatic intrusion of the primary teeth may cause damage to the underlying, developing, permanent teeth (Figure 22-13). The damage can be from the physical trauma or from the infection of the traumatized teeth. The damage is determined when the permanent teeth erupt.

Displaced Teeth

Lateral or extrusive displacement of primary teeth should be repositioned by the dentist as soon as possi-ble. The roots of primary teeth go through resorption faster after an injury and if the teeth are mobile. If infec-tion occurs, the teeth are removed.

After the teeth are repositioned, they are held in place with a splint (Figure 22-14). The splint is left in place for two to four weeks in order to stabilize the teeth. Often with these injuries, the periodontal liga-ment is damaged extensively. The teeth are monitored for vitality and assessed for endodontic treatment.

Avulsed Teeth

An **avulsed tooth** has been completely removed from the mouth. Primary avulsed teeth are not replaced because infection or ankylosis (**ANG**-kill-loh-sis) may occur. Ankylosis is the fusion of bone and cementum. Permanent teeth that have been avulsed should be replaced as soon as possible after the injury. Instruct

FIGURE 22-13 Traumatic intrusion. *(Courtesy of Dale Ruemping, DDS, MSD)*

FIGURE 22-14 Child with teeth in a splint. *(Courtesy of Steve Gregg, DDS)*

the parents to replant the tooth immediately. The success rate is relatively high if this is done. If the tooth cannot be replanted, instruct the parent to place the tooth in milk, saliva, saline, or water and transport the patient and tooth to the dental office immediately. Caution should be taken with the avulsed tooth to place it carefully in liquid and not rinse it off.

Replacing an Avulsed Tooth

1. The tooth is kept moist and the site in the mouth is examined.
2. Local anesthetic is administered.
3. X-rays are taken.
4. The blood clot is removed from the alveolus.
5. The avulsed tooth is cleaned off in a saline solution and then inserted into the alveolus.
6. A splint is placed to retain the tooth in position.
7. Antibiotics, analgesics, and chlorhexidine rinses are prescribed.
8. Endodontic treatment may be required later.

CHILD ABUSE

Child abuse and neglect is a serious problem that all health professionals face. The dental office provides an opportunity for children who are abused to be observed and for the abuse to be reported. The entire dental team needs to be aware of the types of child abuse and the signs of abuse.

The types of child abuse include physical abuse, sexual abuse, neglect, and emotional abuse. The injuries associated with child abuse that might be evident in the dental office include fractured teeth and jaw bones, lacerations around the labial frenum, missing teeth with no explanation, and bruises or scars on the lips. Marks on the child's arms, legs, and neck may also be noticed by the dental team. Lack of personal hygiene or appropriate clothing for the season, extensive caries, and lack of response to the need for the child to receive dental treatment are concerns to the dental team and should be noted and followed if the child's health and welfare are continually compromised.

The Law and Reporting Child Abuse

The laws regarding reporting child abuse may differ from state to state, but most require the dentist to report suspicious signs of abuse. The laws are designed to protect children and provide help for families.

Reports should include:

▶ The nature of the concern

▶ Description of the injury, including type, color, size, characteristics, and location

▶ X-rays and color photographs

▶ Child's name, age, address, sex, and date of birth

▶ Parents' or caregivers' names

▶ Physician's name

▶ Child's and caregiver's explanations of the injury

Report the findings to a social service agency, the local police department, or a child protective service. The dentist may be asked to appear in court and/or file the report.

CHAPTER SUMMARY

The scope of the pediatric treatment for the child patient includes restoring and maintaining the primary, mixed, and permanent dentition and applying preventive measurs for dental caries, periodontal disease, and malocclusion. The primary focus of the pediatric dental practice is preventive treatment and dealing with the compromised child patient. The whole staff needs to enjoy working with children and be sincere and honest in their actions and feelings. To be effective in the management of children, the dental team must keep upbeat, motivated, and aware.

The role of the dental assistant in the pediatric practice will vary considering the areas of responsibility. One part the assistant is involved in is the management of the child. Another part is the skills the assistant performs at chairside. Depending on the state, when the assistant works independently, he or she assumes the authority role and must maintain control of the child. The dental assistant is also an educator, both with the child and the parents.

CASE STUDY

On Friday afternoon, Mrs. Anderson brought her daughter, Noelle, four years old, to Dr. Bryan's office for emergency treatment. Noelle had fallen and hit her face. Her maxillary left central incisor was pushed into the alveolus so that only the incisal third of the tooth was exposed. Noelle had seen Dr. Bryan for an exam when she was three years old.

Case Study Review

1. What is the condition of Noelle's teeth called?

2. At what stage of tooth eruption is Noelle likely to be? What could happen to Noelle's teeth as a result of the physical trauma? Are the permanent teeth affected?

3. Because Noelle had only been in the office for one visit when she was three, would behavior management be a consideration?

To complete your study of this chapter, work the review activities that follow. Also, refer to the software that accompanies this text.

REVIEW QUESTIONS

Multiple Choice

1. The best age range for introducing dental care in the dental office is
   a. two to six years old.
   b. four to eight years old.
   c. six to ten years old.
   d. ten to twelve years old.

2. Fear that is based on a person's own personal experiences is called
   a. objective fear.
   b. subjective fear.
   c. intraverted fear.
   d. extraverted fear.

3. If the pulp of a primary tooth has been exposed, which of the following procedures would be indicated?
   a. Pulpectomy.
   b. Pulpotomy.
   c. Apexification.
   d. Root canal.

4. Stainless steel crowns are indicated for all of the following *except*
   a. following a pulpotomy procedure.
   b. hypoplastic or hypocalcified teeth.
   c. incipient decay.
   d. extensive carious decay.

5. Tongue thrusting
   a. pushes the tongue against the posterior teeth.
   b. pushes the tongue against the anterior teeth when swallowing.
   c. pushes the tongue against the palate when swallowing.
   d. pushes the tongue against the floor of the mouth.

CRITICAL THINKING

1. Think of an office theme or design that would be attractive to children. Would there be any maintenance the assistant would be responsible for?

2. List three behavior management techniques that would be effective with a young patient who is visiting the dental office for the first time.

3. A five-year-old child comes into the dental office with bruising on the upper arms and cuts around and inside the mouth. List some steps that may be taken in the pediatric dental office with a suspected child abuse case.

Periodontics

OBJECTIVES

The student should strive to meet the following objectives and demonstrate an understanding of the facts and principles presented in this chapter:

1. Describe the scope of periodontics.

2. Identify members of the periodontal team and their roles.

3. Describe the stages of periodontal disease.

4. Explain the diagnostic procedures involved in the patient's first visit to the periodontal office.

5. Identify and describe periodontal instruments and their uses.

6. Describe non-surgical procedures and the dental assistant's role in each procedure.

7. Explain surgical procedures and dental assisting responsibilities.

8. Identify the types of periodontal dressing and how they are prepared, placed, and removed.

9. Describe periodontal maintenance procedures and the patient's role relating to each.

KEY TERMS

bone resorption (p. 489)

bruxism (p. 485)

calculus (p. 484)

coronal polish (p. 495)

curette (p. 490)

electrosurgery (p. 492)

frenectomy (p. 499)

furcation (p. 485)

gingival grafting (p. 498)

gingivectomy (p. 496)

gingivitis (p. 485)

gingivoplasty (p. 496)

hoe scaler (p. 490)

interdental knives (p. 491)

mucogingival surgery (p. 498)

occlusal equilibration (p. 488)

osseous surgery (p. 498)

ostectomy (p. 498)

osteoplasty (p. 498)

periodontal dressing (p. 498)

periodontal flap surgery (p. 498)

periodontal knives (p. 491)

periodontal pocket (p. 488)

periodontal probe (p. 489)

periodontal probing (p. 488)

periodontitis (p. 485)

periodontium (p. 484)

periosteal elevators (p. 493)

plaque (p. 488)

pocket marking pliers (p. 493)

prophylaxis (p. 495)

recession (p. 488)

root planing (p. 495)

scaling (p. 495)

sickle scalers (p. 490)

surgical scalpel (p. 492)

tooth mobility (p. 488)

ultrasonic instruments (p. 491)

INTRODUCTION

The periodontist specializes in diseases of the tissue around the root of the tooth. This specialty deals with symptoms, probable causes, diagnosis, and treatment of periodontal disease.

THE PERIODONTAL TEAM

The team in a periodontal office includes the periodontist, dental assistants, dental hygienists, and business office staff.

▶ The periodontist coordinates treatment with the general dentist in the overall care of the patient. The periodontist screens the patient, performs the surgical care, and provides continual care according to the patient's needs.

▶ The dental assistant performs chairside assisting duties and the expanded functions allowed by state dental practice acts, including placing and removing periodontal dressing, removing sutures, and performing coronal polishes. The dental assistant takes radiographs, makes impressions for study models, places sealants, and administers fluoride treatments. The dental assistant also gives pre- and postoperative instructions and prepares the treatment room for surgery. These functions are in addition to treatment room preparation and maintenance and sterilization procedures. The dental assistant is involved in educating and motivating the patient throughout the treatment. In some offices, the dental assistant also may perform laboratory tasks, such as pouring study models or making periodontal splints.

▶ The dental hygienist performs traditional hygiene procedures and, depending on the state dental practice act, may also administer local anesthetic. In a periodontal practice, the hygienist often sees patients who have more advanced periodontal disease; therefore, their responsibilities include deep curettage, root planing, and clinical examination procedures.

PERIODONTAL DISEASE

Evidence of periodontal disease has been noted in ancient history studies. Ancient human skulls demonstrate evidence of bone destruction, and early civilizations told of treatment methods such as using wire to tie loose teeth together. According to the American Academy of Periodontology, three out of four adults will experience, to some degree, periodontal problems at some time in their lives. Periodontal disease occurs in children and adolescents with marginal gingivitis and gingival recession, which are the most prevalent conditions (Figure 23-1).

FIGURE 23-1 View of patient with mild gingivitis.

Periodontal disease involves the **periodontium**, which represents the tissues that support the teeth and includes the following:

▶ **Gingiva**—Tissues that surround the teeth.

▶ **Epithelial attachment**—Area at the bottom of the sulcus where the gingiva attaches to the tooth.

▶ **Sulcus**—Space between the tooth and the free gingiva. In healthy mouths, the sulcus is 1 to 3 mm deep.

▶ **Periodontal ligaments or membranes**—Fibers of connective tissue that surround the root of the tooth and attach the cementum to the bone.

▶ **Cementum**—Hard surface that covers the dentin on the root of the tooth.

▶ **Alveolar bone**—Bone that forms the socket that encases the root of the tooth.

Symptoms of Periodontal Disease

The symptoms of periodontal disease include bleeding gums, loose teeth (mobility), inflamed gingiva, abnormal contour of the gingiva, periodontal pocket formation, malocclusion, halitosis, pain and tenderness, and recession and discoloration. All of these symptoms may be present or the symptoms may vary (Figure 23-2A).

Causes of Periodontal Disease

Local irritants are a significant cause of periodontal disease. One irritant, **bacterial plaque**, is a common cause of the inflammation of the gingival tissues. The bacterial plaque forms around the margin of the gingiva and, if left undisturbed, mineralizes and appears as a yellow or brown deposit on the teeth. This hard deposit is called **calculus** (tartar) (Figure 23-2B). If plaque and calculus

FIGURE 23-2 (A) View of patient with unhealthy gingival tissues—advanced gingival inflammation. (B) Unhealthy gingival tissues and lingual calculus.

are not removed, they continue to develop and grow on both supragingival and subgingival surfaces.

Poor Oral Hygiene. Poor oral hygiene results in the buildup of plaque and calculus. Lack of daily brushing and flossing leads to plaque and debris buildup on the teeth and appliances. (Proper brushing and flossing techniques are discussed in Chapter 2, Oral Health and Nutrition.)

Improper Nutrition. Improper nutrition leads to overall poor health, which often is evident in the gingival tissues. Eating a balanced diet, including foods that keep teeth strong and the tissues free of disease, can aid in maintaining a healthy mouth.

Malocclusion. Malocclusion can be a factor in periodontal disease. Improper tooth alignment and occlusion can lead to plaque and calculus formation in areas where food and debris are not removed easily. Also,

patients with sensitive teeth or who need dental restorations will favor these areas and alter chewing patterns, putting additional pressure on periodontal structures.

Stress. Stress can lead to bruxism (grinding of the teeth), which puts pressure on the teeth and surrounding tissues. Problems with the periodontium during times of stress may be evident because the patient may not eat healthy foods or maintain oral hygiene properly.

Systemic Factors. Systemic factors, including hormonal imbalances, hereditary predisposition, and certain diseases and medications, are often reflected in the gingival tissues. Examples include hormonal changes due to pregnancy, diabetes, cardiovascular disease such as hypertension, patients at risk for bacterial endocarditis, blood diseases such as leukemia, HIV infection, genetic conditions such as Down syndrome, emotional disorders, systemic drugs such as Dilantin or immunosuppressants, and thyroid deficiencies.

Types of Periodontal Disease

There are two main classifications of periodontal disease: gingivitis and periodontitis. Through clinical research and improved technology, the understanding of periodontal disease has broadened in scope. Considering the course and characteristics of the disease, more classifications have been added (see Tables 23-1 and 23-2).

Gingivitis. Gingivitis is inflammation of the gingival tissues. It is common in all ages. Causes may include buildup of plaque and calculus, poor-fitting appliances, and poor occlusion, and the condition may occur in association with certain systemic diseases (scurvy), hormonal changes (pregnancy), or prolonged drug therapy (phenytoin, which is an anticonvulsant drug). The tissues become reddish in color, interdental papilla may be swollen and bulbous, and tissues may bleed after brushing and flossing. Gingivitis precedes periodontitis but does not always progress to it. Proper brushing and flossing can reverse this condition in some cases by removing the plaque.

Periodontitis. Periodontitis involves the formation of periodontal pockets. This occurs when margins of the gingiva and periodontal fibers recede and the supporting bone becomes inflamed and destroyed. There is an increase in tooth mobility as the pockets become deeper, and there may be furcation (area where the roots divide) involvement in multi-rooted teeth.

Acute Necrotizing Ulcerative Gingivitis. Acute necrotizing ulcerative gingivitis (ANUG) occurs most frequently in young adults sixteen to thirty years old. Causes include stress, smoking, inadequate diet, and poor oral hygiene. Characteristics of this form of

TABLE 23-1 CLASSIFICATION OF PERIODONTAL DISEASE

Classifications	Characteristics	Contributing Factors
Gingivitis common forms		
Chronic gingivitis	Common in adults and children. Redness, gingival bleeding, changes in the contour of the gingiva, edema, enlargement, loss of tissue tone. No radiographic changes are detected in the periodontium in gingivitis.	Predominately caused by plaque accumulation.
Necrotizing ulcerative gingivitis (also known as NUG, acute necrotizing ulcerative gingivitis [ANUG])	People aged sixteen to thirty are mainly affected. Severe inflammation of the marginal gingiva, bleeding, acute pain, necrosis and ulceration of the interdental papilla, foul breath, and craterlike depressions in the crest of the interdental papilla.	Poor oral hygiene, stress, poor diet, and smoking.
Gingivitis associated with hormonal changes (e.g., pregnancy, puberty, steroid therapy, or birth control medication).	Sudden onset. Gingival inflammation, enlargement of the papillae, and bleeding.	Results from an exaggerated response to bacterial plaque. Response to elevated levels of hormones or steroids.
Gingivitis attributed to the effects of certain drugs (e.g., phenytoin and cyclosporin).	Gingival overgrowth or hyperplasia. Changes in size and contour of the gingiva lead to increased plaque accumulation and inflammation.	Link between bacterial plaque and drug-induced gingival overgrowth.
Linear gingival erythema (HIV-G or now known as LGE)	Patients with AIDS. Severe erythema (redness and inflammation along the marginal gingiva. Extends to the attached gingiva. Some bleeding and pain.	Immunodeficiency virus.
Periodontitis		
Adult periodontitis	Onset in mid-twenties. Slow progression. Gingival inflammation, periodontal pockets, bone loss, and eventual tooth mobility. Classified as early, moderate, or advanced depending on the degree or severity of bone loss. Treatment includes non-surgical and surgical procedures followed by regular maintenance therapy.	Poor oral hygiene, genetic factors, malpositioned teeth, and stress.
Early-onset periodontitis, such as prepubertal periodontitis and juvenile periodontitis	Rare occurrence. Prepubertal periodontitis affects the primary or mixed dentition. Severe gingival inflammation, rapid bone loss, mobility, and tooth loss. Juvenile periodontitis occurs around puberty. Females are affected more than males. Severe and rapid bone loss that begins with the incisors and first molars. Sparse plaque and calculus buildup for degree of destruction.	Usually genetic basis.

gingivitis are inflamed gingiva, metallic taste, bad breath, pain, and hemorrhage of the tissues. This condition is also known as Vincent's disease and trench mouth. It appears in individuals in the same unhealthy state and frequently occurs in college students around the time of final examinations (because of stress).

TABLE 23-2 PERIODONTAL DISEASE STAGES

Periodontal disease is caused by plaque, the colorless, sticky film of bacteria that constantly forms on the teeth. The bacteria in plaque produce by-products that can irritate the gums and, over a period of time, seriously damage the structures that support the teeth.

Healthy Tissues	Gingivitis	Early Periodontitis	Moderate Periodontitis	Advanced Periodontitis
Gum is firm, fits tightly to teeth, and does not bleed.	Gum tissue may be inflamed, swollen, and bleeds easily during brushing, flossing, or when your dental professional examines you.	Continued inflammation, loss of gum attachment and bone support.	Supporting gum and bone tissue have deteriorated, tooth loosens.	Severe destruction of tissue and bone, causing tooth loss.

PERIODONTAL DIAGNOSTIC PROCEDURES

 The first appointment with the periodontist is often an information-gathering appointment. After completing the medical dental history, the patient is seated in the treatment room for an extraoral and intraoral examination. Radiographs and impressions are taken and a periodontal screening is completed. Developing rapport with the patient is essential for successful treatment. The patient must have confidence in the dentist and the staff. The patient has responsibility in the treatment of periodontal disease and should be educated and motivated. Information to share with each patient includes following oral hygiene instructions, diet suggestions and modifications, personal habit changes, and routine office visits.

Medical Dental History

The medical dental history gives the operator and the patient the opportunity to learn about each other. The operator gains information about why the patient is seeking treatment; if there is a systemic condition such as tuberculosis, HIV, AIDS, or diabetes; how the patient feels about his or her teeth; previous dental treatment; and if the patient has any oral habits that have contributed to the present condition. The patient has the opportunity to ask questions of the dentist and gain an understanding of what is involved with periodontal treatment. The patient's history must be accurate and complete. A history checklist should open the way for significant conversation between the patient, the dental assistant, and/or the dentist.

Sample Medical History Form. The following types of questions should be answered by the patient.

1. Chief complaints:

   ▶ Why did you come to the periodontist?

   ▶ Specifically, what area(s) of your mouth is (are) causing you concern?

   ▶ Do you currently have pain in or near your ears?

   ▶ Does any part of your mouth hurt when clenched?

   ▶ Are there any areas in your mouth that have unhealed or inflamed sores?

2. Medical history:

   ▶ Are you ill at this time? If so, what is (are) your ailment(s)?

   ▶ Are you currently undergoing any medical treatment(s)? If so, what kind(s)?

   ▶ Are you taking any medication(s)? If so, what kind(s)?

   ▶ Have you ever had adverse responses to any type(s) of antibiotic? If so, what type(s)?

   ▶ Have you ever had adverse responses to any type(s) of anesthetic? If so, what type(s)?

   ▶ Are you pregnant?

   ▶ Are you allergic to anything?

   ▶ Do you have any of the following?
   Rheumatic fever
   A heart murmur
   Cardiovascular disease
   Hepatitis
   Kidney infection
   Tuberculosis
   Diabetes
   AIDS
   HIV

   ▶ Do you have, or have you ever had, problems with any of the following?
   Prolonged bleeding
   Allergies

Oral symptoms related to pregnancy, menstruation, or menopause

▶ Do you have any oral conditions present? If so, how long have they been present and has there been any treatment for them?

3. Oral history:

▶ Have you had any extractions? Have you had any restorations?

▶ Do you have any problems after dental treatment, such as bleeding, pain, or swelling?

▶ Do you have any problems with your teeth, such as bleeding gums, pain, mobility, or sensitivity?

▶ Do you have difficulty with your joints when eating or opening and closing your mouth?

4. Oral habits:

▶ Do you have any habits such as grinding, clenching, or mouth breathing?

▶ Do you smoke?

▶ Do you use alcohol or drugs?

5. Family history:

▶ Does anyone in your family have a history of periodontal disease?

6. Oral hygiene:

▶ Which brushing technique do you use?

▶ Do you floss? If so, how often?

▶ What type of toothbrush do you use?

▶ Do you use any other oral hygiene aids? If so, what kinds?

Clinical Examination

The clinical examination includes an extraoral examination of the face and neck; an intraoral examination of the tongue, palate, buccal mucosa, the teeth, the oropharynx area; and the periodontal examination.

Extraoral Examination. The extraoral examination includes observation of the skin and lips and palpation of the lymph nodes and the temporomandibular joint.

Intraoral Examination. The intraoral examination combines viewing and palpating the tissues in the oral cavity. The operator looks for abnormalities in color, size, texture, and consistency of all tissues. The intraoral examination is inclusive of an oral cancer screening. The condition of the teeth and any prosthetic appliances are examined, noting any areas that might cause or contribute to periodontal disease. Any necessary treatment is recorded on the patient's chart.

Periodontal Examination. The periodontal examination is a thorough examination of the periodontium using periodontal charts. The periodontal charts depict the condition of the patient's periodontal tissues. The charting is completed either manually or on a computer. The oral cavity is examined, and information is gathered by the operator while the dental assistant records the information on the periodontal chart.

▶ **Patient oral hygiene** is evaluated and the amount of **plaque** and calculus present is determined. This evaluation includes both supragingival and subgingival deposits.

▶ **Periodontal probing** measures the depth of the **periodontal pocket** with a periodontal probe (refer to Periodontal Instruments—Periodontal Probes). A normal sulcus is 3 mm deep or less. When the depth is greater than 3 mm, it is termed a periodontal pocket. To determine the sulcus depth, six sites are probed and recorded on each tooth. There are three sites on the facial, including mesiofacial, midfacial, and distofacial, and three sites on the lingual, including mesiolingual, midlingual, and distolingual. The periodontal probe is inserted into the sulcus until the operator feels resistance. Tactile sensation indicates the level of the epithelium attachment. The calibrations on the probe measure the depth of the pocket. These are recorded on the chart.

▶ **Tooth mobility** measures movement of the tooth within the socket. The mobility test is accomplished by pushing the tooth in a buccolingual direction using the handle ends of two instruments or by using the automatic device for assessing mobility. Mobility is usually recorded using a scale of 0 to 3: 0 = normal, 1 = slight or 1 mm, 2 = moderate or 2 mm, and 3 = severe or 3 mm.

▶ **Furcation involvement** measures destruction of interradicular bone in the furcation area of multi-rooted teeth. A curved instrument is inserted in the furcation to determine the amount of involvement.

▶ **Appearance of the gingiva** is evaluated in terms of color, size, shape, texture, position, consistency, bleeding, and amount of exudate (pus).

▶ **Bleeding** is the amount of blood present during probing. It is a major indicator of inflamed gingiva.

▶ **Recession** is the loss of the gingival tissue exposing the underlying cementum/dentio, usually seen on the facial surface.

▶ **Occlusion** is evaluated and described. The occlusal bite relationship is checked with articulating paper or wax to identify areas that show excessive biting or chewing force.

Occlusal equilibration is the process of alleviating areas with excessive force. Once these "spots" have been determined, burs, discs, and stones are used to reduce and restore occlusion without interference.

Radiographic Interpretation

Radiographs are useful tools when evaluating the periodontium for periodontal disease. The radiographs show the teeth and the level and position of the alveolar bone. When periodontal disease is present, the alveolar bone recedes both vertically and/or horizontally. **Vertical bone resorption** is found on individual teeth on the interproximal surface (Figure 23-3A). **Horizontal bone resorption** occurs when there is equal crestal bone loss on the mesial and distal surfaces of the proximal teeth (Figure 23-3B).

Periapical x-rays supplemented with bite-wing radiographs are most commonly taken, and the x-rays must be as dimensionally accurate as possible. Usually, a full-mouth series is taken for comparisons throughout the mouth.

Presentation of the Treatment Plan

After gathering all the periodontal diagnostic information, the periodontist determines the appropriate treatment plan for the patient. The patient is scheduled for a consultation appointment. During this appointment, the prognosis (anticipated outcome) of the patient's condition and the treatment sequence are explained. Charts, radiographs, study models, and photographs are used to educate the patient. The patient's role in the treatment is discussed. The patient must be actively involved in the treatment and motivated to follow the home-care plan and keep treatment appointments. Once all questions are answered and the treatment plan is understood, appointments and financial arrangements are completed.

PERIODONTAL INSTRUMENTS

Periodontal instruments are designed to probe, scrape, file, and cut the hard surfaces of the teeth, alveolar bone, and soft tissues of the gingiva. These instruments must be kept sharp. Usually, the hygienist or a specially trained assistant is responsible for maintaining periodontal hand instruments. There are both manual and automatic methods for sharpening the edges of periodontal instruments to the angles required.

Periodontal Probes

The **periodontal probe** is the primary instrument used in the periodontal examination (Figure 23-4). This is a **calibrated instrument** used to measure the depth of periodontal pockets. The probe is also used to measure areas of recession, bleeding, or exudate. The calibrations on the periodontal probe are in millimeters and vary depending on the manufacturer and the operator's preference. These markings may be indentations or color coded for easy reading. The probe may be flat, oval, or round in cross-section but must be thin enough to fit easily into the gingival sulcus.

FIGURE 23-3 (A) Vertical bone loss shown on x-ray, on the mesial of the maxillary left first bicuspid (#12). (B) Horizontal bone loss shown on x-ray between the maxillary right molar, bicuspids, and cuspid (#s 3, 4, 5, and 6).

FIGURE 23-4 Variety of periodontal probes.

A computerized probe system detects and stores information on pocket depth, recession, furcation involvement, and mobility. The information is shown on a computer screen and can be printed out.

Explorers

Explorers are used to detect and locate calculus, tooth irregularities, faulty margins on restorations, and furcation involvement. The explorer gives the operator the best tactile information for assessment.

The explorers used in periodontics are supplied in a variety of shapes, similar to those also used in general dental procedures. The working ends are thin and sharp. They may be curved or at near right angles to adapt to the curves of the tooth surfaces.

Sickle Scalers

Sickle scalers are sharp hand instruments that are used to remove hard deposits such as supragingival (above the gingiva) and subgingival (below the gingiva) calculus from the teeth. Scalers are supplied in a variety of shapes and angulations to access all surfaces of the teeth. The working end of a scaler has two sharp edges that come to a point (Figure 23-5). The handles are often large and are ribbed, serrated, or knurled. Sometimes, the metal handles are covered with color-coded rubber grips to prevent muscle fatigue and for better control of the instrument (Figures 23-6A through C).

Curettes

The curette is a hand instrument used for removing subgingival calculus, smoothing the root surface, and removing the soft tissue lining of the periodontal pocket. The working end has a cutting edge on one or both sides of the blade and the end is rounded, not pointed like the scaler (Figure 23-5). The curette is a finer instrument that is designed to adapt to the curves of the root surfaces. There are two basic curettes: **universal curettes**, which are used throughout the mouth, and **Gracey curettes**, which are supplied in a set of several instruments that are designed and angled to be used in specific areas (Figure 23-7). The curette handles are similar to those on the scalers.

Working end of a scaler ——— Working end of a curette

FIGURE 23-5 Cross-section of a scaler and a curette.

FIGURE 23-6 Types of periodontal scalers. (A) Combination instrument with a sickle on one end and a Jacque on the other. (B) The Shephard's hook. (C) A Jacque.

Hoe Scalers

The **hoe scaler** has a blade bent at a 90° angle at the end of the working end. This cutting edge is beveled and sharp. The hoe scaler is placed in the periodontal pocket to the base and then pulled toward the crown of the tooth with even pressure to plane and smooth the root surface (Figure 23-8B).

Chisel Scalers

Chisel scalers are used most often in the anterior of the mouth. The blade of the chisel is slightly curved and the cutting edge is beveled (Figure 23-8A).

FIGURE 23-7 Types of periodontal curettes: Gracey curettes. (A) No. 5-6. (B) No. 7-8. (C) No. 9-10. (D) No. 13-14.

Files

Periodontal files are supplied in a variety of blade shapes and shank angulations (Figure 23-8C). They are used in a pulling motion interproximally to remove calculus and for root planing. Files are also used to remove overhanging margins of dental restorations.

Ultrasonic Instruments

Ultrasonic instruments are used to remove hard deposits, stains, and debris during scaling, curettage, and root planing procedures. They are used as an adjunct to manual scaling procedures. Ultrasonic units generate high-power vibrations to a handpiece with a variety of tips (Figure 23-9). These vibrations cause the calculus to fracture and be dislodged. Because ultrasonic vibrations cause heat, the units have cooling systems that circulate water through the handpieces and out openings near the tips. The water spray cools and also flushes the area. It is beneficial for a dental assis-

tant to be present to evacuate the volume of water and debris. Although the ultrasonic units are effective and fast, care must be taken to prevent injury to the tissues and the teeth.

Periodontal Knives

Periodontal knives or gingivectomy knives are used to remove gingival tissue during periodontal surgery. The knives most commonly used are the broad-bladed Kirkland knives (Figure 23-10A). These knives are kidney-shaped and sharp around the entire periphery of the blade. They are supplied as either single- or double-ended instruments.

Interdental Knives

Periodontal knives that are used to remove soft tissue interproximally are called **interdental knives**. The Orban No. 1 and 2 are very popular interdental knives. These spear-shaped knives have long, narrow blades with cutting edges on both sides of the blade (Figure 23-10B).

FIGURE 23-8 Periodontal (A) chisel, (B) hoe, and (C) file. *(Courtesy of Miltex Instrument Co., Inc., Lake Success, NY)*

FIGURE 23-9 Ultrasonic scaling unit.

FIGURE 23-10 Gingivectomy knives. (A) Kirkland broad-blade knife. (B) Orban interdental knife.

Surgical Scalpel

The **surgical scalpel** is used for periodontal surgical procedures to remove gingival tissue. The surgical scalpel is also known as the Bard-Parker scalpel. The scalpel has two components: a sterilizible metal or plastic handle and a disposable blade. The blades come in different shapes and sizes. Disposable scalpels are also available (Figure 23-11).

Electrosurgery

The **electrosurgery** setup consists of a control box, foot-operated on-off controls, one terminal plate that is placed behind the patient's back or shoulders, and another terminal that is a probe with various cutting tips that the dentist uses for the surgery. The electro-

FIGURE 23-11 (A) Surgical knife. Bard-Parker and blades. (B) Blade remover. (C) Disposable scalpels. *(Courtesy of Miltex Instrument Co., Inc., Lake Success, NY)*

surgery unit uses tiny electrical currents to incise the gingival tissue and also coagulate the blood during the procedure (Figure 23-12). The dental assistant must keep the oral evacuator near the surgical site to remove the debris and odors.

Pocket Marking Pliers

Pocket marking pliers are used to transfer the measurement of the pocket to the outside of the tissue so the operator can see the depth level of the pocket. The pocket marking pliers have one straight, thin beak that is placed in the pocket and another that is bent at a right angle at the tip. When the beaks are pinched together, the gingival tissue is perforated, leaving small, pinpoint markings (Figure 23-13).

Periosteal Elevators

Periosteal elevators are used to reflect soft tissue away from the bone. The elevators are usually double ended, with one long, tapered end and one round, bladed end (Figure 23-14).

FIGURE 23-14 Various periosteal elevators.

Periodontal Scissors, Rongeurs, and Forceps

Periodontal scissors are used during periodontal surgery, mainly to remove tags of tissue and to trim margins. There are other uses and many varieties, but most often the blades are long and very thin.

Soft tissue rongeurs or nippers are hinged pliers used to shape the soft tissue (Figure 23-15A).

Tissue forceps are used to retract tissue or to hold the tissue in place. They are designed similar to hemostats, except the beaks are curved near the end at right angles to each other (Figure 23-15B).

(A)

FIGURE 23-12 Electrodes used with an electrosurgical unit. *(Courtesy of Macan Engineering and Manufacturing Co.)*

(B)

FIGURE 23-13 Pocket marking pliers.

FIGURE 23-15 (A) Soft tissue rongeurs. (B) Tissue forceps.

NON-SURGICAL PERIODONTAL PROCEDURES

Principles of Periodontal Procedures

For periodontal treatment that is effective and efficient with minimal discomfort to the patient or stress to the operator, the following principles are followed:

▶ Comfortable position for the operator and the patient
▶ Effective pain control for the patient
▶ Use of a dental assistant to maintain the operating field for clear vision, good illumination, and retraction

▶ Maintain instruments properly (sharp and in order for use during the procedure)
▶ Correct instrument grasp, fulcrum, and instrument adaptation

Occlusal Adjustment

Occlusal adjustment or equilibration is a procedure that involves adjustment of the occlusal surface to eliminate detrimental forces and to provide functional forces for stimulation of a healthy periodontium. The adjustment procedure is performed quadrant by quadrant and may require several appointments to fully equilibrate the patient's whole mouth.

PROCEDURE

23-1 Occlusal Adjustment

The procedure is performed by the periodontist. It involves marking the patient's bite and adjusting the occlusal surfaces of the teeth. The dental assistant prepares the articulating paper or wax; maintains the operating field; and changes burs, discs, and stones in the handpiece.

EQUIPMENT (Figure 23-16)

FIGURE 23-16 Occlusal equilibration armamentarium.

▶ Basic setup: mouth mirror, explorer, cotton pliers
▶ Cotton rolls and 2 × 2 gauze sponges
▶ Saliva ejector, HVE tip, air-water syringe tip
▶ Articulation forceps and articulating paper and/or occlusal wax

▶ Low-speed handpiece
▶ Diamond burs, various discs and stones
▶ Polishing wheels and discs

PROCEDURE STEPS (*Follow aseptic procedures*)

1. Seat and prepare the patient for the occlusal adjustment procedure.

2. Prepare the articulating forceps with paper, or prepare to transfer the wax. Dry the quadrant with the air syringe or a gauze sponge.

3. The periodontist places the articulating paper over the occlusal surfaces and instructs the patient to bite down and grind the teeth side to side.

4. The articulating paper is removed, and the colored marks left by the paper are evaluated. The markings indicate how teeth in the maxillary and mandibular arches occlude.

5. Change burs, discs, and stones as requested by the periodontist. Transfer the handpiece to the periodontist, and use the air-water syringe and the evacuator to keep the area clean and clear during the adjustments procedure.

6. This process is repeated until the teeth occlude evenly over the quadrant.

7. Each quadrant is evaluated and adjusted.

Scaling and Polishing

The purpose of **scaling** is to remove plaque, calculus, and stains from the surfaces of the teeth. The deposits above the gingival margin, supragingival deposits, and those just below the gingival margin are removed with scalers and curettes. After this, the coronal surfaces of the teeth are polished with rubber cups, brushes, an abrasive, porte polishers, and dental tape. This procedure is called a **prophylaxis** and can be performed by the dentist or the dental hygienist. Depending on the state dental practice act, dental assistants can remove supragingival deposits and/or perform the **coronal polish**.

In a routine prophylaxis, deposits from above and just slightly below the gingival margins are removed. In a peri-odontal scaling, the subgingival deposits are more extensive and involve removal of irritants from deep pockets and smoothing of the root surface (Figure 23-18).

Root Planing

After the plaque and calculus are removed from the periodontal pocket and the root surface, the cementum is often rough and irregular. This provides a surface ideal for accumulation of plaque and calculus formation. The roughness is removed by **root planing**. This is a process of planing or shaving the root surface with curettes and other periodontal instruments to leave a smooth root surface. For the patient's comfort, anesthetic is given during this procedure.

P R O C E D U R E

23-2 Scaling, Curettage, and Polishing

This procedure is done by the periodontist or the dental hygienist. A dental hygiene assistant assists during this procedure. Responsibilities include instrument transfer, rinsing the oral cavity, evacuation with the HVE, removing debris from instruments, retraction, and maintaining patient comfort.

EQUIPMENT (Figure 23-17)

FIGURE 23-17 Scale and polish (prophylaxis) tray setup.

▶ Basic setup: mouth mirror, explorer, and cotton pliers

▶ Saliva ejector, HVE tip, and air-water syringe tip

▶ Cotton rolls and gauze sponges

▶ Periodontal probe

▶ Scalers: Jacque and Shepherd's hook

▶ Curettes: Universal and Gracey

▶ Dental floss and dental tape

▶ Prophy angle—rubber cups and brushes

▶ Prophy paste

▶ Optional—disclosing solution or tablets

PROCEDURE STEPS (Follow aseptic procedures)

1. The operator examines the oral cavity.

2. The operator uses scalers and curettes to remove calculus and debris from around the teeth. Often, the operator cleans all surfaces of the teeth in one quadrant before moving to the next quadrant.

3. After all the calculus has been removed, the operator polishes the teeth with prophy paste, rubber cup, and brush.

NOTE: Some practices use a prophy jet (spray salt-water) as an alternative to the rubber cup polish (see polishing of the coronal surfaces of the teeth in Chapter 28, Advanced Chairside Functions).

4. The operator uses dental tape and prophy paste to clean the interproximal areas. Then, the entire mouth is flossed and rinsed.

Gingival Curettage

Gingival curettage, also known as soft tissue curettage, is a procedure that involves scraping the inner gingival walls of the periodontal pockets to remove inflamed tissue and debris. This is accomplished with curettes and ideally is performed after the scaling and root planing of the tooth. By removing diseased tissue and irritants, the edema is reduced and the gingival tissue may begin to heal itself (Figure 23-18).

Postoperative Treatment

▶ **Oral hygiene**. The patient is taught good brushing and flossing techniques. Periodontal aids such as interproximal brushes, soft wooden tips, and/or bridge threaders are selected to assist the patient in cleaning large interdental spaces or around fixed appliances. Videos, pamphlets, and various other aids are used to motivate and educate the patient.

▶ **Antibacterial therapy**. Antimicrobial mouth rinses and antibiotic regimens are used in addition to routine treatments. Fluorides also are prescribed because they have bactericidal effects against the formation of plaque.

▶ **Diet and smoking**. Patients should be advised to avoid spicy foods, citrus fruits, and alcoholic beverages and to otherwise follow a normal diet. Smoking should be stopped, because the smoke irritates the tissues and delays the healing process.

SURGICAL PERIODONTAL PROCEDURES

The accepted rationale for periodontal surgery has been to arrest the disease process, reduce the periodontium to a level that is easier for the patient to keep

(A)   **(B)**

FIGURE 23-18 Placement of instruments on tooth for scaling. (A) Supragingival scaling. (B) Subgingival scaling.

clean, and perform effective scaling and root planing procedures.

Gingivectomy

A **gingivectomy** is the surgical removal of diseased gingival tissue that forms the periodontal pocket. The pocket must be eliminated to prevent the accumulation of debris and bacteria. This surgical procedure reduces the height of the gingival tissue, which provides visibility and access in order to remove irritants and smooth the root surface. This promotes the healing process and makes it easier for the patient to access the area during cleaning.

The gingivectomy procedure involves marking the pocket depths with pocket marking pliers and then excising the gingival tissue with periodontal knives, a scalpel, surgical scissors, or electrosurgery. After the tissue is excised, calculus and necrotic root tissue are removed and smoothed with scalers and curettes. The area is rinsed gently and covered with a gauze sponge until the hemorrhage is controlled. Once the blood clots have formed, a periodontal dressing is placed to promote healing, reduce the chance of infection, and prevent disturbance to the area.

Gingivoplasty

Gingivoplasty is reshaping the gingival tissue to remove deformities such as clefts, craters, and enlargements. A gingivoplasty does not involve the removal of periodontal pockets; it is completed to recontour the gingiva and often immediately follows a gingivectomy. A gingivoplasty is performed with periodontal knives, a scalpel, rongeurs, rotary diamonds, curettes, and surgical scissors. The gingival margin is tapered and thinned, creating a scalloped edge. Interdental grooves are contoured.

Postoperative Treatment Following Surgery

▶ **Oral hygiene.** Normal brushing and flossing should be completed in areas not involved in the surgery. Brush only the biting surfaces of the teeth involved in surgery. Gently rinse the mouth with warm saltwater after twenty-four hours.

▶ **Diet.** Avoid hot, spicy foods and citrus foods; eat soft foods; and chew on the healthy side of the mouth so that the periodontal dressing is not disturbed.

▶ **Pain.** The patient can expect mild to moderate discomfort, and medication should be prescribed.

▶ **Swelling and bleeding.** Some swelling may occur. Place an ice pack over the area for ten minutes and remove for ten minutes. Repeat as needed. Some seepage and bleeding may occur and is normal; however, if it persists, call the dentist.

PROCEDURE

23-3 Gingivectomy

This procedure is performed by the periodontist in order to remove diseased gingiva and clean the periodontal pockets. The dental assistant prepares the instruments and materials, prepares the patient, and performs assisting responsibilities during the procedure. According to state dental practice acts, the dental assistant may place and remove the periodontal dressing.

EQUIPMENT

▶ Basic setup: mouth mirror, explorer, cotton pliers
▶ Periodontal probe
▶ Cotton rolls and gauze sponges
▶ Saliva ejector, HVE tip, air-water syringe tip, surgical aspirator tip
▶ Anesthetic setup
▶ Pocket marker
▶ Periodontal knives—broad bladed and interproximal
▶ Scalpel, blades, and diamond burs
▶ Scalers and curettes
▶ Soft tissue rongeurs and surgical scissors
▶ Hemostat
▶ Suture needle and thread
▶ Periodontal dressing materials

PROCEDURE STEPS (Follow aseptic procedures)

1. The anesthetic is administered to anesthetize the tissues and reduce the blood flow to the area.

2. The periodontist examines the patient's periodontal chart, and then the area is examined with a periodontal probe.

3. The depths of the pockets are marked with pocket markers (Figures 23-19A and B).

4. The broad-bladed knife or scalpel is used to incise the marked gingiva. Evacuate the area and transfer instruments (Figure 23-19C).

5. Interdental knives are used to remove interproximal tissue. Scissors, rongeurs, and burs are used to remove tissue tags. Have gauze ready to receive any tissue from instruments and to clean the area of debris.

6. After the tissue is removed, the periodontist scales and planes the root surfaces. Irritants are removed and the surfaces are smoothed to promote healing. Continue to pass instruments and evacuate the area. A sterile saline solution may be used to irrigate the area.

7. If sutures are needed, they are placed at this time. Prepare the suture needle and thread and have them positioned in a hemostat, ready to pass to the dentist. Retract tissue as needed.

8. After the sutures are placed and the area is irrigated with the sterile saline solution, a periodontal dressing is prepared and placed. Assist the periodontist with the suture placement, evacuate the area, and prepare the periodontal dressing.

9. After the placement of the dressing is completed, the patient is given postoperative instructions and dismissed. Make sure the patient does not have any debris on his or her face, give postoperative instructions, and dismiss the patient.

FIGURE 23-19 A gingivectomy procedure. (A) and (B) Marking the pocket depth with the pocket marker. (C) Incising the marked tissue with periodontal knives.

Periodontal Flap Surgery

Periodontal flap surgery involves surgically separating the gingiva from the underlying tissue. The gingiva is incised with a scalpel and then separated with a periosteal elevator. Once the tissue is retracted, the periodontist has good visibility and access to bone, tooth, and the tooth roots (Figure 23-20).

The design of the flap depends on the objectives of the surgery and the periodontist. The amount of exposure necessary for the surgery and the repositioning of the flap are important considerations. The periodontist exposes an area large enough to remove the irritants completely with the periodontal instruments. The appearance of the gingiva after the surgery depends on the proper repositioning of the flap. The tissue is positioned to heal in a manner that leaves as little evidence of the surgery as possible.

When the flap is retracted, the diseased tissue and debris are removed, the roots are planed, and the alveolar bone is trimmed and contoured. The area is rinsed with a saline solution and the flap is repositioned and sutured. A **periodontal dressing** may be applied to protect the surgical site.

Osseous Surgery

Osseous surgery removes defects/deformities in the bone caused by periodontal disease and other, related conditions. Two types of bone surgeries that correct the deformities are **osteoplasty**, reshaping the bone, and **ostectomy**, removal of bone.

Osseous surgery can be either **additive** or **subtractive**. During additive osseous surgery (sometimes called augmentive surgery), bone or bone substitute is added to fill in areas. This is a bone grafting (moving tissue from one area to another) procedure.

During subtractive osseous surgery, the bone is removed with chisels, rongeurs, files, diamond burs, and stones.

After the bone has been grafted or removed and contoured, the flap is repositioned and sutures are placed. The area is rinsed gently and blotted dry before a periodontal dressing is placed (Figure 23-21).

Mucogingival Surgery

Mucogingival surgery is reconstructive surgery on the gingiva and/or mucosa tissues. The surgeries may involve covering exposed roots, increasing the width of the gingival tissue, and reducing frenum or muscle attachments. Periodontal disease can cause negative changes in the gingiva, and mucogingival surgery improves these areas. Two common examples of mucogingival surgery are gingival grafting and the frenectomy.

Gingival Grafting

During a **gingival grafting** procedure, tissue is taken from one site and placed on another. Often, tissue from the palate is used for the graft. The procedure involves

FIGURE 23-20 Flap surgery to exposed impacted tooth. (A) Incision is made. (B) Retracting the flap of tissue. *(Courtesy of Gary Shellerud, DDS)*

FIGURE 23-21 Osseous surgery. Alveolar bone is exposed. *(Courtesy of Gary Shellerud, DDS)*

PROCEDURE

23-4 Osseous Surgery

This procedure is performed by the periodontist. It involves removing and recontouring diseased and defective bone tissue. The extent of the periodontal disease process determines the amount and type of surgery performed.

EQUIPMENT

▶ Basic setup: mouth mirror, explorer, cotton pliers

▶ Periodontal probe

▶ Cotton rolls and gauze sponges

▶ Saliva ejector, HVE tip, air-water syringe tip, surgical aspirator tip

▶ Anesthetic setup

▶ Scalpel and blades

▶ Periodontal knives—broad bladed and interproximal

▶ Tissue retractor

▶ Periosteal elevator

▶ Diamond burs and stones

▶ Rongeurs, chisels, and files

▶ Scalers and curettes

▶ Hemostat and surgical scissors

▶ Suture setup

▶ Periodontal dressing materials

PROCEDURE STEPS (*Follow aseptic procedures*)

In osseous surgery, a flap of soft tissue is incised and reflected to expose the bone for reshaping and/or removal. This procedure is performed by the periodontist.

1. After the anesthetic is administered, the soft tissue is incised and loosened from the underlying bone. Transfer instruments and maintain good visibility for the operator.

2. The tissue flap is reflected and stabilized with tissue retractors. Retract and hold the tissue.

3. Once the bone is exposed, the diseased bone tissue is excised. Scalers and curettes are used to remove calculus and diseased tissue and the roots are planed. Transfer instruments, rinse the area with a sterile saline solution as needed, evacuate, and keep the instruments clean by removing debris from instruments with the gauze sponge.

4. The bone is shaped and contoured using diamond burs and stones, rongeurs, chisels, and files.

5. The tissue flap is replaced and positioned over the alveolar bone, then sutured in place. Prepare the suture and stabilize the tissue with tissue forceps during the suturing procedure.

6. Prepare the periodontal dressing materials and assist the operator in the placement. In some states, the dental assistant is allowed to place and remove the periodontal dressing.

7. Remove any debris from the patient's face, give postoperative instructions, and dismiss the patient.

---

preparation of the site of the graft by eliminating any periodontal pockets and exposing a bed of connective tissue. Then, a graft (section of tissue) is obtained from the donor site, often the palate area. This graft is positioned carefully and sutured securely in place. The donor site is covered with a periodontal dressing or another protective material until it is healed, which usually takes one to two weeks (Figure 23-22).

Frenectomy

The **frenectomy** is a complete removal of the frenum, including the attachment to the underlying bone. The frenum may be removed is if it is attached too close to the marginal gingiva. The procedure involves incising the frenum and removing a triangular section. The periodontal fibers are separated and cut to the bone. The labial mucosa is then sutured to the apical periosteum. The periodontal dressing is prepared and placed over the suture site.

PERIODONTAL DRESSING

Periodontal dressings or packs are placed after periodontal surgical procedures. The dressings do not have any medicinal qualities; they are bandages used to protect the tissue during the healing process.

FIGURE 23-22 Gingival graft. (A) Gingival recession shows need for a graft. (B) Graft positioned and sutured in place. (C) Graft after healing period. *(Courtesy of Gary Shellerud, DDS)*

The purposes of the periodontal dressing include:

▶ Minimizing postoperative infection and hemorrhage

▶ Protecting the tissues during mastication

▶ Covering the surgical site in order to reduce pain due to trauma or irritation

▶ Providing support for teeth that are mobile

Types of Periodontal Dressings

There are different materials used for periodontal dressings. The most common types are the zinc oxide-eugenol materials and the non-eugenol materials.

Zinc Oxide-Eugenol Materials. The zinc oxide-eugenol materials are supplied in a powder (zinc oxide) or liquid (eugenol) form that can be mixed before the procedure and stored for later use. Some offices mix the material, wrap it in wax paper, and then freeze it until needed.

The presence of eugenol in this dressing can cause an allergic reaction. The area becomes red and a burning sensation is experienced by the patient.

Non-Eugenol Materials. The non-eugenol materials come in a two-paste system: one tube of base material and one tube of accelerator. The two pastes are dispensed in equal portions on a paper pad and mixed together prior to placement.

The non-eugenol dressings do not cause sensitivity problems, and some non-eugenol dressing materials have bacteriostatic agents added.

PERIODONTAL MAINTENANCE PROCEDURES

Periodontal surgery does not end the need for periodontal treatment. The patient determines the success of the treatment by being committed and following the designed therapy. Periodontal disease is an ongoing process, but continual care maintains the status of periodontal health after surgery. Dedicated home oral-hygiene routines and periodic visits to the dentist are necessary for successful periodontal care.

Once the patient has accepted the treatment plan, plaque-control techniques are taught by the dental assistant and/or the hygienist. As the patient continues through treatment, the patient's hygiene skills and personalized intraoral aids are evaluated and adjusted according to the patient's individual needs. After surgery, the patient is instructed to keep the area as clean as possible in order to enhance the healing process. After the periodontal dressing is removed, interdental cleaners, floss, and water irrigators may be used to remove plaque and debris. When the tissues have healed sufficiently, the patient can begin the oral hygiene regimen prescribed.

23-5 Preparation and Placement of the Non-Eugenol Periodontal Dressing

The periodontist routinely places the dressing, but in some states the dental assistant is allowed to place and remove the periodontal dressing. The dressing is placed after the surgery to protect the tissues and promote the healing process.

EQUIPMENT

▶ Basic setup: mouth mirror, explorer, and cotton pliers

▶ Gauze sponges

▶ Non-eugenol periodontal dressing material (base and accelerator)

▶ Paper pad and tongue depressor

▶ Lubricant

▶ Instrument to contour dressing (spoon excavator, sickle scaler)

PROCEDURE STEPS *(Follow aseptic procedures)*

1. After the hemorrhaging is controlled, the patient's lips are coated lightly with Vaseline.

2. The dressing materials are dispensed into equal lengths and mixed with a tongue blade until homogeneous. (Using a paper pad and tongue blade make cleanup easier). The material is allowed to set for two to three minutes until the tackiness is gone (Figure 23-23A).

3. Lubricate gloved fingers with Vaseline so the putty-like material can be handled easily.

4. The dressing comes with a retardant to slow the setting time, if necessary; it can be molded easily for three to five minutes and worked for fifteen to twenty minutes.

5. The dressing is molded into a thin strip slightly longer than the length of the surgical site. Divide the strip into two equal lengths, one for the facial surface and one for the lingual surface (Figure 23-23B).

6. To begin the placement, form the end of one strip into a hook shape. Wrap this hook around the distal of the most posterior tooth (Figure 23-23C).

(A)

(B)

FIGURE 23-23 Preparation and placement of the periodontal dressing. (A) Mixing the materials. (B) Preparing the materials for placement. *(continued)*

(continued)

P R O C E D U R E   **2 - 5** *continued*

7. Adapt the rest of the strip along the facial surface, gently pressing the pack into the interproximal areas (Figure 23-23D).

8. The second strip is applied to the lingual surface in the same manner. The pack is wrapped around the last posterior tooth and then adapted to the lingual surface, moving toward the midline.

9. The pack should cover the gingiva evenly without interfering with occlusion or the tongue movements.

10. Check the dressing for overextensions. These areas are removed with a spoon excavator or scaler. Gently press the instrument into the dressing to detach the extra material. Smooth the pack and evaluate it for an even thickness.

11. Ask the patient how the pack feels. Instruct the patient to move his or her tongue, cheeks, and lips to mold the pack. Make any adjustments to ensure that the dressing is securely in place, trimmed, and contoured.

12. Give the patient instructions about the periodontal dressing, including:

    ▸ The pack is kept on for one week after surgery.

    ▸ The pack will harden in a few hours and then withstand normal chewing stresses.

    ▸ The pack may chip and break off during the week but should remain intact as long as possible. If there is pain when pieces of the pack come off or the pack becomes rough, the patient should call the office.

    ▸ The patient should brush the occlusal surface of the teeth involved in the surgery and continue to brush and floss the rest of the teeth as normal.

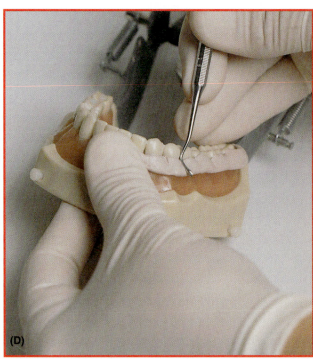

FIGURE 23-23 *(continued)* (C) Placing the dressing on the tissue. (D) Contoured dressing.

PROCEDURE

23-6 Removal of the Periodontal Dressing

This procedure is performed by the periodontist or the dental assistant depending on the expanded functions. The patient has worn the dressing for a week to ten days. The patient's mouth is examined before removing the dressing to check for areas where the dressing may have come loose or come off completely.

EQUIPMENT

▶ Basic setup: mouth mirror, explorer, and cotton pliers

▶ Saliva ejector, HVE tip, air-water syringe tip

▶ Gauze sponges and tissue

▶ Instruments to remove the dressing (spoon excavator, sickle explorer, surgical hoe)

PROCEDURE STEPS *(Follow aseptic procedures)*

1. After seating the patient, the surgical site is evaluated and the dressing is removed.

2. A surgical hoe or a spoon excavator is inserted along the margin. Lateral pressure is applied to pry the dressing away from the tissue (Figure 23-24).

3. The pack may come off in large pieces and then scalers and floss can be used to remove any par-

FIGURE 23-24 Removal of the periodontal dressing.

ticles from the interproximal areas and tooth surfaces. Cotton pliers are used to remove particles of dressing that are embedded in the surgical site.

4. Gently rinse the entire area with warm water to remove any debris. The air-water syringe can be used carefully.

▮ CHAPTER SUMMARY

Periodontal disease is as old as the human race. According to the American Academy of Periodontology, three out of four adults will experience, to some degree, periodontal problems at some time in their lives. Periodontal disease occurs in children and adolescents, with marginal gingivitis and gingival recession being the most prevalent conditions.

The dental assistant performs chairside assisting duties and the expanded functions allowed by the state Dental Practice Act, including placing and removing periodontal dressing, removing sutures, and performing coronal polishes. The dental assistant takes radiographs, makes impressions for study models, places sealants, and administers fluoride treatments. The assistant also gives pre- and postoperative instructions and prepares the treatment room for surgery. These functions are in addition to treatment room preparation and maintenance and sterilization procedures. The dental assistant is involved in educating and motivating the patient throughout the treatment. In some offices, the dental asisstant may also perform laboratory tasks, such as pouring study models or making periodontal splints.

CASE STUDY

Melissa Moore is forty-two years old. She has been Dr. Sanchez's patient for fourteen years. Melissa has her teeth examined and cleaned every six months. Over the years, she has developed several teeth with pocket readings of between six and eight. At Melissa's last cleaning appointment, the hygienist explained that she found over ten areas with periodontal probing readings of over six and areas where the tissues bleed easily. Melissa is in good general health but has been taking medication to reduce anxiety for the past six months.

Case Study Review

1. Are Melissa's periodontal readings within the normal range?

2. What questions should be asked in reference to the change in her condition in such a short period of time?

3. Explain how stress could affect Melissa's periodontal health.

 To complete your study of this chapter, work the review activities that follow. Also, refer to the software that accompanies this text.

REVIEW QUESTIONS

Multiple Choice

1. The periodontium includes:
   a. gingiva, epithelial attachment, cementum, sulcus, enamel, and pulp chamber.
   b. gingiva, enamel, cementum, dentin, sulcus, and periodontal ligaments.
   c. gingiva, epithelial attachment, sulcus, periodontal ligaments, cementum, and alveolar bone.
   d. periodontal ligaments, sulcus, gingiva, salivary glands, and mucous membrane.

2. Periodontal disease is a virus that can be transmitted from one individual to another.
   a. This is a true statement.
   b. This is a false statement.

3. One periodontal instrument is used to remove sub-gingival calculus and smooth the root surface. The working end is rounded at the end and has cutting edges on both sides of the blade. This instrument is a
   a. hoe.
   b. file.
   c. scaler.
   d. curette.

4. The procedure to remove calculus and debris from the tooth and periodontal pocket is known as
   a. root planing.
   b. scaling and curettage.
   c. polishing procedure.
   d. occlusal adjustment.

5. Periodontal surgery that involves the recontouring of the alveolar bone is called
   a. mucogingival surgery.
   b. gingival grafting.
   c. osteoplasty.
   d. ostectomy.

Critical Thinking

1. What are the signs and symptoms of periodontal disease?

2. Name the periodontal disease that occurs in young adults and is the result of stress, inadequate diet and sleep, and poor oral hygiene.

3. Patients must take an active part in the treatment of periodontal disease. List several means the dental assistant uses to aid the patient.

Fixed Prosthodontics

OBJECTIVES

The student should strive to meet the following objectives and demonstrate
an understanding of the facts and principles presented in this chapter:

1. Define the scope of fixed prosthodontics.

2. Explain considerations the dentist must make when recommending various prostheses to a patient.

3. Describe various types of fixed prostheses and their functions.

4. Describe dental materials used in fixed prostheses.

5. Explain the involvement of the laboratory technician in the fabrication of
   fixed prostheses.

6. Describe the role of the dental assistant in all phases of fixed prosthodontic treatment.

7. Explain techniques for retaining the prosthesis when there is little or no
   crown on the tooth.

8. Describe implant retainer prosthesis.

9. Explain techniques for maintaining fixed prostheses.

KEY TERMS

INTRODUCTION

Fixed prosthodontics is the specialty that deals with replacement of missing teeth or parts of teeth with extensive restorations. The restorations or **prostheses** (artificial parts for missing tissues) are fabricated in a dental laboratory from detailed impressions taken in the dental office. When finished, the prostheses are cemented permanently in the patient's mouth.

Fixed prostheses replace missing teeth and tooth structures which:

▶ Restores masticatory function

▶ Improves esthetics and, often, self-esteem

▶ Improves speech

▶ Promotes good oral hygiene

▶ Prevents further movement of the teeth because of support of the prostheses

The fixed prosthesis becomes part of the natural dentition and is maintained with routine brushing and flossing techniques. The main disadvantages are the expense of the prosthesis and the time involved in preparing the tooth, taking the impression, fabricating the restoration, and permanently cementing it in place. The restorations routinely take at least two appointments to complete. Dental insurance may cover some of the expense of prosthetic restorations.

There are several advantages of having a permanent restoration: The restoration is secure in the mouth, it is esthetic, and it restores function for many years. These advantages outweigh the initial monetary expense and time commitment.

The **prosthodontist** receives additional education and clinical practice to specialize in fixed and removable prosthodontic procedures. Patient cases include general **fixed prosthetic** procedures that are difficult, involved, and extensive. Such cases might include patients who have had extensive surgery due to cancer of the mouth. The patients are referred by general dentists and other specialists to the prosthodontist.

There are many types of fixed prostheses and a variety of materials used for their preparation, fabrication, and cementation.

PATIENT CONSIDERATIONS

When a patient needs fixed prosthodontic treatment, the dentist performs an examination that includes:

▶ A medical and dental history

▶ Examination of the intra- and extraoral tissues

▶ Radiographs

▶ Impressions for study models (diagnostic casts)

▶ Intraoral photographs taken with the intraoral camera

▶ Extraoral photographs

Patients who are candidates for fixed prostheses should have healthy supportive tissues and be motivated to maintain the prostheses. Sometimes, patients need to have periodontal or orthodontic treatment prior to the fixed prosthodontic treatment.

Case Presentation

With less complicated cases, the dentist presents the treatment to the patient at the time of the examination. Other cases require time for the dentist to make the diagnosis and treatment plan before the patient is scheduled for the case presentation.

At the case presentation, the dentist recommends the type of prosthesis and explains what is involved in treatment, including the number of appointments and what the patient can expect. The dentist uses study models, radiographs, pictures of completed cases, samples of various dental prostheses on models, pamphlets, educational videos, and computer images in the presentation. The computer-imaging component shows the patient before and after images (Figure 24-1).

When presenting the treatment choices to the patient, the dentist or the office manager explains the cost of the prosthesis, whether insurance will cover any of the treatment, and the number of appointments required.

TYPES OF FIXED PROSTHESES

Fixed prostheses are **indirect restorations**, meaning they cannot be placed directly in the mouth after the

FIGURE 24-1 Computerized imaging system shows the patient before and after views of the prostheses.

tooth is prepared like amalgam or composite restorations, which are **direct restorations**. Instead, impressions are taken and then the fixed prostheses are fabricated in a dental laboratory. The indirect restorations are designed to replace missing tooth structure in a variety of ways, including full crowns, partial crowns, inlays, onlays, bridges, and veneers.

Crowns

Crowns cover teeth with extensive decay or breakdown. The prepared tooth is covered with an anatomically shaped and fitted crown. Crowns are constructed of different materials or a combination of materials. The tooth may require a full crown, which is often referred to as a **full-cast crown** (Figure 24-2). A full crown covers the entire coronal surface of the tooth. Sometimes, the tooth is broken down so badly that means to retain the

full crown on the tooth are required. (Retention is discussed later in this chapter.)

A **partial crown** is a cast restoration that covers three or more, but not all, surfaces of a tooth. A **three-quarter crown** normally is prepared so that the mesial, distal, and lingual surfaces are reduced but the facial surface is left intact (Figure 24-3). The incisal or occlusal surface of the tooth is also reduced.

Inlays and Onlays

Inlays and onlays are restorations that replace missing tooth structure within the tooth. **Inlays** cover the area between the cusps in the middle of the tooth and the proximal surfaces that are involved (Figure 24-4A). Inlays are MOD (mesio-occluso-distal), MO (mesio-occlusal), DO (disto-occlusal), or O (occlusal). **Onlays** are like inlays except they include the cusp ridges of the tooth (Figure 24-4B). Inlays and onlays are also cast restorations that are made of a variety of materials. The extent of lost tooth structure and the preparation determine which type of cast restoration is best suited to restore function and preserve the strength of the tooth.

Bridges

A bridge is a restoration that spans the space of a missing tooth or teeth. The bridge is divided into units, and each unit of a bridge represents a tooth. A bridge may replace one or more adjacent teeth in the same arch. The missing tooth is replaced by a **pontic**, which can be designed in a variety of forms. Two common pontics are the hygienic (free cleansing/sanitary) and cosmetic (ovate). The hygienic pontics allow for space between the tissue and pontic, usually seen in the posterior area. The cosmetic pontics are tooth colored and fill in the entire space to the gingival tissue.

FIGURE 24-2 (A) Porcelain fused to metal crown. (B) Full porcelain crown.

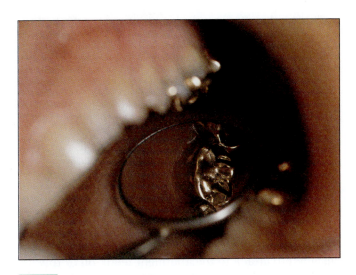

FIGURE 24-3 Three-quarter gold crown.

FIGURE 24-4 (A) Gold inlay restorations. (B) Gold onlay restoration on mandibular first molar.

Porcelain-fused-to-metal bridge

(A)

FIGURE 24-5 (A) Three unit bridge abutments, pontics, and retainers. (B) Maryland bridge.

The teeth adjacent to the pontic are called **abutments**. Crowns, inlays, or onlays may be placed on the abutment teeth to support and provide stability for the pontic (Figure 24-5A).

Bridges are made of a variety of materials to meet the patient's esthetic and functional needs. After the bridges have been fabricated, they are permanently cemented in the patient's mouth. Bridges also can be retained by one or two teeth on the same side. This type of bridge is known as a cantilever bridge.

The **Maryland bridge**, or resin-retained fixed bridge, is used to replace one tooth. The abutment teeth have very little tooth structure removed during the preparation. The bridge consists of a pontic with extensions (retainers) of varying shapes. The extensions are designed to attach to the abutment teeth, on or toward the lingual surface. The retainers of the Maryland bridge are roughened by electrolytic etching to increase

their bonding to the natural tooth structure (Figure 24-5B).

The preparation of the teeth for the Maryland bridge is usually minimal. The impressions are taken and temporaries may be placed. The laboratory procedures are the same for all cases except the electrolytic etching of the inside of the bridge retainers. The cementation steps are as follows:

1. The dental dam is placed to protect the tissues from the acid etching.

2. The abutment teeth are cleaned with pumice and water, then rinsed and dried thoroughly.

3. The prepared surfaces of the teeth are acid etched for thirty to sixty seconds, rinsed thoroughly, and dried.

4. A dual-cured composite cementing material is applied to the etched surfaces of the bridge retainers and the etched tooth surface.

5. The bridge is positioned on the abutment teeth.

6. Once the material has set, excess cement material is removed.

Veneers

Veneers are thin layers of tooth-colored material that cover much of the facial surface. They are used to cover badly stained teeth and to reshape the anatomy of teeth. Veneers improve appearance with very little removal of tooth structure. Examples include:

▶ Full crown on anterior maxillary teeth—Covered with veneers for a natural appearance (Figure 24-6).

▶ Tetracycline stains on the maxillary anterior teeth—Veneers cover the stain for improved appearance (Figure 24-7).

(A)

(B)

FIGURE 24-7 (A) Patient with tetracycline staining. (B) Patient with tetracycline staining after direct resin veneers have been placed. *(Courtesy of Kerr Corporation)*

▶ Diastema (an abnormal space between two adjacent teeth in the same arch) on maxillary central incisors—Veneers close the space (Figure 24-8).

Veneer procedures are changing constantly as technology progresses. There are many types of veneers, materials used, and techniques. Direct resin veneers, indirect resin veneers, and porcelain veneers are three types.

Direct Resin Veneers. **Direct resin veneers** are made in the dental office directly on the patient's tooth. This procedure requires one appointment. In preparation for the veneer procedure, little, if any, tooth structure is removed. The tooth is etched, adhesive is applied, and opaquers and body shade are placed. The incisal shade follows. The shade can be varied between the incisal edge and body of the veneer. The veneers are contoured and finished. Generally these materials are light cured and require routine polishing and periodic maintenance.

(A)

(B)

FIGURE 24-6 Veeners on anterior teeth. (A) Before placement. (B) After placement. *(Courtesy of George J. Velis, DDS)*

FIGURE 24-8 (A) Patient with diastema between two central incisors and (B) Patient with diastema after indirect resin veneers have been placed. *(Courtesy of George J. Velis, DDS)*

Indirect Resin Veneers. **Indirect resin veneers** require two appointments. At the first appointment, the tooth is prepared and an impression is taken. The impression is sent to the laboratory for fabrication of the veneer. During the second appointment, the veneer is bonded in place. The indirect resin veneers do not bond well to resin cement. They lack strength and wear at a greater rate than porcelain veneers.

Porcelain Veneers. **Porcelain veneers** are similar to indirect resin veneers in that they require two appointments and are fabricated in the dental laboratory. Porcelain veneers are natural in appearance and are durable. The technique for the porcelain veneer is sensitive to shade selection and gingival margin adaption if the veneer is to look natural and adapt well.

P R O C E D U R E

24-1 Porcelain Veneers

This procedure is performed by the prosthodontist and is completed in two appointments. During the first appointment, the tooth is prepared and impressions are taken; at the second appointment, the porcelain veneer is applied. Between appointments, the impressions are sent to a dental laboratory, where the porcelain veneer is fabricated.

EQUIPMENT (*For the preparation appointment*)

▶ Basic setup: mouth mirror, explorer, and cotton pliers

▶ Cotton rolls, 2 × 2 gauze

▶ HVE tip, air-water syringe tip

▶ Anesthetic setup

▶ High-speed handpiece and assorted burs

▶ Shade guide

▶ Spoon excavator

▶ Low-speed handpiece with prophy angle, rubber cup, and pumice

▶ Retraction cord and placement instrument

▶ Bite registration materials

▶ Alginate impression materials for model of opposing arch

▶ Final impression materials (polysiloxane or polyether)

▶ Temporary veneer (optional)

▶ Laboratory prescription form

(continued)

P R O C E D U R E   2 4 - 1 *continued*

PROCEDURE STEPS (*Follow aseptic procedures*)

Preparation Appointment (First Appointment)

1. A bite registration and an opposing arch impression are taken.

2. The teeth are cleaned with rubber cup and pumice to remove extrinsic stains. A shade is selected by the dentist to determine how light the patient wants the veneers and to estimate how light the finished shade will be.

3. The teeth are prepared according to the design of the veneer. The incisal edge and the cervical margin are prepared carefully so that the finished veneer is even with the gingival crest or just slightly subgingival.

4. The retraction cord is placed to achieve hemostasis and ensure visualization of the margins.

5. A final impression is taken with a dimensionally stable material such as polysiloxane or polyether.

6. Temporary veneers are placed if necessary, although most patients do not require temporary veneers.

7. The retraction cord is removed after the temporary veneers are placed.

8. The patient is informed that the gums will be tender for several days because of the retraction cord placement.

9. The patient is dismissed.

Laboratory Fabrication

1. The impressions are sent to the dental laboratory with a laboratory prescription.

2. The laboratory follows the dentist's prescription regarding length of veneer, shade, thickness, and texture. (Color photos of the patient are helpful in the designing and shading process.)

3. The laboratory fabricates the veneers and returns them to the office.

EQUIPMENT: (*For the cementation appointment*)

▶ Basic setup: mouth mirror, explorer, and cotton pliers

▶ Cotton rolls, 2 × 2 gauze, cheek and lip retractors

▶ Saliva ejector, HVE tip, air-water syringe tip

▶ Porcelain veneers from the laboratory

▶ Low-speed handpiece with prophy angle, rubber cup, and pumice

▶ Silane coupling agent and small applicator (brush)

▶ Retraction cord and placement instrument

▶ Chlorhexidine soap

▶ Plastic or ultrathin metal strips

▶ Etchant and applicator

▶ Bonding agent and curing light

Cementation Appointment (Second Appointment)

1. The second appointment should be scheduled as close as possible to the first appointment because the patient is often without temporary coverage. The laboratory should be scheduled ahead of time so the turnaround time is minimal.

2. Complete a preliminary cleaning of the teeth with pumice to remove plaque and stains.

3. The veneers are tried on the tooth and adjustments are made with finishing diamonds. (The veneers are very fragile and require careful handling.)

4. Once all adjustments are completed, clean and dry the inside of the veneers thoroughly. Acid etchant is used to clean and decontaminate the inside surface of the veneer.

5. Apply a thin layer of silane coupling agent (this material allows bonding to porcelain).

6. Place the light-cured bonding agent in the veneers. Make sure there are no air bubbles. The material fills the veneer and is spread evenly. The veneers are then placed in a light-protected area or box until the teeth are prepared.

7. Prepare the teeth for bonding by placing a retraction cord on the facial surface. Clean the facial surface with chlorhexidine soap and a prophy cup or brush.

8. Isolate the teeth being bonded with cotton rolls, cheek and lip retractors, a saliva ejector, and plastic or ultrathin metal strips.

9. Etch the teeth to be bonded, following the directions of the specific adhesive system.

10. Apply the adhesive to the teeth being bonded.

11. Seat each veneer in the correct position.

(continued)

12. In some cases, the veneer is spot cured and excess cement is removed.

13. Light cure each veneer in place.

14. Remove excess cement with a scalpel.

15. Contour and refine the margins with finishing diamonds or burs (Figure 24-9).

16. Polish the veneers with rubber wheels, cups, and polishing paste.

FIGURE 24-9 Finishing porcelain veneer margins with a diamond bur. *(Courtesy of Kerr Corporation)*

TYPES OF MATERIALS USED FOR FIXED PROSTHESES

The materials used for the construction of fixed crowns, bridges, inlay, onlays, and veneers depends, among other considerations, on their locations in the mouth, the strength required, the amount of tooth structure, and esthetics (natural-looking teeth are the current trend, while at one time having gold showing was very prestigious). Because patients want tooth-colored restorations, more porcelain and composite materials are being used.

Gold Casting Alloys

Gold used in crowns, inlays, and onlays is not pure gold but a combination of metals. When two or more metals are combined, they form an **alloy**. Pure gold is too soft for use in cast restorations, so other metals, such as platinum and palladium, are added, along with iron, tin, or zinc, to form **dental casting alloy**.

Restorations made of gold alloy include full gold crowns, inlays, and onlays. These are fabricated mainly for the posterior teeth where they are not as visible. Gold crowns are also fabricated with tooth-colored veneers. The veneers may cover the entire crown or just the facial surface. Crowns that have veneers are known as **porcelain-fused-to-metal crowns**, or ceramo-metal crowns (Figure 24-10).

These porcelain-fused-to-metal crowns are very popular and are commonly used where strength and esthetics are needed. They resist fracture, abrasion, and discoloration. These crowns are used in all areas of the mouth for single-tooth restorations or for bridges. The disadvantages are that the tooth requires more reduction to allow for the thickness of the porcelain and the porcelain is abrasive and can wear down natural teeth or metal restorations.

Tooth-Colored Cast Restorations

Tooth-colored cast restorations are made either of porcelain or composite resin. There is an increase in the use of these materials because of the cosmetic appearance they provide. Porcelain is used for inlays, bonded veneers, porcelain-fused-to-metal crowns, and bridges. Porcelain cast restorations require at least two appointments and are more expensive than the gold cast restorations. Porcelain, a type of ceramic, resembles natural tooth structure but is not as strong when used alone. Porcelain is susceptible to fracture under occlusal stresses, but with resin-bonding techniques, this aspect has improved. Restorations that are solely porcelain are used mainly on single teeth and rarely for fixed bridges.

Composite resin indirect technique restorations are fabricated in a dental laboratory. Inlays, onlays, and veneers are made from impressions taken at the first appointment; then, the dental laboratory creates the restorations from composite resin material. This material is heated and placed under pressure. These restora-

FIGURE 24-10 Bridge with full gold crown on second molar and metal crown with porcelain facing on pontic and anterior abutment (second bicuspid). *(Courtesy of Clifton O. Caldwell, Jr., DDS, FICD, FACD)*

FIGURE 24-11 Composite resin inlays on patient's left mandibular. *(Courtesy of George J. Velis, DDS)*

tions are stronger than direct composite resin restorations and are bonded in place during the second appointment (Figure 24-11).

ROLE OF THE LABORATORY TECHNICIAN

The dental laboratory technician and the dentist work closely to give the patient quality restorations. The relationship between the laboratory and the dental office is critical. Good communication and clearly defined expectations are essential.

The laboratory technician performs the following procedures in fixed prosthesis construction: making custom trays, pouring impressions, articulating stone casts (models), preparing wax patterns, investing, and casting gold alloy restorations. The laboratory technician also constructs porcelain and porcelain-fused-to-metal restorations and fabricates the prosthesis according to the dentist's prescription and from the impressions sent from the dental office.

It is important that the impression materials be handled properly and that everything needed is sent to the laboratory. The dental assistant often is responsible for having everything ready for the laboratory pickup.

ROLE OF THE DENTAL ASSISTANT

The dental assistant is very involved in all stages of fixed prosthodontic treatment. It is important to understand the sequence of the procedure and the different types of restorations when assisting the dentist. The dental assistant explains the steps of the procedure to the patient, answers questions, and gives postoperative and home-care instructions.

The dental assistant is responsible for preparation of equipment and supplies needed for both appointments. Each tray setup is arranged according to the sequence of the procedure, with auxiliary instruments and materials close at hand. The procedures require many different types of dental materials, including alginate, bite registration materials, final impression materials, retraction cord, temporization materials, and final cements. The dental assistant prepares and/or utilizes these materials throughout the procedure.

The dental assistant assists the dentist in all aspects of the procedure, from selecting the shade of the tooth to general chairside assisting. In some states, the qualified dental assistant can perform procedures such as placing the retraction cord, placing and removing temporaries, taking preliminary impressions, and removing excess cement. The dental assistant also coordinates the patient's appointments and the laboratory schedule. In some offices, the dental assistant may perform some laboratory functions, such as making custom trays and pouring study models.

The Fabrication of the Prosthesis in the Dental Laboratory

Once the case is in the dental laboratory, there are several steps to fabricate the prosthesis, depending on the number of units and the types of materials used. These basic steps give the dental assistant an idea of the steps involved in the fabrication.

Laboratory steps include:

▶ Pouring the alginate impression of the opposing arch in plaster

▶ Pouring the final impression to make a master model and die (replica of the prepared tooth)

▶ Creating a wax pattern on the die

▶ Investing and preparing the wax pattern for casting

▶ Casting the die once the invested material and the metal are heated to the desired temperature

▶ Casting the crown in gold alloy to prepare for the porcelain veneer to be made

▶ Painting porcelain on the crown in layers and then curing it in an oven at high temperatures

▶ Finishing and polishing the porcelain-fused-to-metal crown

RETENTION TECHNIQUES

Often, the teeth being restored with a fixed prosthesis have substantial loss of tooth structure due to decay, fractures, or large, deteriorated restorations. Also, root canal therapy may be required before the crowns and bridges are made.

P R O C E D U R E

24-2 Preparation for a Porcelain-Fused-to-Metal Crown

This procedure is performed by the prosthodontist and the dental assistant. Like the porcelain veneer procedure, this process involves two appointments. The following procedure includes the steps in the preparation appointment, including retention procedures, and the steps in the cementation appointment.

EQUIPMENT (Figure 24-12)

FIGURE 24-12 Tray setup for the preparation appointment (armamentarium).

▸ Basic setup: mouth mirror, explorer, and cotton pliers

▸ Cotton rolls, gauze, dental floss, articulating paper, and forceps

▸ HVE tip, saliva ejector, and three-way syringe tip

▸ Anesthetic setup

▸ Dental dam setup

▸ High-speed handpiece with a selection of diamonds, discs, and burs

▸ Irreversible hydrocolloid (alginate) impression materials

▸ Spoon excavator, scaler, plastic filling instrument, and cement spatula

▸ Tooth shade guide (optional)

▸ Retention materials depending on the amount of tooth structure retained—core buildup materials and postretention pins (optional)

▸ Gingival retraction cord and placement instrument

▸ Final impression materials and tray (stock or custom tray)

▸ Bite registration materials

▸ Crown and collar scissors

▸ Provisional (temporary) coverage materials

▸ Low-speed handpiece with burs, discs, and stones

▸ Laboratory prescription and container for impressions (off-tray item)

PROCEDURE STEPS *(Follow aseptic procedures)*

1. The patient is given local anesthetic. Prepare the syringe, transfer the syringe to the prosthodontist and, during the administration of the anesthetic, observe the patient.

2. Alginate impressions are taken for fabrication of certain types of temporaries and also for a model of the opposing arch. Select the trays, mix the irreversible hydrocolloid, and take the impressions. The impressions are stored properly until needed and/or poured in plaster or stone.

3. While waiting for the anesthetic to be effective before the tooth is prepared, the tooth shade is selected. A **shade guide** is used to match the natural teeth.

NOTE: This is a very important step for the esthetics of the crown and the appearance of the patient. The shade guide includes a variety of shades, and the shades can be variegated to match the varying shading of the patient's natural teeth (Figure 24-13A).

Moisten the shade guide and hold it close the natural teeth under natural light (Figure 24-13B). Record the information on the patient's chart and on the laboratory prescription.

(continued)

P R O C E D U R E   **2 4 - 2** *continued*

FIGURE 24-13 (A) Shade guide. (B) Matching the shade sample to the patient's natural teeth.

4. Crowns are prepared with the high-speed handpiece and various diamonds and burs. (The tooth must be reduced to accommodate the thickness of the metal and porcelain materials and to have enough strength.)

5. The margins of the preparation are either finished in a **chamfer** or **shoulder** preparation. The chamfer provides adequate bulk and extends easily into the gingival sulcus. The shoulder provides a ledge that is sometimes beveled (Figure 24-14). Prepare and transfer the high-speed handpiece, then evacuate and maintain the operating field with the air-water syringe. Retract and exchange instruments as needed.

The abutment teeth are prepared for full crowns by tapering margins of the preparation to the crown of the tooth. This preparation design allows for the placement and withdrawal of the finished restoration.

6. Once the tooth is prepared, the gingival tissue is retracted from the preparation so that a detailed impression can be made of the margins. The margins of the preparation must be detailed in the impressions so that the finished crown fits snugly and securely on the tooth. The retraction cord is placed around the prepared tooth and pushed into the sulcus with a plastic filling instrument or a retraction cord-condensing instrument (Figure 24-15).

FIGURE 24-14 Examples of cavity margin on the preparation—chamfer, shoulder, and shoulder with beveled edge.

FIGURE 24-15 Placing retraction cord around the prepared tooth.

(continued)

(Gingival retraction techniques are discussed in detail in Chapter 28, Advanced Chairside Functions.) In some states, the dental assistant is permitted to place the gingival retraction cord. Transfer a piece of retraction cord in cotton pliers to the prosthodontist. Then, transfer the appropriate cord-condensing instrument. The retraction cord remains in place for five minutes.

7. The prosthodontist selects the tray and impression material to be used. There are a variety of materials that are suitable for final impressions (see Chapter 27, Laboratory Materials and Techniques). The tray and syringe are selected and prepared and the materials are mixed.

8. Transfer cotton pliers to remove the retraction cord. Transfer the syringe material and receive the cotton pliers and cord. The prosthodontist removes the retraction cord, receives the syringe, and dispenses the material around the margins of the preparation (Figure 24-16A). During this time, mix and load the heavier material into the tray. The prosthodontist places and holds the tray with the impression material in the patient's mouth. Once the prosthodontist has seated the tray, move the light from the patient's face and clean up the impression materials. The final impression is rinsed, disinfected, and placed in a plastic laboratory container (Figure 24-16B).

9. The **bite registration**, also called the occlusal registration, is taken after the final impression is completed. The purpose of the bite registration is to record the way the patient occludes the maxil-lary and mandibular teeth. There are many types of materials that can be used to record the bite of the patient, including wax and vinyl polysiloxane materials (Figure 24-17). Prepare the materials and transfer them to the prosthodontist, who places the tray and takes the bite impression. In some states, the dental assistant legally can take the bite impression. After the bite registration is taken, rinse the patient's mouth. The materials are rinsed, disinfected, and placed in a plastic laboratory container.

The provisional restoration is very important in crown and bridge construction. The temporary retains the teeth in the same position so that the adjacent and opposing teeth do not shift position. The temporary protects the prepared tooth so that the patient can function normally. Between appointments, the temporary should look natural and be acceptable to the patient. Usually, the patient wears the temporary for seven to ten days, sometimes longer depending on the extent of the prosthetics.

There are many types of temporary techniques and materials available (see Chapter 27, Laboratory Materials and Techniques). Some temporary crown forms are preformed, while others are custom made for each patient (Figure 24-18). The provisional must be fitted to the tooth in order to protect the margins, maintain the space, and be esthetically pleasing.

10. After trimming and contouring the temporary, it is polished and cemented with temporary cement.

(A) (B)

FIGURE 24-16 (A) The dental assistant receives the syringe with the light-bodied impression material and transfers the tray with the medium- to heavy-bodied impression material to the dentist. (B) Final impression.

(continued)

P R O C E D U R E   24-2 *continued*

FIGURE 24-17 Materials used to take the bite registration.

The dental assistant either assists the prosthodontist or makes the temporary restoration depending on the expanded functions laws. When assisting with the temporary, prepare the materials and trays as dictated by the technique. Some temporaries require crown and bridge scissors and crimping and contour pliers, while others need burs, discs, and stones to contour and finish. Transfer and receive the instruments and keep the area rinsed and dried. Once the temporary is completed, mix the temporary cement and place some in the crown. Transfer the bite stick for the patient to bite on, then transfer a 2 × 2 gauze sponge to wipe off any excess.

11. Once the cement is dried, the bite stick is removed and a scaler is used to remove excess dry cement. Transfer dental floss to check the interproximal contacts.

12. Hold articulating paper in articulating forceps for the patient to bite on to test the bite. If adjustments are needed, transfer the low-speed handpiece with finishing burs. The patient's mouth is rinsed and evacuated before the patient is dismissed.

FIGURE 24-18 Different types of preformed temporaries.

13. After the patient has been dismissed, the patient's impressions and models and the laboratory prescription are ready for the laboratory pickup (Figure 24-19). The following information is usually included on the laboratory prescription:
    ▶ Patient's name
    ▶ Description of the prosthesis
    ▶ Types of materials the prosthodontist wants the prosthesis to be constructed from
    ▶ The shade or shading desired
    ▶ The prosthodontist's name, license number, address, telephone number, fax number, and signature
    ▶ The date when the case will be back in the dental office

FIGURE 24-19 A laboratory prescription. *(Courtesy of Dr. Randall Stephens)*

P R O C E D U R E

24-3 Cementation of Porcelain-Fused-to-Metal Crown

The following procedure is performed by the prosthodontist and the dental assistant. The temporary is removed, the permanent prosthesis is evaluated, and the final cementation is completed.

EQUIPMENT (Figure 24-20)

FIGURE 24-20 Tray setup for the cementation appointment.

▶ Basic setup: mouth mirror, explorer, and cotton pliers

▶ Cotton rolls, gauze, dental floss, articulating paper, and forceps

▶ HVE tip, saliva ejector, and air-water syringe tip

▶ Low-speed handpiece with finishing burs, discs, and stones

▶ Anesthetic setup

▶ Spoon excavator and scaler

▶ Plastic filling instrument (PFI)

▶ Orangewood bite stick (crown remover, crown seater, and mallet are optional)

▶ Final cementation materials (glass ionomer cement, polycarboxylate cement, resin cements, or zinc phosphate cement)

▶ Porcelain-fused-to-metal crown from laboratory

PROCEDURE STEPS (*Follow aseptic procedures*)

1. The day before the patient's appointment, make sure the laboratory has completed the crown and that it is in the office.

2. Once the patient arrives for the appointment, prepare him or her and explain the treatment. Prepare the topical and local anesthetic, then transfer the syringe and observe the patient. Once the anesthetic is placed, rinse and evacuate the mouth.

3. The provisional coverage is removed with a crown remover, scaler, and other instruments that fit under the margin of the temporary.

4. Once the temporary is removed, the excess cement is removed. The dental assistant either assists during this stage of the procedure by transferring instruments and keeping the area clean and free of debris or removes the temporary and excess cement as part of the expanded functions. Once the temporary is removed, rinse and dry the area and prepare the crown.

5. The cast crown is positioned on the preparation. If there is difficulty in the seating of the crown, a bite stick and/or mallet may be used. The occlusion, the margins, and contacts are all evaluated and adjustments are made, if necessary. If the porcelain is adjusted, it is sent back to the laboratory to be refinished. Transfer instruments, dental floss, and articulating paper and forceps. Keep the area clean and dry and transfer the low-speed handpiece with finishing burs, discs, and stones. If the casting has to be returned to the laboratory, disinfect the crown and prepare it for return to the laboratory.

6. Before cementing the crown, the area is isolated with cotton rolls and protective liners and/or a cavity varnish is placed.

7. The permanent cement is mixed according to manufacturer's directions and placed in the crown and on the prepared tooth (Figure 24-21).

(continued)

PROCEDURE   24-3   *continued*

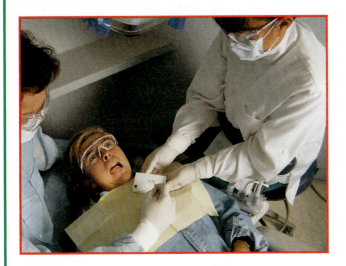

FIGURE 24-21 Dental assistant passes the final cement and crown for cementation.

FIGURE 24-22 Crown permanently cemented. Excess cement around the margins being removed.

8. Once the crown is seated on the tooth, the patient bites on a bite stick or crown seater until the cement hardens. Prepare the permanent cement when the prosthodontist is ready and place some cement in the crown. Pass the plastic filling instrument and place cement on the preparation. Receive the PFI and transfer the crown and the bite stick for the patient to bite down on.

9. After the cement has hardened, it is removed with a scaler, excavator, or an explorer (Figure 24-22). The

patient's mouth is rinsed and evacuated. Dental floss is used to remove excess cement interproximally.

10. The patient is given instructions for brushing and flossing the area and told to call the office if there are any questions or problems. Document the procedure and dismiss the patient.

The dentist improves the retentive capability of the tooth if the tooth being restored will not retain the restoration alone. There are several options for building up the tooth including core build-ups, retention pins, and post-retained cores.

Core Buildups

A core buildup is treatment performed for vital teeth that have very little crown structure. For this procedure, the dentist removes any decay and defective restoration and then builds a core that supports and provides more retention for the cast restoration.

The core buildup or **retention core** is made of amalgam, composite, or a silver alloy/glass ionomer combination (Figure 24-23). These materials come in powder/liquid, syringe, or capsule form and are set chemically or light cured.

Retention Pins

The dentist often places **retention pins** for additional retention of the core buildup. The pins are placed

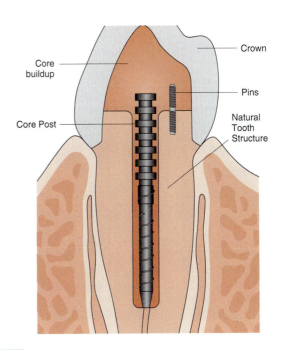

FIGURE 24-23 Tooth with core post, core buildup, and pins.

Core buildup

Core Post

Crown

Pins

Natural Tooth Structure

strategically depending on the amount of buildup needed and the type of restoration. Pins are placed before the core material. The core buildup material surrounds the pins (Figure 24-24).

Pins often come in kits with various sized pins, drills, and a hand driver or mechanical placement device (Figure 24-25). The drills are used in a low-speed handpiece to drill holes for the specific pins. The pins are retained in the drilled holes.

FIGURE 24-24 Pins placed in a prepared tooth for support and retention.

FIGURE 24-25 (A) Retention pins kit. (B) Close-up of pins (maxillary restorative pins). *(Courtesy of Coltène/Whaledent, Inc.)*

Post-Retained Cores

Post-retained cores are often the treatment of choice when the tooth is non-vital and has root canal therapy (Figure 24-26). A portion of the root canal filling is removed and a post is fitted in the canal and cemented in place. The posts are made of materials such as titanium, titanium alloy, gold plated metal, and stainless steel. They come in different sizes and are often purchased in a kit. The kits contain various sized posts, drills, reamers used to prepare the tooth, and wrenches or keys for hand placement.

Once the post is fitted in the root canal, it is cemented in place. Core buildup materials are then placed around the post. The tooth is then ready for preparation of the prosthesis.

IMPLANT RETAINER PROSTHESES

After six months, the dental implants have been in place long enough for the osseointegration process to be substantial. A fixed prosthesis stage can begin. Retainers that cover the implant may be a crown or part of a bridge. The abutments are fabricated in the dental laboratory and are either screw retained or cement retained (Figure 24-27).

The screw-retained prosthesis uses one screw to attach the abutment to the implant and a second screw to attach the abutment to the prosthesis. Sometimes, a

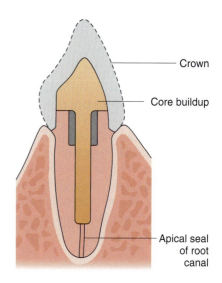

Crown

Core buildup

Apical seal of root canal

FIGURE 24-26 A core post in place in a non-vital tooth.

FIGURE 24-27 (A) Screw-retained implant prosthesis. (B) Cement-retained implant prosthesis.

composite restoration is placed over the screw for esthetic purposes.

The cement-retained prosthesis uses transitional cement to cement the prosthesis to the abutment. Transitional cement is used so that, in case of problems with the implant, the entire system can be retrieved. The abutment is screwed into the implant like the screw-retained prosthesis.

MAINTENANCE OF FIXED PROSTHODONTICS

The patient is given home-care instructions on how to properly maintain the new crown or bridge and is instructed to call the office if the restoration comes loose or falls out.

Fixed Prostheses Maintenance

Maintenance of the fixed prosthesis should become part of the patient's daily regimen. Brushing and flossing are continued. Depending on the patient's individual needs, various aids can assist in cleaning hard-to-reach areas. Toothbrushes should be soft and multi-tufted and have heads small enough to reach all areas in each quadrant. Dental floss works well under bridgework. A bridge threader can be used with the floss to clean under the pontic and along the abutment teeth. Inter-

proximal brushes and tips are designed for removal of plaque around the fixed prosthesis.

Dental Implant Maintenance

Dental implants require maintenance just like fixed prostheses. Plaque builds up on the implant and needs to be removed routinely. The patient should be advised of the aids available, and a home-care regimen should be recommended. The toothbrush selected should be soft with multi-tufted nylon brush. There are numerous aids to choose from to use as adjuncts to the toothbrush, including threading systems, dental floss, interproximal brushes, water irrigators, and antimicrobial rinses.

There are several dental flosses that work well on dental implants or are designed specifically for implants. The floss is a wider band of ribbon to wrap around the implant and is moved in a back-and-forth motion (shoe-shine motion) (Figure 24-28).

Interproximal brushes provide easy access around the implant due to their small heads (Figure 24-29). The brushes must be plastic coated to prevent damaging the titanium surface of the implant. The brushes remove plaque and stimulate the gingival tissues to increase the blood flow in the surrounding areas. The interproximal brush is inserted interdentally and angled toward the occlusal or incisal surface. A gently rotating motion of the brush is suggested for around the implant, near the gingival margin.

FIGURE 24-28 Dental floss used for dental implants.

FIGURE 24-29 Interproximal brush: one piece and handle with disposable brush.

Water irrigators are available to remove debris and plaque from around the dental implant. The patient should be advised, however, to use the irrigators at the lowest pressure setting in order to prevent damage to the tissues. The gentle spray should be directed interproximally and kept at a horizontal level along the gingival margin. The spray should not be directed into the gingival sulcus.

Antimicrobial rinses are recommended for many dental implant patients. There are a number of different rinses available, such as chlorhexidine gluconate and phenolic compounds. The rinses are used once or twice daily depending on the type. The chlorhexidine gluconate rinses are safe and aid in the fibroblast attachment to the implant surface.

CHAPTER SUMMARY

Fixed prosthodontics is the specialty that deals with replacement of missing teeth or parts of teeth with extensive restorations. There are many types of fixed prostheses and a variety of materials used for preparation, fabrication, and cementation. The dental assistant is very involved in all stages of fixed prosthodontic treatment. It is important to understand the sequence of the procedure and the different types of restorations when assisting the dentist.

The goal of this chapter is to assess the more common procedures to give the dental assistant the background and sequence to assist the dentist. The restorations routinely take at least two appointments to complete. The assistant explains the steps of the procedure to the patient, answers questions, and gives postoperative and home care instructions.

CASE STUDY

Ann Arthur is unhappy with the appearance of her anterior teeth. The maxillary and mandibular incisors are a dull, medium-yellow shade. There is a slight diastema (space) between the maxillary central incisors. Ann has considered treatment for several years and has scheduled an appointment for next week. She does not work but has dental insurance through her husband's insurance plan.

Case Study Review

1. What are the two concerns Ann has about her anterior teeth?

2. What treatment options are available?

3. Once a treatment plan is in place, how might financial information, such as insurance, be considered by the business staff?

To complete your study of this chapter, work the review activities that follow. Also, refer to the software that accompanies this text.

REVIEW QUESTIONS

Multiple Choice

1. Which of the follow prosthetic restorations covers only the area between the cusps on the occlusal surface of the tooth?
   a. Three-quarter crown.
   b. Inlay restoration.
   c. Onlay restoration.
   d. Veneer restoration.

2. The part of a dental bridge that replaces the missing tooth is called the
   a. abutment.
   b. pontic.
   c. connector.
   d. retainer.

3. Materials used to fabricate crowns and bridges include all of the following *except*
   a. gold alloy.
   b. porcelain.
   c. composite resin.
   d. amalgam.

4. During the preparation appointment, the retraction cord is
   a. placed after the tooth is prepared but before the final impressions are taken.
   b. placed after the final impressions are taken.
   c. placed before the tooth is prepared.
   d. placed with the temporary restoration.

5. All of the following materials are needed during the preparation appointment *except*
   a. alginate.
   b. gingival retraction cord.
   c. bonding agent.
   d. temporary cement.

Critical Thinking

1. What are the expanded functions in your state that relate to the fixed prosthodontic procedures?

2. Name the types of restorations that are fabricated of gold alloy, porcelain-fused-to-metal, or porcelain.

3. Name possible techniques for building up a crown that is badly broken down.

Removable Prosthodontics

OBJECTIVES

The student should strive to meet the following objectives and demonstrate an understanding of the facts and principles presented in this chapter:

1. Define removable prostheses and list the reasons for using them.

2. Describe the patient considerations related to removable prosthetic treatment.

3. Explain the dental assistant's role in removable prosthetic treatment.

4. Outline the steps of the diagnostic appointment and list the materials needed.

5. Describe the consultation appointment and the materials required for the case presentation.

6. Describe the advantages and disadvantages of the partial denture, the components, and the appointment schedule.

7. Describe the complete denture, the patient considerations, and the appointment schedule.

8. Explain the types and steps of denture reline procedures.

9. Describe the procedure for a denture repair.

10. List the steps to polish a removable prosthetic appliance.

11. Explain the overdenture and the advantages and disadvantages related to it.

KEY TERMS

abutment (p. 527)

anatomical (p. 532)

baseplate (p. 534)

bite rim (p. 534)

border molding (p. 535)

centric occlusion (p. 536)

connectors (p. 528)

denture base (p. 529)

framework (p. 528)

muscle trimming (p. 535)

non-anatomical (p. 532)

overdenture (p. 541)

partial dentures (p. 526)

prostheses (p. 526)

relined (p. 539)

rests (p. 528)

retainer (p. 528)

vertical dimension (p. 534)

INTRODUCTION

Removable prosthodontics, like fixed prosthodontics, refers to the replacement of missing teeth and tissues with artificial structures, or **prostheses**. The difference is that with removable prosthodontics, the prosthesis can be removed from the mouth by the patient for cleaning, examination, and repair. Removable prosthodontics involve two types of prosthesis: **partial dentures** and **complete (full) dentures**.

The partial denture replaces one or more teeth in one arch and is retained and supported by the underlying tissues and remaining teeth.

The complete denture replaces all the teeth in one arch. A full denture is retained and supported by the underlying tissues of the gingiva and oral mucosa, the alveolar ridges, and the hard palate. In some cases, teeth are retained in the arch or implants are placed to support the denture.

The goals of removable prosthodontics are to restore lost functions, stabilize the arch, and improve esthetics. The lost functions include the ability to masticate food properly and to have clear speech. With removable prosthodontics, the patient regains these functions, improves appearance, and, within a short adjustment period, becomes very comfortable and confident with the prosthesis.

Most patients prefer to have fixed prostheses, but in some cases it may not be the treatment of choice due to existing conditions, such as unhealthy bone structure, not having the motivation to maintain good oral hygiene, or financial restrictions. Removable prosthodontics offers an alternative that restores function and esthetics for the patient.

Prosthodontics is a specialty that requires additional training upon completion of dental school. The routine prosthodontic procedures are performed by the general dentist as well as the prosthodontist. The prosthodontist may see patients who need surgery as a result of cancer, patients who have been in accidents involving severe facial/jaw trauma, or patients with anomalies such as cleft lip or cleft palate.

PATIENT CONSIDERATIONS

Good communication between the patient and the prosthodontic staff is required for successful removable prosthodontics. The patient should be in good health, have a positive attitude, and be cooperative. The patient's mental and physical capabilities must be such that he or she can adapt to wearing the prosthesis and be able to maintain good oral hygiene. Impaired health may contribute to a lack of muscle coordination, which is needed to place and remove the partial prosthesis or to retain a denture in place. If the patient is in poor health, it is often reflected in the oral cavity. Also, the added stress of a new appliance may lower the resis-

tance of unhealthy tissue and complications may occur. Fluctuations in the patient's weight may alter the fit of the prosthesis, and it may need to be relined.

Some patients are very conscientious and require patience and understanding during the time of adjustment. There are also pamphlets and videos available to inform patients about their new prostheses (Figure 25-1).

THE DENTAL ASSISTANT'S ROLE

The dental assistant's main functions are to prepare materials, record measurements and details for the fabrication of the denture, give patient education and support, and perform some laboratory procedures. The procedures in removable prosthodontics do not require many instrument exchanges, and the dental assistant does not continually maintain the oral cavity throughout the appointment with the air-water syringe and the HVE. The steps in removable prosthodontics involve as many extraoral as intraoral procedures.

THE DIAGNOSIS AND TREATMENT PLANNING

The first appointment for a removable prosthesis is to examine the patient. A medical history is taken or reviewed to determine the patient's state of health. The dentist may also talk with the patient to determine how the patient feels about his or her existing oral condition and about the prospect of having a partial or full denture. The dentist examines the patient's remaining teeth and tissues.

After a prophylaxis, preliminary impressions for study models and working casts are taken. (Review Chapter 27, Laboratory Materials and Techniques, for more information on taking alginate impressions.) Radiographic films are exposed and processed by the dental

FIGURE 25-1 Patient going to have full dentures placed—and how they will look after the dentures are placed and a natural look is restored.

assistant as part of the diagnostic aids. Photographs are made of the patient, including full face, frontal view, profile view, and a close-up. The patient is then scheduled for a consultation appointment in a few days.

THE CONSULTATION APPOINTMENT

The patient is seated in an area designed for patient consultations. The following aids are ready to help the patient better understand what is involved in treatment:

▶ Study models of the patient's mouth

▶ Radiographs mounted on a viewbox

▶ Patient's photographs

▶ Visual aids to explain the types of removable prostheses (this may include pamphlets, models, pictures, or video programs)

▶ Proposed treatment plan

The dental assistant has all of the items prepared so that the dentist can explain the diagnosis, the proposed treatment plan, and the prognosis to the patient. The dentist answers any questions and concerns expressed by the patient. As with other dental procedures, a cost estimate is prepared and presented to the patient, along with the number of appointments the procedure will require. The treatment plan may involve restorative dentistry, periodontal treatment, endodontic treatment, or surgical procedures. These procedures must be completed and the patient must be completely healed before prosthodontic preparation can begin.

When the patient has accepted the treatment plan, a suitable financial plan is approved and insurance information is gathered. Often, the dental office takes insurance information at the first appointment and then contacts the insurance company for information on the patient's coverage. This information is presented at the consultation appointment. The necessary appointments are then made for treatment.

THE REMOVABLE PARTIAL DENTURE

Partial dentures are designed to restore missing teeth and to preserve the remaining hard and soft tissues of the arches. The partial distributes the forces of mastication between the abutment teeth and the alveolar mucosa. The **abutment** is a natural tooth that becomes part of the support for the partial. The abutment teeth must be in good condition or be restored to withstand the stresses of chewing with a partial denture.

Advantages of a Removable Partial

The following are reasons a partial denture may be part of a patient's treatment plan when he or she has missing teeth.

▶ Partial dentures are repaired and adjusted easily. If teeth are lost in the dental arch, they can be added to the partial denture.

▶ When there are no teeth for a distal attachment, the removable partial denture is one treatment choice to restore function to that quadrant.

▶ Partial dentures require fewer intraoral procedures than fixed protheses. This means fewer appointments and less chair time for the patient.

▶ Maintaining good oral hygiene of the abutments and the appliance is easier for the patient because the prosthesis is removable.

▶ The partial restores the mesial-distal contacts between the teeth and the anterior-posterior continuity of the arch. This provides support that teeth standing alone do not have; therefore, the arch is stabilized.

▶ The partial maintains a proper occlusal plane by preventing supra-eruption of the teeth on the opposing arch.

▶ The removable partial makes it unnecessary to reduce tooth structure. The partial appliance can be fitted to children and adolescents and is replaced easily to compensate for the growth of a child.

▶ When several teeth are missing in both quadrants of an arch, a removable partial denture is designed to restore lost dentition in the long span.

▶ The removable prostheses may be designed to support periodontally involved teeth.

▶ Compared to the fixed prostheses, the partial prostheses is a less expensive treatment.

Considerations for a Partial Denture

Before choosing the partial denture as the treatment, the dentist must consider several factors. There must be a number of sufficiently positioned teeth in the arch in order to support and stabilize a removable prosthesis. To retain the appliance, there must be adequate root structure of the remaining teeth, and the alveolar bone and mucosa must be evaluated to determine whether they can support the partial denture. Another consideration is whether the patient exhibits interest in and is motivated to adjust to the partial denture. The patient must also maintain good oral hygiene, especially around the teeth to which the partial is attached.

Components of a Removable Partial Denture

The components of the removable partial denture are the metal framework, rests, connectors, retainers, denture base, and artificial teeth (Figure 25-2). Partial dentures are designed for individual patients without set patterns.

FIGURE 25-2 Mandibular partial denture. (A) Denture base. (B) Denture teeth. (C) Connectors (lingual bar). (D) Occlusal rest.

The Metal Framework. The metal **framework** is the skeleton of the removable partial (Figure 25-3A) to which the remaining units (such as the rests, connectors, and retainers) are attached. Part of the framework is a mesh or loop area that is designed to retain the acrylic base material. The acrylic portion of the partial denture surrounds the framework.

The Rests. The **rests** are the part of the removable partial denture that contacts a tooth to provide vertical and horizontal support. The rests control the position of the partial in relationship to the supporting structures. To provide the best support, the rests are placed as close as possible to the center of the tooth so that they can direct functional forces to the long axis of the tooth. These rests are positioned on the occlusal, incisal, or cingulum (lingual) surfaces. (Figures 25-3A, B, and C)

The Connectors. The **connectors** unite the various parts of the partial into one unit, hold the working parts in the proper position, and distribute the stresses. They are divided into major and minor connectors. The **major connectors** connect the left and right quadrants of the partial. On the mandibular, the major connector is often a lingual bar or plate. On the maxillary, the major connector is a palatal bar or strap or a complete palatal plate (Figure 25-4). A **stress-breaker**, or **hinge**, may be built into the partial. This is a metal device that relieves pressure on the abutment teeth. The stress-breaker is like a hinge that gives some release to the occlusal stresses during mastication.

The **minor connectors** connect the major connectors with the other units of the partial, such as the clasps and rests. They maintain the integrity of the arch by an anterior-posterior bracing action. The minor connectors protect against food impaction by filling the tooth-tissue junctions.

The Retainer. The **retainer** is sometimes called a clasp. The retainer contacts the abutment teeth and

FIGURE 25-3 Partial denture with: (A) metal framework, (B) Placement of clasp with rest on the tooth. (C) Partial in place.

prevents the partial from moving. The position of the prosthesis is controlled by the retainer and its relationship to the remaining teeth and supporting structures. The retainer designs are usually either circumferential or bar type. The **circumferential-type clasp** (retainer) encircles and adapts to the contours of the abutment

FIGURE 25-4 A major connector for maxillary-palatial strap.

FIGURE 25-5 Circumferential clasp.

tooth (Figure 25-5). The **bar-type clasp** extends from a gingival direction toward the occlusal.

Denture Base. The denture base is most often made of acrylic resin with fibers to give a natural appearance. It rests upon the oral mucosa, providing coverage and stability. This portion of the partial is sometimes referred to as the saddle. The denture teeth are held in the denture base.

Artificial Teeth. The artificial teeth are made of either acrylic resin or porcelain. They come in a variety of shapes (molds), sizes, and shades. The artificial teeth are secured to the denture base by pins or holes on the undersides of the teeth.

Partial Denture

The abutment teeth where the metal framework of the partial rests must be prepared before the final impressions are taken. The occlusal surfaces of the teeth are reduced to allow for clearance of the metal framework of the partial between the arches. This surface must be

contoured so that the partial denture will be held firmly in place. The buccal and lingual surfaces are prepared to allow the partial to be inserted and removed without binding. If the teeth cannot be contoured adequately with burs, discs, and stones, they are prepared for fixed crowns before the partial denture is fabricated.

After the abutment teeth have been prepared, the dentist takes final impressions and a bite registration. These are sent to the dental laboratory with a laboratory prescription form. The dental laboratory follows the dentist's instructions and constructs an appliance that consists of the cast framework and the denture teeth set in the wax bite rim (Figure 25-6). The partial denture is **articulated** on the models to simulate how the appliance will occlude and mesh in various jaw positions. The laboratory then sends the partial to the dental office for the try-in and any adjustments. See Table 25-1 for the appointments for a partial denture.

FIGURE 25-6 Metal framework with wax bite rims ready for placement of denture teeth.

TABLE 25-1 APPOINTMENTS FOR A PARTIAL DENTURE

Appointment	Procedure
Examination	Prophylaxis is completed, preliminary impressions are taken, and radiographs and photographs are taken.
Consultation	Treatment is explained to the patient and treatment choice is decided.
Final impressions	Abutment teeth are prepared, final impressions are taken, bite or occlusal registration is taken, and the shade and mold of artificial teeth are selected. Note: Sometimes restorative, periodontal, endodontic, or surgical procedures must be completed before the final impressions can be completed.
Try-in and adjustment	The framework is placed in the patient's mouth and adjustments are made accordingly.
Delivery	The partial is seated in the patient's mouth and instructions are given regarding how to place and remove the partial and oral hygiene techniques.
Adjustment	As needed, the adjustments are made.

P R O C E D U R E

25-1 Final Impressions for a Partial Denture

This procedure is performed by the dentist. After preparing the materials needed for the final impressions, the dental assistant greets and seats the patient. A protective drape is placed on the patient and the procedure is explained to him or her.

EQUIPMENT

▶ Basic setup: mouth mirror, explorer, and cotton pliers

▶ Mouthwash

▶ Custom tray (refer to Chapter 27, Laboratory Materials and Techniques) or stock tray

▶ Contouring wax for the impression trays

▶ Impression materials—spatula and mixing pad or dispensing gun and tips

▶ Wax or silicone bite registration materials

▶ Tooth shade and mold guides

▶ Laboratory prescription form

▶ Disinfectant and container for impressions and bite registration

PROCEDURE STEPS *(Follow aseptic procedures)*

1. The dentist examines the oral cavity and tries the custom or stock tray in the patient's mouth. Sometimes, wax is placed on the borders of the tray to secure a contoured fit. Once the tray is prepared, an adhesive is painted on the inside of the tray.

2. The final impression material is prepared and placed in the tray according to the manufacturer's directions.

3. Once the final impression is completed, receive the final impressions and either disinfect them right away or set them aside to disinfect after the procedure is completed.

4. The occlusal or bite registration is taken. When completed, it is also disinfected in preparation for the laboratory. Prepare the materials being used for the bite registration. Soften the wax in warm water and then fold it several times before placing it in the patient's mouth. Mix other materials on a paper pad and place them on a quadrant tray. Then, place them in the patient's mouth or dispense them directly into the oral cavity with a dispensing gun and tip. After the bite materials set and they are removed from the mouth, disinfect them and put them with the final impressions.

5. The shade of the artificial teeth is taken with a moistened shade guide under natural light. This can be completed at any point in the appointment sequence. Once the shade is determined, record it on the laboratory prescription and the patient's chart. Assist the dentist in the shade determination and the recording.

6. The dentist completes the laboratory prescription with the details of the partial denture design. Make sure the patient's face is clean of impression materials and debris and then dismiss him or her.

THE COMPLETE DENTURE

The complete denture is also called the full denture. When all the natural teeth are lost, a denture is fabricated to restore function and improve esthetics for the patient. (A person is said to be **edentulous** when he or she has no teeth remaining.) The denture is supported by the alveolar bone and the oral mucosa. The shapes and conditions of the tissues determine how much support the denture will have.

Considerations for the Complete Denture

▶ There is extensive bone loss and lack of support for remaining teeth in the arch.

▶ The patient has exhibited lack of motivation and/or the ability to maintain the remaining teeth.

▶ The remaining teeth have gross decay, periodontal disease, or abscesses.

▶ The patient is edentulous.

▶ The patient lacks the financial means to have alternative treatments, including dental implants and fixed prostheses.

Necessities for Successful Denture Treatment

Dentures are not like natural teeth. They are prosthetic appliances that the patient has to adjust to. For the

PROCEDURE

25-2 Try-In Appointment for a Partial Denture

This procedure is performed by the dentist. The dental assistant prepares the materials and the patient.

EQUIPMENT

▶ Basic setup: mouth mirror, explorer, and cotton pliers

▶ Hand mirror for patient viewing

▶ Articulating paper and forceps

▶ Adjusting instruments, including wax spatula, pliers, and a heat source

▶ Low-speed handpiece with burs, discs, and stones

▶ Contour pliers

▶ Partial denture from the laboratory

PROCEDURE STEPS *(Follow aseptic procedures)*

1. The appliance is placed in the patient's mouth and adjustments are made accordingly. If adjustments are made to the denture base and/or the position of the teeth, prepare the spatula by warming it in the heat source (alcohol torch or Bunsen burner) and transfer it to the dentist. Transfer the articulating paper and evaluate the occlusion. If adjustments are needed, transfer the handpiece and burs.

2. The patient is given a hand mirror for viewing. Dismiss the patient and disinfect the partial to prepare it for the laboratory.

patient to have success with dentures, he or she should have a positive attitude about the procedure and about wearing dentures. Dentures take time and patience to adjust to, and the patient who understands this will be more successful wearing dentures. Educate the patient so that he or she can prepare mentally. There are many pamphlets and videos available to explain to the patient what he or she can expect and how to function when wearing a denture.

The patient should be in good health. When a patient is in poor health, it is often reflected in the oral cavity. The added stress of a denture may lower the resistance of unhealthy tissues. Also, if there is weight loss or gain, the way the denture fits may change and a reline of the denture may be required. Impaired health may contribute to a lack of muscle coordination, which is needed to retain the denture in place.

The patient should have healthy alveolar ridges and oral mucosa. These tissues will be under stress from the denture and, if the denture does not fit properly, degeneration can occur at a much faster rate.

Components of the Complete Denture

 The denture has two basic components: the **base** and the **denture teeth** (Figure 25-7). The external surface of the denture resembles natural tissues and extends over the retro-molar pad on the mandible or the maxillary tuberosity area on the maxilla. The external surface is smooth and polished, while the internal surface matches the contours of the oral mucosa and the alveolar bone. The denture teeth are

articulated to occlude with the natural or artificial teeth of the opposing arch.

Denture Base. The base is made of denture acrylic and may have a metal mesh embedded in the acrylic for additional strength. The acrylic resins are pigmented to shade the base to resemble the normal gingiva; often, fibers are part of the acrylic to give the denture a natural appearance. The base covers the alveolar ridge and gingival tissues. The denture teeth are embedded in the denture base, just like the partial denture.

Denture Teeth. The denture teeth used in construction of the denture are made of porcelain or acrylic resin. The porcelain teeth are more resistant to stain and wear but are more brittle than the resins. They may wear away the opposing natural tooth structure, so

FIGURE 25-7 Full denture: denture base, artificial teeth, tissue side of the denture and occlusal view.

P R O C E D U R E

25-3 The Delivery Appointment for a Partial Denture

This procedure is performed by the dentist with the assistance of the dental assistant. The partial denture will be returned from the laboratory in a sealed container.

EQUIPMENT

▶ Basic setup: mouth mirror, explorer, and cotton pliers

▶ Partial denture

▶ Articulating paper and forceps

▶ Low-speed handpiece and acrylic burs and finishing burs

PROCEDURE STEPS *(Follow aseptic procedures)*

1. The preparations for the patient are completed.

2. The materials and equipment are similar to the try-in appointment with the exception of the wax adjustment instruments.

3. The patient is seated. If the patient has an old appliance, it is removed and placed in a cup with water.

4. The dentist seats the new partial denture (Figure 25-8) and makes any necessary adjustments. Rinse the partial denture and hand it to the dentist for insertion. Articulating paper is used to check the patient's occlusion. If adjustments are needed, transfer the low-speed handpiece with finishing or acrylic burs. Transfer contouring pliers for adjustments to the metal clasps.

5. The dentist instructs the patient on how to insert and remove the partial denture. Explain the care of the partial and the supporting teeth. Also explain that it may take several days to adjust to the partial and sore spots that may appear. If the patient has any problems or questions, instruct him or her to call the office for an appointment right away.

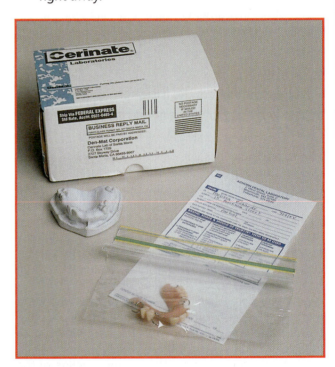

FIGURE 25-8 Complete partial denture returned from the dental laboratory.

they are used more often when the opposing teeth are also porcelain. The porcelain teeth sometimes have a "clicking" sound when the patient is eating or talking.

The acrylic resin (plastic) teeth have the advantage of greater resistance to breakage. They are quieter and bond more efficiently to the denture base. The adjustments require less time, because the acrylic teeth can be polished in the office whereas the porcelain teeth must go back to the laboratory to be refinished. The acrylic resin teeth are used when the patient has natural opposing teeth and in patients with poor ridges.

The porcelain teeth are secured in the denture base by mechanical means of pins on the anterior teeth and diatoric holes on the posterior (Figure 25-9A). The plastic teeth adequately bond to the denture base material and do not require mechanical retention.

Posterior denture teeth are either **anatomical** or **non-anatomical**. The anatomical teeth resemble natural teeth, with cusps and developmental grooves. The non-anatomical teeth do not have detailed anatomy on the occlusal surface but are concave and somewhat flat. The non-anatomic occlusals are designed for additional strength for patients with too little alveolar ridge to retain dentures.

Denture teeth come in sets for the anterior and for the posterior. The anterior set includes six teeth: two cuspids, two laterals, and two central incisors. The posterior set includes eight teeth: four bicuspids and four molars. These sets have matching shades and molds (shapes) (Figure 25-9B).

Immediate Dentures

The sequence of the appointments for the complete denture depends on whether the patient is edentulous or has remaining teeth. When the patient is edentulous, he or she may already have a complete denture. This denture may have to be replaced with a new denture for better fit and retention, or the denture may have broken or been lost.

When the patient has remaining teeth, he or she will need to have the teeth extracted before receiving the denture. In this situation, there are two treatment sequences:

1. The patient can have all remaining teeth extracted and the alveolar bone shaped and contoured (alveoplasty). The patient waits for four to six months for the tissues and the alveolar bone to heal before the denture construction begins. The *advantage* of the sequence is that the tissues have healed and the alveolar ridge has resorbed to a stable position before impressions for the denture are started and the denture is fabricated. The *disadvantage* is that the patient is without teeth for the healing period. Esthetics and diet restrictions are concerns for the patient.

2. In the second treatment sequence, the patient has only the posterior teeth extracted—The anterior teeth remain. The construction of the denture begins as soon as the hard and soft tissues of the posterior areas have healed completely. When the dentures are completed, the anterior teeth are extracted and the denture is inserted. This is called an **immediate denture**. The *advantages* of the immediate denture are that the patient is never without teeth, the dentist and the laboratory have the patient's remaining teeth to reproduce the original appearance, there are no extreme diet restrictions, and the denture acts as a compress and bandage to protect the extraction sites. The *disadvantages* include no anterior try-in to evaluate the fit, the alveolar ridge changes after the extractions and alveoplasty, the denture needs to be relined in four to six months, and, because of the reline and the two appointments with the oral surgeon, this process is more costly to the patient.

The following sequence of appointments takes into consideration when the patient is having the surgery appointments. Most patients elect to have the immediate denture sequence, and those additional appointments are noted in the procedure descriptions. For a brief overview of the appointments for a complete denture, see Table 25-2.

Examination and Diagnosis Appointments for the Complete Denture

The examination appointment for complete dentures is similar to that of the examination for the partial denture.

(A)

(B)

FIGURE 25-9 (A) Porcelain teeth showing pins and diatoric holes. (B) Sets of denture teeth showing shade and mold.

TABLE 25-2 APPOINTMENTS FOR A COMPLETE DENTURE (BRIEF OVERVIEW)

Appointments	Procedure
Examination	An oral exam is completed. Preliminary impressions and radiographs are taken. The patient is asked to bring photos for the next appointment.
Consultation	Treatment is explained to the patient. Discussion of the treatment includes both the dentist's and the patient's responsibilities.
Oral surgery	During the appointment, the posterior teeth are removed and the alveolar bone is contoured.
Final impressions	When the healing of the posterior extractions are complete, the patient returns to the dental office and final impressions are taken.
Jaw relationships	The jaw relationship is determined with baseplates and bite rims.
Denture delivery	The patient is scheduled for surgery to have the anterior teeth extracted and the immediate denture seated.
First follow-up (scheduled several days after the patient receives the denture)	With the immediate denture, the patient is seen the next day in the dental office.
Adjustments	As needed, adjustments are made.

The dentist completes a detailed examination of the condition of the tissues, the shapes and sizes of the ridges, the retromolar and tuberosity areas, the frenum attachments, and the undercut areas. Radiographs and preliminary impressions are taken. Current photographs are made and the patient is asked to bring in other photographs for reference to create a natural appearance for the patient.

Preparation of the diagnosis, treatment plans, and the financial estimate are similar to those of the partial denture prosthesis preparation.

Denture Construction Between Appointments

Between the consultation and the final impressions appointment, the alginate impressions are poured in plaster or stone. On these models, custom acrylic trays are constructed. In the case of an immediate denture, the custom trays are fabricated to allow space for the anterior teeth present in the mouth and the posterior edentulous areas.

Between the final impression appointment and the measurements appointment at the dental laboratory, the master cast is poured in stone from the final impressions. The master cast is used to construct a **baseplate**. A baseplate is a preformed, semi-rigid, acrylic resin material that temporarily represents the denture base.

On the baseplate, several layers of baseplate wax are attached (Figure 25-10). This wax is called the **bite rim**. The bite rims represent the space provided by the teeth

in normal occlusion. It gives the **vertical dimension** for the denture and establishes the position of the mandible to the maxilla. In the natural dentition, the length of the crowns of the teeth determine the distance between the upper and lower jaws. This distance is called the vertical dimension.

If the patient is receiving an immediate denture, the baseplate and bite rims are fabricated to fit over the posterior areas only. The patient's existing anterior teeth are used for jaw relationships and measurements.

FIGURE 25-10 Baseplates and bite rims made in the dental laboratory from the final impressions.

PROCEDURE

25-4 Final Impression Appointment

This procedure is performed by the dentist. Materials are prepared and transferred to the dentist by the dental assistant.

EQUIPMENT (Figure 25-11)

FIGURE 25-11 Tray setup for final impressions for a complete denture with custom trays.

▶ Basic setup: mouth mirror, explorer, cotton pliers

▶ HVE tip, air-water syringe tip

▶ Cotton rolls and gauze

▶ Mouthwash for patient to rinse with prior to impressions being taken

▶ Custom tray (see Chapter 27, Laboratory Materials and Techniques)

▶ Compound wax and Bunsen burner for border molding the rims of the trays

▶ Laboratory knife to trim border molding

▶ Impression materials—spatulas and mixing pads or dispensing gun and tips

▶ Laboratory prescription form

▶ Disinfectant and container for impressions and bite registration

PROCEDURE STEPS (*Follow aseptic procedures*)

1. The final impressions are taken after custom trays have been fabricated from the casts taken at the examination appointment. The custom trays are inserted into the patient's mouth and evaluated for fit.

2. The impression compound is heated and placed along the borders of the custom tray (Figure 25-12). The tray is cooled and then placed in the patient's mouth. With the tray in the patient's mouth, the lips, cheeks, and tongue are moved to establish accurate length for the periphery and adjacent tissues to be included in the final impression. This is called **border molding**, or **muscle trimming**.

3. Final impression materials are prepared and placed in the custom trays. The maxillary impression must include the tuberosities, frenum attachments, and other landmarks of the arch. The mandibular impression must include retromolar pads, oblique ridge, mylohyoid ridge, and frenum attachments.

4. Once the material has set, it is removed from the patient's mouth. The mouth is then rinsed thoroughly.

5. This procedure is repeated with the opposing arch if a full denture is being fabricated for both arches.

6. The impressions are disinfected and sent to the dental laboratory with the prescription form.

7. After the impressions have been taken, the patient is dismissed.

FIGURE 25-12 (A) Custom tray that has been border molded to fit the patient for final impression.

P R O C E D U R E

25-5 Jaw Relationship Appointment

This procedure is performed by the dentist. During this appointment, the measurements, shape, and shade of the denture are determined. The dental assistant prepares equipment and materials and assists the dentist throughout the procedure.

EQUIPMENT (Figure 25-13)

FIGURE 25-13 Tray setup for a jaw relationship appointment.

▶ Basic setup: mouth mirror, explorer, and cotton pliers

▶ HVE tip and air-water syringe tip

▶ Hand mirror

▶ Laboratory knife, #7 wax spatula, Bunsen burner

▶ Shade guide

▶ Millimeter ruler and boley gauge

▶ Baseplates and bite rims

▶ Face bow

▶ Photographs of the patient, showing the shapes and shades of the teeth

▶ Laboratory prescription form

▶ Disinfectant

PROCEDURE STEPS *(Follow aseptic procedures)*

1. The baseplates and bite rims are inserted into the patient's mouth. The dentist determines and marks the midline of the maxillary and mandibular arches.

2. The bite rims represent the teeth and give the vertical dimension. The dentist adjusts the wax bite rims with the laboratory knife and wax spatula until the patient has a natural lip drape and the correct amount of tooth and gingiva is visible when the patient is talking and smiling and the lips are in a resting position. The cuspid lines are determined to position cuspids at the corners of the mouth.

3. The **centric occlusion** is determined when the jaws are closed in a position that produces maximal contact between the occluding surfaces of the maxillary and mandibular arches. The jaw relationships are determined by evaluating how the mandible relates to the maxilla. The patient moves the mandible as far backward (retrusion) and forward (protrusion) as possible, and then as far to the right and then the left (lateral movement). Specially designed baseplates and materials assist in determining these measurements. Once determined, the information is used to articulate the casts to duplicate the normal motions of the patient. The laboratory technician constructs the complete denture in wax and with artificial teeth from these records.

4. After the jaw relationships are determined, the denture teeth are selected and the arrangement of the anterior teeth are discussed with the patient. The proper shade is determined using the shade guide and natural light. The shade guide is compared with the patient's complexion and remaining natural teeth or photographs to achieve a natural look. Usually, the age of the patient indicates the shade range (the teeth stain and become darker with age). The shape (mold) of the teeth is determined by evaluating the remaining natural teeth or from photographs. Sometimes, the shape of the patient's face also is used to guide the selection.

5. Because patients are concerned about the natural appearance of the teeth, some patients want to duplicate the arrangement of the teeth, including spaces, overlapping, and so on. Other patients want to correct the alignment of the natural teeth in the new denture. Spending a little more time at this point and having clear communication with the patient to determine what the expected outcome is often pays off when the patient receives the denture and is pleased with the appearance.

PROCEDURE

25-6 The Try-In Appointment

This procedure is performed by the dentist. The dental assistant prepares the patient, the instruments, and materials and coordinates with the dental laboratory.

EQUIPMENT AND SUPPLIES

The equipment and supplies are the same for the try-in appointment as they are for the jaw relations and measurement appointment.

PROCEDURE STEPS *(Follow aseptic procedures)*

1. The "try-in" denture is disinfected before being placed in the patient's mouth.

2. The patient is seated and the denture is inserted into the patient's mouth. The dentist and/or the dental assistant spends a few minutes talking with the patient. This allows the patient time to adjust to the denture.

3. The denture is evaluated for esthetics, retention, and comfort. The occlusion is checked with articulating paper.

4. The dentist makes adjustments to the position of the teeth. The shade can be changed by the dental laboratory technician in the dental laboratory, if necessary.

5. Once the dentist and the patient are satisfied with the denture, it is disinfected and placed back on the articulator to be returned to the laboratory.

Once the baseplate and bite rims are constructed, they are sent back to the dental office for the patient's next appointment.

Denture Construction Between Appointments—Laboratory Procedures

Between appointments, the laboratory prepares a try-in denture. Denture teeth are mounted in the wax bite rim. They are positioned according to the dentist's directions, but the position can be altered at the try-in appointment (Figure 25-14).

Denture Construction Between Appointments—Final Laboratory Procedures

The denture is returned to the laboratory for final processing. This is a multi-step process that converts the wax try-in denture to a denture with an acrylic resin base and plastic or porcelain teeth. A dental flask is utilized for this process (Figure 25-16). The dental assistant should visit the dental laboratory and observe the steps involved in processing a denture to better understand and visualize the steps involved.

Denture Adjustments Appointments

After receiving the immediate denture, the patient returns to the office the next day. The denture is

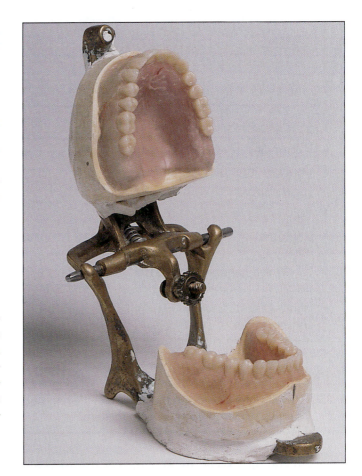

FIGURE 25-14 Wax bite rims with denture teeth on articulator ready for try-in appointment.

P R O C E D U R E

25-7 The Delivery Appointment for the Complete Denture

This procedure is performed by the dentist. The dental assistant prepares the patient and coordinates with the dental laboratory. The dentures come back from the laboratory in a container that keeps them moist.

EQUIPMENT: (Figure 25-15)

FIGURE 25-15 Tray setup for seating completed dentures.

▶ Basic setup: mouth mirror, explorer, and cotton pliers

▶ HVE tip and air-water syringe tip

▶ Dentures from the laboratory

▶ Hand mirror

▶ Articulating forceps and paper

▶ High-speed handpiece and diamond and finishing burs

▶ Low-speed handpiece and assorted acrylic burs and discs

▶ Home-care instructions pamphlet, denture brush and container to place dentures in when they are not in the patient's mouth

PROCEDURE STEPS (*Follow aseptic procedures*)

1. The patient is seated and the appliances are removed and placed in a container to keep them moist.

2. If the patient is receiving an immediate denture, the denture is inserted after the extractions and alveoplasty. If there are more than simple extractions, the patient is scheduled with an oral maxillofacial surgeon. The dental laboratory sends the denture to the surgeon's office instead of to the dentist's office before the patient's surgery.

3. The new denture is inserted into the patient's mouth and the patient is given a few minutes to adjust. Then, the dentist begins the examination.

4. The patient's occlusion is evaluated and, if adjustment is needed, burs and discs are used. The denture is removed from the patient's mouth and the dentist uses a low-speed handpiece and acrylic burs to reduce any high spots on the inside of the base (the part of the denture that is against the tissues) of the denture. Sometimes after the adjustments, the denture needs to be polished in the laboratory. If this process is necessary, the denture must be disinfected before replacing it in the patient's mouth.

5. The dentist evaluates the retention of the denture and the jaw relationships by having the patient demonstrate various facial expressions, swallowing, chewing actions, and speaking.

6. The patient learns to insert and remove the denture and daily maintenance of the denture (see Table 25-3).

7. The patient is given instructions to call the office with any questions or problems and is scheduled for an adjustment appointment in a few days. The patient is dismissed. As a courtesy, often the dentist or dental assistant calls the patient the following day to check on the patient's progress with the new denture.

removed and the tissues are examined. If any areas are uncomfortable to the patient at this time, the dentist performs minor adjustments. Because of the swelling and tenderness from the surgery, the dentist will not remove too much of the denture surface at this time. The patient is taught how to insert and remove the dentures and oral hygiene techniques. He or she is rescheduled in a couple of days for any adjustments.

FIGURE 25-16 Dental flask and investment material used with denture teeth to fabricate the denture base.

The patient returns to the office after wearing the denture for several days. The dentist evaluates the tissues and may smooth rough areas, relieve pressure spots, and adjust the occlusion. The amount of adjustment varies with every patient, and this process may require several appointments over a period of time until the denture is comfortable.

The occlusion is adjusted with the burs, stones, and discs on the cusps of the denture teeth. The pressure spots are relieved on the tissue surface of the denture base. Pressure indicator paste is placed on the internal surface of the denture and then inserted into the patient's mouth. Pressure areas are marked and the dentist then uses acrylic burs and stones for the adjustments.

DENTURE RELINE

The tissue side of the denture bases may need to be **relined** to improve the fit of the denture and the comfort of the patient. After a period of time, the supporting tissues often shrink and change in size because of the pressure put on them by the complete or the partial denture. The denture relining adds a new layer of acrylic to the inside of the denture (Figure 25-17). This procedure can be done in the dental office (chairside) or sent to the dental laboratory.

The chairside (soft) reline saves the patient time and makes it possible for the patient to never be without the denture. This reline process is a temporary solution, because the soft reline is not as durable and will not last as long as the laboratory reline. The laboratory reline takes more time, and the patient may be without the dentures for a day. The laboratory reline replaces the tissue side of the denture.

Tissue Conditioning

Sometimes the tissues are irritated and inflamed due to an ill-fitting denture. These tissues must be healed before a denture reline is completed. This process is called **tissue conditioning**. A temporary soft lining material is placed in the denture to relieve the pressure and allow the tissues to heal. The healing usually takes several weeks and then the denture can be relined.

TABLE 25-3 HOME-CARE INSTRUCTIONS

Keep the denture moist when not wearing it in order to prevent dimensional change.
Do not use abrasive dentifrice on the acrylic because it is easily abraded.
Do not clean acrylic dentures in hot water, because the acrylic can be deformed and distorted when exposed to high temperatures.
Dentures have low thermal conductivity, so the patient will notice a decrease in thermal changes to the tissues under the acrylic denture base.
Rinse thoroughly twice a day and after eating, if possible.
Use a soft denture brush and toothpaste designed for partials and dentures.
Remove the denture and rinse the oral cavity daily.
Denture adhesives are not needed with a well-fitting denture. As the tissues change and the denture does not adapt as well, adhesives will fill in the spaces so retention is increased.
Commercial cleaners are available for overnight soaking. Use warm water with these products.
The patient may want to fill the sink with water or place a washcloth in the sink in case the denture or partial is dropped.

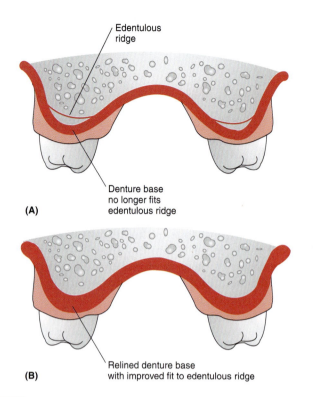

FIGURE 25-17 (A) An ill-fitting denture. (B) Fit with denture reline.

FIGURE 25-18 Dental lathe to polish prosthesis, rag wheel, and tripole.

DENTURE REPAIR

The denture may need repair from time to time. Sometimes a denture tooth becomes loose or is lost or the denture is dropped and fractured. When the patient brings the denture or partial to the office for repair, the dental assistant should disinfect it before the repair process begins. Some of the repairs can be completed in the dental office, but other, more complex repairs must be sent to the dental laboratory. The patient may need to be seen by the dentist if an impression is needed or, in some cases, the dentures can be left at the office for repairs. The repairs often do not take long and the patient returns later in the same day or the next day to pick up the denture. Sometimes the patient is seen by the dentist for minor adjustments.

POLISHING THE REMOVABLE PROSTHESES

After the dentist has adjusted the tissue surface of the removable prosthesis with acrylic burs, discs, and stones, it may need to be polished to smooth the surface. The polishing can be accomplished on a dental lathe with rag wheels, pumice slurry, and various other polishing agents, such as Tripole or a paste of tin oxide and water (Figure 25-18). Care must be taken not to overheat the denture, because the denture base has a relatively low heat-transfer temperature. If the denture

is overheated, it may be distorted, which affects the fit and the appearance of the denture. Also, the plastic teeth should be protected because they will abrade easily. Once the polish is complete, the prosthesis is washed in soap and water, disinfected, and stored in water until it is delivered to the patient. For each patient, separate burs, rag wheels, and pumice should be used to maintain infection control. Burs and rag wheels can be sterilized. The pumice is mixed with a disinfectant and green soap mixture and should be changed daily or after each use, if possible.

THE OVERDENTURE

Over time, the pressure applied during mastication on the mucosa and the supporting underlying alveolar bone causes the bone to shrink/absorb. The denture is not as stable, and retention becomes a problem for the

FIGURE 25-19 Overdenture supported with abutments (roots are restored with a cast-gold post and dome-shaped core combination). *(Courtesy of Clifton O. Caldwell, Jr., DDS, FICD, FACD)*

PROCEDURE

25-8 Denture Relining

This procedure is performed by the dentist. The dental assistant prepares the patient and the materials. The reline materials are available in either hard or semi-soft materials. There is a variety to choose from, depending on the dentist's preference.

EQUIPMENT

▶ Basic setup: mouth mirror, explorer, and cotton pliers
▶ Low-speed handpiece with acrylic burs
▶ Chairside reline materials
▶ Mouth rinse

Chairside Relining

PROCEDURE STEPS *(Follow aseptic procedures)*

1. Clean the denture by placing it in an ultrasonic unit for a few minutes.

2. The dentist uses acrylic burs to roughen the tissue side of the denture.

3. The material is mixed according to manufacturer's directions and then placed in the clean denture, covering the entire tissue surface. The materials have low thermal reaction and cure directly in the patient's mouth.

4. The patient rinses with mouthwash to clean saliva and debris from the tissues.

5. The denture is inserted into the patient's mouth and the patient is asked to bite until the material reaches the initial set stage. Explain to the patient that sometimes the tissue will have a slight burning sensation from the acrylic material during the setting time.

6. The denture is removed to complete the setting process.

7. Excess material is trimmed away and the denture is polished. Follow routine disinfecting before the denture is inserted into the patient's mouth.

Laboratory Relining

The patient's denture is prepared in the same manner as it is for the chairside relining procedure. The following are the impression and laboratory steps. The tray setup is the same as that in the chairside relining, except for the type of materials used. Often, the denture or partial is used as the tray for the impression materials. A variety of impression materials, including polysulfides, polyethers, and silicone, are used to take the impression.

PROCEDURE STEPS *(Follow aseptic procedures)*

1. The impression material is mixed and placed in the denture (tray) according to the manufacturer's directions. The material should cover the entire tissue surface of the denture evenly and without excess.

2. The denture is inserted into the patient's mouth and positioned firmly. The patient should occlude and hold until the material is set.

3. After the material sets, the denture is removed from the patient's mouth, disinfected, and prepared to be sent to the dental laboratory. The laboratory prescription is completed and the patient is dismissed.

4. The dental laboratory processes the impression materials into an acrylic resin base that is fused to the denture.

5. The patient returns to the dental office as soon as the laboratory can process the denture. The turnaround time varies from hours to several days. The procedure is scheduled with the laboratory to minimize the time the patient is without the denture.

6. When the patient returns to the office, the denture is seated and adjustments are made as needed.

patient. An **overdenture** can be fabricated to prevent or reduce this problem. The patient with overdentures has shown less alveolar bone loss.

To fabricate an overdenture, the dentist saves certain parts of the patient's remaining teeth or places dental implants in the dental arch on which the denture will attach. Instead of the denture base resting on the

mucosa and the alveolar bone, the denture is supported by the retained prepared teeth or the dental implants (Figure 25-19).

The retained teeth are endodontically treated and prepared with posts and cores or with special prefabricated attachments. The tissue side of the denture is constructed with part of the attachment aligned with the implant or retained tooth. There are various types of attachments, including magnets and a "snap" design.

The *advantages* include retention and stability of the denture, especially if the patient does not have much alveolar ridge to retain a denture to begin with. The *disadvantages* include an increase in the cost and time involved because of the surgeries, endodontic treatment, and restorative procedures. Also, the patient must maintain the retained teeth and/or the dental implants. Plaque control is essential to prevent bone loss around the implants and the retained teeth and to inhibit root caries on the retained teeth. The patient must be diligent and motivated for the success of the overdenture.

CHAPTER SUMMARY

Removable prosthodontics, like fixed prosthodontics, refers to the replacement of missing teeth and tissues with artifical structures, or prostheses. With removable prosthodontics, however, the prosthesis can be removed from the mouth of the patient. Most patients prefer to have fixed prostheses, but in some cases it may not be the treatment of choice due to existing conditions.

The dental assistant's main functions are to prepare materials, record measurements and details for the fabrication of the denture, provide patient education and support, and perform some laboratory procedures. The procedures in removable prosthodontics do not require many instrument exchanges, and the assistant does not continually maintain the oral cavity throughout the appointment with the air-water syringe and the HVE. The steps in removable prosthodontics involve as many extraoral as intraoral procedures. The dental assistant has all of the items prepared so that the dentist can explain the diagnosis, the proposed treatment plan, and the prognosis to the patient.

CASE STUDY

Julie Davidson has been told by Dr. Jacobson that she needs a maxillary full denture. Mrs. Davidson has had problems with her teeth over the years because of advanced periodontal disease. She is an office manager for a group of physicians. Julie is very conscientious about her appearance and apprehensive about wearing dentures.

Case Study Review

1. What denture procedure would allow Julie to continue to function with her natural teeth while her maxillary denture is fabricated?

2. What types of patient information are available?

3. To prepare the patient for the denture procedure, what should the dental assistant be considering?

 To complete your study of this chapter, work the review activities that follow. Also, refer to the software that accompanies this text.

REVIEW QUESTIONS

Multiple Choice

1. Removable prosthodontics includes all of the following procedures *except*
   a. partial denture.
   b. full denture.
   c. crown and bridge.
   d. immediate denture.

2. Parts of the partial denture that contact the teeth to provide vertical and horizontal support are
   a. connectors.
   b. rests.
   c. retainers.
   d. denture bases.

3. Denture teeth are made of
   a. porcelain.
   b. plastic.
   c. both porcelain and plastic.

4. When the jaws are closed to produce the maximum contact, what can be determined?
   a. Vertical dimension.
   b. Centric occlusion.
   c. Vertical occlusion.
   d. Horizontal dimension.

5. All of the following are correct home-care instructions for a patient just receiving a full denture *except*
   a. rinse the denture twice a day and after eating, if possible.
   b. use a soft denture brush and toothpaste designated for dentures.
   c. place water or a washcloth in the sink in case the denture is dropped while cleaning it.
   d. use hot water when cleaning the denture in order to remove bacteria.

Critical Thinking

1. What types of materials can be used to take the final impression for a partial denture?

2. During which complete denture appointment must the baseplates and bite rims be ready for use?

3. When would a patient be a good candidate for an overdenture? What is an overdenture?

Restorative and Laboratory Materials and Techniques

Chairside Restorative Materials

OBJECTIVES

The student should strive to meet the following objectives and demonstrate an understanding of the facts and principles presented in this chapter:

1. Explain the types of dental restorative materials.

2. List dental standards and organizations responsible for those standards.

3. Explain the role of the dental assistant.

4. List and explain the properties of dental materials.

5. List the types of materials used to restore cavity preparations.

6. Identify the types of dental cements. Explain their properties, composition, uses, and manipulation.

7. Describe bonding agents and their manipulation.

8. Identify the types of direct restorative materials and where they are used.

9. Describe the steps of cavity preparation.

10. Identify cavity preparation terminology.

11. Explain the properties, composition, and manipulation of dental amalgam.

12. Identify the armamentarium and steps of an amalgam procedure.

13. Explain the composition of composite resins.

14. Explain the properties and manipulation of various composite restorations.

15. Identify the armamentarium and steps of a composite restoration.

16. Explain the use of glass ionomer/resin restorative materials.

KEY TERMS

acid etchant (p. 561)

adhesives (p. 563)

alloy (p. 567)

amalgam (p. 567)

base (p. 551)

bonding agents (p. 563)

calcium hydroxide (p. 552)

cavosurface margin (p. 565)

composite (p. 574)

compules (p. 574)

corrosion (p. 549)

dimensional change (p. 549)

dual-cured materials (pp. 561–562)

ductility (p. 549)

exothermic (p. 552)

flow (p. 550)

galvanism (p. 550)

glass ionomer (p. 552)

light cured (p. 551)

liner (p. 551)

luting (p. 551)

malleability (p. 549)

mechanical retention (p. 550)

microleakage (p. 550)

primer (p. 576)

(continued)

INTRODUCTION

In dentistry, there is a wide variety of material used. Although some materials have been around for a long time, there are constant changes and new products always being introduced. The dental team is updated by attending seminars and dental conferences and through local sales representatives.

Generally, the materials are divided and categorized according to their functions. Some materials have a broad spectrum of uses. After the tooth has been prepared and the decay removed, certain materials are utilized to restore the tooth. Dental materials are regulated and tested for function and safety before they become available for use. The American Dental Association and the Food and Drug Administration regulate dental materials. The ADA Council on Dental Materials, Instruments, and Equipment is responsible for the information and testing of dental materials and periodically publishes a listing of certified dental materials in the *Journal of the American Dental Association* and in the *Clinical Products in Dentistry: A Desktop Reference.*

The ADA, in cooperation with the government, sponsored research on more than fifty types of dental materials. From this research, specifications and standards were established. These standards are updated continually and used to evaluate new materials. If a material meets the specification requirements, the **ADA Seal of Certification** is awarded. This certifies that the material has reached the criteria established by the ADA and the U.S. government and is safe and effective.

For new types of dental materials, the ADA Council conducts the Acceptance Program for evaluation. **The Seal of Acceptance of the ADA** indicates that the material has proven to be safe and effective through biological, laboratory, and clinical evaluation, but there are no physical standards or specifications by which the material can be measured for certification.

There are also federal and international organizations that develop standards for materials, instruments, and equipment produced around the world. These are the Fédération Dentaire Internationale and the International Standards Organization (ISO).

The Role of the Dental Assistant

The dental assistant's role when working with dental restorative materials depends on the expanded functions of the individual state practice acts that regulate the practice of dentistry. The general chairside dental assistant prepares and mixes the material while the dentist places the material in the oral cavity. Some states allow the dental assistant to perform these responsibilities in addition to placing the material in the oral cavity.

Knowledge of the properties of the dental material is necessary in order for the dental assistant to properly prepare and manipulate the materials. The dental assistant's knowledge of dental materials also is beneficial for patient education and protection. Expanded-function dental assistants must understand and be competent in the placement and finishing of the materials.

PROPERTIES OF DENTAL MATERIALS

Replacing natural tooth structure has presented a number of challenges. The oral cavity environment and functions create complex situations. Properties that are considered for dental materials include:

Acidity

Acidity is viewed in two ways:

1. Consider the natural acidity of the oral cavity. The acidity (pH) of the mouth varies greatly. The normal pH of the oral cavity is around neutral (pH 7.0). Some foods are acidic, such as citrus fruits, and some bacteria found in the plaque are also acidic. The saliva aids in reducing the acidity of the mouth, but dental materials are subject to varying amounts of acid. How the materials react to the changing acidity levels determines their use in the oral cavity.

2. The second consideration is that the acidity of the materials may cause irritation to the gingival tissues or damage to the pulp. These materials can be used successfully in the mouth, but care is taken to prepare them carefully and/or place them following manufacturer's directions.

Adhesion

Adhesion is the force or attraction that holds unlike substances together. Adhesion involves physical or chemical forces. Chemical adhesion is quite strong and more desirable, but the physical adhesion is more common. Adhesion is a way to attach solid structures together. An example of physical adhesion is the dental plaque adhering to the tooth. Chemical adhesion is found with certain dental cements.

Biting Forces

Biting Force

The average biting force for a person with natural dentition varies from 130 to 170 pounds on the molars and progresses downward to about 40 pounds on the incisors. When force is applied on an individual tooth, this represents about 25,000 pounds per square inch (psi) on a single cusp or a molar.

Dental materials are subject to various types of biting forces. Natural dentition can withstand much more force than prostheses such as dentures and bridges. **Force** is defined as any push or pull on an object. The result of force on an object is resistance. The reaction of the object to resist the external force is called **stress**. Forces can cause stress over a large area, such as a quadrant, or over a small area, such as the occlusal surface of a tooth. Enough stress can be placed on an object to cause a change. This change or deformation is known as **strain**.

There are three types of stress and strain (Figure 26-1):

1. *Tensile*—Pulls and stretches a material. Under tensile stress and strain, the structure tends to be elongated. An example of tensile stress and strain are wires that are pulled in opposite directions or elastic bands (rubber) used in orthodontics. The ability of a material to withstand forces of tensile stress without failing is known as **ductility**.

2. *Compressive*—Pushes or compresses the material together. An example of compressive stress and strain is chewing or biting. The ability of a material to withstand compressive stresses without fracturing is known as **malleability**.

3. *Shearing*—Slides one part of a material parallel to another part in a back-and-forth motion. An example of shearing stress and strain is **bruxism**, or grinding of the teeth.

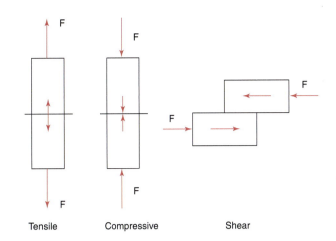

FIGURE 26-1 Tensile, compressive, and shearing stress and strain.

Corrosion

Corrosion is the result of chemical or electrochemical attacks of the oral environment on pure metal, such as gold, or an alloy, such as amalgam. Components of food and/or saliva react with the metals and cause deep pitting and roughness. Sometimes the metals become dull and discolored. This effect is referred to as **tarnish** (Figure 26-2).

Dimensional change

Dimensional change in a material can occur from a variety of causes, such as the setting process of a material or exposure to heat or cold. The change in a material usually is measured in a percentage of the original length or volume. If an impression material goes through dimensional change, the permanent restoration may not fit on the tooth because the impression material does not represent the exact dimensions of the prepared tooth.

FIGURE 26-2 Amalgam restoration showing corrosion and tarnish. *(Courtesy of Dr. Gary Shellerud)*

Elasticity

Some materials have the property of **elasticity**, which is the ability to be distorted or deformed by an applied force and then return to its original shape once the force is removed. Rubber bands exhibit this property, but if they are stretched for too long or too far, they reach their *elastic limit* and will not return to their original shape.

The *elastic modulus,* or modulus of elasticity, is a measure of the stiffness of a material below the elastic limit. This is a measure of how a material can resist deformation or change.

Flow

Flow, or creep and slump, is a continuing deformation of a solid. Under a constant force, certain materials change and deform. Examples of materials where flow is a factor are dental waxes and certain impression materials. Amalgam is subject to flow under constant compressive forces.

Galvanism

When two different metals are present in the mouth there is potential for the creation of small electrical shocks. This is known as **galvanism**. The oral fluids act as a carrier between the two metals to cause an electrical shock. This can occur when a gold restoration in one arch contacts an amalgam restoration in the opposing tooth in the opposite arch. The same shock happens if an individual bites a piece of tin foil and it contacts a tooth with a restoration.

Hardness

The resistance of a material to scratch or indent is known as the material's hardness. There are various ways to measure the hardness of a material. Dental materials that can be dented or scratched will show wear.

Microleakage

When saliva and debris from the oral cavity seep between the tooth structure and the restorative materials this is known as **microleakage**. The dentist prepares the cavity and places materials to prevent microleakage, but some microleakage still occurs. Recurrent decay and tooth sensitivity are some of the problems resulting from microleakage (Figure 26-3).

Retention

Retention in dentistry is one means by which materials and surfaces are attached to one another. Different types of retention methods are used with the various types of restorative materials. The materials that are placed directly into the cavity preparation (direct

FIGURE 26-3 Microleakage around the margins of an amalgam restoration.

restorative materials) such as amalgam and composites are retained in place by mechanical means. **Mechanical retention** includes preparing the walls of the cavity preparation to be convergent (slanted in), by roughening the tooth surface with etchant, or by placing retentive grooves in the cavity walls.

Retention for indirect restorations such as gold inlays or crowns is accomplished with bonding agents and cements. Cements and bonding agents may be retained to the tooth surface by mechanical or chemical means. **Chemical retention** involves a chemical reaction between the tooth surface and the material.

Solubility

When a material is **soluble**, it dissolves in fluid. The solubility of a dental material is one factor used to determine the success of the material in the oral cavity. A material that is soluble may be useful as a base or liner where it is not exposed to the oral fluids. If the material is exposed to the saliva, it dissolves and exposes the tooth structure.

Thermal Properties

One **thermal property** that is important to consider is **thermal conductivity**. This is the ability of material to transmit heat. With some materials heat transmits rapidly, while with others the process is very slow. Thermal conductivity of a material is a consideration when it is placed near the dental pulp because a material that has a low rate of thermal conductivity offers more protection. Materials are placed in layers over the pulp to protect it from thermal changes. For example, the patient with a denture can drink hotter coffee because the denture base material has low thermal conductivity; thus, it protects the tissues under the denture.

Thermal expansion is another consideration of dental materials. With temperature changes materials expand and contract. When materials are used in the oral cavity, they must expand and contract at a rate close to that of the tooth structure. Dimensional changes that occur from thermal expansion and contraction can lead to microleakage and sensitivity of the tooth.

Viscosity

Viscosity of a material is the ability of liquid to flow. The thicker the material, the less it flows; therefore, it is said to be more viscous than a thin material that flows easily. Honey that is cool is thick and viscous, but when heated, it becomes less viscous. Materials that are more viscous do not spread easily over a surface. For example, if a cement is viscous, it will not flow over the tooth surface to produce adequate retention.

Wettability

The ability of a material to flow over a surface is **wettability**. This is an important property when applying certain dental materials. Wettability can be demonstrated by observing the shape of a drop on a solid material (Figure 26-4). If the drop spreads out (forming a low contact angle), the solid is readily wetted by the liquid. If the drop beads (forming a high contact angle), there is poor wetting of the solid. An example of this is with pit and fissure sealants—They should have good wettability to cover the grooves of the occlusal surface (Figure 26-4).

TYPES OF RESTORATIVE DENTAL MATERIALS

Dental materials used to restore the teeth can be divided into two sections:

1. Liners, bases, cements and bonding agents—Materials to prepare the teeth for the actual restorative materials

2. Amalgam and composite restorative materials

These materials are mixed at chairside by the dental assistant as indicated by the dentist, following manufacturer's instructions and the dentist's preferences. It is the dental assistant's responsibility to maintain the materials and the mixing equipment.

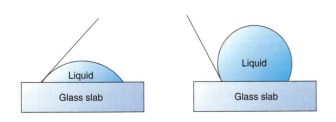

FIGURE 26-4 Example of "wettability" of a material.

DENTAL CEMENTS

Dental cements usually come in a powder/liquid form, a two-paste system, a capsule, or a dispensing syringe. Most of these materials are mixed manually, but a few of the powder/liquid cements come in capsules that are mixed mechanically. Cements are mixed in a precise ratio to attain a specific consistency, ranging from a liquid solution to a putty consistency.

Dental cements set or cure by either **self-curing** (chemical reaction between two materials) or by means of a curing light (**light cured**). The light-cured materials are becoming very popular because the operator has more time to place and manipulate the materials before curing them. These materials are sensitive to overhead lights, however, and must be protected from light if dispensed ahead of time.

There are several terms used in conjunction with dental materials. Knowing these terms assists in understanding the uses and functions.

▶ **Luting**—Bonding or cementing together. Dental cements may be used as luting agents to bond inlays, bridges, and so on to teeth.

▶ **Permanent luting cement**—A long-term cementing agent.

▶ **Temporary luting cement**—A short-term cementing agent.

▶ **Intermediate luting cement**—A material that lasts six months to a year.

▶ **Liner**—A material that is placed in a thin layer on the walls and floor of the cavity preparation. The liner protects the pulp from bacteria and irritants.

▶ **Base**—Applied in a putty or thick layer between the tooth and the restoration to protect the pulp from chemical irritation, temperature changes, electrical protection, and mechanical injury. Bases are strong enough to be placed under restorative materials and to support the materials from occlusal stresses.

▶ **Sedative** or **palliative effect**—Soothing effect a material may have on a tooth. The sedative or palliative material may relieve pain but does not provide a cure for the problem.

▶ **Varnish**—A thin layer of material that is placed to seal the walls and floor of the cavity preparation.

Uses of Dental Cements

There are many types of dental cements, and each type of cement can have several uses (see Table 26-1 for the types of the cements and their uses). Some cements are combined with other materials to modify or expand their functions. Examples are the reinforced zinc oxide eugenol cements and the glass ionomers.

TABLE 26-1 DENTAL CEMENTS AND FUNCTIONS

Types of Cements	Uses or Functions
Zinc phosphate	Permanent cementation of crowns, inlays, onlays, bridges, and orthodontic bands and brackets. An insulating base.
Zinc oxide eugenol	Temporary cementation of crowns, inlays, onlays, and bridges. A temporary restoration and a low-strength base (palliative base). Also a periodontal dressing after periodontal surgery. Root canal sealer.
Reinforced zinc oxide eugenol	Permanent cementation of crowns, bridges, inlays, and onlays. An insulating base and temporary restoration.
Polycarboxylate	Permanent cementation of crowns, bridges, inlays, onlays, and orthodontic bands and brackets. A high-strength base and a temporary restoration.
Glass ionomer	Permanent cementation of crowns, bridges, inlays, onlays, and orthodontic bands and brackets. A high-strength base and a low-strength liner. A permanent bonding liner for composites. Also a root canal sealer, restorative material, and core buildup material.
Calcium hydroxide	A low-strength liner.
Varnish	A thin liner.
Resin cement	Permanent cementation of cast crowns, bridges, inlays, onlays, and endodontic posts. Cementation of ceramic or composite inlays and onlays, cementation of resin-bonded bridges, and cementation of orthodontic bands.

Zinc Phosphate Cement

Zinc phosphate cement is one of the oldest cements, and while it does have some disadvantages, it is still a reliable choice for a luting and base cement. It comes in a powder/liquid form, and there are several different brands available.

Composition. The zinc phosphate powder is primarily zinc oxide with a small amount of magnesium oxide and pigments. The powder is available in shades of white, yellow, and gray. The liquid is a solution of phosphoric acid in water buffered by agents to slow down the setting reaction. Because the liquid is acidic and irritating to the pulp, the tooth must be protected with bases or liners before the cement is placed.

When the powder and liquid are mixed together, a chemical reaction occurs and heat is released. The reaction is called **exothermic**. As heat is produced, the reaction speeds up even more. There are specific guidelines to follow when mixing zinc phosphate cement in order to minimize the temperature rise and slow the reaction process. This provides reasonable working time and allows for maximum incorporation of powder.

Properties. When mixed, the zinc phosphate cement is high in strength and reaches two-thirds of this strength in less than an hour. Zinc phosphate sets (hardens) in five to nine minutes and has a long mixing time of up to two minutes. The viscosity is affected by the mixing time and the temperature. Zinc phosphate bonds to the tooth by means of mechanical interlocking.

Manipulation Considerations. When the zinc phosphate powder is mixed with the liquid, there is an exothermic reaction. The zinc phosphate cement is mixed on a cool glass slab to dissipate (spread) the heat of the mix. The slab is cooled in cold water and then dried completely. Any moisture left on the slab affects the properties of the cement. The glass slab should be clean and free of scratches and dried cement. A stainless steel cement spatula is used to mix the powder into the liquid. The spatula also should be cool.

The bottle of powder is gently shaken, and the powder and liquid should be the same brand and type of cement. The powder and liquid may come in dispensing bottles, or they may need a scoop for the powder and a dropper for the liquid. The powder is placed on one side of the slab and then proportioned for mixing. Then the liquid is dispensed on the slab (Figure 26-5). The powder usually is divided into differently sized sections for easier mixing. Follow manufacturer's instructions.

As mentioned, one objective in mixing the cement is to dissipate the heat from the exothermic reaction. If the heat is dissipated, the setting reaction is slowed and more powder can be incorporated to make the cement stronger. To accomplish this, several mixing techniques are used:

▶ The glass slab is cooled.

▶ The first increment of powder is mixed into the liquid for ten to fifteen seconds before more powder is brought into the mix.

▶ Spatulate the mix slowly when incorporating the powder into the liquid.

▶ Mix slowly over a large area of the slab, wiping both sides of the spatula.

Of all the cements, mixing zinc phosphate is most critical and each procedural step must be followed. When zinc phosphate cement is mixed to a luting consistency, the cement is creamy and follows the spatula about one inch above the mixing slab. When zinc phosphate cement is mixed to a base consistency, the cement is like thick putty.

FIGURE 26-5 Zinc phosphate powder dispensed and divided into portions and liquid being dispensed.

PROCEDURE

26-1 Mixing Zinc Phosphate Cement

This procedure is completed by the dental assistant for the dentist. The equipment and materials are prepared and the material is mixed and passed to the dentist. Sometimes the dental assistant places the cement in the cast restoration while the dentist places material on the prepared tooth.

EQUIPMENT AND SUPPLIES

▶ Zinc phosphate powder and liquid (dispensers, if needed)

▶ Cooled glass slab

▶ Flexible stainless steel cement spatula

▶ 2 × 2 gauze sponge

▶ Timer

▶ Plastic filling instrument

PROCEDURE STEPS (Follow aseptic procedures)

1. Shake the powder before removing the cap.

2. Place an appropriate amount of powder on one end of the slab. The amount of powder to be used is determined by the powder-liquid ratio and the amount of cement required for the pro-

cedure. For example, it would take less cement to cement a crown than a bridge.

3. Level the powder with the flat side of the spatula blade into a layer about 1 mm thick.

4. Divide the powder according to the manufacturer's instructions. One suggestion is to divide the powder into two equal portions with the edge of the spatula; divide each of these portions into quarters, then two sections into eighths and one of the eighths into sixteenths.

5. Gently shake the liquid. Dispense the liquid from a dropper bottle onto the opposite side of the glass slab. Hold the liquid vertical while dispensing to produce uniform drops. Recap to avoid spilling and evaporating the liquid.

6. Incorporate one small portion of powder into the liquid, following specific manufacturer's directions on mixing times. Use the flat side of the spatula blade to wet the powder particles (for about fifteen seconds).

7. Hold the spatula blade flat against the glass slab. Using a *wide sweeping motion,* spatulate the powder and liquid over a *large area of the glass slab* (Figure 26-6).

(continued)

FIGURE 26-6 Mixing zinc phosphate powder and liquid. As powder is incorporated, larger area of glass slab is used.

(A)

(B)

FIGURE 26-7 (A) Demonstration of luting consistency. Spatula lifts cement one inch from glass slab. (B) Base consistency—thick putty. NOTE: Most of the glass slab was used and there is excess powder to facilitate the base to be picked up and manipulated.

8. Adding small amounts of powder will help neutralize the acid, control the setting time, and achieve a smooth consistency of the mix. Incorporate each increment of powder thoroughly into the mix before adding more powder.

9. The mix will appear watery at first and then, as more powder is incorporated, the mix will become creamy. Gather all particles of powder and liquid from around the edges of the mix from time to time.

10. Turn the spatula blade on edge and gather the mass to check the consistency.

11. Continue to add additional increments to the mix until the desired consistency is reached and within the prescribed time.

12. Gather the entire mass into one unit on the glass slab.

13. The consistency for luting (cementing) will be creamy. It will follow the spatula for about one inch as it is lifted off the glass slab before breaking into a thin thread and flowing back into the mass (Figure 26-7A).

14. The consistency of the base should be putty-like, and the base should be able to be rolled into a ball or cylinder with the flat side of the spatula (Figure 26-7B).

15. Once the cement has been mixed to the desired consistency, wipe off the spatula with a 2 × 2 gauze. Hold the glass slab under the patient's chin, and pass the plastic filling instrument.

16. Wipe the spatula and the glass slab off with a moistened 2 × 2 gauze.

17. To clean the glass slab and spatula, soak them in water or a solution of bicarbonate of soda to loosen the hardened cement and then sterilize/disinfect accordingly.

Zinc Oxide Eugenol Cement

Zinc oxide eugenol cement, often referred to as ZOE, is another cement that has been used for many years. It is noted for its sedative or soothing effect on the dental pulp (refer to Table 26-1 for the variety of uses zinc oxide eugenol has). The functions of this cement are diverse because of additives that enhance the properties. There are two types: **type I** is not as strong and is used for temporary restorations and cementation; **type** II has been reinforced and is stronger and can be used for permanent cementation.

One of the type II zinc oxide eugenol cements is different from the rest in function. It is called an **Intermediate Restorative Material (IRM)**. This material is placed in the patient's mouth and lasts up to one year. This material comes in a powder/liquid form and in capsules (Figure 26-9). It is used when a tooth cannot be restored immediately, during illness, when the patient is moving, and because of economic reasons.

PROCEDURE

26-2 Mixing Zinc Oxide Eugenol Cement— Powder/Liquid Form

This procedure is completed by the dental assistant when the dentist signals. The equipment and materials are prepared and the material is mixed and passed to the dentist. The dental assistant follows the manufacturer's directions for specific information on proportions, incorporation technique, and the mixing and setting times.

EQUIPMENT AND SUPPLIES

▶ Zinc oxide eugenol cement

▶ Dispensers that go with the specific material

▶ Paper pad or glass slab

▶ Cement spatula

▶ Timer

▶ Plastic filling instrument

▶ 2 × 2 gauze sponges

▶ Alcohol or orange solvent

PROCEDURE STEPS *(Follow aseptic procedures)*

1. Fluff the powder before removing the cap.

2. Place the powder on the mixing pad according to manufacturer's directions. Replace the cap to avoid spilling and contamination.

3. After swirling, place the liquid on the paper pad. Hold the dispensing dropper perpendicular to the mixing pad and dispense the drops. Dispense near the powder but not touching it.

4. Incorporate the powder into the liquid in divided increments or all at once, according to manufacturer's directions.

5. Spatulate with the flat part of the blade and with an even pressure to wet all the particles of the powder. With some cements, a firm pressure is required to accomplish this.

6. Gather up the powder and liquid from the edges of the mix.

7. Gather up the entire mass into one unit on the slab to test the consistency.

8. The consistency for temporary luting will be creamy, like frosting (Figure 26-8).

9. The consistency for an insulating base or IRM will be putty-like and can be rolled into a ball or cylinder.

10. Once the material has been mixed to the desired consistency, wipe the spatula with a 2 × 2 gauze. Hold the pad under the patient's chin and pass the plastic filling instrument.

11. Receive the plastic filling instrument and wipe it off. The top page of the paper pad is removed and folded to prevent accidental contact with the cement.

12. To clean material that has hardened on the spatula or glass slab, wipe it with alcohol or orange solvent.

FIGURE 26-8 ZOE temporary luting cement's consistency.

Composition. Zinc oxide eugenol comes in several forms, including power/liquid, two-paste systems, capsules, and syringes or capsules. The powder for the conventional (type I) zinc oxide eugenol cement is zinc oxide, resin, zinc acetate, and an accelerator. The liquid, eugenol, is sometimes mixed with other oils, such as clove oil. The reinforced (type II) zinc oxide eugenol cement includes the addition of alumina and polymers (resins) to the powder, and ethoxybenzoic acid is added to the eugenol. There are non-eugenol zinc oxide

P R O C E D U R E

26-3 Mixing Zinc Oxide Eugenol Cement— Two-Paste System

This material is often used for temporary luting of provisional coverage. The dental assistant dispenses and mixes the material according to manufacturer's directions. The dental assistant assists the dentist during the placement of the temporary. Sometimes the dental assistant places the cement in the provisional coverage of the tooth, if this procedure is included in expanded function regulations.

EQUIPMENT AND SUPPLIES

▶ Two-paste zinc oxide eugenol (accelerator and base)

▶ Paper pad

▶ Cement spatula

▶ 2 × 2 gauze sponge (moistened)

▶ Plastic filling instrument

PROCEDURE STEPS (*Follow aseptic procedures*)

1. Dispense the amount of material required for the procedure. This is equal lengths of the accelerator and the base. They usually are placed parallel to each other on the paper pad.

2. Gather the materials and mix into a homogenous mass. Spread over a small area, then gather. Repeat the process. The material should be a creamy mix that follows the spatula up for an inch (luting consistency).

3. Wipe both sides of the spatula and then gather all the material into one area.

4. Wipe off the cement spatula with the moist 2 × 2 gauze sponge.

---

cements available for patients who are sensitive to eugenol. The non-eugenol cements (type I) are formulated with other oils.

Properties. Zinc oxide eugenol has several properties that affect the selection of this material. ZOE is very soluble in the mouth and dissolves quickly. The reinforced ZOE has the strength required for permanent cementation and retention, but it is not as strong as zinc phosphate. The pH of the zinc oxide eugenol cements is neutral. With the sedative effect on the tooth, these materials do not require a protective base or liner.

FIGURE 26-9 IRM-Type II (ZOE) comes in powder, liquid, and capsules.

Zinc oxide eugenol materials are not used under composites or acrylic restorations because the eugenol is not compatible with these materials. The eugenol retards the setting process.

Manipulation Considerations. Most of zinc oxide eugenol materials are mixed on a paper pad with a stainless steel cement spatula. A glass slab may be used to control the setting time. Gently shake the powder before dispensing and swirl the liquid. Usually these materials have specific powder dispensers and liquid droppers. Care should be taken not to allow the eugenol into the rubber bulb of the dropper. The eugenol breaks down the rubber, thereby contaminating the liquid.

The type of material being mixed determines whether the powder is incorporated into the liquid in increments or brought in all at once. Usually, the mixing time is thirty to sixty seconds. All of the powder is mixed into the liquid to produce a uniform, smooth, creamy mix. Zinc oxide eugenol cements set quickly in the mouth because of the moisture and the warmth.

Some ZOE cements are two-paste systems. With the two-paste systems, one is an accelerator and the other is a base. They are dispensed in equal lengths on a paper pad. The two pastes are different colors and are mixed until a uniform color is achieved, which takes about ten to fifteen seconds.

The setting time ranges from three to five minutes in the oral cavity for most zinc oxide eugenol materials.

They are mixed to either a luting or base consistency depending on the use and the specific material.

Polycarboxylate Cement

Polycarboxylate cement, also known as zinc polycarboxylate, is used for permanent cementation and as an insulating base. This cement is said to be "kind" to the pulp and was the first cement that had the ability to chemically bond to the tooth structure. There are several brands of polycarboxylate cement, and the cement comes in a powder/liquid form.

Composition. The powder of the polycarboxylate cement is similar to the zinc phosphate with zinc oxide as the main component. The liquid is what makes this cement different; it is a viscous solution of polyacrylic acid and water. The powder comes in a bottle with a specific dispenser, and the liquid comes in a squeeze bottle or a calibrated syringe (Figure 26-11).

Properties. Polycarboxylate cement sets in three to five minutes and does not exhibit exothermic heat. This material bonds chemically to the tooth structure and mechanically to the restoration. The strength of polycarboxylate is similar to the reinforced ZOE and less than zinc phosphate cement. The material may appear quite viscous, but it flows readily when applied to a surface. The polycarboxylate cement is much less irritating

PROCEDURE

26-4 Mixing Polycarboxylate Cement

The dental assistant prepares and mixes the polycarboxylate materials to the desired consistency. The amount of materials dispensed depends on the size of restoration and the number of units involved.

EQUIPMENT AND SUPPLIES

▶ Polycarboxylate powder and liquid and a dispenser for the powder

▶ Paper pad or glass slab

▶ Flexible stainless steel spatula

▶ 2 × 2 gauze sponge (moistened)

▶ Timer

▶ Plastic filling instrument

PROCEDURE STEPS (*Follow aseptic procedures*)

1. The powder is fluffed before dispensing with the dispensing scoop.

2. The powder is measured and dispensed on one side of a paper pad or a glass slab.

3. Uniform drops of liquid are placed toward the opposite side of the powder. Follow manufacturer's directions for the appropriate number of drops per scoop of powder.

4. Incorporate from three-fourths to all of the powder into the liquid and use a folding motion while applying some pressure to wet all the powder. Mix quickly until all the powder is incorporated. (Because the liquid is thick, it is harder to incorporate the powder.)

5. The mix will be slightly more viscous than zinc phosphate cement and is glossy. Gather all the cement, wiping both sides of the spatula.

6. For luting consistency, the mix will follow the spatula up one inch.

7. For a base consistency, the same amount of powder is used, but the liquid ratio is decreased. The mix for the base should be glossy, but the consistency is tacky and stiff.

8. The mix must be used immediately before it becomes dull and stringy. (Figure 26-10)

9. The cleanup is done immediately by wiping the spatula with a wet 2 × 2 gauze or by soaking the spatula with the dried cement in a 10 percent sodium hydroxide solution. The paper pad sheet is removed, folded, and disposed of. (Fold the paper pad to prevent touching the cement and spreading it onto instruments and the patient's face.)

FIGURE 26-10 The powder and liquid show cobwebs when cement is mixed for too long.

FIGURE 26-11 Polycarboxylate powder and liquid in dispensing syringe. *(Courtesy of ESPE)*

to the pulp, with reactions similar to zinc oxide eugenol cement.

Polycarboxylate materials have a shelf life because of the water in the liquid. If the liquid discolors and becomes thick, it should be discarded.

Manipulation Properties. The polycarboxylate cements are mixed on a paper pad or a glass slab with a stainless steel cement spatula. The powder is fluffed before the dispenser is used. The viscous liquid is dispensed from a squeeze bottle or a calibrated syringe. The liquid bottle is held perpendicular and squeezed until a drop begins to fall. The size of the drop varies because of this dispensing technique and the viscosity of the liquid. The syringe improves the accuracy of dispensing the liquid.

Polycarboxylate cements are mixed in thirty to sixty seconds and have a short working time of about three minutes. The material loses its shine and becomes stringy or forms "cobwebs." At this point, the cement should not be used.

Glass Ionomer Cement

Glass ionomer cement is one of the newer cement systems. This cement is diverse in its applications; thus, there is more than one type of glass ionomer material.

▶ **Type I**—A finer grain glass ionomer used for cementation of crowns and bridges because it chemically bonds to the tooth structure. Type I is also used for orthodontic bonding and pit and fissure sealant.

▶ **Type II**—A coarser grain glass ionomer that comes in various shades for use in selected restorations, such as Class III and V and pediatric restorations (discussed later in this chapter).

▶ **Type III**—Glass ionomer used as a liner and dentin bonding agent.

▶ **Type IV**—Reinforced or admixtures of glass ionomers. Silver or amalgam filings are combined with the glass ionomer material to be used for crown and core buildups.

FIGURE 26-12 Glass ionomer cements, various brand names.

Glass ionomer cements come in numerous brands. It comes in powder/liquid, paste systems, syringes, and capsule forms. The glass ionomers come in both self-curing and light-curing materials (Figure 26-12).

Composition. Glass ionomer powder is a silicate glass powder containing calcium, aluminum, and fluoride (calcium fluoroaluminosilicate glass). The liquid is an aqueous solution (the solution contains water) of polyacrylic acid.

Properties. Glass ionomer material is strong enough to act as a supportive base and is similar to zinc phosphate cement in strength. The material mechanically and chemically bonds to the tooth structure. The material releases fluoride ions, which prevent secondary decay by strengthening the tooth structure. Glass ionomers have non-irritating qualities similar to polycarboxylate cements. The complete setting reaction of the glass ionomers takes up to twenty-four hours.

Manipulation Considerations. Glass ionomer cements are mixed on a paper pad or a cool glass slab. The paper pads are preferred for easy cleanup, but glass slabs may be used to retard the setting action. The materials should be mixed quickly following manufacturer's directions because of the water content of the liquid. Water evaporation affects the properties of the cement.

Although many properties are the same as those of the polycarboxylate cements, the liquid of the glass ionomers is not as viscous and is therefore easier to dispense and mix. The powder is dispensed first using the scoop and the amount indicated in the manufacturer's instructions. The liquid is dispensed just prior to manipulation. The mixing time is usually thirty to sixty seconds. The working time for the material is about two minutes.

The tooth must be completely isolated, cleaned, and dried before the cement is placed. The glass ionomer cement sets in the mouth in about five minutes.

PROCEDURE

26-5 Mixing Glass Ionomer Cement

This procedure is completed by the dental assistant. The equipment and materials are prepared and mixed when the dentist indicates. The material must be used immediately after it is mixed. This material requires that the tooth be clean of debris and dry, so the dental assistant should rinse and evacuate and then isolate the area before beginning to mix the cement.

EQUIPMENT AND SUPPLIES

▶ Glass ionomer materials and appropriate dispensers

▶ Paper pad or cool glass slab

▶ Flexible stainless steel spatula

▶ 2 × 2 gauze sponges (moistened)

▶ Timer

▶ Plastic filling instrument

PROCEDURE STEPS *(Follow aseptic procedures)*

1. Fluff the powder and, using the recommended scoops, place the appropriate number of scoops on the paper pad or glass slab.

2. Swirl the liquid and then place the specified number of drops on the pad near the powder. Replace the cap on the liquid immediately to prevent evaporation. (Figure 26-13)

3. Divide the powder into halves or thirds and then draw the sections into the liquid one at a time.

4. Mix over a small area until all the powder is incorporated. The cement should be creamy and glossy for the luting consistency and tacky and stiff for the base consistency.

5. Once the cement has obtained the final consistency, wipe off the spatula with a 2 × 2 gauze. Hold the paper or glass slab under the patient's chin and pass the plastic filling instrument to the dentist.

6. To clean up, remove the top paper, fold it, and dispose of it. The instruments are wiped after use for easier cleanup.

7. Glass ionomer capsules are also available for use. They are activated by placement in an "activator" or dispenser to break the seal between the powder and liquid in the capsule.

8. The capsules are then placed in an amalgamator to be mixed (triturated) for a specific amount of time, usually ten seconds. Follow manufacturer's directions.

9. Insert the capsule in the appropriate dispenser and pass it to the dentist for dispensing the material needed.

10. To clean up, the capsule is discarded and the activator and the dispenser are disinfected.

FIGURE 26-13 Dispensed glass ionomer powder and liquid.

Calcium Hydroxide Material

Calcium hydroxide is a cement that is used as a low-strength base under any restoration. It is used for indirect or direct pulp capping procedures (near or direct pulp exposures). This material has a therapeutic effect on the pulp. The area is sealed with the calcium hydroxide so that secondary dentin may form.

Calcium hydroxide comes in powder/liquid, a two-paste system, or a one-paste system. The form many offices use is the two-paste system: catalyst and base (Figure 26-14). Calcium hydroxide comes in a self-curing and a light-curing formula.

Composition. Calcium hydroxide has complicated formulas with several ingredients in addition to calcium hydroxide. The light-cured calcium hydroxide formula also contains a polymer resin.

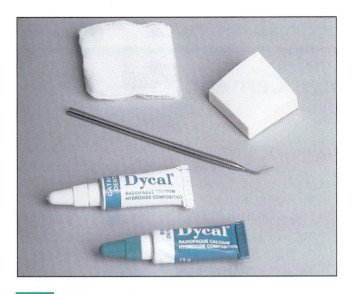

FIGURE 26-14 Calcium hydroxide material, paper pad, and small balled instrument used to mix and place the material.

Properties. Calcium hydroxide is low in strength and is placed in a thin layer near or over the pulp. It is easy to mix and place. The cement has low thermal conductivity but is usually not used in a thick enough layer to provide thermal protection. An insulating base is often placed over the thin layer of calcium hydroxide.

Manipulation Considerations. The two-paste system is mixed on a small paper pad with a metal spatula, an explorer, or a small ball-ended instrument. The base and the catalyst of the two-paste system come as a set and cannot be interchanged with those of other calcium hydroxide paste systems.

This material is dispensed in equal portions and mixed for about ten to fifteen seconds. The setting times vary from two to seven minutes.

Cavity Varnish

Cavity varnish is a material used to seal the dentin tubules that are exposed during an amalgam cavity preparation. This thin liquid is placed on the surface of the dentin only. There are various types of varnish, and some come with solvents.

Composition. Cavity varnishes are resin solutions of different compositions. The **copal varnish** contains organic solvents (ether, acetone, or chloroform) and is used only under amalgam restorations because the solvent material in the varnish may interfere with the setting action of composite and resins. The **universal varnishes** do not have the organic solvent and may be used under all restorations.

Properties. Varnishes are placed in a thin layer over the dentin tubules. The varnishes do not exhibit any

P R O C E D U R E

26-6 Mixing Calcium Hydroxide Cement— Two-Paste System

This material is dispensed and mixed by the dental assistant. It is often the first step in restoring the cavity preparation.

EQUIPMENT AND SUPPLIES

▶ Calcium hydroxide two-paste system

▶ Small paper pad

▶ Small ball-ended instrument or explorer

▶ 2 × 2 gauze sponge

PROCEDURE STEPS (*Follow aseptic procedures*)

1. Dispense small and equal amounts of both the catalyst and base onto the paper pad.

2. Wipe off the ends of the tubes and replace the caps.

3. Mix the two materials together using a circular motion.

4. Mix until the materials are a uniform color within the ten to fifteen second mixing time.

5. Use a 2 × 2 gauze to remove excess material from the mixing instrument.

6. Pass the instrument to the dentist and hold the paper pad close to the patient's chin.

7. Wipe off the instrument with a gauze for the dentist between applications.

8. Receive the instrument, wipe it off, tear and fold the top page of the paper pad, and dispose of it.

P R O C E D U R E

26-7 Preparing Cavity Varnish

The materials needed for application of cavity varnish are prepared by the dental assistant. Depending on expanded function laws, the dental assistant applies the varnish or assists the dentist during placement.

EQUIPMENT AND SUPPLIES

▶ Cavity varnish and solvent (Figure 26-15)

▶ Two cotton pliers

▶ Cotton pellets or pieces of cotton rolled into small, football-shaped balls, or a small brush

▶ Cotton roll

PROCEDURE STEPS (*Follow aseptic procedures*)

1. Clean and dry the cavity preparation.

2. Prepare cotton pellets for application of two layers of varnish. The pellets must be small in order to apply the varnish on the dentin surface.

3. Remove the cap from the varnish bottle. Holding the two cotton pellets in the pliers, dip them into the varnish until they are moistened. Then, replace the cap on the varnish.

4. Place the cotton pellets on a 2 × 2 gauze and dab off the excess varnish.

5. Using one pellet, apply the varnish to the cavity preparation. Coat the surface of the preparation.

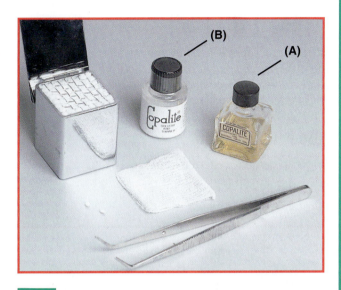

FIGURE 26-15 (A) Varnish and (B) solvent with materials needed for placement. Cotton pellets and cotton pliers for dipping into the varnish.

6. Allow the first coat to dry, and then apply a second coat in the same manner.

7. Dispose of the cotton pellets and clean the cotton pliers with solvent before sterilizing them.

8. To prepare the cotton pellets one at a time, two separate cotton pliers must be used to avoid contamination.

---

strength and do not provide any thermal insulation. The cavity varnishes are insoluble in the oral fluids and reduce leakage around the margins of restorations, thereby preventing microleakage. Varnish also prevents penetration of the acids from some cements into the dentin. These materials are non-acidic and non-irritating.

Manipulation Properties. Cavity varnishes often are placed in two layers for greater protection and to prevent voids. Recap the varnish immediately to minimize evaporation of the varnish. The cavity varnish comes with a separate bottle of solvent. If the varnish becomes too thick, solvent can be added. The solvent also can be used to clean the applicator and to remove any varnish on the external tooth surfaces.

Cavity varnish is not mixed; it is placed directly on the tooth with one of various types of applicators, such as small cotton pellets or brushes.

Resin Cement

Resin cements have multiple uses with a wide variety of procedures, including permanent cementation of cast metal restorations and porcelain/resin restorations and veneers, orthodontic brackets, and endodontic posts. Resin cements may be supplied in a two-paste system, powder/liquid set, or syringe. The manufacturer may supply the **acid etchant** gel or liquid with the material. Some of these materials may be shaded to complement the translucency of the crown or inlay.

There are three types of resin cements: self-curing (chemical), light cured, and dual cured. **Dual-cured**

P R O C E D U R E

26-8 Placing Resin Cement—Dual-Curing Technique

This procedure is done by the dental assistant for the dentist. The equipment and materials are prepared, and the material is mixed and passed to the dentist. Because this material is dual curing, a curing light and eye protection are needed.

EQUIPMENT AND SUPPLIES

▶ Resin cement system (Figure 26-16)

▶ Paper pad

▶ Stainless steel spatula

FIGURE 26-16 Resin cements system. *(Courtesy of Kerr Corporation)*

▶ Plastic filling instrument

▶ Curing light and protective shield or glasses

▶ 2 × 2 gauze sponges

PROCEDURE STEPS *(Follow aseptic procedures)*

1. Clean and dry the tooth and isolate the area with cotton rolls.

2. Pass the etchant to the dentist.

3. Wait the required time for the etchant and rinse the tooth thoroughly.

4. Lightly air dry the tooth and apply the adhesive.

5. Dispense and mix the two components together to a homogeneous, creamy mixture.

6. Hold the pad close to the patient and pass the placement instrument. The dentist places the material on the tooth and restoration.

7. Hold a 2 × 2 gauze to remove any excess materials.

8. Receive the placement instrument and prepare the curing light.

9. Either the dental assistant or the dentist holds the curing light and uses the protective shield when the light is activated.

10. Clean up immediately. Wipe any excess cement off the instruments and discard disposable items.

---

materials contain chemicals for a self-curing as well as a light-curing reaction. The self-cured materials are used with metal or metal combination materials and endodontic posts; the light-curing materials are used with porcelain/resin restorations, veneers, and orthodontic brackets.

Composition. The resin cements are similar to composites in composition. Variation comes with individual products adjusted for different functions. The resin matrices are BIS-GMA (bisphenol A-glycidyl methaceylate) or dimethacrylate resin diluted with low-viscosity monomers. The resin cements are more fluid than direct filling composites because the amount of filler particles are reduced to create low viscosities for cementation purposes.

Properties. Most resin cements are radiopaque and exhibit adequate strength and wear resistance for lut-

ing. These materials are insoluble in oral fluids but are irritating to the pulp; thus, a protective cement is required. Some of the products contain fluoride.

Manipulation Considerations. Resin cements do not adhere to metal or ceramic materials; these materials must be roughened with etchants to produce mechanical bonding or the tissue surfaces of ceramics are treated with a silane coupling agent to produce a chemical bond with the resin cements. Sometimes, a wire mesh or undercuts may be added to the tissue side of the prosthesis to aid in retention.

Self-cured materials come with an initiator and an activator. These are mixed on a paper pad for twenty to thirty seconds. Excess cement must be removed before the material is set completely to prevent any marginal leakage. Light-cured materials come in syringes and must be cured for at least forty seconds. Dual-cured materials come in two component systems that are mixed together for twenty to thirty seconds. Once mixed, these materials begin to set slowly, allowing for placement of the cement on the prosthesis and the prosthesis to be seated in the oral cavity. Once in position, the visible light unit is activated to harden the cement.

BONDING AGENTS

Bonding agents are also known as **adhesives** and **bonding resins**. These materials are used to improve the retention between the tooth structure (enamel and dentin) and the restoration. These materials come in many forms and are often complete systems (Figure 26-17). These materials bond enamel and dentin to porcelain, resins, precious and non-precious metals, composites, and amalgam.

The bonding materials are low-viscosity resins that may or may not contain fillers. Some of the bonding agents contain additives with adhesive enhancers, and some contain fluoride. These materials are mainly light cured or dual cured.

Enamel Bonding

Adhesion of dental materials to enamel is accomplished by acid etching with phosphoric acid. This solution alters the surface of the enamel and creates microscopic undercuts between the enamel rod (Figure 26-18). Low-viscosity, unfilled resin bonding agents then penetrate into these undercuts and mechanically lock into them. The restorative material then bonds to this layer and becomes a solid unit. Bonding to enamel is required before placement of composite restorations, pit and fissure sealants, veneers, resin-cemented crowns and bridges, and orthodontic brackets.

FIGURE 26-17 Bonding agents and systems.

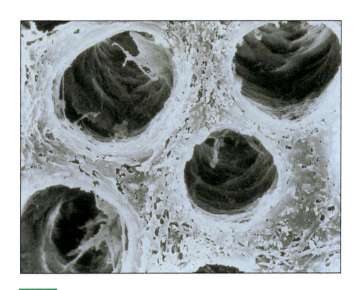

FIGURE 26-18 Microscopic view of etched enamel. *(Courtesy of Kerr Corporation)*

The acid etching process involves the use of thirty to forty percent phosphoric acid solution. The etchant comes in liquid or gel form and is supplied in bottles or syringes. The liquids are placed with small cotton pellets, sponges, brushes, or disposable applicators.

Dentin Bonding

Dentin bonding is more of a challenge than enamel bonding. Some of the obstacles include:

▶ Dentin has a high water content, which can interfere with the bonding to the tooth.

▶ The composition of the dentin is more organic than inorganic and contains water. These factors make dentin difficult to bond to.

▶ Dentin is directly above the pulp, so the operator must take care not to injure the pulp.

▶ When the dentin is cut with a bur during the cavity preparation, it forms a **smear layer**. This layer of debris lies on the cavity floor and walls and prevents contact between the intact dentin and the bonding agent/adhesive.

The current dentin bonding materials use an etchant to remove the smear layer, because the smear layer is not attached firmly and is unreliable. When the smear layer is removed, the adhesives achieve a mechanical bond with the dentin. Many of the bonding agents are suitable for both enamel and dentin surfaces because of the application of the acid etchant.

RESTORATIVE DENTISTRY

Restorative dentistry, also known as operative dentistry, involves various materials and techniques. There

26-9 Placing Etchant

The dental assistant prepares the materials and isolates the area. The dentist places the etchant. When the allotted time has passed, the dental assistant thoroughly rinses the tooth.

EQUIPMENT

▶ Acid etchant, usually a thirty to forty percent solution

▶ Isolation materials (rubber dam or cotton rolls)

▶ Applicator (syringe, cotton pellets, or small applicator tips)

▶ Dappen dish

▶ Air-water syringe

▶ Timer

PROCEDURE STEPS *(Follow aseptic procedures)*

1. Isolate the area.

2. Clean the surface thoroughly.

3. Prepare the etchant applicator or syringe.

4. Place the etchant on the surface for fifteen to thirty seconds depending on manufacturer's directions.

5. Rinse the tooth after the designated time for fifteen to twenty seconds with the air-water syringe and evacuate thoroughly for ten to twenty seconds.

NOTE: The etched surface will have a frosty appearance. This surface needs to be isolated until the cementation is complete. If saliva or other fluids contact the surface, the etching process must be repeated.

26-10 Placing Bonding Agent

Steps in the application of bonding agents vary with manufacturers, so follow the directions that come with the product. The dental assistant prepares the materials for each step and keeps the area dry and free of debris (sometimes, cavity cleaners are used).

EQUIPMENT AND SUPPLIES

▶ Bonding system that contains acid etchant, primer or conditioner, adhesive material

▶ Applicators (disposable tips or brushes)

▶ Dappen dish

▶ Isolation means

▶ Air-water syringe

▶ Curing light and shield

▶ Timer

PROCEDURE STEPS *(Follow aseptic procedures)*

1. If the cavity preparation is near the pulp, place calcium hydroxide or glass ionomer lining cement over the area.

2. The etchant is placed on the enamel and the dentin for the specified amount of time, usually fifteen to twenty seconds. Usually, the etchant is placed on the enamel first and then the dentin, because the dentin is more sensitive to the etchant.

3. Rinse the tooth as soon as the time is up. Continue to rinse for at least five to ten seconds. Move quickly to prevent bacterial contamination of the dentin.

4. If the bonding involves both the enamel and dentin, a primer step is included. The primer or conditioner is placed with a brush or an applicator. This material wets the dentin and penetrates the dentin tubules.

5. The bonding resin is then applied, and the curing light is used to harden the material.

6. Cleanup involves disposing of applicator tips or brushes.

are many reasons why a tooth needs to be restored, including decay, fracture, abrasion, esthetics, and attrition. Restorative materials such as amalgam and composites are used to restore the tooth. These materials are called direct restorative materials because they are mixed and placed directly in the cavity preparation in one appointment.

Reasons for restoring teeth include:

▶ Arresting the loss of tooth structure. Stopping the decay process early allows the preparation to be conservative and small restorations to be stronger.

▶ Preventing the recurrence of decay by placing margins that can be reached easily for cleaning. This is known as **extension for prevention.**

▶ Restoring the contour of the tooth (the shape and design of the crown of the tooth). The proper contour prevents food impaction and gingival irritation.

▶ Restoring the function of the tooth and establishing occlusion with opposing teeth for mastication of food.

▶ Restoring or improving the esthetic look of the teeth.

Classification

Dental caries are classified to simplify the examination, charting, diagnosis, and patient communication. There are several ways to classify cavities and restorations (see Chapter 7, Dental Charting). The classifications include Black's classification, which identifies areas of decay according to the surfaces they are located on, such as Class I for occlusal caries on the posterior teeth and Class III for dental caries on the mesial or distal of anterior teeth where the incisal edge is not involved. Another classification is according to the number of surfaces involved, for example simple, compound, and complex. A third method of classifying dental caries is according to whether the caries are pit and fissure areas or smooth surface areas.

Cavity Detection

Cavities can be detected with radiographs, probing with an explorer, or the use of a special dye. This dye detects caries by distinguishing between good, sound, hard dentin and dentin that is infected with bacteria and softened. The dye is placed in the preparation early in the procedure to keep from removing too much tooth structure. The dye is applied for about ten seconds and then rinsed off. Burs and spoon excavators usually remove all the stained dentin. This process is repeated until no caries remain. This material also can be used to identify cracks and root canals.

Cavity Cleaners/Disinfectants

Cavity cleaners/disinfectants can be used in the cavity preparation. Like any body wound, the cavity should be cleaned and disinfected to reduce bacterial growth under restorations that can lead to sensitivity. This step is completed before the tooth is etched.

Cavity Preparation Identification

Once the tooth is prepared, there are terms used to describe the inside of the cavity preparation. Knowledge of these terms helps the dental assistant better communicate with the dentist and also understand the details of the cavity preparation.

The preparation of the tooth forms walls, lines, and angles. A **wall** is the side or floor of the cavity preparation. The wall is named according to the surface of the tooth it is nearest to, such as the buccal wall or distal wall. The internal wall that runs parallel to the long axis of the tooth is the **axial wall.** The wall that overlies the pulp is the **pulpal wall** or **floor.** The wall nearest the gingiva that is perpendicular to the long axis of the tooth is the **gingival wall.**

Lines are formed when two surfaces meet and form a **line angle.** The line angles are named according to the two surfaces, such as the distopulpal line angle or axiogingival (Figure 26-19). (Note that the names of the two surfaces are usually joined with an "o" between the words.) In the "corners" of the cavity preparation, three lines (surfaces) come together to form **point angles.** The point angles are named by joining the names of the walls, such as the mesiolinguopulpal line angle or the distobuccopulpal point angle (Figure 26-20).

The **cavosurface margin** is the angle that is formed by the junction of the wall of the preparation and the untouched surface of the tooth (Figure 26-21). The sealing of this margin is critical to prevent marginal leakage. Sometimes, this margin is beveled (slanted) during the preparation.

The Elements of Cavity Preparations

The cavity preparation is a systematic cutting of the tooth structure that depends on the location of the

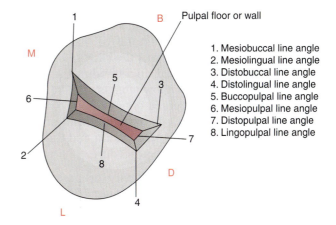

1. Mesiobuccal line angle
2. Mesiolingual line angle
3. Distobuccal line angle
4. Distolingual line angle
5. Buccopulpal line angle
6. Mesiopulpal line angle
7. Distopulpal line angle
8. Lingopulpal line angle

FIGURE 26-19 Cavity preparation line angles (looking down on occlusal view).

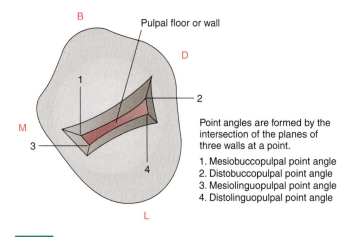

FIGURE 26-20 Cavity preparation point angles.

Point angles are formed by the intersection of the planes of three walls at a point.

1. Mesiobuccopulpal point angle
2. Distobuccopulpal point angle
3. Mesiolinguopulpal point angle
4. Distolinguopulpal point angle

1. Buccogingival line angle
2. Linguogingival line angle
3. Buccoaxial line angle
4. Linguoaxial line angle
5. Axiogingival line angle
6. Gingivobuccoaxial point angle
7. Gingivolinguoaxial point angle
8. Buccodistal line angle
9. Linguodistal line angle
10. Distopulpal line angle
11. Linguopulpal line angle
12. Buccopulpal line angle
13. Distobuccopulpal point angle
14. Distolinguopulpal point angle
15. Additional line angle, the pulpoaxial line angle is formed by the intersection of the pulpal and axial walls
16. Pulpolinguoaxial point angle
17. Pulpobuccoaxial point angle
18. Cavosurface margin

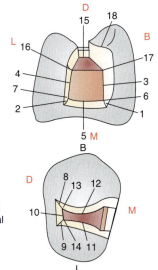

FIGURE 26-21 Cavity preparation line angles, point angles, and cavosurface margin. (Top figure is view from mesial, bottom figure is view from occlusal.)

decay, the extent of the decay, the amount of lost tooth structure, and the type of restorative material to be used. When the dentist prepares the cavity, some basic considerations are followed. Understanding these steps helps the dental assistant know what is coming next so he or she can be prepared to change burs, rinse and evacuate the oral cavity, mix materials, and so on. It also keeps the focus on the preparation and the dental assistant more involved in the procedure.

The Cavity Preparations. Cavity preparations include the following considerations (Figure 26-22):

▶ **Outline form**—Designates the overall shape of the cavity preparation. The outline form is determined by the extent of the decay, the type of restorative material, and the retention of this material.

FIGURE 26-22 Steps of cavity preparation. Opening cavity with bur, outline cavity, and refining and finishing cavity preparation.

▶ **Resistance form**—The internal shape of the cavity that protects the tooth and the restoration from the stresses of mastication.

▶ **Retention form**—The internal shape of the cavity walls that retains the restoration. In an amalgam preparation, the walls of the preparation are often slightly undercut to form mechanical locking of the amalgam and the cavity preparation.

▶ **Convenience form**—The alteration to the cavity preparation that is necessary for instrumentation during the preparation and the insertion of the restorative materials. This is usually beyond the outline form and opens the tooth for the dentist to have enough space to prepare the cavity properly.

▶ **Finishing** or **refinement of the cavity preparation**—The final planing of the cavity walls before the placement of the restoration.

▶ **Cleansing** or **debridement of the cavity preparation**—The spraying and rinsing of the cavity preparation to remove the debris. The dental assistant uses the spray from the air-water syringe and the HVE to cleanse the area.

AMALGAM RESTORATIVE MATERIALS

After the cavity has been prepared and the liners and bases have been placed, the tooth is ready to be restored. One of the most common restorative materials is dental **amalgam**, which has been used for many years. Dental amalgam is an effective, long-lasting, and comparatively inexpensive restorative material. Amalgam is a combination of an alloy with mercury. An **alloy** is the combination of two or more metals.

Dental amalgam is pliable when first mixed, so it is easily placed in the cavity preparation. It is carved before hardening to resemble tooth structure. This material is used on the posterior teeth because of its strength and because it is not esthetically pleasing.

Composition

Dental amalgam is composed of silver, tin, copper, and zinc (optional) to form an alloy. This alloy is mixed with mercury to form the amalgam. The ADA has specifications that regulate the composition of dental amalgam (see Table 26-2 for the characteristics of each of the alloy components).

Types of Dental Amalgam

The dental amalgam consists of a low copper and high copper alloy. The metals for the alloys are prepared in several ways to produce the lathe cut (comminuted particles) and spherically shaped particles. The way these metals are prepared affects their properties. The low copper alloys are available with comminuted and spherical particles. The high copper alloys are supplied as comminuted, spherical, or combination particles (admix).

TABLE 26-2 DENTAL ALLOY COMPOSITION

Silver	**40 to 70 percent**	**High copper amalgam**
	68 to 72 percent	**Low copper mix**
	• Used to form the metallic compound with mercury (Hg) that determines the dimensional changes that occur during hardening.	
	• Increases strength of restoration.	
	• Increases expansion.	
	• Is slow to amalgamate.	
	• Hardens rapidly.	
	• Tarnishes easily.	
	• Decreases setting time.	
Tin	**22 to 30 percent**	**High copper amalgam**
	26 to 37 percent	**Low copper amalgam**
	• Aids in the amalgamation (chemical combining) of the alloy with the mercury because of its strong affinity for mercury.	
	• Reduces expansion during setting.	
	• Reduces strength.	
	• Setting time is slower.	
	• More susceptible to corrosion (conventional alloy).	
	• Tends to weaken the amalgam.	
Copper	**12 to 30 percent**	**High copper amalgam**
	4 to 5 percent	**Low copper amalgam**
	• Increases strength and hardness.	
	• Increases expansion of amalgam during hardening.	
	• Reduces flow of finished restoration.	
	• Resists corrosion (high copper).	
	• Reduces marginal failure (high copper).	
Zinc	**0 to 1 percent**	**For both high & low copper amalgam**
	• Used to minimize the oxidation of the other metals present in alloy during manufacturing. Zinc is a scavenger and reacts with oxygen, preventing it from combining with silver, tin, or copper. NOTE: Should moisture contamination occur during manipulation or condensation of the amalgam, delayed expansion may occur. Zinc-containing dental amalgams are particularly sensitive to moisture. Zinc reacts with water to form the zinc oxide and hydrogen gas that may cause the unwanted and excessive expansion of the set amalgam restoration.	

The spherical alloys have smoother surfaces that require less mercury when mixed. These alloys are also easier to condense and have improved carving and polishing properties. The combination alloys adapt better to the cavity preparation and produce better contacts with the adjacent teeth.

Mercury

Dental **mercury** is a very toxic chemical and must meet the specifications listed by the ADA. Dental professionals are aware of the hazards and safety measures when working with dental mercury to prevent problems from occurring.

Mercury is the only metal that is in a liquid state and vaporizes (particles of mercury scatter and float freely in the air) at a relatively low room temperature. Mercury is absorbed through the pores of the skin and through inhalation. Some potential sources of mercury contamination in the dental office are:

1. Mercury leaking out of a capsule during trituration
2. Mercury vapor that may occur during triturating and dispensing
3. Polishing an amalgam restoration
4. Removal of hardened amalgam restoration
5. Contacting amalgam during the procedure
6. Carpeting in the treatment rooms could retain amalgam particles and vacuuming these surfaces disperses the mercury through the air
7. Scraps of amalgam left in an open container

Studies have revealed that in most dental offices, the level of mercury vapor is well below the maximum safe environmental concentration levels. Another study testing the blood mercury level in dentists displayed a reading well below the level at which symptoms begin to show.

There has been some concern about the level of mercury in patients with numerous amalgam restorations. Recent studies have shown that these patients ingest a very low amount of mercury from the amalgam fillings, well below what they would ingest from food, water, and the atmosphere. A very small number of people are at possible risk of allergic reactions to mercury. The reaction manifests as a skin reaction that appears after the placement of an amalgam restoration. Including questions on the medical history is a step of prevention. Because of the concerns, the dentist and the dental assistant should stay current with the studies and the ADA recommendations.

The ADA recommends that a program of mercury hygiene be established at each dental practice. Potential office hazards involving mercury can be eliminated by practicing appropriate mercury hygiene. The guidelines should include:

1. Wear disposable gloves, a face mask, and glasses when working with amalgam.

2. Educate all personnel regarding the potential hazards of mercury and good mercury hygiene practices.

3. A no-touch technique should be used when handling mercury. If the skin is exposed, wash with soap and water, and rinse under running water.

4. Use capsules containing a measured amount of mercury and alloy.

5. Use an amalgamator with a protective cover to reduce the chance of any mercury vapor being released and to confine mercury that might be sprayed from an ill-fitting capsule.

6. Store mercury and amalgam scraps in capped, unbreakable jars containing used x-ray fixer, finely divided sulfur, glycerin, or mineral oil.

7. Carpeting in the dental treatment rooms is not recommended. Carpeting retains mercury, which is difficult to retrieve.

8. Use water spray and high-volume evacuation when cutting old amalgams or polishing new restorations. Wear a mask during these procedures.

9. Avoid working with mercury or amalgam near a heat source, such as the autoclave.

10. Handle mercury only over impervious surfaces. The area should have a continuous lip to retain any spillage.

11. The office should have proper ventilation to reduce the possibility of mercury vapor inhalation. Change the air filter frequently.

12. Office personnel should have periodic urinalyses to check for any mercury in the body.

13. Monitor the dental office to determine mercury levels.

14. Keep a mercury spill kit if the office uses large quantities of mercury in the case of a spill. Clean up any mercury scraps or spills immediately, following OSHA recommendations (Figure 26-23).

Forms of Dental Alloy

Dental alloy is purchased in disposable capsule form. The **capsule** contains a premeasured amount of alloy and mercury and sometimes a **pestle**. The pestle, a small pellet, is made of metal or plastic and aids in the mixing of the alloy and mercury. In the capsule, a thin membrane separates the alloy and the mercury until they are mixed. Some capsules come with activators to break the membrane or the capsules are twisted or compressed before being mixed. The capsules are most often plastic and come with screw-type or friction-fit caps. Disposable capsules are color coded to distinguish single, double, and triple mixes (Figure 26-24).

FIGURE 26-23 Mercury spill kit.

FIGURE 26-24 Examples of amalgam capsules.

Properties

The strength of amalgam is not adequate to withstand occlusal forces alone. The preparation is designed so that the remaining tooth structure sustains the forces to the amalgam. Proper manipulation of amalgam is important in the overall strength and success of the restoration.

Amalgam is subject to dimensional change, such as expansion and contraction. The amount of expansion and contraction is controlled by the composition of the alloy and manipulation techniques.

Another property of amalgam is the ability of the material to **creep**. Creeping is a change in the material when under a constant load.

Amalgam restorations are subject to tarnish and corrosion in the oral cavity. Tarnish is the discoloration of the surface, and corrosion is the deterioration of the surface. The combination (admixed) and the spherical high copper amalgams are less susceptible to corrosion. Careful finishing and polishing of amalgams reduces tarnish and corrosion.

Manipulation

Trituration is the mechanical means of combining (mixing) the dental alloy and mercury. **Amalgamation** is the actual chemical reaction that occurs between the alloy and the mercury to form the silver amalgam. Specially designed machines used to triturate (amalgamate) the alloy and mercury are called dental **amalgamators** or **triturators**. These machines have cradles to hold the capsules, cradle covers, timers, and variable speed controls (Figure 26-25). Each amalgamator must be set for the type of dental alloy used. Usually, trituration of the alloy and mercury is ten to fifteen seconds. This produces a homogeneous and uniform mix. Follow the manufacturer's directions and the alloy specifications.

Trituration of the amalgam is an important step in the success of the restoration. The quality of the mix is determined by the mixing time, the speed of the amalgamator, and the force being applied during the trituration. Varying conditions in the trituration process can cause some problems. If the amalgam is mixed too long (overtriturated), it will be soupy before hardening and difficult to remove from the capsule. If the amalgam is undermixed (undertriturated), it will be crumbly and dull in appearance and the strength of the amalgam will be reduced.

Amalgam Bonding

Amalgam bonding agents are now available and used in many restorations to bond the amalgam to the tooth surface (Figure 26-29). The amalgam bonding increases the retention of the restoration and decreases marginal leakage. The bonding agent is a low viscosity resin, similar to those discussed earlier in this chapter. The procedure describes the application of bonding agents.

FIGURE 26-25 Kerr amalgamators. *(Courtesy of Kerr Corporation)*

P R O C E D U R E

26-11 Using the Dental Amalgamator

This procedure is completed by the dental assistant. The materials and equipment are prepared before the procedure begins. The type of amalgamator and capsules vary.

EQUIPMENT

▶ Amalgamator

▶ Premeasured capsule of dental alloy and mercury

▶ Amalgam well, dappen dish, or squeeze cloth

▶ Amalgam carrier/condenser

▶ Scrap container for excess amalgam

PROCEDURE STEPS (Follow aseptic procedures)

1. Assemble materials for the procedure. Select trituration time and speed for the type of alloy and amalgamator.

2. Prepare the capsule by twisting the cap, squeezing the capsule, or using an activator.

3. Insert the capsule into the cradle (prongs) of the amalgamator. Place one end first, then slide the other end down into place. Practice placing the capsules into the cradle with one hand (Figure 26-26A).

4. Close the cover of the amalgamator.

5. Activate the amalgamator for the prescribed time and speed (Figure 26-26B). (The timer will automatically switch off after the prescribed trituration time.)

6. Lift the cover and remove the capsule.

7. Open the capsule and empty the amalgam into an amalgam well. Avoid touching the amalgam with gloved hands. Use cotton pliers, if necessary. A well-mixed amalgam will have a glossy appearance with a smooth, velvety consistency.

8. Reassemble the capsule and place it to the side.

9. Hold the carrier and load the amalgam (Figure 26-27).

10. Pack the carrier, applying pressure so that the cylinder is packed tightly. Wipe excess material from the end of the carrier on the sides of the amalgam well.

11. Pass the amalgam carrier to the dentist and prepare to exchange a condenser for the carrier. When practicing, dispense the amalgam from the carrier into a dappen dish and evaluate the mix. The cylinders of amalgam should be smooth and shiny.

(A)

(B)

FIGURE 26-26 (A) Placing capsule in the amalgamator. (B) Activating the amalgamator timer.

P R O C E D U R E   2 6 - 1 1 *continued*

FIGURE 26-27 Loading an amalgam carrier.

12. Repeat the loading and dispensing of all the material. Toward the end of the manipulation, the amalgam becomes harder to load into the carrier because it begins to set. This is the stage that takes practice in order to become proficient.

FIGURE 26-28 Placing amalgam scrapes in a sealed container.

13. To clean up, expel any excess amalgam into the appropriate container. The instruments are cleaned and sterilized (Figure 26-28).

The placement of the amalgam follows immediately, before the bonding agent sets.

NOTE: Other retention methods are discussed in Chapter 24, Fixed Prosthodontics, including the placement of retention pins and core buildups.

FIGURE 26-29 Amalgam bonding materials.

Complete Amalgam Procedure

The sequence of the procedure is for a complete amalgam restoration. The steps include administrating anesthetic; placing the rubber dam; placing liners and bases; assembling the matrix and wedge; and mixing, placing, condensing, and finishing the amalgam restoration. This gives the dental assistant an overall view of assisting during an amalgam procedure. Many of these steps, such as placing the rubber dam, are discussed in detail in other chapters because they can be performed by an expanded function dental assistant. These steps are indicated with EF after the procedure.

COMPOSITE RESTORATIVE MATERIALS

Composite restorative materials dominate the field of esthetic restorations. These materials have natural appearances and were used primarily for anterior restorations but are being developed as esthetic restorations for the posterior teeth. Composite materials also are used for veneers of the anterior teeth that have been stained or that have some erosion. (These procedures are discussed in Chapter 24, Fixed Prosthodontics.)

Technology is expanding the types of materials available as alternatives to dental amalgam. With concerns over the mercury in amalgams and the desire for the

P R O C E D U R E

26-12 Amalgam Restoration—Class II

This procedure is completed by the dentist and the dental assistant. The tooth is prepared with the dental handpiece and assorted burs. Once the tooth is prepared, it is restored with dental amalgam.

EQUIPMENT AND SUPPLIES (Figure 26-30)

- Basic setup: mouth mirror, explorer, cotton pliers
- Air-water syringe tip, HVE tip, and saliva ejector
- Cotton rolls, gauze sponges, pellets, cotton tip applicators, and floss
- Topical and local anesthetic setup
- Rubber dam setup
- High- and low-speed handpieces
- Assortment of dental burs
- Spoon excavator
- Hand cutting instruments (hatches, chisels, hoes, and gingival margin trimmers)
- Base, liner, varnish
- Paper pad, cement spatula, and placement instrument
- Matrix retainer, matrix bands, and wedges
- Locking pliers or hemostat
- Amalgam capsules
- Amalgam well
- Amalgam carrier and condensers
- Amalgamator
- Carving instruments
- Articulating paper and forceps

PROCEDURE STEPS *(Follow aseptic procedures)*

1. Greet and prepare the patient for the procedure. Review the medical history.

2. Prepare for the administration of the topical and local anesthetic. Dry the injection site and apply topical anesthetic (Expanded Function—EF). Prepare the syringe and summon the dentist. Transfer the mirror and explorer for the dentist to examine the tooth before beginning the procedure. When the dentist is ready, transfer a 2×2 gauze in one hand and the syringe in the other. The dentist replaces the needle cap and places the syringe on the tray. After the injection, rinse and evacuate the patient's mouth.

3. Prepare the rubber dam materials and equipment to assist the dentist in the placement (EF).

4. Transfer the mouth mirror and the high-speed handpiece with a bur. Position the HVE tip and maintain visibility throughout the procedure by retracting the cheek and tongue, keeping the mirror clear with the air-water syringe, and evacuating the site (Figure 26-31). Transfer and receive instruments at the den-

FIGURE 26-30 Amalgam procedure tray setup armamentarium.

FIGURE 26-31 Cavity being prepared by the dentist with the dental assistant evacuating and keeping the mirror dry and clean.

(continued)

PROCEDURE 26-12 *continued*

tist's signals. Instruments used at this point may include the explorer, the excavator, hatchets, hoes, angle formers, gingival margin trimmers, and chisels.

5. When the preparation is finished, transfer a cotton pellet with a cavity cleaning preparation to clean the inside of the tooth (EF). The area is then rinsed and dried. At the dentist's direction, mix the cavity liner (calcium hydroxide or glass ionomer), prepare the varnish and the base (glass ionomer, polycarboxylate, zinc phosphate, or modified ZOE), and transfer them to the dentist for placement. If the materials are light cured, hold the light tip near the material to be cured and, with the protective shield in place, activate the light to cure the material.

6. Assemble the matrix retainer and the band into the correct position according to the tooth being restored and transfer it to the dentist (EF). After the matrix is placed, transfer the wedge in cotton pliers (locking is best) or in a hemostat. The dentist places the wedge. (Refer to Chapter 28, Advanced Chairside Functions, for more information.)

7. When the dentist is ready, prepare the amalgam capsule by twisting the cap, squeezing the capsule together, or placing it in an activator, then placing the capsule in the amalgamator. The amalgamator is set for the specific type of amalgam material and the size of the mix. When the amalgam material has been mixed, remove the capsule from the amalgamator and place it in the amalgam well or a dappen dish. The amalgam is loaded into the amalgam carrier. If the carrier is double ended, both ends are filled and the loaded carrier is passed to the dentist (Figure 26-32). The carrier and the condenser are used alternately until the restorative material fills the cavity. In some offices, the dental assistant loads the carrier and, at the dentist's direction, places the amalgam in the cavity preparation, eliminating the exchanging of instruments and allowing the dentist to focus on the condensing of the amalgam. After the last exchange, transfer the dentist an explorer to loosen amalgam from the matrix band. While the dentist is using the explorer, clean up any amalgam scraps from the carrier and the well and place them in a sealed container.

8. Receive the explorer and transfer carving and finishing instruments at the dentist's signals. Operate the HVE tip near the site to evacuate any amalgam particles. After the dentist completes the preliminary carving, pass the cotton pliers to remove the wedge and then receive the wedge, pliers, and matrix retainer. The cotton pliers may be used again to remove the matrix band. Receive the cotton pliers and band and then transfer the carver of the dentist's choice for finishing the carving of the anatomy in the restoration.

9. The rubber dam is carefully removed at this time (EF). Transfer the clamp forceps, receive the forceps with the clamp, and transfer scissors to cut the interseptal dam. Receive the scissors, frame, napkin, and dam material. Rinse and evacuate the patient's mouth.

10. Dry the area and transfer the articulating paper, positioned on the forceps, to the dentist. The assistant may be instructed by the dentist to place the articulating paper over the restoration. The patient is instructed to gently tap the teeth together (Figure 26-33). Additional carving and checking the occlusion are continued until the dentist is satisfied and the patient is comfortable.

11. The restoration is wiped off with a wet cotton roll to remove any blue marks left by the articulating paper. Rinse and evacuate the patient's mouth thoroughly and clean any debris from the patient's face. The patient is cautioned not to chew on the side of the restoration for a few hours and is then dismissed.

FIGURE 26-32 Loaded carrier, ready for use.

FIGURE 26-33 Articulating paper for patient to gently close onto to check the occlusion.

natural appearance of teeth, there is ongoing research and development with composite restorative materials. Composites, glass ionomers, and porcelain materials are used for esthetic restorations.

These direct restorative materials are inserted into the cavity preparation and then self-cured, light cured, or dual cured. They come in syringes or single-application cartridges (**compules**) and have a variety of shades or shade modifiers. The location and the size of the cavity determines which material the dentist chooses.

Composition

Composite restorative material is composed of the following components:

▶ An organic polymer matrix, such as dimethacrylate, identified as BIS-GMA or urethane dimethacrylates.

▶ Inorganic filler particles, such as quartz, silica, and lithium aluminum silicate.

▶ Organic silane coupling agents. The inorganic filler particles are treated with an organic silane coupling agent to provide a bond between the inorganic fillers and the resin matrix.

Barium, strontium, zinc, or zirconium may be added to make the composite material more radiopaque.

The composites are classified according to the type, amount, and size of the filler particles, but all are referred to as composite resins. Composite particles are fine, microfill, and combinations of the fine and microfill filler particles, called **hybrids**. The filler particles can make up as much as 84 percent of the composite material by volume.

▶ **Fine composites** (macrofill) contain filler particles that range in size from 1 to 3 microns. These materials are used for Class IV restorations because they are strong enough to resist fracture and are esthetically pleasing. They do not polish to the same high finish as the microfill and the hybrids.

▶ **Microfill composites** contain fillers that range in size from 0.01 to 0.1 microns. They are used as a cosmetic filling material for Class III and V restorations. Microfills are also used for direct veneers and diastema closures. Some microfills are reinforced for Class IV restorations and the occlusal portion of Class I and II restorations. Microfill composites are esthetic restorations that resist wear due to abrasion and polish well, leaving a high-luster finish.

▶ **Hybrid composites** contain more than one type of filler particle, usually glass and silica. The glass particles are in the 1 to 3 micron range, and the silica is 0.04 micron. These composites are stronger and less likely to fracture in high-stress areas than the microfill composites. The hybrids combine the strength and

esthetics of the other composites to make a restoration that is strong and polishable.

Properties of Composites

The properties of the composite resin materials vary depending on the type and size of the filler. These aspects of the composites are being researched and improved for a strong, esthetic, long-lasting restoration. Overall, the composites exhibit the following properties:

▶ Resistant to fracture.

▶ Occlusal wear resistance is improving.

▶ These materials have good esthetics to match to the tooth structure.

▶ Some composites are radiopaque, making them more visible on radiographic film.

▶ The composites bond efficiently to the dentin and the enamel.

▶ The composites are often placed in layers to reduce the effect of polymerization (setting) shrinkage.

▶ The composite resins have adequate strength for specified applications. The strength requirement varies for different classifications of cavities. For example, the anterior Class III and V cavities do not require high strength but require color stability. The posterior Class I and II must exhibit enough strength to withstand occlusal stresses, but appearance is not as critical. All composite restorations require a smooth finish to reduce the potential for plaque and debris accumulation and for staining.

▶ Expansion and contraction rates of the composite materials are similar to the tooth structure.

Manipulation Considerations

To bond the composite material and the tooth structure, the cavity preparation is acid etched for thirty to sixty seconds. The etchant is rinsed completely and the surface is dried. After etching, the tooth has a chalky, dull appearance. Adhesion of the composite to the etched surface is rated high, but it can be further improved by the use of a bonding agent. Bonding agents are applied as described previously to both the enamel and the dentin. The composite then adheres to the bonding agent.

Shrinkage of composites can be minimized by placing the composite in small layers in the cavity preparation. After each layer is placed, it is light cured to the hardened form. The layering of the composite is also a method to modify the shade of the restoration. The layers can be composed of different types of composites with varying properties to enhance the qualities of the material.

PROCEDURE

26-13 Composite Restoration—Class III

This procedure is completed by the dentist and the dental assistant. The tooth is prepared with the dental handpiece and assorted burs. Once the tooth is prepared, it is restored with composite.

EQUIPMENT AND SUPPLIES (Figure 26-34)

FIGURE 26-34 Composite procedure tray setup.

▶ Basic setup: mouth mirror, explorer, cotton pliers

▶ Air-water syringe tip, HVE tip, and saliva ejector

▶ Cotton rolls, gauze sponges, cotton pellets, cotton tip applicators, and dental floss

▶ Topical and local anesthetic setup

▶ Rubber dam setup

▶ High- and low-speed handpieces

▶ Assortment of dental burs (including diamond and cutting burs)

▶ Spoon excavator

▶ Hand cutting instruments (dentist's choice may include binangle chisel and Wedelstaedt chisel)

▶ Base and liner with mixing materials and placement instruments

▶ Etchant and applicator, if necessary (usually comes with composite system)

▶ Primer (usually comes with composite system)

▶ Composite materials, including a shade guide

▶ Composite placement instrument (plastic filling instrument)

▶ Curing light with protective shield

▶ Celluloid matrix strip and wedges

▶ Locking pliers or hemostat

▶ Finishing burs or diamonds

▶ #12 scalpel

▶ Abrasive strips

▶ Polishing discs

▶ Lubricant

▶ Articulating paper and forceps

PROCEDURE STEPS (Follow aseptic procedures)

1. The patient is seated and prepared for the procedure. Confirm the procedure and review the medical history.

2. Rinse the patient's mouth, dry the injection site, and place the topical anesthetic (EF). Prepare the syringe. When the dentist comes in, remove the topical anesthetic applicator and transfer the mouth mirror and explorer to the dentist. After receiving the mirror and explorer, the anesthetic syringe is transferred to the operator. Following the administration of the local anesthetic, rinse the patient's mouth.

3. The shade is determined for the composite material before the placement of the rubber dam (Figure 26-35). Under natural light, the dentist compares a shade guide to the patient's teeth. A shade or combination of shades is selected to match the patient's teeth as closely as possible. The shade is recorded on the patient's chart for further reference.

4. The dental dam is placed by the dental assistant or with the dental assistant helping the dentist.

(continued)

P R O C E D U R E   26-13 *continued*

FIGURE 26-35 Determining the shade before the procedure begins.

5. Transfer a mirror, high-speed handpiece, and bur to the dentist. Maintain visibility throughout the procedure by cleaning the mirror, retracting the tissues, and evacuating the area. During the cavity preparation, transfer instruments and change burs as indicated by the dentist.

6. When the cavity preparation is complete, rinse and dry the preparation. How close to the pulp the cavity preparation is determines the type of base or liner needed for protection. Mix the appropriate materials, usually a calcium hydroxide or glass ionomer liner, and hold the mixing pad, applicator, and 2 × 2 gauze near the patient's chin. After each application, wipe the instrument. If the materials need the light for the curing process, the curing light is prepared and positioned.

7. Transfer a brush or applicator tip containing the acid etching materials to the dentist, who applies it to the cavity preparation. The etchant is rinsed thoroughly after the recommended time.

8. The celluloid matrix strip is placed by the dentist. If required, a plastic wedge is also placed (the plastic wedges permit light curing of the bonding agent and the composite).

9. The bonding material is placed according to manufacturer's instructions. With some bonding resins, a **primer** or conditioner is placed before the bonding material.

10. Most composites are applied in a single-application syringe, which can be used to place the material directly into the cavity preparation. Sometimes, a composite placement instrument is used for placement. The matrix is held around the tooth to restore contour. If the material is light cured, it is placed in incremental layers and light cured after each layer is placed. The self-curing composites are mixed and placed in the cavity preparation. Within a few minutes, the material begins to chemically set.

11. Transfer cotton pliers to remove the wedge and the matrix strip. After receiving these items, an explorer is transferred to check the restoration.

12. Transfer the low-speed handpiece with finishing bur to the dentist. When the dentist is using the handpiece, use the air syringe. Finishing burs, diamonds, and abrasive discs may be used to finish the composite restoration. Abrasive strips may be used to smooth the interproximal areas. Composite polishing points, discs, and cups are then used to smooth the restoration (Figure 26-36).

13. The dental dam is removed carefully and the oral cavity is rinsed.

14. Transfer the mirror and explorer to the dentist for examination, dry the tooth, receive the mirror and explorer, and pass the articulating paper. The occlusion is checked and any high marks are removed. The patient's mouth is rinsed and the patient is given postoperative instructions.

FIGURE 26-36 Polishing burs and abrasive strip for composites.

Composites are mainly packaged as one-paste systems that are light cured. The paste may come in a syringe for multiple applications or in single-dose cartridges that are used with a syringe (Figure 26-37). The pastes also come in a variety of shades. A specific shade guide comes with the composite systems to assist in the selection of a shade that matches the patient's natural dentition.

The pulp can be protected with a cavity liner before the acid etching, bonding, and composite placement steps.

Often, a plastic or Teflon-tipped filling instrument is used to place and shape the composite. These instruments come in various sizes and shapes to aid in adapting the composite material to the cavity preparation.

Modifications

Procedure 26-13 is for a Class III restoration. Some modifications to the procedure may be required for Classes I, II, IV, and V. Most of the procedures are similar, but there are a few changes or considerations.

Classes I and II. Classes I and II are posterior restorations. The shade selection is not as critical with these restorations as it is with the anterior classes. The Class I restoration does not require a matrix, because only the occlusal surface is involved. With the Class II restorations, some operators prefer the clear matrix band, which is used with a retainer, and wedges, which facilitate the light-curing process.

Some anatomy may be carved into the composite before the final curing. Discs may be difficult to use in some areas, but diamonds, finishing burs, and polishing points are used to smooth and finish the restoration.

Class IV. Class IV anterior restorations involve the proximal surface and the incisal edge. In some cases,

retention pins are required because of the amount of lost tooth structure. The pins are positioned once the tooth is prepared, before the placement of the composite material.

A matrix strip or preformed celluloid crown form can be used to mold the composite (Figure 26-38). If the celluloid crown form is used, the dentist places the composite into the cavity preparation in layers, curing after each step. A crown form is filled partially and placed over the cured resin in the preparation to form the incisal angle of the restoration. The crown form is prepared with a small hole placed in the incisal edge to prevent air from being trapped. Excess material is removed, and the curing light is used to harden the composite.

After the material is cured, the crown form is removed and the final shaping and finishing are completed with finishing burs, polishing discs, and strips.

Class V. Class V gingival one-third restoration may not require a matrix strip. A precontoured matrix may be used, or a matrix may not be used at all. The restorative materials can be placed in the cavity preparation and shaped with a plastic or composite filling instrument, then light cured. Finishing should be minimal with these restorations.

GLASS IONOMER RESTORATIONS

Type II glass ionomer materials are used as an esthetic restoration most often in non-stress bearing restorations. Examples include restoring the gingival one-third and root surface cavities. These materials are not suitable for areas that require strength or where esthetics are critical.

Resin Ionomers

The combination of the composite resins and glass ionomers have improved the qualities of the glass ionomer restorations. They are used for Class III and V

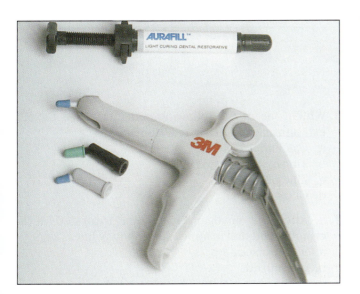

FIGURE 26-37 Composite syringes and cartridges.

FIGURE 26-38 Celluloid matrix strip with metal clip.

restorations. They come in various shades and are light-cured materials.

The technique for placement is similar to that for composites, with the following exceptions. The tooth is conservatively prepared with no need for mechanical retention or bevels. A retraction cord may be placed with the Class V preparations to expose the entire margin of the cavity preparation. The preparation is cleaned with a chlorhexidine soap solution. Follow the manufacturer's directions on the finishing and polishing of the restoration. Some need to be kept moist or have lubricants placed when polishing. A layer of light-cured enamel bonding agent is applied over the finished restoration.

CHAPTER SUMMARY

The general chairside assistant prepares and mixes the material, while the dentist places the material in the oral cavity. Some states allow the assistant to also place some of the materials in the oral cavity. Knowledge of the properties of the dental material is necessary for the dental assistant to properly prepare and manipulate the materials. The dental assistant's knowledge of dental materials is beneficial for patient education and protection. Expanded-functions dental assistants must understand and be competent in the placement and finishing of the materials.

CASE STUDY

Charlotte Larson needs to replace several restorations in her maxillary molars. Over the years, she has had numerous amalgam restorations placed throughout her mouth. Although Charlotte has never had any trouble, she is concerned after reading articles about restorations containing mercury. She also is interested in more natural-looking restorations.

Case Study Review

1. List some of the concerns Charlotte may have read regarding restorations containing mercury.

2. What information could the dental assistant give to Charlotte in response to her concerns? What resources are available for information?

3. Are there any alternative restorative materials available for Charlotte?

 To complete your study of this chapter, work the review activities that follow. Also, refer to the software that accompanies this text.

REVIEW QUESTIONS

Multiple Choice

1. The reaction of the object to resist external force is called
   a. strain.
   b. stress.
   c. shearing.
   d. elasticity.

2. All of the following are uses of dental cements except
   a. permanent luting.
   b. high-strength base.
   c. temporary filling.
   d. permanent restoration.

3. Which one of the following cements, when mixed, exhibits an exothermic reaction?
   a. Calcium hydroxide.
   b. Zinc oxide eugenol.
   c. Zinc phosphate.
   d. Glass ionomer.

4. If, after the amalgam has been triturated, it is crumbly and dull in appearance, it may have been
   a. undermixed.
   b. overmixed.
   c. exposed to moisture before mixing.
   d. mixed at too high a speed.

5. Of the composite materials, the material that finishes to the highest luster and resists wear due to abrasion is the
   a. fine fill composite.
   b. microfill composite.
   c. hybrid composite.

Critical Thinking

1. Give two examples of thermal conductivity relating to dentistry.

2. How is the amount of powder and liquid that is dispensed determined?

3. Would cavity varnish be placed under or over calcium hydroxide? Explain your answer.

Laboratory Materials and Techniques

OBJECTIVES

The student should strive to meet the following objectives and demonstrate an understanding of the facts and principles presented in this chapter:

1. Identify the materials used in the dental laboratory and perform the associated procedures.

2. Demonstrate the knowledge and skills needed to prepare, take, and remove alginate impressions and wax bites.

3. Demonstrate the knowledge and skills necessary to prepare reversible hydrocolloid impression material for the dentist.

4. Demonstrate the knowledge and skills necessary to prepare elastomeric impression materials such as polysulfide, silicone (polysiloxane and polyvinyl siloxanes), and polyether for the dentist.

5. Demonstrate the knowledge and skills necessary to use gypsum products such as Type I: Impression plaster; Type II: Laboratory or model plaster; Type III: Laboratory stone; Type IV: Die stone; and Type V: High-strength die stone.

6. Demonstrate the knowledge and skills necessary to pour and trim a patient's alginate impression (diagnostic cast).

7. Identify the use of a dental articulator for dental casts or study models.

8. Identify the different classifications and uses of waxes used in dentistry.

9. Demonstrate the knowledge and skills necessary to fabricate acrylic tray resin self-curing and light-curing custom trays, vacuum-formed, and thermoplastic custom trays.

10. Demonstrate the knowledge and skills necessary to contour prefabricated temporary crowns and to fabricate and fit custom temporary restorations.

KEY TERMS

accelerates (p. 591)

articulator (p. 606)

calcination (p. 596)

catalyst (p. 591)

distortion (p. 591)

exothermic reaction (p. 596)

gel (p. 582)

gypsum (p. 596)

homogenous (p. 611)

imbibition (p. 582)

irreversible hydrocolloid (p. 582)

monomer (p. 609)

polymer (p. 609)

polymerization (p. 591)

polysulfide (p. 591)

reversible hydrocolloid (p. 590)

silicones (p. 591)

sol (p. 582)

study models (p. 587)

syneresis (p. 582)

thermoplastic (p. 609)

undercuts (p. 609)

INTRODUCTION

A number of materials are used by dental assistants specifically in the dental laboratory that are not used in the dental treatment room. Some other materials are used initially in the treatment room and then taken by the dental assistant to the laboratory, where a second procedure is completed. Many of the models are taken to an in-office dental laboratory, where the laboratory technician completes the procedures or the models are sent out to a commercial dental laboratory for additional procedures to be completed.

Any dental assistant who has skills in performing laboratory duties is an asset to his or her employer. The better cross-trained the dental team members are, the better the dental office functions. A number of basic functions in the dental laboratory are routinely performed by the dental assistant, such as pouring and trimming study models, fabricating custom trays, and fabricating provisional temporaries. To accomplish these procedures, the dental assistant must understand the materials that are used, the properties of each material, and the steps in each procedure.

HYDROCOLLOID IMPRESSION MATERIALS

Impressions are taken to reproduce an accurate three-dimensional duplicate of an individual's teeth and surrounding tissues. The impression makes a negative reproduction where gypsum material can be poured and therefore creates a completed positive model. Varying degrees of accuracy can be obtained depending on the type of impression material and gypsum used. The operator gives directions to the dental assistant on the type of model that is desired. Models can be used for many purposes. One of the most common models that the dental assistant will make is the study cast or primary model. Normally, the impression material used is irreversible hydrocolloid, which is commonly called alginate.

Alginate (Irreversible Hydrocolloid) Impression Material

Alginate is a generic name used for a group of **irreversible hydrocolloid** impression materials. Alginate is used when less accuracy is needed. One of the most common areas in which alginate is used is in making diagnostic casts or study models. Alginate impression material is used routinely in making opposing models for fixed and removable prosthetics, orthodontic appliances, mouth guards, bleach trays, provisional restorations, and custom trays.

Alginate material's primary ingredient is potassium alginate, therefore giving the generic name to the material. **Potassium alginate** is extracted from seaweed and kelp, which is a marine growth found primarily off the coastline of Japan. This material readily dissolves in water to form a viscous **sol** (liquid). Added to this potassium alginate is a calcium sulfate which, through a chemical reaction, forms a **gel** (solid). To control the setting time and allow for the material to be placed in a tray and into the patient's mouth, trisodium phosphate is added. Without this retarder, the material would be set before it could be inserted into the patient's mouth. A retarder slows the setting of the material. To increase the strength and stiffness and make up the bulk of the material, fillers are used. Some of the fillers that may be in alginate are diatomaceous earth, zinc oxide, color, and flavoring. The fillers constitute from one-half to three-quarters of the total composition of the material. A small amount of **potassium titanium fluoride** is added to the material to counteract a specific action of the alginate where it tends to soften the surface of the gypsum products, not allowing it to fully set on the surface.

Advantages and Disadvantages of Alginate. Alginate has a number of advantages that allows it to be widely used in the dental office. They include:

▶ Ease of manipulation

▶ Minimal equipment required

▶ Economical

▶ Meets the requirements for accuracy for a number of applications

▶ Rapid setting

▶ Comfort for the patient

▶ Can be used for both teeth and tissue impressions

▶ Withdraws over **undercuts** (recessed areas that are wider on the bottom than on the top) because of its elastic properties

The disadvantages of alginates primarily come from the loss of accuracy due to atmospheric conditions. If the impression is stored prior to pouring, it is susceptible to dimensional change due to loss or gain of water. If the impression looses water content due to heat, dryness, or exposure to air, it causes shrinkage. This condition is known as **syneresis** (sin-er-**EE**-sis). If the reverse happens and the impression takes on additional water and causes swelling, the impression will have a dimensional enlargement, known as **imbibition** (im-bah-**BIH**-shun). The material also can cause some tissue distortion due to its thickened consistency. Another disadvantage is that it is not as precise or accurate as some of the other materials on the market.

Setting Time for Alginate. The time from which the alginate powder material is mixed with water until it is completely set is called the **gelatin time**. The gelatin time is different depending on the type of material used. Most of the materials come in two types: Type I is a fast-set alginate and Type II is a regular-set alginate. The gelatin time for both is broken into two different increments. The first is the working time, where the dental assistant mixes the material to the desired consistency, loads it into the tray, and inserts and positions the tray into the patient's mouth. The working time for the regular set is approximately one minute and less than that for fast set. The second phase is the setting time, where the material remains in the patient's mouth and sets until the chemical reaction is completed, the gel is formed completely, and the tray is removed from the patient's mouth. Type I for both the working and setting times ranges from one to two minutes. Type II normally ranges from two to four and one-half minutes for both working and setting times. The setting times can be altered. The most convenient way to control the setting time is to adjust the temperature of the water. The suggested temperature of water to be used is room temperature (70°F or 21°C). If the temperature of the water is higher, there are shorter working and setting times. If the water is cooled, the working and setting times are longer. Warm weather causes the alginate to set more rapidly as well. Some offices refrigerate the water during hot humid times.

The choice of whether to use Type I or Type II is made according to the preference of the operator and the conditions of the patient needing the impression. The outcome of both materials is the same. Cases in which the slower material Type II is beneficial would be where the operator is working alone or the tray is going to be difficult to insert into the oral cavity in the correct position in the patient's mouth. The faster set, Type I, is beneficial where the patient is a child or where the patient has a problem with gagging and the tray needs to be removed as rapidly as possible for patient comfort.

Alginate Packaging, Storage, and Shelf Life.
Normally, alginate is purchased in air-tight plastic canisters the size of coffee cans (Figure 27-1). The powder may be inside, in a foil or plastic bag, to be placed in the container when ready for use. Along with the powder are the measuring devices for the powder and the water. Some of the canisters have built-in areas on the outside for the water-measuring devices. This makes it convenient for the dental assistant. Alginate can be bought in premeasured sealed bags, but it is much more costly and normally unnecessary because measuring the powder is not a difficult procedure.

It is important that alginate not be stored in an area that can have temperatures over 120°F because it causes loss of strength and lower resistance to deformation. If kept in an area where moisture can contaminate it, the material will demonstrate erratic setting times. Optimum storage is in a cool, dry place. Keeping the lid screwed tightly in place while not in use aids in prevention of unintentional moisture contamination. The normal shelf life for alginate materials is not more than one year.

Alginate Powder/Water Ratio.
All the alginate materials come with their own specific measuring devices for both the powder and the water. First, read

FIGURE 27-1 Foil bags and a plastic canister of alginate with measuring devices.

the manufacturer's directions for dispensing the material. The dispensing of each material may be slightly different. For instance, some of the materials direct that the powder be fluffed with the lid on prior to putting it into the powder scoop, while others may indicate that the powder should be packed into the scoop. This makes a definite difference regarding the amount of powder that is used. The water measure is normally a plastic cylinder with lines on it to indicate the amount of water for each scoop of powder. Normally, it takes two scoops of powder to two increments of water for each mandibular impression. Three of each is normally needed for the maxillary impression. (These can alter depending on the size of the patient's arches.)

It is important that the correct amounts of both powder and water are used. If a lower water-to-powder ratio transpires, a stiffer, thicker mix is produced. Along with being more difficult to use, the material has decreased detail, decreased ability to pull from undercuts, decreased flexibility, increased tissue displacement, rapid setting time, increased strength, and a mix that is not as uniform in consistency. If a higher water-to-powder ratio is used, the impression has a decreased resistance to deformation, decreased strength, and increased setting time. Both increases and decreases in spatulation affect the setting time and decrease the strength of the material.

Bowls and Spatulas Used for Alginate Impressions.
The operator can use a flexible rubber bowl and stiff spatula to mix alginate or a disposable bowl with built-in water measuring lines. The flexible rubber bowl allows easy mixing of the alginate but must be sterilized or disinfected after use. The disposable bowl comes with a disposabe spatula that can be used for mixing alginate at one end and mixing plaster at the other end. The disposable bowl and spatula can be thrown away and they eliminate the aseptic procedures required after contamination of the rubber bowl and spatula (Figures 27-2A and B).

(B)   Alginate bowl

FIGURE 27-2 (A) Bowl-Away and Spat-Away disposable bowl and spatula used for mixing alginate and plaster. (B) Bowl-Away and Spat-Away show the water measuring lines in the mixing bowl and the different ends of the disposable spatula: one for alginate and one for plaster. *(Courtesy of Millennium Advantage Products 1-888-798-5373)*

Trays Used for Alginate Impressions. Several trays are available for alginate impressions (Figure 27-3). Most commonly used are the perforated trays that come in metal and plastic. The trays have holes in them

FIGURE 27-3 An assortment of alginate trays.

for the material to ooze through and lock the impression material in the tray. If not using the perforated trays, the material may stay in the patient's mouth as the tray is removed. The impression then has to be retaken due to loss of accuracy from the flexible material coming loose from the rigid tray. Some operators use a rim lock tray in place of the perforated tray. The rim lock tray has a border around the top of it to aid in holding the material in place. This tray has no perforations in it. Both the perforated tray and the rim lock tray come in plastic and metal. The metal trays can be cleaned and reused after sterilization.

Whichever tray is used, the operator must make sure that the tray fits correctly in the patient's mouth. Selecting the correct tray is essential to obtaining an accurate impression. The trays come in several sizes. The operator first examines the patient's mouth and identifies a sterilized or disposable tray that he or she thinks will fit. The trays should be tried in the patient's mouth to ensure a correct fit and the proper comfort for the patient. The tray should extend 2 or 3 mm beyond the last molar area and below both the lingual and facial tooth surfaces. Keep in mind that there should be enough room for 2 mm of the alginate material between the tray and all surfaces of the teeth and tissue. If the size of the tray seems appropriate but the tray does not extend over the last molar area, utility wax strips can be used. The wax is placed in layers until the desired length is achieved. The wax also can be placed around the border of the tray to lengthen it on the lingual and facial areas and to provide more comfort for the patient (Figure 27-4). The process of placing the wax around the border of the tray is called **beading**.

Taking Alginate Impressions for Diagnostic Casts (Study Models).
In some states, dental assistants are allowed to take the alginate impressions, while in other states, the dental assistant can select the tray, mix the material, load the material into the tray, and pass the tray for the dentist to place in the patient's mouth.

FIGURE 27-4 Alginate tray with beading wax on the periphery. This aids in tray extension and comfort for the patient.

PROCEDURE

27-1 Preparing for an Alginate Impression

This procedure is performed by the dental assistant in the states where it is allowed. The materials are prepared and the alginate impression is taken on the maxillary and mandibular arches.

EQUIPMENT AND SUPPLIES

▶ Flexible spatula/broad blade or disposable spatula

▶ Flexible rubber bowl(s) or disposable bowl

▶ Alginate material with water and powder measuring devices

▶ Water

▶ Impression tray(s)

PROCEDURE STEPS (*Follow aseptic procedures*)

Patient Preparation

1. Health history is reviewed.
2. The patient is seated in an upright position with a patient napkin in place.
3. The patient's mouth is rinsed with water or mouth rinse to remove any food debris and to aid with removing thick saliva.
4. The procedure is explained to the patient.
5. The impression trays are tried in the oral cavity to determine the correct size.

Material Preparation

1. Wax is placed around the borders of the impression trays, if necessary, to extend the borders of the trays or to provide additional patient comfort (Figure 27-4).
2. The impression water (room temperature) is measured for the mandibular model, normally two calibrations of the water measurement device

supplied by the manufacturer. The water is placed in the flexible mixing bowl. NOTE: Place the water in the bowl first to ensure that all the powder is incorporated into the mixture.

> Taking the mandibular model first allows the patient to build confidence and feel more secure prior to the maxillary impression, which often causes more gagging.

3. Fluff the powder prior to opening the powder canister, if the manufacturer's directions indicate.
4. Fill the measure of powder by overfilling and then leveling off with the spatula (use the flat blade, not the edge blade of the spatula) to get an accurate measure. Dispense two corresponding scoops into a second flexible rubber bowl.
5. When ready, place the powder in the water.
6. Mix the water and powder first with a stirring motion. Then, mix by holding the bowl in one hand, rotating the bowl occasionally, and using the flat side of the spatula to incorporate the material through pressure against the side of the bowl (Figure 27-5). The mixing for Type I fast set is thirty to forty-five seconds; Type II regular set is one minute.
7. Upon completion, the mixture should be homogeneous and creamy. When the material is mixed correctly, load it into the impression tray. On the mandibular tray, the material should be loaded from both lingual sides (Figure 27-6). Use the flat side of the blade to condense the material firmly into the tray. If necessary to further smooth the surface, take a gloved hand, moisten, and smooth the top.

FIGURE 27-5 Mixing the alginate material in a flexible rubber bowl, pushing on the sides of the bowl to eliminate the incorporation of air bubbles.

FIGURE 27-6 Loading the mandibular alginate tray from the lingual side to eliminate air spaces.

PROCEDURE

27-2 Taking an Alginate Impression

Refer to Procedure 27-1, Preparing for an Alginate Impression, to identify the needed PPE, equipment, and supplies.

PROCEDURE STEPS (Follow aseptic procedures)

1. Facing the patient, retract the right cheek slightly.

2. Use the excess alginate material to rub onto the occlusal surfaces of the teeth in order to obtain more accurate anatomy.

3. Invert the impression tray so that the material is toward the teeth.

4. Turn the tray so that it passes through the lip opening with one side of the tray entering first, using the other hand to retract the opposite corner of the mouth.

5. When the tray is completely in the patient's mouth, center it above the teeth.

6. Lower the tray onto the teeth, placing the posterior area down first, leaving the impression tray slightly anterior.

7. Have the patient raise the tongue and move it side to side to ensure that the lingual aspect of the alveolar process is defined in the impression.

8. Pull out the lip from the center with other hand.

9. Finish placing the impression tray down and, as it is done, push slightly toward the posterior area with the tray. This pushes the impression material down into the patient's anterior vestibule area, therefore producing a good esthetic model. One area that often lacks detail in the impression is the anterior segment. By leaving the tray slightly anterior and pushing the tray toward the posterior and making sure the lip is out of the way, this problem can be overcome.

10. Allow the lip to cover the tray. It should be close to the handle portion of the tray.

11. Hold it in the patient's mouth with two fingers on the back of the tray, one on the right side, one on the left side, until set (Figure 27-7). Check the excess material around the edges of the impression tray, or in the bowl, to determine if the mate-

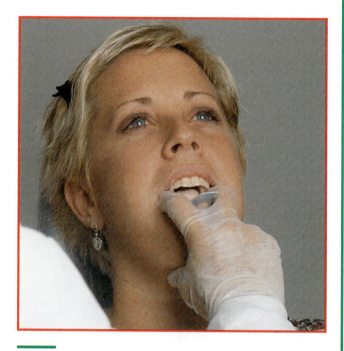

FIGURE 27-7 Holding the mandibular alginate tray in the patient's mouth, maintaining a stable force while the material is setting.

rial is set. The material should feel firm and not change shape when pushed.

12. The maxillary alginate impression is loaded from the posterior, making sure that the material completely fills the tray without voids (Figure 27-8A). Smooth the material (Figure 27-8B). Take a small amount of alginate out from the palate area to prevent the impression material from going down the patient's throat after insertion (Figure 27-8C). Place some alginate on the occlusal surfaces of the maxillary teeth.

13. Place the maxillary tray in the patient's mouth by turning the tray so that it passes through the lip opening with one side of the tray entering first, using the other hand to retract the opposite corner of the mouth (Figure 27-8D). Raise the tray to the maxillary arch and hold out the lip prior to seating the tray in place. Hold it in position until the material is set in the bowl (Figure 27-8E).

(continued)

PROCEDURE 27-2 continued

FIGURE 27-8 (A) Load the maxillary alginate tray from the posterior area. (B) Smooth the material. (C) Remove a small amount of alginate from the palate area prior to seating the tray in the patient's mouth. This aids in less material going down the back of the patient's throat. (D) Insert the tray into the mouth with one side first and then rotate the entire tray into the patient's mouth. (E) Hold the tray in position until the material is set.

Wax Bite Registration

A wax bite registration is taken to establish the relationship between the maxillary and the mandibular teeth. It can be used to verify the occlusal relationship when trimming the diagnostic casts (**study models**). Normally, wax that is formed in a horseshoe shape is used, but the flat sheets of utility wax can be used as well.

Other materials are used in taking a bite. Polysiloxane impression material, specifically designed for occlusal registration, can be dispensed using a dispensing gun and cartridge tip. It is dispensed directly onto the occlusal surface, and the patient is asked to close in the normal biting position and remain closed until the material sets, normally within two minutes. The set material is removed, disinfected, stored, and used to establish the patient's occlusal relationship.

Accuracy of an Alginate Impression

▶ The tray covers all the necessary areas.
▶ The tray is centered on the central incisors.
▶ The tray is not pushed down or up too far, allowing the teeth to penetrate through the material to the tray.
▶ The impression is not torn.
▶ The impression is free of bubbles and voids.
▶ The impression shows sharp anatomic detail of all the teeth and tissues.
▶ The impression has a good "peripheral roll" and includes all the vestibule areas.
▶ The mandibular impression shows good detail in the retramolar area and shows lingual frenum and the mylohyoid ridge area.
▶ The maxillary impression shows good detail in the tuberosities and palate areas.

P R O C E D U R E

27-3 Removing the Alginate Impression

Refer to Procedure 27-1, Preparing for an Alginate Impression, to identify the needed PPE, equipment, and supplies.

PROCEDURE STEPS (*Follow aseptic procedures*)

1. When the material is completely set, remove it from the mouth by first loosening the tissue of the lips and cheek around the periphery with fingers to break the suction-like seal.

2. Place fingers of the opposing hand on the opposite arch to protect the adjacent arch as the tray is being removed.

3. Remove the tray in an upward or downward motion (depending on the arch) with a quick snap. Turn it to the side to allow it to be removed from the oral cavity.

4. Remove any excess alginate material from the patient's mouth with the evacuator and have the patient rinse. Check the patient's face for any excess alginate material. If present, give the patient a tissue and mirror to remove the material.

5. Check the impression for accuracy (Figure 27-9).

6. Rinse the impression gently with water to remove saliva or blood.

FIGURE 27-9 The alginate impression is checked for accuracy after removal from the patient's mouth.

7. Spray with approved surface disinfectant.

8. If there is a time lapse (maximum of twenty minutes) prior to pouring, wrap the alginate impression in an air-tight container or a moist towel and place it in a plastic bag labeled with the patient's name. If the impression is placed in a wet towel for an extended period of time, imbibition (taking up of additional moisture) may occur.

P R O C E D U R E

27-4 Disinfecting Alginate Impressions

This procedure is performed by the dental assistant immediately after removing the alginate impressions from the patient's mouth and caring for the patient.

EQUIPMENT AND SUPPLIES

▶ Approved disinfectant

▶ Covered container

PROCEDURE STEPS (*Follow aseptic procedures*)

1. Rinse the impressions gently under tap water to remove any debris, blood, or saliva.

2. Spray the impressions with an approved disinfectant (See Chapter 9, Infection Control).

3. If not pouring immediately, place the impressions in a covered container.

4. Label the container with the patient's name.

27-5 Taking a Bite Registration

This procedure is performed by the dental assistant under the direction of the dentist or by the dentist with the dental assistant assisting.

EQUIPMENT AND SUPPLIES

▶ Bite registration wax or wax horseshoe or polysiloxane and extruder gun and disposable tips

▶ Laboratory knife

▶ Warm water or torch

PROCEDURE STEPS *(Follow aseptic procedures)*

1. The patient remains seated in an upright position with a patient napkin in place after the impressions are taken.

2. The procedure is explained.

3. The bite registration wax is tried in to determine correct length. If correction is needed, the laboratory knife is used to trim off the excess.

4. The patient is instructed to practice biting to establish occlusion.

5. The bite registration wax is heated in warm water or with a torch to soften.

6. The wax is placed on the mandibular occlusal surface of the patient. If using polysiloxane, the bite registration material is extruded from the disposable tip directly onto the occlusal surface of the mandibular teeth (Figure 27-10A).

7. The patient is instructed to bite together gently in the correct occlusion.

8. The wax will cool in one to two minutes while the patient keeps the teeth together in occlusion. If using polysiloxane, the patient gently occludes until the material sets (Figure 27-10B).

9. The wax or polysiloxane bite is then removed gently without distortion.

10. The wax or polysiloxane bite registration is disinfected, labeled and stored for use during trimming of the diagnostic casts (Figure 27-10C).

(A)

(B)

(C)

FIGURE 27-10 (A) Bite registration material is extruded from the tip directly onto the occlusal surface of the mandibular teeth. (B) Patient gently occludes until material sets. (C) Wax bite, or polysiloxane bite, taken on a patient for use in establishing the patient's occlusion.

Reversible Hydrocolloid Impression Material (Agar-Agar)

One of the first impression materials that has good detail and is used for final impressions is **reversible hydrocolloid** impression material, sometimes referred to as agar-agar. The composition for this material is somewhat similar to alginate in that the main component is derived from seaweed and kelp. It also has fillers, additives, coloring, and flavoring. The unique difference between reversible and irreversible hydrocolloid material is the setting reaction. The setting of the irreversible hydrocolloid (alginate) is accomplished by a chemical reaction. Reversible hydrocolloid changes from a gel to a sol and back again due to thermal reaction. The material begins in a gel (solid) state and, after boiling in a hydrocolloid conditioner unit for ten minutes, it becomes liquid and remains in that state for hours if placed in a water storage bath of 150°F or 66°C until the operator is ready to use it. Five minutes before taking the impression, the tray material is moved into a water bath of 110°F or 45°C. It is further cooled in the mouth as cool water flows through the water trays, connected to hoses at the dental unit. Most units have two water connectors where the hoses can be attached.

Advantages and Disadvantages of Reversible Hydrocolloid.

The primary advantage of using reversible hydrocolloid is the accuracy of the impression. The accuracy is more precise and more detailed than that for alginate, irreversible hydrocolloid, and reversible hydrocolloid can be used for impressions for crown and bridge construction. This material can be used for impressions for both teeth and tissue. It is more economical than many materials on the market for final impressions, after the initial equipment has been purchased.

The disadvantage is the additional equipment needed to prepare the material. In addition, reversible hydrocolloid can lose accuracy due to atmospheric conditions. The preparation and setting time is increased to ten minutes. This material was used widely in earlier years and now has declined some, due to the emergence of a number of elastomeric materials available with similar accuracy.

Reversible Hydrocolloid Packaging and Equipment.

The tray material is supplied in collapsible plastic tubes (Figure 27-11). The syringe material is supplied in either cylinders in a jar or syringe carpules. Both materials come in several colors and strengths. Special water-cooled trays and attachment hoses to circulate the water must be used with this material.

A hydrocolloid conditioner unit is used to prepare the material for use. This electric unit has three compartments (Figure 27-12). As with all equipment and material, read the directions and specific time for the material to be placed in each compartment. Normally, a timer is built into the conditioner. Each compartment in the conditioning unit is filled with clean water. The first com-

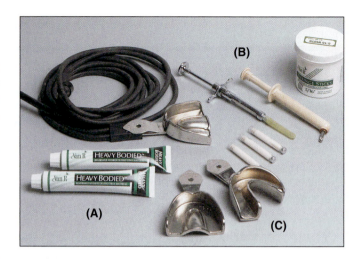

FIGURE 27-11 Hydrocolloid. (A) Tubes. (B) Syringes and cartridges. (C) Trays used with the hydrocolloid conditioning unit to obtain final impressions.

partment on the left, facing the unit, is for boiling the material. The tubes are placed, with the lids tight and upside down, in the unit. The syringe material is placed in a holding case for the cartridges or inside the boiling syringes if cylinders are used. The material must stay in the syringes or tubes or it will disperse throughout the water and be unusable. There, the material is boiled for ten minutes. The digital machines can be set to start the timer for ten minutes as soon as the boiling temperature is reached. If not using a digital machine, the dental assistant has to monitor the boiling temperature and time carefully. After the boiling process is complete, the temperature drops to the preset storage temperature.

The second compartment is the storage compartment. After the tubes and syringe material is boiled, it is

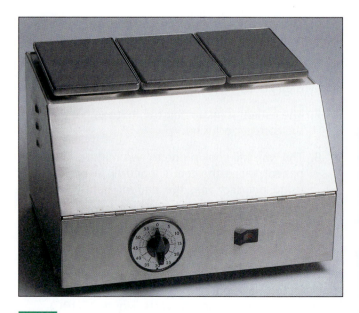

FIGURE 27-12 Hydrocolloid conditioning unit with boiling bath, storage bath, and conditioning bath. *(Courtesy of Van R)*

moved to the middle compartment for storage. In this compartment, the temperature is set to maintain the material in a liquid state. The material can stay in this compartment for hours or days before use.

The third compartment on the right, facing the unit, is for the tray material only. The material is placed in a water-cooled tray and then placed in the compartment to be tempered for five minutes. This cools the material so that it does not burn the patient's mouth upon insertion. The syringe material remains in the fluid state to get into the crevices around the prepared tooth and obtain the necessary anatomy on the adjacent teeth. Because of the small opening in the syringe, the amount coming from the syringe cools rapidly as it is used.

The hydrocolloid conditioner unit requires very little maintenance. The compartments should be emptied and rinsed out on a regular basis and then wiped with a soft cloth and refilled with clean water. A condition cleaner can be placed in the compartments and left for one hour to remove any buildup. The cleaner is then rinsed out prior to placing clean water in the compartments.

ELASTOMERIC IMPRESSION MATERIALS

Elastomeric impression materials have rubber-like qualities and are used for areas that require precise duplication. The materials in this classification are not as affected by the atmospheric changes as the hydrocolloids. They are more elastic and rubber-like when set, therefore allowing the removal from the mouth to take place without tearing and distortion. **Distortion** is a dimensional change in shape. There are three primary groups of materials in this classification: polysulfide, silicone (polysiloxane and polyvinyl siloxanes), and polyether. Each group has slightly different properties and characteristics, even though they all have the elastic qualities. All the materials have a catalyst and base that are mixed together to start the chemical self-curing process. The **catalyst** is the ingredient that **accelerates** or starts the process of setting the material. The process by which the catalyst and accelerator begin to cure and the material changes from a paste to an elastic, rubber-like material is called **polymerization**. The accelerator is dispensed as a paste from a small tube or in liquid form from a bottle with a dropper. The **base** that makes up the volume of the material is normally dispensed in a paste. Often, the tube openings of base and catalyst are different sizes, with the catalyst tube opening being smaller. Many of the materials are now dispensed in an "extruder gun" with a mixing tip. The mixing tip brings together the correct amount of each material and dispenses it, premixed (Figure 27-13). If this technique is used, there is no need for a mixing pad and spatula. A new tip is required for each application and the material must be purchased in special cartridges.

FIGURE 27-13 Extruder gun cartridge and tips used in mixing and dispensing material.

Polysulfide

Polysulfide impression materials have been around a long time and may be called mercaptan or rubber-base materials. They are supplied in two pastes: a base and a catalyst. The base is the larger tube and the white color of the two pastes. It is made from liquid polysulfide polymer (thiodol polysulfide rubber) with filler added. The dark brown accelerator is made from lead peroxide. These pastes can be purchased as light (syringe material), regular, heavy, and extra heavy (tray material).

The advantages of the polysulfide material include relative stability after the final set has been achieved, good accuracy, sharpness of detail, and a relatively long shelf life (several years). It is advisable to pour the polysulfide impression within an hour, but impressions have been known to be left for days prior to pouring with no noticeable change in dimension. The disadvantages of polysulfide are the odor (it smells like sulfur because of the base), taste, staining (it permanently stains cloths because of the accelerator), and the relatively long setting time (ten minutes is required from the start of the mix to the setting of the material prior to removal from the patient's mouth). The time can be accelerated slightly due to increased temperature, moisture, and an increased amount of accelerator.

Silicone (Polysiloxane and Polyvinal Siloxanes)

One material group that has had the greatest growth has been the silicones. A number of new materials have emerged onto the market from this group. **Silicones** have the advantages of polysulfide without the disadvantages. They are more expensive than the polysulfide, however. Advantages of the material include high accuracy, no shrinkage, dimensional stability, high tear resistance, no taste, and no odor.

P R O C E D U R E

27-6 Taking a Polysulfide Impression

This procedure is performed by the dentist with the dental assistant assisting. This procedure can be a four- or six-handed procedure. Everyone should wear some protective overclothing. Polysulfide is a material used in taking final impressions for which extreme accuracy is required.

EQUIPMENT AND SUPPLIES

▶ Two rigid, tapered, laboratory spatulas

▶ Paper pad, provided by the manufacturer

▶ Two pastes each (two syringes, two trays) from the same manufacturer (a base and an accelerator of the syringe material and a base and an accelerator of the tray material)

▶ Impression syringe with tip in place and plunger out of the cylinder

▶ Custom tray that has been painted with corresponding adhesive and permitted to dry

PROCEDURE STEPS *(Follow aseptic procedures)*

1. Health history is reviewed.

2. The patient is seated in an upright position with a patient napkin in place and a large drape over the clothes.

3. The patient's mouth is rinsed with water or a mouth rinse to remove any food debris and aid with removing thick saliva.

4. The procedure is explained to the patient.

5. The material is mixed concurrently by two individuals. The syringe material is mixed slightly ahead of the tray material.

6. Dispense the accelerator onto the pad in a long, even line about four inches long. If more material is needed, additional lines can be placed together on the paper pad. NOTE: Be sure to wipe the end of the tube before placing the lid back on to prevent mess and sticking of the top.

7. Dispense the base onto the pad in a long, even line the same length as the accelerator (Figure 27-14). Additional lines can be dispensed, but they should not touch the accelerator until the

FIGURE 27-14 The polysulfide material is dispensed and ready to mix. The lines are of equal length, but the amount of material is different.

operator wants the process of polymerization to begin.

8. When ready, the individual with the syringe material begins the mixing by first gathering up the accelerator with the spatula and placing it in the base material. Spatulate the pastes together with broad sweeps. After a minute has lapsed, the individual mixing the tray material begins the same process.

9. When the mix is homogeneous and lacks brown or white streaks, it is completely mixed. This process takes from forty-five seconds to one minute.

10. The syringe material is then loaded into an impression syringe using the back portion or the working end nozzle of the barrel and pushing the syringe over the material repeatedly to force the material into the chamber (Figure 27-15). When the material is in the syringe chamber, wipe the edges quickly and place the plunger in the syringe. Extrude the material slightly to make sure it is working and pass it to the dentist.

11. The tray material is mixed to the same consistency and within the same time frame. The bulk of the tray material is picked up by the spatula and loaded into the impression tray and spread evenly.

(continued)

P R O C E D U R E   2 7 - 6 *continued*

FIGURE 27-15 Loading the mixed polysulfide syringe material into the syringe for placement directly around the prepared tooth.

The tray is then transferred to the dentist after the syringe has been used. The mixing and loading (working time) must be completed within four minutes.

12. The impression must remain in the patient's mouth, held by the operator or the dental assistant, for six minutes in order to achieve a final set.

13. Cleanup is accomplished after the material has reached the rubber stage. The material peels off the spatula. The paper pad normally has a corner for the spatula to fit under to aid in removing the soiled top sheet (Figure 27-16). The disposable impression syringe and paper sheet can be disposed of and the spatula sterilized.

14. The removal of the tray is done in much the same manner as was the alginate. Remove the impression after releasing the seal, taking care to protect the opposing teeth from the quick snap.

FIGURE 27-16 The polysulfide material provides for easy cleanup after it is set. The paper pad has a precut corner to allow the easy insertion of the spatula for cleanup and disposal.

The material comes in a number of different forms. It is available in putty form for making a custom tray, in tubes of base and accelerator (catalyst) for injection, and regular and heavy type for impressions. It also is available in the cartridge form to be used with the mixing tip and extruding gun (automix cartridge system).

The putty material comes in two different colors. Each container of putty has a colored scoop that is used for either the base or the catalyst (Figure 27-17). Do not mix up the scoops because doing so will contaminate the material and cause the polymerization process to start, making the material hard and useless. The material is dispensed with an equal volume of base and catalyst putties. The putty is much like Silly Putty used by children. It is kneaded and mixed quickly until a homogeneous color is achieved. This mixing takes about thirty seconds. Mixing putty with latex gloves will adversely affect the set of some materials—Read the directions. The silicone is placed in the tray, covered with a thin plastic sheet, and placed in the patient's mouth or over the model. It takes about three minutes for the material to harden. Remove the plastic, and a custom tray is ready for the impression material. The putty material is not suitable for detailed impressions.

FIGURE 27-17 Two scoops of the putty or putty and tube of accelerator are dispensed for easy incorporation.

P R O C E D U R E

27-7 Taking a Silicone (Polysiloxane) Two-Step Impression

This procedure is performed by the dentist with the dental assistant assisting. Silicone (polysiloxane) is a material used in taking final impressions for which extreme accuracy is required.

EQUIPMENT AND SUPPLIES

▶ Spatula

▶ Paper mixing pad

▶ Vinyl overgloves

▶ Two containers of putty (one base and one catalyst) with color-coordinated scoops or one putty base and liquid dropper of catalyst (Figure 27-18)

▶ Stock tray with adhesive painted on the interior

▶ Plastic sheet for use as a spacer

▶ Extruder gun, mixing tip with intraoral delivery tip or injection syringe (Figure 27-18)

▶ Cartridges of impression material (light-body or wash material)

PROCEDURE STEPS *(Follow aseptic procedures)*

Patient Preparation

1. Health history is reviewed.

2. The patient is seated in an upright position with a bib in place.

FIGURE 27-18 Extruder gun, mixing tips, and cartridges of impression material. *(Courtesy of Kerr Corporation)*

3. The retraction cord is placed around the prepared tooth.

4. The procedure is explained.

Preliminary Putty Impression

1. Place on vinyl gloves.

2. Either equal scoops of the putty are mixed together or putty base and drops of catalyst are mixed together. The putty must be kneaded together until a homogenous mixture is obtained within the manufacturer's recommended time. Normally, this time is thirty seconds. The mixture must be one even color with no streaks.

3. After the material is mixed, pat it into a patty and load it into the prepared tray. With a finger, make a slight indentation where the teeth are located.

4. Place the plastic spacer sheet over the material and insert it into the patient's mouth. The objective is to create 2 mm of space for the final syringeable viscous impression material.

5. The setting of the putty takes about three minutes. The tray is then removed from the patient's mouth, the spacer is removed, and the putty is checked for accuracy and left to set further.

Final Impression

1. After the tooth has been prepared, the area cleaned and dried, the retraction cord placed, and the doctor indicates that he or she is ready for the final impression, prepare the material.

2. The tray with the preliminary impression is ready with the spacer removed. The extruder gun is prepared and loaded with the light-body or wash material.

3. The syringe (light-body) material is extruded through the mixing tip and placed in the preliminary impression (Figure 27-19).

4. The tip is wiped off and an intraoral delivery tip placed on for direct injection around the prepared tooth after the retraction cord has been removed. The extruder gun is transferred to the

(continued)

P R O C E D U R E   2 7 - 7 *continued*

FIGURE 27-19 The syringe material is extruded from the extruding gun into the prepared tray.

dentist. Instead of using the intraoral delivery tip, some dentists prefer to use an injection syringe, which can be loaded with the mixing tip.

5. The tray is seated by the dentist immediately into place and held steady for three to five minutes, depending on the material used.

6. After the material has set, the impression tray is removed after releasing the seal and taking care to protect the opposing teeth from the quick snap.

7. Immediately rinse the impression under water and lightly air blow dry. Disinfect according to manufacturer's directions.

8. Impressions should be poured immediately but can be poured up to weeks later and still remain dimensionally stable.

When ready for the impression, the tray is loaded by the operator squeezing the dispenser handle of the extruding gun and engaging the plunger. The plunger enters the cartridge and extrudes the material through the mixing tip and into the putty material in the impression tray. The syringe material can also be injected from the mixing tip into the impression syringe for use around the sulcus of the tooth. When ready, the tray is placed in the patient's mouth and immobilized until set (three and one-half minutes for a fast set and five minutes for a regular set). The impression is removed after the seal is loosened and the opposing teeth are protected. The impression is run under cold water and sprayed with disinfectant. The impression is very stable and can be poured weeks later. The total time from mixing to the final set is from four to six minutes.

Light-cured impression materials are also available. The advantage of this material is that the setting time is controlled by the operator. The disadvantage is that it is sometimes difficult to move the curing light over the complete surface of the material. A clear-plastic impression tray must be used. The light must hit all areas in order to bring about the curing. The light acts as a catalyst to set up the material.

Polyether

Polyether is another impression material used for crowns and bridges. It has excellent accuracy and dimensional stability. It is supplied in tubes as pastes, a larger one for the base and the smaller one for the catalyst. The material comes only in regular body and is stiffer than many of the other materials. It can be used for both the custom tray and the syringe. If used for a custom tray, a tray is chosen that is the correct size, painted with adhe-

sive, and allowed to dry for one minute. The material is dispensed on a paper pad, supplied by the manufacturer, one inch per tooth involved in the impression. Equal lengths of material are placed on the pad, not equal amounts (Figure 27-20). This material is then mixed by placing the catalyst in the base in a figure-eight motion and obtaining a homogenous mixture free of streaks. The mixing should not take longer than thirty seconds. When mixing is complete, the material is loaded onto the spatula and into the tray. The tray is seated by the dentist in the patient's mouth. After about two minutes of holding the impression in the patient's mouth, agitate the tray in

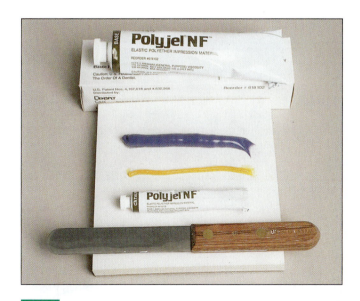

FIGURE 27-20 Polyether impression material is dispensed on the paper pad, ready to be mixed. The material is of equal lengths, not equal amounts.

all directions to make room for the final polyether impression material after the teeth are prepared. Remove the tray after three minutes.

To take the final impression after the teeth are prepared with polyether, dispense the material in a similar manner. Less material is needed because of the volume already in the preliminary tray. If a less viscous impression material is desired by the dentist, a thinner (or body modifier) can be added to the mixture. The catalyst and the modifier are mixed into the base material. The material is loaded into an injection syringe, and the excess material is placed in the preliminary impression (Figure 27-21). The impression tray is then reinserted into the patient's mouth and held for four minutes to obtain an accurate impression. This technique can be accomplished in a one-step technique as well, eliminating the preliminary tray.

After the tray is loosened from the mouth and removed with a quick snapping motion, protecting the opposing arch, it is rinsed with cold water and then completely air dried. The impression can be disinfected with a 2 percent solution of glutaraldehyde for ten minutes.

GYPSUM MATERIALS

Several different **gypsum** materials are used when pouring an impression to make a model. It is important to identify the application for the material prior to determining the type of gypsum product to use. Gypsum materials vary in strength, dimensional accuracy, resistance, reproduction detail, water/powder ratio, and setting times.

The primary types of gypsum that are used in dentistry are:

▶ Type I: Impression plaster

▶ Type II: Model or laboratory plaster

FIGURE 27-21 Mixed polyether is loaded into a syringe.

▶ Orthodontic stone/combination of Type II: Model or laboratory plaster and Type III: Laboratory stone

▶ Type III: Laboratory stone

▶ Type IV: Die stone

▶ Type V: High-strength, high-expansion die stone

During the process of manufacturing the various types of plasters and stones, the gypsum product (which is mined as a hard rock) is ground to a fine powder. It is then heated in large, cylindrical kettles equipped with agitators. The heating is controlled accurately and is continued until a specific amount of the water is driven out of the gypsum. This process is known as **calcination**. Several methods of calcination are used to derive the different stones and investment die stones. During this process, the gypsum, which is a calcium sulfate dihydrate (where there is one molecule of calcium sulfate to two molecules of water), is changed to a hemihydrate powder (one water molecule to every two molecules of calcium sulfate). Because both plaster and stone are white in color, yellow, blue, and pink pigments are added to the stone to make it easier to distinguish which material is being used.

The strengths of the gypsum products are determined by the calcination process and the water/powder ratio needed to incorporate the mixture. Plaster (beta hemihydrate) is gypsum particles that are larger and more irregular than the particles of stone (alpha hemihydrate) that have undergone further processing and transformed into more dense particles. It is important to follow the manufacturer's directions when mixing gypsum products. One of the chief obstacles to overcome when mixing gypsum products is the incorporation of the air and wetting each particle. Plaster particles are more irregular and require more water to wet each surface of each particle. The ratio of water to powder for plaster is 50 mL of water to 100 grams of powder; stone requires only 30 mL of water to 100 grams of powder. Die stones require even less water because the particles are smaller, less irregular, and more dense.

Incorporating the water is an important step in mixing the gypsum products. Using a flexible rubber bowl and a stiff spatula allows the operator to stir the viscous material and press against the sides of the bowl to eliminate any unnecessary air bubbles. Avoid whipping the powder and the water together, because doing so increases the air in the mixture. It should be mixed to a creamy, putty-like consistency. A grainy mixture will not pour into the impression. The incorporating and spatulating procedure should take about one minute. Overspatulating causes a breakdown of crystals and soft spots in the model.

Gypsum becomes set when the plaster or stone transforms back to the dihydrate through a chemical reaction. This process gives off heat, called an **exothermic reaction**. The temperature of the water increases or decreases the setting time. The hotter the water, the more rapidly the material sets. There are retarders such as borax and sodium citrate that can be added to the material to slow down the set. Potassium sulfate accelerates the setting time. The manufacturers add small concentrations of the retarders or accelerators to cause a decrease or an increase in the setting rate of the gypsum.

It is important to have the correct water-to-powder ratio. If less water is incorporated, the model can have greater setting expansion. It will have increased strength and hardness but may result in a thick mixture that becomes a dry, crumbly mass that cannot flow into the impression. At this stage, more water cannot be added to the mixture. It will need to be disposed of and a new mixture made. If too much water is incorporated into the mixture, the model will be weak, slow setting, and filled with air spaces. A plaster model will set in ten to twenty minutes and can be determined by feel. If the heat has dissipated, the model is set. It goes through a cycle and heats up and seems to perspire; then, the heat diminishes and the model is cool and dry. The final set occurs after twenty-four hours when the model reaches the optimum hardness. The gypsum powder is measured by weight and the water is calibrated by volume.

All gypsum products are packaged in some type of plastic bag or container to ensure that they do not become contaminated with moisture. If contaminated, the properties and the setting reaction may be altered. These plastic bags are normally further packaged in a cardboard box for easier handling.

Plaster

Plaster (plaster of paris) is a white gypsum referred to as beta-hemihydrate. It was one of the first gypsum products available to dentistry. It is the weakest and least expensive of the gypsum products. It is calcinated in an open kettle method, and the result is particles that are rough, irregular, and porous. The final product is a powder that, when mixed with water, reverts to a gypsum product or a dihydrate. Plaster takes more water to incorporate the powder into it. After the model dries and the water evaporates, the areas where the water was become air bubbles. This is the primary reason that plaster is weaker than stone. Stone is more compact and requires less water, therefore making a stronger model. Plaster is used in areas where detail and strength are not as important. Plaster is used to pour up study models, for opposing models, in mounting study models and casts, and for repairing casts.

Type I: Impression Plaster

Impression plaster (modified Type II: laboratory or model plaster) was used to take impressions prior to the newer, easy-to-manipulate impression materials now on the market. The plaster (Type I), mixed with a water-to-powder ratio of 60 mL of water to 100 grams of powder, is placed in the mouth carefully on the area to be duplicated, and then the operator must wait for the plaster to set. After the set (usually four to five minutes), the material is broken apart and reassembled in the laboratory. Because the material is so rigid, it fractures and breaks easily. Today, the material is rarely used for impressions. It is used primarily to mount casts on an articulator because of its quick setting time.

Type II: Laboratory or Model Plaster

Model plaster is used routinely in the dental office by the dental assistant to pour diagnostic casts or study models. It is slightly stronger than the Type I: impression plaster, because it requires a water-to-powder ration of 50 mL of water to 100 grams of powder, making the material less porous.

Type III: Laboratory Stone

Type III: laboratory stone is stronger than plaster and is used where more strength is needed. It requires 30 mL of water to 100 grams of powder, therefore making it denser, harder, and stronger. It is normally yellow in color due to the manufacturer's added pigments, more expensive than plaster, and referred to as alpha-hemihydrate. It is used for study models (diagnostic casts) that require more strength, working casts, and models for partial and full dentures.

Orthodontic Stone

Orthodontic stone is a mixture of laboratory or model plaster and laboratory stone. This white stone allows for a stronger model to be used for the diagnosis and treatment of orthodontic cases.

Type IV: Die Stone

Type IV: die stone is calcinated by autoclaving in the presence of calcium chloride. This modified alpha-hemihydrate is referred to as die stone. A die is a positive replica of the prepared tooth made from stone. It requires much less water (less than 24 mL to 100 grams of powder) to incorporate its small, uniform particles. More stone with less water and air makes the model strong and resistant to abrasion. It is used most often for dies or where a very strong model or cast is needed.

Type V: High-Strength, High-Expansion Die Stone

Recently, the ADA added a new material to its list of gypsum products. Type V: die stone requires from 18 to 22 mL of water to 100 grams of powder, making it the strongest accepted gypsum product available for use in the dental office.

Water-to-Powder Ratio Recommendations

Type I: Impression plaster	100 grams powder	to	60 mL water
Type II: Laboratory or model plaster	100 grams powder	to	50 mL water
Type III: Laboratory stone	100 grams powder	to	30 mL water
Type IV: Die stone	100 grams powder	to	24 mL water
Type V: Die stone	100 grams powder	to	18–22 mL water

P R O C E D U R E

27-8 Pouring an Alginate Impression with Plaster

This procedure is performed the dental assistant in the dental laboratory.

EQUIPMENT AND SUPPLIES (Figure 27-22)

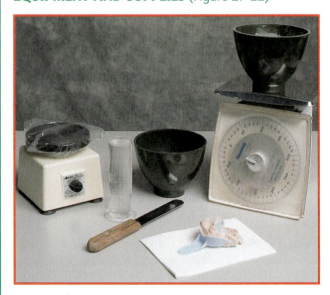

FIGURE 27-22 Equipment needed to pour plaster.

▶ Spatula, metal with rounded end and stiff, straight sides

▶ Two flexible rubber mixing bowls

▶ Scale

▶ Plaster (100 grams)

▶ Gram measuring device

▶ Water measuring device (calibrated syringe or vial)

▶ Vibrator with paper or plastic cover on the platform

▶ Room-temperature water

▶ Alginate impression (disinfected)

PROCEDURE STEPS (*Follow aseptic procedures*)

Mixing the Plaster

1. Measure 50 mL of room-temperature water into one of the flexible mixing bowls (Figure 27-23).

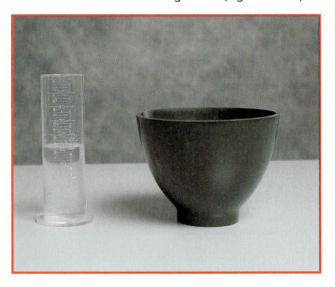

FIGURE 27-23 Measure 50 mL of water into a flexible mixing bowl.

(continued)

P R O C E D U R E   **2 7 - 8** *continued*

2. Place the second flexible mixing bowl on the scale and set the dial to zero. This allows the plaster powder to be weighed (Figure 27-24).

3. Weigh out 100 grams of plaster in the second rubber bowl.

4. Add the powder from the second bowl to the water of the first bowl. Placing the water in first allows for all the powder to become incorporated into the mixture. Allow several seconds for the powder to dissolve into the water.

5. Use the spatula to slowly mix the particles together. The initial mixing should be completed in twenty seconds. The total mixing procedure should take about one minute.

6. Turn on the vibrator to medium or low speed.

7. Place the rubber bowl on the vibrator platform, pressing lightly.

8. Rotate the bowl on the vibrator to allow the air bubbles to rise to the top surface (Figure 27-25). The mixing and vibrating should be completed within a couple of minutes. The mixture is ready if the spatula can cut through it and it stays to the sides without changing positions. It will appear like whipped cream with a smooth, creamy texture (Figure 27-26). Another way to check whether the powder/water is in correct ratio is to place a

spoonful on the spatula and turn it upside down. If the material remains in place, the mixture is ready.

NOTE: If the spatula is held sideways, any mixture will fall from it.

FIGURE 27-25 The vibrator brings the air bubbles to the surface of the plaster.

FIGURE 27-24 Measure 100 grams of plaster powder for pouring an alginate impression.

FIGURE 27-26 The consistency of plaster should allow for it to retain its position as the spatula slides through it.

P R O C E D U R E

27-9 Pouring an Alginate Impression for a Study Model

This procedure is performed by the dental assistant in the dental laboratory immediately after mixing the plaster. The impression is ready to pour, the excess moisture is removed, and a laboratory knife has been used to eliminate any excess impression material that will hamper the pouring of the model.

EQUIPMENT AND SUPPLIES

▶ Metal spatula (stiff blade with rounded end) or disposable spatula

▶ Mixed plaster from Procedure 27-8, Pouring an Alginate Impression with Plaster

▶ Vibrator with paper towel or plastic cover on platform

PROCEDURE STEPS *(Follow aseptic procedures)*

1. Use the vibrator at low or medium speed.

2. Hold the impression by the handle with the tray portion on the platform of the vibrator. Allow a small amount of plaster to touch the most distal surface of one side of the arch in the impression (Figure 27-27).

3. When the plaster touches the impression that is on the vibrating platform, it flows down the back of the impression and into the anatomy of the teeth. Continue to add small increments of the plaster in the same area as the plaster flows around toward the anterior teeth and to the other side of the arch. (Using this technique allows the air to push ahead of the plaster material and eliminates bubbles. This produces a model that has detailed anatomy qualities.)

4. Add the plaster in this manner until it flows out the other side of the impression and fills the anatomic portion of the model. Rotating the impression

FIGURE 27-27 The mixed plaster is vibrated into the alginate impression, starting at the posterior area of an arch and continuing to fill from that area while the material rotates around to the opposite side of the arch.

around on the platform of the vibrator aids in allowing the material to travel around the arch.

5. After the anatomy portion is filled with plaster, use larger increments to fill the entire impression, off the vibrator. When filled, place lightly on the vibrator to coalesce (combine). Overvibration can cause bubbles to form.

6. If a two-pour method is to be used, small blobs should be left on the top of the plaster so that it can attach to the art portion of the model. (A flat surface may break apart at a later date.)

Trimming and Finishing Diagnostic Casts

The diagnostic casts (study models) are used to present the case to the patient. It is important that they have an attractive appearance. Not only are they part of the

patient's permanent record, but they are also a direct reflection of the type of work the office performs for the patient. They can be trimmed in a geometric form that is pleasing in appearance. Standard guidelines are used in trimming the casts.

PROCEDURE

27-10 Pouring the Art Portion of a Plaster Study Model Using the Two-Pour Method

This procedure is performed by the dental assistant in the dental laboratory after the anatomical portion of the study model has set.

EQUIPMENT AND SUPPLIES

▶ Metal spatula (stiff blade with rounded end) or disposable spatula

▶ Flexible rubber bowl or disposable bowl

▶ Vibrator with a paper towel or plastic cover on the platform

▶ Paper towels

▶ Plaster

▶ Calibration measurement device

▶ Room-temperature water

▶ Water measuring device

PROCEDURE STEPS (*Follow aseptic procedures*)

1. After pouring the anatomical portion of the impression, allow it to set for five to ten minutes.

2. Wipe the rubber bowl and spatula with paper towel and dispose of the material. Wash, clean, and ready the rubber bowl and spatula for a second pour of plaster.

3. The ratio of powder to water can be altered to create a thicker mix, which is desirable for bases. If pouring the bases or art portion of both the maxillary and the mandibular casts, use 100 grams of powder to 40 mL of water. If pouring only one model, mix half the amount of powder and water.

4. Mix the plaster in the same manner as before. It will appear much thicker. This part of the model is not as crucial as the anatomical portion. Areas that have bubbles can be repaired easily.

5. Gather the plaster on the spatula and place it on a glass slab or a paper towel (Figure 27-28). It is important to allow the material to mass upward and not to spread out like a pancake.

6. After all the material is on the paper towel, invert the poured anatomy portion onto the base material.

7. Hold the tray steady and situate the handle so that it is parallel to the paper surface or glass slab. It is important to get a base that is even and uni-

FIGURE 27-28 Plaster is gathered to make a base. It must have enough body so that it does not flatten out.

form in thickness. This makes it easier to trim the model later.

8. Carefully drag the excess plaster up over the edges of the cast, filling in any voided areas (Figure 27-29). Try not to cover any margins of the impression tray while doing this. This locks the plaster onto the tray and may cause the cast to fracture when removing the impression material and the tray.

NOTE: If using a one- or single-pour method, the base is poured immediately after the anatomical portion is poured. The two-pour method allows the material to initially set in the anatomical portion prior to inverting it and allows even the slightest plaster to flow from any crucial areas.

FIGURE 27-29 The operator must smooth out the plaster sides of the base after the filled impression is inverted on it.

27-11 Removing the Plaster Model from the Alginate Impression

This procedure is performed by the dental assistant in the dental laboratory after the study model has set.

EQUIPMENT AND SUPPLIES

▶ Laboratory knife

▶ Maxillary and mandibular plaster models, set in the alginate impressions

PROCEDURE STEPS *(Follow aseptic procedures)*

1. Allow the plaster to set for forty to sixty minutes before removing the impression material and the tray. The exothermic heat should be gone from the plaster material to indicate it is set.

2. Using a laboratory knife, gently remove any plaster that is up on the margin of the tray (Figure 27-30).

3. Holding the handle of the impression tray, lift the tray straight upward.

4. If the tray does not come off, identify the area that is holding it back. Remove the necessary plaster in that area to release the tray and impression material. Be sure to lift in an upward motion

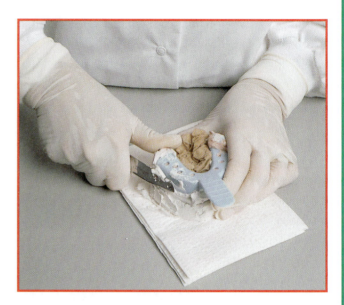

FIGURE 27-30 Use a knife to remove the remaining plaster on the impression prior to removing it from the model.

to remove the tray. Wiggling side to side or lifting sideways may fracture the teeth and anatomical portion of the cast.

Two-thirds of the trimmed model is made from the anatomic portion of the cast (Figure 27-31). The anatomic portion includes the teeth, the mucosa, and frenum attachments and is about one inch wide. This area was duplicated from the oral cavity. The remaining one-third is the base or the art portion of the cast. This portion is trimmed in a geometric form with specific angles and is about one-half inch wide. When maxillary and mandibular models are trimmed and in occlusion, they should have an overall height of three inches.

NOTE: The grinding stone on the model trimmer can be cleaned with a brush and the water increased to run over the surface. Shut off the machine and clean the guide table and the reservoir beneath where the plaster accumulates. If this is allowed to build up, the water will back up and cause water to splash out while trimming.

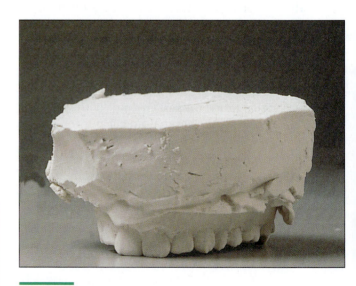

FIGURE 27-31 The anatomic portion of the cast after trimming will make up two-thirds of the model.

PROCEDURE

27-12 Trimming Diagnostic Casts/Study Models

This procedure is performed by the dental assistant in the dental laboratory after the study model has set, been separated from the alginate impression, and prepared for trimming.

EQUIPMENT AND SUPPLIES

▶ Safety glasses

▶ Maxillary and mandibular models

▶ Two flexible rubber mixing bowls

▶ Laboratory knife

▶ Pencil

▶ Measuring straight edge

PROCEDURE STEPS *(Follow aseptic procedures)*

1. If the maxillary and mandibular plaster models are dry, soak them in rubber mixing bowls for five minutes prior to trimming. The trimming wheel on the model trimmer is more effective if the models are wet prior to trimming.

2. Place on safety glasses and adjust the model trimmer so that the water runs freely over the grinding wheel when the trimmer is on.

3. Invert the models so that the teeth are resting on the counter. Evaluate whether the base is parallel to the counter (Figure 27-32). Keep in mind that the art portion is one-half inch when completed.

4. Turn on the model trimmer and trim the base so that it is parallel to the occlusal plane. The model

trimmer works best if light, even pressure is used when applying the models to the grinding wheel. Hold the model as level as possible during this procedure (Figure 27-33).

5. Rest hands on the table of the model trimmer and keep fingers away from the grinding wheel.

6. The model may have to be returned to the counter for re-evaluation and then again to the model trimmer to achieve a parallel surface. Trim both models to this stage.

NOTE: Move the models back and forth once across the grinding surface as the model comes off the grinding wheel. This eliminates the circular grinding marks made as the wheel rotates.

7. Place the models together in occlusion (a wax bite may be necessary) and again evaluate whether the objective of obtaining parallel models has been achieved. If not, grind to get the models to this stage. All other cuts will be off if this stage is not achieved, because this flat surface is laid on the model trimming table guide to grind the other areas.

FIGURE 27-32 The base of the model should be parallel to the counter before proceeding to trim the study model.

FIGURE 27-33 The base of the study model is trimmed as the operator maintains even pressure on the trimming wheel.

(continued)

8. When the cut maxillary and mandibular models as a pair are parallel, keep them in occlusion and evaluate which posterior teeth are the most distal: the maxillary or the mandibular. When that has been determined, take that model and draw with pencil a line behind the retromolar area indicating where to trim (Figure 27-34).

9. Place the base surface of that model on the model trimmer table guide and cut the posterior area at a right angle with the base up to the indicated lines (Figure 27-35).

10. Put the two models back into occlusion and place the cut model on the top, whether it is the maxillary or the mandibular. Place the opposite base on the model trimmer table guide holding the models together and trim the posterior at a right angle to the base (Figure 27-36). The trimmed model acts as a guide to follow while trimming. When small particles of plaster are trimmed off the first base, it indicates that they are trimmed to the same plane. To evaluate this, the models are taken off the grinding wheel and placed on their backs (Figure 27-37). The occlusal plane is at a right angle to the counter. If the models stay in

FIGURE 27-34 A pencil line is drawn from 2 mm distal from the last molar to 2 mm distal from the molar on the opposite side of the arch. This establishes a cutting line for the back cut.

FIGURE 27-36 The models are placed together to trim the back cut.

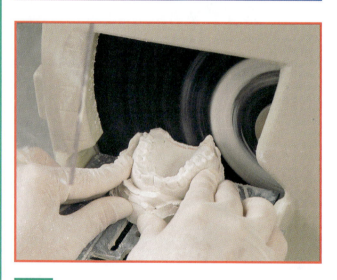

FIGURE 27-35 The posterior of the base of the model is cut at a right angle to the base.

FIGURE 27-37 The models are placed on their backs on a hard, flat surface in occlusion to verify whether the back cuts are correct.

(continued)

P R O C E D U R E   2 7 - 1 2 *continued*

occlusion, the objective has been met. If they fall apart and out of occlusion, then place them back onto the grinding wheel until they stay in the correct position.

11. The top, bottom, and back now are trimmed. Left to trim are the heel, side, and anterior cuts. The first to be cut are the side angles. Take the pencil and mark the following areas: outward from the middle of the mandibular premolars to the edge of the model and the maxillary cuspids in the same manner. Draw a line running parallel to the teeth at the greatest depth of the buccal vestibule, from the molars to the premolars. This line will be about 5 mm from the buccal surface

of the teeth. Mark both sides of the maxillary and the mandibular models in this manner.

12. Place the model base back on the model trimmer table guide and trim the model to the pencil lines on both sides (Figure 27-38). Repeat this procedure with both models.

13. Mark with pencil a dot at the midline of the maxillary model in the vestibule area. Using the straight edge of the measuring device, draw a line from the dot to the canine/cuspid line on each quadrant (Figure 27-39). Cut both of the anterior cuts, forming a pointed area at the midline and the center of both cuspids. If the teeth are highly

FIGURE 27-38 The vestibule or side area is cut at the deepest area. A line can be drawn to establish a proper cut line.

FIGURE 27-40 The maxillary anterior area is cut in a point, bringing both cuspid cuts to the midline between the maxillary central incisors.

FIGURE 27-39 A line is drawn from the midline of the central incisors to the middle of the cuspid to establish a cut line for the anterior.

FIGURE 27-41 A rounded line is drawn on the mandibular from cuspids to cuspids to indicate where the cut should be made.

(continued)

irregular, adjustments may have to be done. After the lines are drawn, make sure that the cuts will not trim away the protruding teeth. If it appears that this may happen, move the lines out on each side to accommodate this. The model should appear symmetrical (Figure 27-40).

14. The mandibular model is marked in a rounded manner from the middle of the canine/cuspid on one side to the middle of the canine/cuspid on the other side. A pencil line can be drawn at the depth of the anterior vestibule as a guide for trimming (Figure 27-41).

15. The heel cuts on both the maxillary and mandibular models are three-eighths to five-eighths inches wide and should appear symmetric in length. They can be drawn on the model by turning the base upward and placing an imaginary diagonal line from the cuspid (maxillary) premolar (mandibular) to where the side and back cuts meet. Draw a 90° angle across the base, opposite the anterior area. The heel cuts are small cuts on both the maxillary and the mandibular models that finish the trimming of the models (Figure 27-42).

16. After the models are trimmed symmetrically, a laboratory knife is used to trim the tongue area flat and smooth other areas on the art portion. Take care not to destroy the anatomy of the diagnostic casts. Any air bubbles can be filled with plaster. Use dry plaster on the finger, and push it

into the wet model to fill small air bubbles. To complete the smoothing of the flat surfaces, a fine wet/dry sandpaper can be used under water. Any small beads of plaster can be removed carefully from the surfaces of the teeth.

17. Place the models in a model gloss for 10 minutes or spray with gloss to provide a professional appearance and add strength. The models need to be polished with a dry cloth to buff the surface in order to achieve the desired high gloss.

18. Label both the models with the patient's name and the date the models were taken. In an orthodontic office, the patient's age may also be identified on the models.

FIGURE 27-42 The heel cuts are established on the models and cut.

Trimmed Diagnostic Casts (Study Models) Evaluation (Figure 27-43)

▶ Both maxillary and mandibular models are trimmed symmetrically following specific cut angles indicated.
▶ All the anatomic portion of the model are accurate.
▶ The trimmed models sit on end and maintain occlusion.
▶ Models exhibit a one-half inch base each and a one inch anatomic portion each.
▶ Final finishing is accomplished and the models present a professional appearance.

ARTICULATING CASTS OR STUDY MODELS

An articulator is used to duplicate the patient's occlusion on models (Figure 27-44). An **articulator** is a frame that holds models of the patient's teeth in order

to maintain the patient's occlusion and represent his or her jaws. Articulators can be simple, like hinges that only duplicate the up-and-down motions, or they can be complex, where they are adjustable and can duplicate the side-to-side motions as well as the up-and-down motions.

FIGURE 27-43 Trimmed study models.

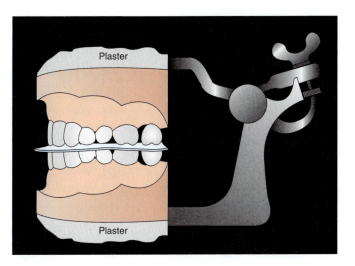

FIGURE 27-44 Articulator.

Articulators can be used to study malocclusion, to wax and carve teeth for crowns and bridges, and to demonstrate to the patient the action that is of concern. They also have a number of other desired uses. The dental assistant may perform the task of mounting models or assist the dentist in this task.

Stephan Articulator

Offices may use a **Stephan articulator**, which allows both the up-and-down motion and has a spring that allows for some lateral movement as well. It has two support bows: one to stabilize the maxillary and one to stabilize the mandibular. The hinge represents the temporomandibular joints. The first step in using this articulator is to trim the models so that they fit within the two bows easily. The top portion of the bases can then be **scored**. To score a model is to make cut marks in the smooth surface so that the added gypsum can adhere. The models are placed within the bows in the correct bite. Normally, the wax bite is used to establish the correct occlusion. The models are then attached to the bows using impression plaster, which flows into the scored area and around the bow. After the plaster has set, the models remain fastened to the articulator and can be opened and the wax bite removed.

DENTAL WAXES

Waxes are among the oldest materials used in dentistry. Over two hundred years ago, impressions were taken of specific areas in the mouth with wax. The waxes are derived from a number of sources, including bees, plants, and minerals. Beeswax has to be refined and bleached to obtain uniformity of color and character. Differences in color and texture may take place if the bee has been feeding on something unusual, for example, plants all yellow in color. Plants in South America and Brazil bring to dentistry a hard wax that is gathered from the fronds of a tree. This wax also is used for polishing automobiles to a high gloss shine. From minerals come petroleum products, such as paraffin wax. In dentistry, only the highest grade of wax is used. It must be uniform and provide consistent results when used.

Groups of Waxes

Waxes are classified into three broad groups: pattern, processing, and impression. Pattern waxes are hard waxes used in crown and bridge casting (inlay wax) and the construction of the baseplate tray (baseplate wax). Processing and impression waxes have many uses in dentistry.

Pattern Wax

Pattern, or inlay, wax normally is supplied in dark-colored sticks (Figure 27-45A). It is used on a die, a positive replica of the prepared tooth made from stone. The wax is melted and applied to the die, making a wax pattern that is used to create the metal and/or porcelain restoration. The composition varies from manufacturer to manufacturer, but most have a certain degree of hardness, toughness, resistance to flaking, and ability to achieve a smooth surface. Desirable properties of inlay wax are that it flows at a temperature slightly above the mouth temperature, it achieves complete burnout at temperatures above 900°F, and it carves away easily without chipping or cracking. These properties are essential in using the lost wax technique of casting. The lost wax technique refers to the wax pattern after the wax is enclosed in investment stone and heated to high temperatures. The high temperatures cause the wax to vaporize, leaving behind a void or an empty space (lost wax) where the melted metal can be invested using centrifugal force.

FIGURE 27-45 Pattern waxes. (A) Inlay wax. (B) Baseplate wax.

The baseplate wax is a hard wax that can be heated to make the initial base on which to form a denture (Figure 27-45B). It comes in Types I, II, and III; Type III is the hardest. Type II is most often used in the fabrication of baseplates.

Processing Wax

Several waxes used in dentistry are in the processing wax classification. Boxing wax is a soft, pliable wax that is used to form a wax box around an impression prior to pouring it with gypsum (Figure 27-46A). It comes in wax strips one and one-half inches wide and can be reused for the purpose of making a ring around the impression to hold the runny gypsum in place until it sets.

Sticky wax is another type of processing wax (Figure 27-46C). It is very brittle at room temperature but when melted with a flame source becomes soft and sticky. It adheres to a number of surfaces, such as metal, gypsum, and porcelain. It is used to hold two fractured pieces together until they can be repaired.

Utility wax, also called periphery or bending wax, is a soft wax that is adhesive and pliable (Figure 27-46B). It does not require additional heat and can be molded to most surfaces. This is the wax used to bead around trays to extend them and assist in patient comfort. This wax is also used for orthodontic patients to cover the brackets and uncomfortable areas until the cheeks and lips can adjust. It is supplied in long ropes or strips and in a number of colors.

Impression or Bite Registration Waxes

Normally containing copper or aluminum particles, impression waxes are used to take bite registrations. They are supplied in horseshoe shapes for obtaining the maxillary and mandibular biting surfaces.

Additional Waxes

Other waxes used in dentistry that are not in the three primary classifications are the study wax and the undercut wax. The study wax is hard wax supplied in blocks used for carving teeth and anatomy (Figure 27-47). Undercut wax is a putty-type wax used to fill in the undercuts prior to the impression being taken.

CUSTOM TRAYS

The dentist may ask for a custom tray for the patient in order to obtain an accurate impression. This may be because a regular stock tray does not fit. The stock tray will not allow a minimum amount space for the material to flow around the prepared area, or it may require that an overabundance of impression material be used to obtain the impression, therefore risking an inferior outcome. In any case, a custom tray can be fabricated to meet the need. Several materials are available to make a custom tray. It can be constructed from self- or light-curing acrylic resin, a vacuum resin, or a thermoplastic material. All materials must be rigid enough to provide subsistence for the material as it is inserted into and removed from the mouth. It is important that the material adapts well during the construction so that the final tray meets the required criteria.

Required Criteria for a Custom Tray

▶ Stable enough to hold the material rigid during placement and removal
▶ Can be smoothed and contoured to the arch
▶ Can be adapted to an edentulous, a partially edentulous, and a full dentition
▶ Can be adapted to allow uniform thickness of impression material in all areas of the arch
▶ Can be altered and contoured to any irregular area
▶ Can be designed so that stops are in the spacer, therefore holding the material in a stable, specifically determined area, providing a more accurate impression

FIGURE 27-46 Processing waxes. (A) Boxing wax. (B) Utility wax. (C) Sticky wax.

FIGURE 27-47 Study wax blocks.

Acrylic Tray Resin Self-Curing Custom Trays

The most common material used to make custom trays is the self-curing acrylic tray resin. It comes in a liquid catalyst (**monomer**) that mixes with a powder (**polymer**) to start the process of curing (**polymerization**). Polymerization occurs when material changes from a plastic pliable state to a rigid state. Once this process starts, it continues until the material is set completely. The material goes through several stages as it is cured. The first stage is after the liquid and the powder are mixed together. This initial set is when the material appears sticky and, if pulled apart, appears to have spider-web strands from particle to particle. The second stage is where the material can be gathered into a ball, kneaded, and contoured to the model. The third stage is where the material goes through an exothermic reaction, giving off a great deal of heat while setting. When the heat has diminished and the material can no longer be shaped, the final set stage is completed. A custom tray should be allowed to set for twenty-four hours prior to use due to the fact that it is still dimensionally unstable.

Acrylic Tray Resin Light-Cured Custom Trays

Acrylic tray resin is supplied in light-cured custom trays. The primary difference between this material and the self-curing is that the setting time is operator controlled. The material stays pliable and workable until a light initiates polymerization. The polymerization process happens quickly. This technique requires special equipment: an oven-like appliance with a special curing light in it. The custom tray is designed and placed in the oven for a quick setting and then is ready for use.

Vacuum-Formed Custom Trays

Like the acrylic tray resin that is light cured, the vacuum-formed custom trays require additional equipment. This unit has a frame that holds the sheets directly under a heating element and, when they are softened, the frame drops the sheet onto the cast as vacuum pressure draws the material to the model. The vacuum-forming unit has other applications in dentistry. Acrylic resin sheets are supplied in several gauges for different applications. The custom tray requires the use of a rigid, heavy, plastic resin.

Thermoplastic Tray Material Custom Trays

Other materials used for making custom trays are the **thermoplastic** beads and buttons. When these small, round beads or buttons are placed in warm water, the thermoplastic reaction takes place. Thermoplastic means that the material becomes soft and pliable when exposed to heat. Once the material is soft, it can be conformed to the model in the desired shape. As the heat dissipates, the material hardens. It is easy to identify when the material is soft enough because it appears clear and then becomes dense when it hardens.

CONSTRUCTING A CUSTOM TRAY

Regardless of the material type used, the custom tray model is prepared in the same manner.

Outlining the Margins of the Tray

If a full custom tray is desired on an edentulous arch, draw a blue line at the bottom of the vestibule area around the facial surface, across the palate area on the maxillary model, around the posterior retromolar area, along the bottom of the vestibule area, and across the opposite posterior retramolar area on the mandibular model (Figure 27-48). From that first marking, make a red line 2 mm upward (toward the ridge). This gives a definite line to follow when adapting the spacer. A **spacer** is placed on the model to allow room in the tray for the impression material. This spacer normally is made of pink baseplate wax, but a commercial nonstick molding material may be used (especially when using the vacuum-formed custom tray because of the heating element) or a moist paper towel can be used. When the spacer is placed, the **undercuts** are filled in. Undercuts are recessed areas in the model that make it impossible to seat or remove the custom tray properly. Undercuts are caused by bubbles in the plaster, cavities, or the shape of the arch or dentition. If using baseplate wax for the spacer, it can be heated with warm water and conformed to the model. Cut it back to the red line in an angle-forming manner (see Procedure 27-13, Constructing a Self-Cured Acrylic Resin Custom Tray). This provides a smoother tissue side to the custom tray and is

FIGURE 27-48 The tray margin is outlined on the stone cast. The deepest area is marked in blue and 1 or 2 mm up from that a red line indicating where the wax spacer is to be located can be drawn.

more comfortable to the patients than a blunt-edge cut. After the spacer is in place, take a warm plastic instrument to lute (secure) the edges of the wax to the cast. After the securing is accomplished, cut into the crest of the wax with a laboratory knife, making small rectangular or round holes. These **stops** (holes on the spacer that allow bumps to be formed on the tissue side of the tray) allow the tray to be seated 2 to 3 mm from the teeth or tissue and to not seat too deeply. This allows an adequate amount of impression material to flow around the prepared teeth or the tissue. There should be a minimum of four stops on an edentulous model, two on each first molar and cuspid area. When making a custom tray for crowns and bridges, the stops should be placed one tooth distal and mesial from the prepared tooth.

The self-curing material is exothermic. It heats up and causes the wax to melt slightly. It is advisable to place a layer of aluminum foil over the wax spacer and into the stops. The foil makes it easier to remove the wax from the tissue side of the tray after the custom tray is made. If foil is not used, a toothbrush and hot water will aid in getting the wax out of the inside (tissue side) of the custom tray.

After the cast is prepared, the custom tray material is mixed according to the manufacturer's directions and formed to the cast. In the doughy stage, the maxillary material can be shaped into a patty and the mandibular can be rolled into a log shape prior to placing the materials on the cast. A handle can be made from the remaining material. It is placed on the anterior of the tray near the midline of the arch. It is secured by wiping the anterior area and the handle area that is to be attached with the resin liquid and then placing it on the custom tray. Because the handle is still soft when it is applied to the cast, it must be held in place until initially set up. Make sure the handle is large and strong enough to allow for leverage in placing and removing the custom tray from the mouth. Remember that the dentist will have his or her fingers and thumb on the handle while performing the procedure, so make sure it can be held easily. When working on edentulous custom trays, the handles should extend upward and outward from the model. If this is not done, the handle is placed so that it protrudes directly through the lip of the patient.

 When the exothermic reaction has completed and the model has cooled (about ten minutes), remove the spacer and evaluate the tray. The inside of the tray does not need to be smooth because the impression material covers this area. Any rough areas on the margins and on the outside of the tray can be smoothed for patient comfort. This can be accomplished by using an acrylic bur in a straight handpiece or with an arbor band on the laboratory lathe. Wear protective glasses when performing either of these trimming procedures. When completed, clean and disinfect the custom tray according to manufacturer's directions and place it in a barrier ready for patient use.

An adhesive is painted on the tissue side of the tray prior to taking the impression. It is normally applied in two coats. The first is allowed to dry and the second is placed ten minutes or so before the impression is taken. This secures the material to the custom tray. Some dentists may want holes placed in the custom tray to further lock the impression material into the tray. This can be accomplished by wearing protective glasses and using a straight handpiece with a round bur to penetrate the custom tray. Either or both techniques will secure the material into the custom tray.

P R O C E D U R E

27-13 Constructing a Self-Cured Acrylic Resin Custom Tray

This procedure is performed by the dental assistant in the dental laboratory on a working cast.

EQUIPMENT AND SUPPLIES

▶ Maxillary and/or mandibular casts

▶ Laboratory knife

▶ Pencil (plain or red and blue)

▶ Wax spatula

▶ Baseplate wax and heating source (warm water or laboratory torch)

▶ Tray resin with measuring devices

▶ Separating medium with brush

▶ Wooden tongue blade and wax-lined paper cup

(continued)

P R O C E D U R E   2 7 - 1 3 *continued*

- ▶ Petroleum jelly
- ▶ Tray adhesive

PROCEDURE STEPS *(Follow aseptic procedures)*

Preparing the Cast

1. Outline the area of the cast for the spacer to be placed (Figure 27-48). This is 2 to 3 mm below the margin of the prepared tooth or 2 to 3 mm above the lowest point in the vestibule if the arch is edentulous.

2. Fill any undercuts in the cast or cover with the spacer material. Heat the spacer material and contour to the pencil line.

3. Using a laboratory knife, trim the wax or spacer to the line using an angled cut instead of a blunt cut (Figure 27-49).

4. Cut the appropriate stops in the spacer (Figure 27-50).

5. Cover the spacer with aluminum foil or paint it with separating medium.

Mixing the Custom Tray Acrylic Self-Curing Resin

1. Measure the powder and the liquid to the correct calibrations on the measuring devices according to the manufacturers' directions.

2. Mix the powder and liquid together in the wax-lined paper cup with the wooden tongue blade until **homogenous** (uniformly mixed).

3. Allow the mixture to go through initial polymerization for two to three minutes. Some manufacturers indicate that a cover be placed over the material during the polymerization.

4. During this time, place petroleum jelly over the cast and on the palms of your hands.

Contouring the Custom Tray Acrylic Self-Curing Resin

1. The material is ready to conform to the tray after the initial set when the material is no longer sticky and can be gathered into a ball. Knead the material to further mix the material and set a small amount aside for the handle (Figure 27-51). This doughy stage allows the material to be formed into a patty for the maxillary arch or a roll for the mandibular arch.

FIGURE 27-49 A wax spacer is trimmed to the indicated line on the working cast.

FIGURE 27-50 Stops are cut into the wax spacer. These allow room for the impression material.

(continued)

P R O C E D U R E   **2 7 - 1 3** *continued*

FIGURE 27-51 The custom tray material is kneaded for use.

2. Place the dough-like patty for the maxillary cast, covering the wax spacer. Contour and adapt it to extend 1 to 2 mm over the wax spacer (Figure 27-52A). Try to complete the adaptation with a rolled edge at the designated area. If unable to accomplish this, a laboratory knife can be used to trim the material back. (Doing this causes rough edges that need to be smoothed back later.)

3. The material set aside for the handle is shaped and a drop of the monomer liquid placed on the tray where the handle is to be adapted and then on the handle where it will be placed on the custom tray. This allows the materials to join together for a better outcome.

4. Place the handle in the midline area of the arch (Figure 27-52B). If making an edentulous custom tray, the handle should come up from the ridge and then outward. A custom tray handle that is made for an area that has teeth can come directly outward.

5. Place the handle and hold it in the proper position until the material becomes firm.

Finishing the Custom Tray Acrylic Self-Curing Resin

1. The setting takes about eight to ten minutes. Remove the custom tray from the cast and take out the spacer material.

2. If foil has been used, the cleaning will not take a great deal of time. If only wax was used, melt it. A wax spatula is used to remove it, along with hot water and an old toothbrush.

3. After the final set (thirty minutes minimum), use an acrylic bur (Figure 27-53) or an arbor band to trim the edges of the custom tray. Do not trim the inside of the tray.

4. Clean and disinfect the custom tray according to the manufacturer's directions. Write the patient's name on the tray.

(A)

(B)

FIGURE 27-52 (A) The custom tray material is adapted to the model over the wax spacer. (B) The handle is attached to the adapted custom tray.

(continued)

P R O C E D U R E **2 7 - 1 3** *continued*

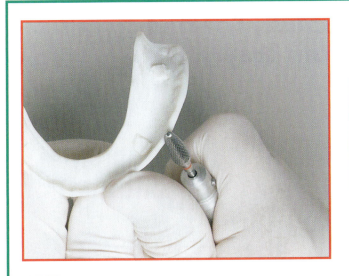

FIGURE 27-53 The custom tray is trimmed with an acrylic bur.

5. Apply the adhesive provided by the manufacturer of the impression material to the inside of the custom tray and along the margins (Figure 27-54).

FIGURE 27-54 The adhesive is applied in a thin coat to the custom tray and allowed to dry.

VACUUM-FORMED TRAY

Trays that are vacuum formed can be used for a number of applications in the field of dentistry. Most often they are used for custom trays, bleaching trays, night guards, mouth guards, and matrices for provisionals. The material comes in several gauges and thicknesses for specific applications (Figure 27-55). Custom tray material is much more thick and rigid than the other applications. All use a vacuum former with a heating element, a cast, and material that can be heated and adapted through vacuum pressure.

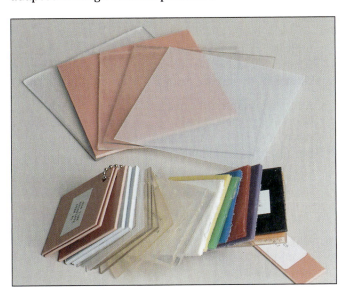

FIGURE 27-55 Various types of vacuum-formed material.

TEMPORARY (PROVISIONAL) RESTORATIONS

After a tooth has been prepared for a crown and prior to the seating of the crown, a temporary restoration must be adapted and temporarily cemented on the tooth to protect it in the interim. These temporary restorations stabilize and protect the tooth for the two days to two weeks it takes to make the crown(s) or bridge(s).

Temporary Restoration Criteria

▶ The temporary restoration is comfortable and esthetically acceptable to the patient.
▶ The temporary restoration remains stable, with proper mesial and distal contacts and occlusal alignment, until the permanent crown is cemented.
▶ The temporary restoration is easily removed, without damaging the tooth, when the permanent restoration is ready for placement.
▶ The temporary restoration fits snugly and accurately along the prepared margin of the tooth. There is less than ½ mm of space between the temporary restoration and the finish line of the margin.
▶ The temporary restoration is contoured in a similar fashion to the original tooth, therefore protecting the gingiva from irritation and interproximal areas from food impaction.

P R O C E D U R E

27-14 Constructing a Vacuum-Formed Acrylic Resin Custom Tray

This procedure is performed by the dental assistant in the dental laboratory on a working cast.

EQUIPMENT AND SUPPLIES

▶ Maxillary and/or mandibular casts

▶ Laboratory knife

▶ Laboratory scissors

▶ Vacuum former with heating element

▶ Acrylic sheets

PROCEDURE STEPS *(Follow aseptic procedures)*

Preparing the Cast

1. The cast is soaked in warm water for up to thirty minutes prior to forming a custom tray on it. This eliminates small air bubbles. (These air bubbles coming to the surface [**percolating**] cause small spaces between the cast and the acrylic sheet. Then, the custom tray does not have the accuracy desired.)

2. Place the spacer, if indicated. (A wax spacer will melt under the heating element, if used.)

3. Mark the desired outer margin of the custom tray.

4. Place the cast on the platform of the vacuum-forming unit.

Contouring the Acrylic Resin Sheets During the Vacuum-Forming Process

1. Select the appropriate acrylic resin sheets to be used for the procedure.

2. Place the acrylic resin sheets between the heater frame and the gasket frame and tighten the anterior knob to secure the material in place. Place the cast on the platform (Figure 27-56).

3. Make sure the heating element is in the correct place above the acrylic resin sheet and turn it on.

4. Watch the resin as it heats. It will begin to sag downward (Figure 27-57). Allow this to continue

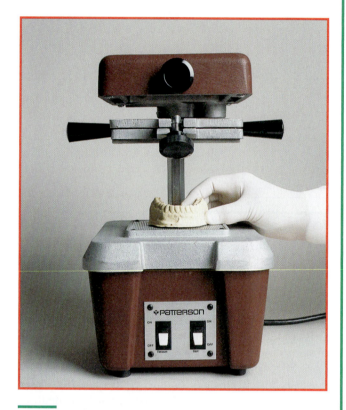

FIGURE 27-56 The resin sheets are secured in place and the cast is placed on the platform of the vacuum-forming unit.

until the resin droops downward about one inch. (Overheating causes air bubbles to form on the surface of the acrylic resin.)

5. After the material is heated properly, take both handles on the frame and pull the frame downward, over the cast. Only touch the handles because the entire area is extremely hot.

6. Turn on the vacuum immediately after the resin sheet is entirely over the cast (Figure 27-58).

7. Turn off the heating unit.

8. Allow the vacuum to continue for one to two minutes in order to cool the resin so it becomes firm again.

(continued)

P R O C E D U R E   **2 7 - 1 4** *continued*

FIGURE 27-57 The resin sheet begins sagging as the material is heated.

FIGURE 27-58 When the resin material has sagged one inch below the holding ring, it is ready to be dropped into position over the cast. The unit is held by the handles to ensure that the operator is not burned.

Finishing the Vacuum-Formed Acrylic Resin Custom Tray

1. After the resin material is cooled, remove it from the vacuum form frame.

2. Separate the resin-formed custom tray from the cast and, using laboratory scissors, trim to the desired form (Figure 27-59).

3. Use a torch to heat and apply a cutout handle section to the custom tray.

4. Clean and disinfect the custom tray according to the manufacturer's directions and write the patient's name on it.

FIGURE 27-59 The vacuum form can be trimmed with scissors.

Types of Temporary Restorations

Temporary restorations, also known as provisional restorations, can be made of a number of materials, both custom and preformed. In many states, the function of fabricating and placing a temporary restoration is delegated to the dental assistant under the supervision of the dentist. Most offices use the preformed aluminum and acrylic crowns, along with the custom acrylic or composite crowns.

Preformed Aluminum Temporary Crowns

Preformed aluminum temporary crowns are supplied in different sizes and anatomic features. They are used on the posterior teeth because they lack esthetic value. Some are made without any anatomy and resemble thimbles with parallel straight sides and flat, occlusal surfaces. More contouring is necessary to adapt this model to the tooth. Others have anatomies similar to the natural teeth and are contoured much like stainless steel crowns. Both the crowns without anatomic features and the ones with anatomic features can be filled with acrylic or composite material to obtain a more custom fit prior to setting the temporary restorations in place over the prepared teeth.

Preformed Acrylic Temporary Crown

Preformed acrylic or plastic temporary crowns are available in different sizes, shapes, and shades

P R O C E D U R E

27-15 Sizing, Adapting, and Seating an Aluminum Temporary Crown

This procedure is performed by the dentist or the dental assistant at the dental unit after a tooth has been prepared for a crown.

EQUIPMENT AND SUPPLIES

▶ Maxillary and/or mandibular selection of aluminum temporary crowns (Figure 27-60)

▶ Millimeter ruler

▶ Basic setup: Mouth mirror, cotton pliers, and explorer

▶ Crown and collar scissors

▶ Contouring pliers

▶ Acrylic or composite temporary material (optional)

▶ Sandpaper discs, rubber wheel, and mandrel

▶ Temporary cement, pad, and spatula

▶ Articulating paper

▶ Dental floss

FIGURE 27-60 Selection of Iso-Form temporary crowns. *(Courtesy of 3M Dental Products Division)*

PROCEDURE STEPS *(Follow aseptic procedures)*

1. Measure the available space for the temporary crown from the mesial to distal with the millimeter ruler. This aids in the selection of a preformed crown having the appropriate mesial and distal contact.

2. Determine the correct crown to try in. The aluminum crown is for the correct tooth in the dentition and the size is chosen according to the measurement taken with the millimeter ruler. (Prevent cross-contamination while taking the crown from the container. Do not use contaminated instruments.) Any crown tried that does not fit must be sterilized before replacing it in the selection tray.

3. Try the selected crown on and check for mesial and distal width. The crown will be above the occlusal plane at this time.

4. The length of the crown is determined by placing the aluminum crown over the prepared tooth and using an explorer to mark the height (Figure 27-61). Another way to accomplish this is to scribe the tooth at the occlusal surface where it aligns with the other teeth on the arch and then taking that amount off the gingival area. Either method shows that the margin of the gingival needs to be trimmed in order to fit.

5. Using a crown and collar scissors (with curved blades), trim the gingival margin. Crowns are never straight across the surface but are longer on the buccal and lingual margins. Use the rounded edges of the scissors to trim.

NOTE: Trimming a small amount at first allows refitting to further check the desired result (Figure 27-62). Taking too much off renders the crown useless. Making several trims to get the desired effect is a better method. Using the scissors in a continuous cutting action gives a much smoother surface. Avoid sharp, uneven edges that cause the patient discomfort around the gingival surface.

(continued)

P R O C E D U R E **2 7 - 1 5** *continued*

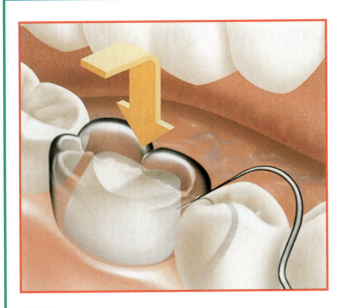

FIGURE 27-61 An explorer is used to establish the height of the temporary aluminum crown. *(Courtesy of 3M Dental Products Division)*

FIGURE 27-62 The aluminum crown is trimmed with crown and collar scissors. *(Courtesy of 3M Dental Products Division)*

6. After the desired length is achieved, use the contouring pliers to invert the gingival edge in an inward manner. This crimping aids in the adaptation of the circumference edge of the aluminum crown to the finish line of the preparation.

7. Smoothing of the rough and jagged edges is accomplished through use of sandpaper discs and a rubber wheel. Check that all edges are smooth and polished (Figure 27-63).

8. Place the aluminum crown on the prepared tooth and check the occlusion with the articulating paper and the contacts with dental floss.

NOTE: If the contacts are weak, use a burnisher on the inside to extend the crown outward to get a better contact.

9. If an acrylic or a composite lining is used, the crown is filled with the material and placed on the prepared tooth. The patient is asked to bite into normal occlusion.

NOTE: The tooth may require light lubrication with petroleum jelly to avoid retention of the material.

The material sets according to manufacturer's directions and is then removed. Any excess material is polished away.

NOTE: Some operators prefer to do this step earlier in the procedure.

10. A final check for marginal fit, contour, and occlusion is done before cementation takes place.

FIGURE 27-63 Smooth the rough and jagged edges of the temporary. *(Courtesy of 3M Dental Products Division)*

P R O C E D U R E

27-16 Cementing the Aluminum Crown

This procedure is performed by the dentist or the dental assistant at the dental unit after the aluminum crown provisional has been prepared, sized, and contoured to the prepared tooth.

EQUIPMENT AND SUPPLIES

▶ Fitted aluminum temporary

▶ Cotton rolls

▶ Temporary cementation material

▶ Mixing pad

▶ Plastic filling instrument

▶ Basic setup: mouth mirror, explorer, cotton pliers

PROCEDURE STEPS *(Follow aseptic procedures)*

1. The prepared tooth is rinsed and dried with cotton rolls in place.

2. The temporary cementation material, such as zinc oxide eugenol, is mixed with a spatula and placed in the aluminum crown.

3. The aluminum crown is placed in position over the prepared tooth and the patient is asked to bite in occlusion until the cement is set.

NOTE: Some operators like the patient to bite on a cotton roll over the aluminum crown while the cement sets.

4. After the cement is set, the excess is removed with an explorer.

5. The contacts are checked with floss and the margins are inspected to determine whether all excess cement has been removed and the crown fits correctly.

6. A final check for occlusion is done with articulating paper.

7. Instructions are given to the patient for care of the temporary aluminum crown.

(Figure 27-64). The advantage of this type of crown is that it is more esthetically pleasing for anterior use. The plastic temporary crown is a form used to match the appropriate shape and contour of the tooth. It is filled with acrylic material and then removed. The preformed acrylic crowns have tabs on the incisal edge for easy placement. These tabs are removed prior to cementation. The preformed acrylic crowns are used more easily because they require little adjustment and can be seated immediately. One disadvantage is that they are shorter in length, or more closely trimmed to the optimum margin length of the prepared tooth. If a patient has had periodontal disease and the crown must be lengthened to cover any areas of recession, the clear-plastic crowns adapt better. They are supplied with longer "necks" on the crown for this purpose.

Custom Acrylic or Composite Temporary Restorations

When making custom acrylic or composite temporary restorations, a matrix is used. The matrix can be direct or indirect. A **matrix** is a form shaped in the pattern of the tooth prior to preparing the tooth

FIGURE 27-64 Preformed acrylic temporary crowns. *(Courtesy of Bosworth Co.)*

PROCEDURE

27-17 Sizing, Adapting, and Seating a Preformed Acrylic Crown

This procedure is performed by the dentist or the dental assistant at the dental unit after the preformed acrylic provisional has been prepared, sized, and contoured to the prepared tooth.

EQUIPMENT AND SUPPLIES

▶ Maxillary and/or mandibular selection of acrylic temporary crowns

▶ Mirror, explorer, and cotton pliers

▶ Acrylic or composite temporary material (optional)

▶ Acrylic bur

▶ Temporary cement, pad, and spatula

▶ Articulating paper

▶ Dental floss

PROCEDURE STEPS *(Follow aseptic procedures)*

Preparing the Preformed Acrylic Temporary Restoration

1. After the tooth has been prepared for a crown, a preformed acrylic temporary restoration is selected and adapted. Choose a crown that has enough width to contact on the adjacent teeth, is long enough to be in proper occlusion, and is the correct shade.

2. Retrieve this crown without cross-contaminating the other acrylic crowns. The tab at the incisal edge allows the operator to try the crown over the prepared tooth (Figure 27-65).

3. If necessary, adjustments are made with an acrylic bur. Polish with a rag wheel and pumice.

4. Take off the tag, place the crown, and check the occlusion with articulating paper.

5. Make adjustments, if necessary, and again polish the adjustment areas for a smooth surface for patient comfort.

Cementing the Acrylic Provisional Crown

1. The prepared tooth is rinsed and dried with cotton rolls in place.

FIGURE 27-65 The acrylic crown is tried over the prepared tooth, holding on to the incisal tab. *(Courtesy of 3M Dental Products Division)*

2. The temporary cementation material, such as zinc oxide eugenol, is mixed with a spatula and placed in the preformed acrylic crown.

3. The preformed acrylic crown is placed in position over the prepared tooth and the patient is asked to bite in occlusion or the operator holds the crown in place until the cement is set.

NOTE: Some operators like the patient to bite on a cotton roll over the preformed acrylic crown while the cement sets.

4. After the cement is set, the excess is removed with an explorer.

5. The contacts are checked with floss and the margins are inspected to determine whether all excess cement has been removed and whether the crown fits correctly.

6. A final check for occlusion is done with articulating paper.

7. Instructions are given to the patient for care of the temporary preformed acrylic crown.

(A)

(B)

FIGURE 27-66 (A) and (B) Temporary matrices. *(Courtesy of 3M Dental Products Division)*

Matrix Used for Direct Technique in Making Temporary Restorations

▶ Alginate impression
▶ Impression material
▶ Freehand (making a block of the material and covering the prepared tooth)
▶ Wax
▶ Thermo-forming beads or buttons

Matrix Used for Indirect Technique in Making Temporary Restorations)

▶ Wax
▶ Thermo-forming beads or buttons
▶ Vacuum-formed shell

A custom acrylic or composite temporary restoration must have good proximal contacts, good occlusal contacts, good food deflection, and good marginal contours (Figures 27-67A through D).

Self-Cure Methyl Methacrylate. There are several categories of materials that achieve the desired outcome of a custom temporary restoration. Each material has advantages and disadvantages. One of the older materials that is routinely used is the methyl methacrylates. The advantages of this material are that it has good physical properties, good esthetics, better color stability than the R'methacrylates, and a lower cost. The disadvantages are the strong odor, high shrinkage, and high exothermic heat given off during the self-cure chemical setting.

Self-Cure R'Methacrylate. The R' (resin) methacrylates have one of the active ingredients, such as vinyl, ethyl, or isobutyl, in place of the methyl. In comparison to the methyl methacrylates, they have lower shrinkage and a lower level of exothermic heat given off during the self-cure chemical setting. They are similar in price per temporary, they are the weakest of the methacrylates, they have poor color stability, and they have the same strong odor that the methyl methacrylates have.

Both the methyl and the R'methacrylates come in a powder and liquid form that is mixed together to form a creamy mix. After mixing, they are allowed to condition for approximately thirty seconds and then are placed in the matrix. A dull surface appears on the top of the material, and it is placed in the mouth over the prepared tooth and held in place for the initial set. It has a rubber appearance at this time. Most manufacturers suggest that the material be taken off and on the prepared tooth during the time of four to six minutes. This is when the exothermic heat is the greatest. The excess can be trimmed off easily with scissors during this time. The final set is from six to eight minutes, and the material

(Figure 27-66). **Direct matrix techniques** (making the matrix directly from the tooth) uses alginate, impression material, freehand (block) technique, wax, thermo-forming beads, or a thermo-plastic button in the matrix. The **indirect matrix technique** (making the matrix on a model or cast) utilizes wax, a vacuum-formed shell, and thermo-forming bead and button matrices.

The alginate and impression materials render more anatomically accurate temporaries. The other materials meet the criteria for a temporary restoration form adequately and may prove to be less costly and more easily made. The utility wax is heated in warm water and then formed over the tooth or model to obtain the shape of the tooth and then cooled. Thermo-forming beads and buttons are heated in hot water and formed on the tooth prior to preparation or on a cast when using the indirect matrix technique. The vacuum-formed shell is made on a vacuum unit using a cast covered with very thin sheets of acrylic resin. After it is heated, this sheet is cut to the desired size for use in making the temporary restoration.

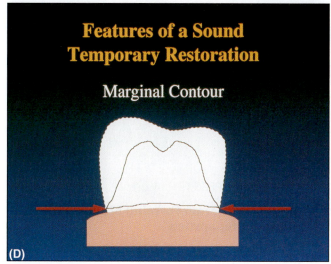

FIGURE 27-67 Criteria for a custom acrylic or composite temporary restoration. (A) Good proximal contacts. (B) Good occlusal contacts. (C) Good food deflection. (D) Good marginal contours. *(Courtesy of 3M Dental Products Division)*

becomes hard plastic. The range of setting time from start to finish is from eight to ten minutes for the materials in these two groups. Many of the newer materials are completed in half the time. The temporary restorations are removed from the matrix and trimmed with an acrylic bur to the desired shape and size (see Figures 27-67A through D for criteria).

After the temporary has been trimmed, it is polished with pumice and a rag wheel. Some of the materials in this category come with glazes. This glaze is applied after the polishing and allowed to dry for five minutes before the temporary is cemented.

Self-Cure Composite Material. Materials in the category of self-cure composite are double the price of the methacrylates. They are much stronger materials because they are made as composites and not plastics. They do not have the odor, the shrinkage, or the exo-

thermic reaction during setting, and they have excellent color stability.

Materials in this category come in two pastes. They are supplied in either two tubes or in a cartridge that fits into extruding guns with auto mixing tips. Both the tubes and the cartridge tips must remain clean and flowing to obtain the correct dispensed amount of the material. If they become clogged with old material, use an explorer to clear the old material out. Dispense a small, pea-shaped amount on the pad before beginning to ensure that everything is working properly.

The material is placed in the matrix and over the prepared tooth for up to two minutes. During the rubber stage (from four to six minutes), it is removed from the mouth to complete curing. The total time from start to finish for this material classification is up to seven minutes. After the material is set, the surface has a greasy layer due to the oxygen in the air, which can be removed

PROCEDURE

27-18 Adapting, Trimming, and Seating a Matrix and Custom Temporary Restoration

This procedure is performed by the dentist or the dental assistant at the dental unit after the tooth has been prepared for a crown.

EQUIPMENT AND SUPPLIES

▶ Basic setup: Mouth mirror, explorer, and cotton pliers

▶ Thermo-plastic buttons/hot water (one possible option for use in making a matrix)

▶ Composite temporary material

▶ Diamond bur

▶ Temporary cement, pad, and spatula

▶ Articulating paper

▶ Dental floss

FIGURE 27-68 The matrix is removed.

PROCEDURE STEPS (*Follow aseptic procedures*)

Making the Thermo-Forming Matrix Prior to the Tooth Preparation

1. Place the thermo-forming matrix buttons in hot water (one button per prepared tooth).

2. Allow the white color of the button to become clear. When that takes place, the material is pliable and able to be adapted.

3. Adapt the material over the tooth and tightly conform it to the tooth area and slightly below the gingival.

4. When the material cools (air can be used to make this more rapid), the matrix appears white and firm. Remove the matrix from the area and set it aside (Figure 27-68).

Preparing the Custom Temporary Restoration

1. After the tooth has been prepared for a crown, coat the teeth with a light application of petroleum jelly.

2. If using the composite self-curing temporary material in two tubes, dispense on the paper pad by holding tubes at a 45° angle.

3. Rotate the end-dispensing handle of the base until a click is heard. (The base is the larger of the two tubes. The smaller of the two holds the catalyst and has two dispensing ends.) Rotate the end-dispensing handle of the catalyst. Two small amounts are expelled. Each click of the dispensing handle is enough material for one temporary.

4. If a shade is being used, mix it with the base. If a mottled effect is desired, mix the shade after the base and catalyst are mixed together.

5. Mix the material together to obtain a creamy substance (about thirty seconds).

6. Place the material in the matrix.

7. Place the matrix over the prepared tooth (manipulation time is about one and one-half minutes).

8. Hold it in place in the mouth for two minutes.

9. Remove it from the mouth and set it aside for two minutes.

10. Remove the crown or bridge from the matrix (Figure 27-69). The additional curing time takes one minute. There are seven minutes total time from start to finish of the set.

(continued)

P R O C E D U R E **2 7 - 1 8** *continued*

FIGURE 27-69 Remove the acrylic bridge from the matrix. *(Courtesy of 3M Dental Products Division)*

FIGURE 27-70 Trimming the temporary.

11. Remove the greasy layer with alcohol or any other organic solvent.

12. Trim with a diamond or an acrylic bur (Figure 27-70).

13. Check the contacts with dental floss.

14. Check the occlusion by having the patient bite on the articulating paper.

15. Check the margins with the explorer and mirror.

P R O C E D U R E

27-19 Cementing the Custom Self-Curing Composite Temporary Crown

This procedure is performed by the dentist or the dental assistant at the dental unit after the temporary restoration has been prepared and is ready to be cemented in place, over the prepared tooth.

EQUIPMENT AND SUPPLIES

▶ Basic setup: Mouth mirror, explorer, and cotton pliers

▶ Cotton rolls

▶ Temporary luting cement

▶ Paper pad

▶ Mixing spatula

▶ Plastic filling instrument

▶ Dental floss

PROCEDURE STEPS *(Follow aseptic procedures)*

1. The prepared tooth is rinsed and dried with cotton rolls in place.

2. The temporary cement material is mixed with a spatula and placed in the custom composite temporary crown.

3. The temporary crown is placed in position over the prepared tooth and the patient is asked to bite in occlusion or the operator will hold the crown in place until the cement is set.

NOTE: Some operators like the patient to bite on a cotton roll over the preformed acrylic crown while the cement sets.

(continued)

P R O C E D U R E   **2 7 - 1 9** *continued*

4. After the cement is set, the excess is removed with an explorer (Figure 27-71).

5. The contacts are checked with floss and the margins are inspected to determine whether all excess cement has been removed and whether the crown fits correctly.

6. A final check for occlusion is done with articulating paper.

7. Instructions are given to the patient for care of the temporary preformed acrylic crown.

FIGURE 27-71 The temporary is placed and the excess cement is removed.

with alcohol or any other organic solvent. The trimming is done with a diamond bur and no polish is necessary. If additional material is required on the temporary, light-cured composite can be used and trimmed accordingly.

Multi-Cured Temporary Materials. Several multi-cured temporary materials are on the market. They have extended working time in the rubbery stage and improved operator control because they can be light cured on demand. They have good strength and are higher in cost. Some of the materials in this group are methacrylates and some are composites having the characteristics of the self-curing materials. The biggest advantage of this group is light-curing control, which allows for a quicker set and unlimited setting time.

CHAPTER SUMMARY

A number of basic functions in the dental laboratory are routinely performed by the dental assistant, such as pouring and trimming study models, fabricating custom trays, and fabricating provisional temporaries. To accomplish these procedures, the dental assistant must understand the materials that are used, the properties of each material, and the steps in each procedure. Any dental assistant who has skills in performing laboratory duties will be an asset to his or her employer. The better crossed-trained the dental team members are, the better the dental office functions.

CASE STUDY

Patrick Norman came into the dental office and wanted to talk to the doctor about a space in the anterior region of his maxillary teeth. After Dr. Smith completed a clinical examination, he asked the dental assistant to make diagnostic casts for further study. After talking to Patrick, the dental assistant found that Patrick has difficulty when anything is placed in his mouth and that gagging is a problem.

Case Study Review

1. What can the dental assistant do to help Patrick with the gagging problem while taking the impressions for the diagnostic casts?

2. What material is used routinely for obtaining preliminary impressions?

3. Would the fast or regular set be more beneficial in this case?

4. Which arch would be taken first? Why?

To complete your study of this chapter, work the review activities that follow. Also, refer to the software that accompanies this text.

REVIEW QUESTIONS

Multiple Choice

1. If an impression loses water content due to heat, dryness, or exposure to air, the condition is known as
   a. imbibition.
   b. syneresis.
   c. distortion.
   d. acceleration.

2. A final impression material that uses water-cooled trays is
   a. polysiloxane.
   b. polysulfide.
   c. reversible hydrocolloid.
   d. silicone.

3. The broad group title that encompasses the hard waxes used in crown and bridge casting (inlay wax) is
   a. pattern.
   b. processing.
   c. impression.
   d. study wax.

4. The liquid catalyst for the self-curing acrylic tray resin is a
   a. polymer.
   b. thermoplastic.
   c. monomer.
   d. spacer.

5. The strongest temporary (provisional) restoration is the
   a. aluminum shell temporary.
   b. self-cure methyl methacrylate temporary.
   c. self-cure R' (resin) methacrylate temporary.
   d. self-cure composite temporary.

Critical Thinking

1. Name several types of final impression material and identify factors that affect usage with each.

2. What are the effects of lower water-to-powder ratio in a mixture of irreversible hydrocolloid?

3. What are some of the advantages of polyether impression material?

Expanded Functions

28

Advanced Chairside Functions

DENTAL DAM

OBJECTIVES

The student should strive to meet the following objectives and demonstrate an understanding of the facts and principles presented in this chapter:

1. Explain the purpose of the dental dam and identify who places the dental dam on a patient.

2. List and explain the advantages and contraindications of the dental dam.

3. Identify the armamentarium needed for the dental dam procedure and explain the function of each.

4. Explain how to prepare the patient for the dental dam placement, explain how to determine the isolation area, and describe and demonstrate how the dental dam material is prepared.

5. List and demonstrate the steps of placing and removing the dental dam.

6. Explain and demonstrate the dental dam procedure for the child patient.

KEY TERMS

anchor tooth (p. 631)

cervical clamps (p. 632)

dental dam clamps (p. 631)

dental dam forceps (p. 633)

dental dam frame (p. 631)

dental dam napkins (p. 631)

dental dam punch (p. 631)

interseptal (p. 633)

inverting (p. 633)

key hole punch (p. 634)

ligature (p. 633)

septum (p. 634)

template (p. 631)

winged clamps (p. 632)

wingless clamps (p. 632)

INTRODUCTION

Dental dam placement is one method used to isolate teeth that are going to be restored. It can be used on almost any patient. The dental dam is a barrier that is applied by the dentist and, in some states, by the dental assistant and the dental hygienist. After the patient has received the anesthetic, the dental dam is prepared and placed. The dental assistant assists the dentist in the placement or places the dental dam before the dentist begins to prepare the tooth. The dam can be placed to isolate one tooth or one or more quadrants.

Advantages of Using the Dental Dam

The advantages of using the dental dam include:

▶ Greater visibility because of the contrast between the tooth and the dental dam material

▶ Greater accessibility to the operating field by retracting the gingiva, the tongue, the cheeks, and the lips

▶ Control of moisture to keep the area dry for better vision and to ensure a dry tooth when bonding agents, etchants, and restorative materials are used

▶ Protection for the patient from swallowing or aspirating debris during the procedure

▶ Protection of the gingiva during acid-etching procedures

▶ Improved patient management and decreased operating time because of limited patient conversation and because a clear, dry field is maintained

▶ Acts as a protective barrier for the patient

▶ Decreased amount of contaminated aerosol exposure

Contraindication to Dental Dam Isolation

Conditions that contraindicate the use of the dental dam include:

▶ Physical conditions of the patient, such as asthma, respiratory congestion, allergies to latex, herpetic lesions, or lesions of the commissures

▶ Concerns the patient might have, such as if the patient is claustrophobic (cannot tolerate the dental dam) or the patient has had or heard of a bad experience with the dental dam (hesitant to have the dam utilized for the dental procedure)

▶ Conditions in the oral cavity, such as partially erupted teeth or malaligned teeth

MATERIALS AND EQUIPMENT

The dental dam procedure requires a variety of instruments and materials. The materials and equip-

ment may be on a separate tray (Figure 28-1), stored at the dental unit, or in a tub for easy use. Materials include the dental dam material, dental dam napkin, dental floss, and tape. Dental dam clamps, forceps, frame, punching guides, and a punch are the specific equipment needed.

Dental Dam Material

The dental dam is a latex or latex-free material that comes in various sizes, weights, and colors selected according to the office preference. The most common sizes of the dental dam are the 5×5 or the 6×6 precut squares. These squares usually come in a box of fifty or more and are lightly powdered on one side to prevent sticking. The dental dam is also available in a continuous roll of five-inch and six-inch widths. This material is cut to the length desired by the operator.

The dental dam is available in different weights (thicknesses), including thin, medium, heavy, extra heavy, and special heavy. The thin or light dental dam materials are passed easily through contacts but tear easily and do not retract the tissues effectively. The medium and the heavy materials are used most often because they do not tear as easily and they provide greater tissue retraction. The heavier the material, the more difficult it is to place interproximally, but the retraction is excellent.

The dental dam is available in various colors (shades), from dark gray or green to lighter pastels. The darker shades provide more contrast with the teeth and make it easier for the operator to see. A scented dental dam is also available and is very pleasing to the patient (in comparison to the latex smell). It may be scented with mint or fruit.

The dental dam material has no definite shelf life but is sensitive to temperature changes and, like other latex

FIGURE 28-1 Dental dam tray setup (labeled). (A) Dental dam punch. (B) Forceps. (C) Frame. (D) Dental dam napkin. (E) Packing instrument. (F) Scissors. (G) Widgets. (H) Clamp. (I) Dental dam. (J) Floss.

rubber, to age. For a longer shelf life, store the dental dam material in the refrigerator.

Dental Dam Napkin

Dental dam napkins are used for patient comfort and to absorb saliva, water, and perspiration. The disposable napkins are made of a soft, absorbent fabric and are pre-cut. They are designed to prevent the dam material from touching the face by covering the area around the mouth and up on the cheeks.

Dental Dam Frame

The **dental dam frame**, or holder, is designed to stretch and secure the dam in place across the patient's face. The frame stabilizes the dental dam and keeps the operating area open. The frames are made of metal or plastic and have small projections around the borders to secure the dental dam.

There are several styles of frames available (Figure 28-2). The metal U-shaped frame is very common and is known as the **Young frame**. It is easy to apply and comfortable for the patient. The Young frame is made of stainless steel and can be autoclaved. The plastic U-shaped frame is also common and is known as the **U-frame**. It is also easy to apply and comfortable for the patient. This plastic frame is radiolucent and autoclavable. The **Ostby frame** is an oval-shaped, plastic frame that was designed to follow the shape of the lower face. There are projections on the outer borders to secure the dental dam. This frame is radiotransparent and can be autoclaved.

Dental Dam Punching Guides

The dental dam may be marked by using a **template** or a **stamp** of the adult and pediatric arches. Both the template and stamp are marked to indicate where the holes for the teeth should be punched. The stamp is used with an ink pad and the dam may be stamped ahead of time.

The template comes in both 5×5 and 6×6 sizes and also can be used to mark the dam ahead of time (Figure 28-3).

The dental dam guides are perfect dental arches, so they will not fit every patient. Instead, the markings act as a guide. They are especially helpful when learning to punch the dental dam, but eventually they become unnecessary and the operator uses the patient's teeth as the guide.

Dental Dam Punch

The action of the **dental dam punch** is similar to that of the paper punch, although the design is much different. The punch has a handle and a working end (see Figure 28-1). The working end of the punch has a **stylus**, which is a sharp projection to punch through the dental dam, and a **punch table** or **plate**. The table has four or five differently sized holes and rotates to facilitate punching holes for the various teeth (Figure 28-4). The punch table should be adjusted so that the hole is centered under the stylus before the punch is made. This prevents damage to the holes of the punch table. When the punch table is rotated, it makes a clicking sound as it adjusts.

Dental Dam Clamps

Dental dam clamps come in numerous designs and sizes to fit around the teeth (Figure 28-5). Their purpose is to stabilize and secure the dental dam material in place. The tooth that the clamp is placed on is often called the **anchor tooth**. The anchor tooth is one or two teeth to the distal of the tooth or teeth being restored.

Dental dam clamps are made of high quality stainless steel and are designed to be used on specific teeth. They are identified by numbers and letters, not by the teeth they are used on. The basic parts to a dental dam clamp include the following (Figure 28-6):

▶ **Bow**—The arched metal joining the two jaws of the clamp together.

FIGURE 28-2 Dental dam frames.

FIGURE 28-3 Dental dam punching guides. (A) Template. (B) Stamp with ink pad.

Hole number 5–Molars, and used for anchor tooth
Hole number 4–Molars
Hole number 3–Cuspids and premolars
Hole number 2–Upper incisors
Hole number 1–Lower incisors

FIGURE 28-4 Punch table with corresponding teeth.

FIGURE 28-5 Assortment of clamps.

▶ **Jaws**—The part of the clamp that expands to fix over the tooth and then releases to fit on the gingival one-third of the tooth. They secure the clamp to the tooth. The jaws are different sizes for different teeth in the arch.

▶ **Forceps holes**—Located on the jaws of the clamp. These holes are where the dental dam forceps attach to the clamp to place and remove the clamp from the tooth.

▶ **Points**—The parts of the jaws that actually contact the tooth. The points are at different widths and angles to fit and secure the clamp on the tooth.

▶ The jaws of the clamp are designed to be winged or wingless. The **winged clamps** have extra projections for better retraction, and they hold the dental dam in place because the wings are angled toward the gingiva. The **wingless clamps** have the letter W in front of the number of the clamp and have no projections.

▶ Some clamps are double bowed. These clamps are called **cervical clamps**. Cervical clamps are used for Class V restorations on anterior teeth. These clamps assist in gingival retraction and often must be stabi-

lized with stick impression compound after the teeth have been exposed. Examples are the SSW 212 or the Hygenic B6 and B5.

▶ Dental dam clamps that have the letter A following the number have jaws that bend sharply downward, toward the gingiva. Clamps without the letter A have jaws that are on a flat plane.

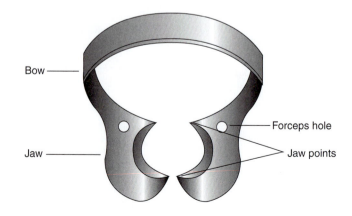

Bow

Forceps hole

Jaw

Jaw points

FIGURE 28-6 Parts of the dental dam clamp.

Selecting the Clamp

The tooth to be clamped must be evaluated before the clamp selection is made. The mesiodistal width at the cementoenamel junction (CEJ) of the tooth must be evaluated in order to select a clamp. The width on the tooth must be about the same as the width between the points of the jaws of the clamp. The faciolingual width at the CEJ of the tooth must also be estimated. This is to ensure that the clamp fits tightly. Once the tooth has been evaluated, a clamp can be selected. To place the clamp, the jaws are opened wide enough to clear the height of contour, which is the widest part of the tooth. Then, the jaws are closed slowly on the tooth to fit tightly at the CEJ. The points should rest securely all around the tooth.

Dental Dam Forceps

Dental dam forceps are used to place and remove the dental dam clamp. The forceps have two beaks that fit into the holes of the jaws of the clamp. Once the beaks are securely in the holes, pressure is applied to the handle of the forceps and the clamp jaws are opened slightly. There is a lock (sliding bar) on the handle that keeps the clamp in this position until it is placed on the anchor tooth. When the handle is squeezed again and the lock is released, the operator has control over the clamp and can make adjustments to the clamp position. As the clamp is placed properly, the tension that expands the clamp is eased and the clamp is secured on the tooth. Once the clamp is stable, the beaks of the forceps are removed from the clamp and the forceps are removed from the mouth.

Dental Floss

Dental floss is used for a variety of reasons with dental dam isolation.

1. A piece of dental floss, about eighteen inches long, is tied to the bow of the dental dam clamp before the clamp is placed. If the clamp slips off the anchor tooth, the floss makes it easy to retrieve. The floss ends are always on the outside of the mouth for quick access. Sometimes, the floss is called a ligature or safety line.

2. The floss is used to ease the dental dam material through tight contacts.

3. The dental floss assists in **inverting**, or tucking, the dental dam material around the teeth to prevent moisture leakage.

4. The clamp stabilizes the dental dam on one end of the arch and dental floss is sometimes used to secure the opposite end. On the distal of the last tooth on the opposite side from the clamped tooth, a piece of floss is placed interproximally and then looped over with a second piece of floss to secure the end of the punched dental dam.

Lubricant

A small amount of lubricant is placed on the back or underside of the dental dam. This facilitates slipping the dam material over the teeth. A water-based dental dam lubricant works better than a petroleum base, such as Vaseline, because it does not leave a film on the teeth, which makes the teeth slippery and makes it difficult to hold the dental dam material in place. For the patient's comfort, a light amount of petroleum jelly or another type of lip lubricant can be applied to the lips prior to placement of the dental dam.

Scissors

Scissors are used to cut the **interseptal** dental dam during removal of the dam from the patient's mouth. **Dental dam scissors** or any small pair of scissors the operator feels comfortable with can be used. When cutting the interseptal dam material, direct the scissors away from the tissues to prevent tearing of the dam material and to completely cut the interseptal dam.

Inverting or Tucking Instrument

The dental floss can be used to invert or tuck the dental dam, but sometimes an instrument is needed to accomplish this step. Some options include a periodontal probe, spoon excavator, or the flat side of the T-ball burnisher. These instruments are used to turn under the edge of the dental dam that is around the tooth. The instrument is started on one side of the tooth and run at an angle to the other side. The edge of the dam is tucked under to assist in keeping the area dry.

Stabilizing Cord

Stabilizing cord is an elastic cord that comes in different sizes and colors (see Figure 28-1). It is stretched and then placed interproximally to secure the dental dam material. The cord is used to stabilize the dental dam placement at the opposite end of the clamp or for individual teeth. For example, instead of using a dental dam clamp, use the stabilizing cord for an anterior dental dam placement.

Ligatures

A **ligature** is a piece of floss or a cord that stabilizes the dental dam in different applications. Ligatures are used in fixed bridge isolation, in bleaching procedures, and on individual teeth isolation. Sometimes, the floss is tied into a slip knot and placed over the tooth, such as in isolation for bleaching a tooth. With some patients, the floss or cord is threaded between the teeth or under the pontics for placement and then tied into place to retain the dental dam material.

PREPARATION BEFORE PLACEMENT OF THE DENTAL DAM

Before the dental dam is placed, the procedure should be explained to the patient and the operator should examine the oral cavity to determine the area of isolation.

Educating the Patient

Patients like to know what is going to happen during their appointments. The dental assistant should explain the purpose of the dental dam and then have the patient acknowledge acceptance of this part of the restorative procedure. If the patient has had the dental dam placed before, ask whether the patient has any questions before beginning the placement. If the patient has not had a dental dam application before, explain how the dam is placed and what to expect before beginning the placement. Some points that might be included are the pressure of the clamp on the tooth, to breathe through the nose, and that the patient can still swallow.

Determining the Area to Be Isolated

Before the dental dam is punched, the area to be isolated needs to be determined and then examined. Follow these steps:

1. Determine the tooth to be restored and then determine the anchor tooth, which is usually one or two teeth distal to the tooth being restored. The number of teeth to be included in the punch is a personal preference. Some operators like only one or two teeth exposed, while others like eight or more teeth to be punched. When learning, a good rule of thumb is to punch to the canine of the opposite quadrant. This is good practice because one of the most difficult aspects of punching the dental dam is accurately punching the curvature of the arch. Once this skill is mastered, the dental dam should be punched precisely for any patient. For example, if tooth #14 was the tooth to be restored, the anchor tooth would be tooth #15 and holes would be punched around the arch to include tooth #6.

2. The size and the shape of the arch are examined so that they can be duplicated on the dental dam as closely as possible to the patient's arch.

3. The area is examined for missing teeth, teeth that are out of alignment, or fixed prosthetics. The dental dam can be punched and placed to accommodate most conditions in a patient's mouth.

4. The area is flossed to identify tight contacts and open spacing.

Dividing the Dental Dam

Select the size and weight dental dam that best suits the patient and the procedure. (Refer to the Materials and Equipment section of this chapter to review the information on the dental dam material.) When preparing the dental dam material for punching, it is first divided into sixths (Figure 28-7). One way to mark the divisions is to fold and then crease the dental dam. This leaves a faint mark on the dam for the operator to use when punching the dam.

To begin, fold the dam in half and then crease the fold. This horizontal line is the division between the maxillary and mandibular arches. With the dam folded in half, fold the dam vertically into equal thirds and crease along each fold. The center third is where the dam will be punched. This represents the width of the arches of most patients. Some operators prefer to divide the dam into thirds only, and some divide the dam into quarters and mark the center point as a reference point before punching.

Punching the Dental Dam

After the dental dam is divided, it is ready to be punched for the placement. There are many places to begin actually punching the dental dam, so it is important for the operator to visualize the patient's arch on the dental dam. Often, the **key hole punch** is punched first. The key punch hole is the largest hole punched in the dental dam. It is the hole that slides over the clamp and onto the anchor tooth. The next holes are punched moving forward, about 3 to 3.5 mm apart. This is the amount of dental dam that slides between the teeth. It is called the **septum**. The punch table is adjusted for the size of the teeth (see Figure 28-4).

FIGURE 28-7 Dental dam divided into sixths.

Maxillary Arch. The maxillary arch is punched in the upper middle sixth portion of the dental dam (Figure 28-8).

▶ Holes punched for the anteriors should be one inch from the top edge of the dam. This assists in positioning the arch.

▶ Variations in this one-inch guide are for patients with full upper lips or mustaches or patients with thin upper lips. The distance is increased or decreased accordingly.

▶ Punch the pattern to follow the patient's arch, leaving 3 to 3.5 mm between each tooth.

▶ The punch includes from one to two teeth distal of the tooth to be restored and then all teeth to the opposite cuspid.

▶ Punch the two centrals first, then continue to punch the remaining teeth. This centers the punch pattern on the dam.

Mandibular Arch. The mandibular arch is punched in the lower sixth portion of the dental dam (Figure 28-9).

▶ The first punch is the key hole punch. Teeth #17 and #32 are punched at the junction of the horizontal half and the vertical third. The more mesial the key punch hole is in the arch, the closer the punch is to the middle and bottom of the dam.

FIGURE 28-9 Mandibular arch punched for mandibular left first molar.

▶ The holes are not punched beginning with the central incisors, one inch from the lower edge of the dam. This would place the top part of the dam over the patient's nose. Instead, the central incisors are usually punched two inches from the lower edge of the dam.

▶ The rest of the punch follows the patient's arch, leaving 3 to 3.5 mm between each tooth.

▶ The punch includes one or two teeth distal of the tooth to be restored and all teeth to the opposite cuspid.

Maxillary and Mandibular Anterior Teeth. When placing the dental dam for the maxillary and mandibular anterior teeth, it is often unnecessary to use a clamp. Dental floss is doubled and a piece of dental dam or stabilizing cord is placed in the distal interproximals of each canine. This is usually enough to hold the dam in place without the placement of a clamp (Figure 28-10).

▶ There is no key punch.

▶ The punches for the two centrals are in the middle third of the dam, one inch from the top edge for the maxillary and two inches from the bottom edge for the mandibular.

Missing or Malpositioned Teeth. Punching for patients who have missing or malpositioned teeth is accomplished by the operator following the patterns of

FIGURE 28-8 Maxillary arch punched for maxillary right first molar.

ment teeth and spaces are left for the number of pontics. Slits are cut between the holes with scissors to allow the bridges to be exposed.

Class V Restoration Placement. For a Class V restoration, the hole is punched facially to its normal position in the arch. A cervical clamp is often used with the Class V restorations, because they retract the gingiva and the dam beyond the borders of the cavity. The lower the cavity is on the facial surface of the tooth, the more the punch hole is moved toward the facial. The largest hole on the punch is used for this clamp, because the double wings allow an additional 1 to 3 mm between adjacent teeth.

Common Errors When Punching the Dental Dam

The curve of the arch should match the arch curve of the patient. Punching the arch too flat or wide results in folds or bunching and stretching on the lingual. Punching the arch too curved or narrow results in folds and stretching on the facial. These errors make tucking the dental dam into the gingival sulcus difficult.

The punch table should be clean and free of previously punched dam material. Also, check for nicks in the holes of the punch table. If there are marks on the punch table or if the stylus does not line up directly, the punched holes may leave a tag of dam material or have a tear around the hole. The dam material will tear more easily when being stretched for placement with either of these errors, and the dam may leak once in place.

The hole spacing should match the space between the patient's teeth. If the holes are too close together, there will not be enough material to seal around each tooth, but the dam will be stretched and gingival tissue will be exposed. If the holes are too far apart, there will be excess material between the teeth. It may be difficult to get all the dam material interproximal when placing the dental dam, and the bunched dental dam material may get in the operator's way during the procedure.

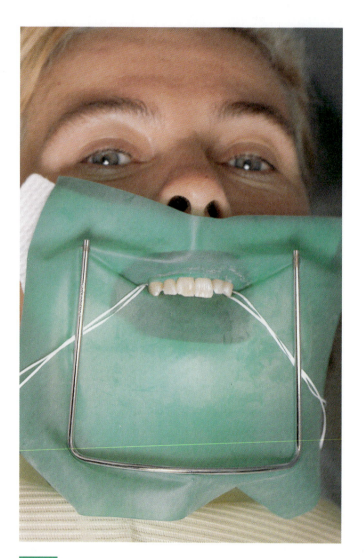

FIGURE 28-10 Maxillary anterior placement with floss used as ligatures.

the teeth in the patients' mouths as the dental dams are punched.

▸ When teeth are malpositioned (out of normal alignment or position), they often are positioned either buccal or lingual of the normal curve of the arch, so the corresponding holes must be positioned either toward the buccal or the lingual to match the arch.

▸ Missing teeth or edentulous areas are accommodated by leaving a space on the dam between holes punched for teeth present in the mouth. So, if tooth #5 is missing, then tooth #4 would be punched, a space would be left, and teeth #6, #7, and so on would be punched.

Bridgework Placement. Patterns for patients with bridgework require punches similar to the punches with the missing teeth. It is impossible to punch holes for the pontics, so the punches are made for the abut-

PLACEMENT AND REMOVAL PROCEDURES FOR THE DENTAL DAM

There are many techniques for placement of the dental dam, and the operator will find through practice which works best. The dental assistant assists the dentist with the dental dam in states where it is not legal for him or her to place the dental dam, but in states where the dental assistant can place the dental dam, the assistant punches the dam, selects the clamp, and places and removes the dental dam without the chairside presence of the dentist.

P R O C E D U R E

28-1 Placing and Removing the Dental Dam

This procedure is performed by the dentist or dental assistant. The patient has been anesthetized before the placement of the dental dam and before the cavity preparation begins. The dental assistant has prepared all equipment and supplies needed for the entire procedure. Only the items needed for the dental dam are listed for this procedure.

EQUIPMENT AND SUPPLIES

▶ Dental dam material (6 x 6 sheets)

▶ Dental dam napkin

▶ Dental dam punch

▶ Assortment of clamps

▶ Dental dam forceps

▶ Dental dam frame

▶ Dental floss

▶ Lubricant

▶ Cotton tip applicator

▶ Tucking instrument (plastic instrument, T-ball burnisher, or spoon excavator)

▶ Scissors

PROCEDURE STEPS *(Follow aseptic procedures)*

Placement of the Dental Dam

1. Inform the patient about the dental dam procedure.

2. Examine the patient's oral cavity to determine the anchor tooth, shape of the arch, tooth alignment, missing teeth, and the presence of crowns and bridges. Also, examine the gingival tissues and check for tight contacts (Figure 28-11).

3. Prepare the dam material by dividing it into sixths and then punch the dam, aligning the stylus and the holes carefully.

4. Center the punch in the upper or lower middle third of the dental dam. Holes are punched according to size of tooth, with the key punch being the largest to accommodate the anchor tooth and the clamp.

FIGURE 28-11 Dental assistant checking the patient's contacts with floss.

5. Holes are punched following the pattern of the patient's arch (Figure 28-12). Lubricate the dental dam on the tissue side of the dam with a water-soluble lubricant.

6. Select the clamp or several clamps to try on the tooth. Things to consider when selecting the clamp include:
   ▶ The clamp design (if it is a winged or wingless clamp)
   ▶ The mesiodistal width at the CEJ of the anchor tooth

FIGURE 28-12 Dental assistant punching the dental dam material.

(continued)

P R O C E D U R E   2 8 - 1 *continued*

- ▶ The faciolingual width at the CEJ of the anchor tooth
- ▶ The height of the occlusal plane of the anchor tooth

7. Attach a safety line on all clamps that are to be tried on. When trying on the clamps, keep the end of the safety line in hand (Figure 28-13).

8. Secure the clamp on the clamp forceps and spread the jaws slightly to lock the forceps.

9. Place the clamp over the anchor tooth. To widen the jaws of the clamp, squeeze the forceps handle slightly to release the locking bar (Figure 28-14).

FIGURE 28-13 Clamp with floss safety ligature and dental dam clamp forceps.

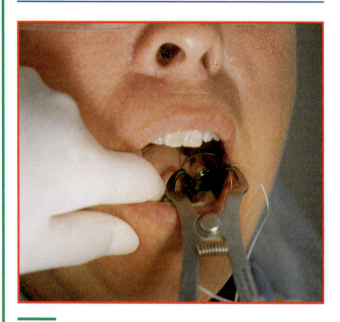

FIGURE 28-14 Dental dam clamp placed on the anchor tooth.

10. Fit the lingual jaws of the clamp on the lingual side of the tooth first. Next, spread the clamp and slide the buccal jaws of the clamp over the height of contour of the buccal surface of the tooth. Release the pressure on the clamp forceps slightly against the tooth to evaluate the clamp, but do not release the clamp from the forceps.

11. The jaw points of the clamp should be at the CEJ, adapting to the gingival embrasures on the buccal and lingual. The clamp should be secure on the tooth, not pinching any gingival tissue. The clamp may be adjusted to the tooth by moving the wrist to the left and right and by putting more pressure on the distal or mesial of the clamp.

12. When the clamp is in place, confirm with the patient that the clamp position is comfortable (Figure 28-15).

13. Place the dental dam over the clamp bow by grasping the dam material and placing the index

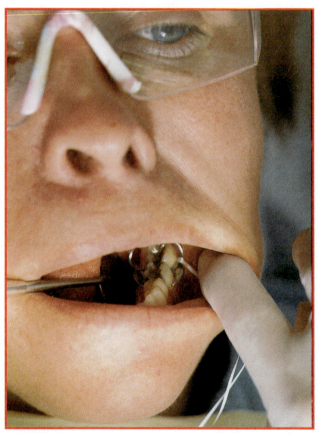

FIGURE 28-15 Evaluate clamp placement and patient comfort.

(continued)

P R O C E D U R E   **2 8 - 1** *continued*

fingers on each side of the key hole punch. Spread the hole wide enough to slip over the clamp. Stretch the hole over the anchor tooth and one side of the clamp, then expose the other clamp jaw so that the entire clamp and anchor tooth are exposed. Pull the safety line through the dam and drape to the side of the patient's mouth.

14. Isolate the most forward tooth, usually the opposite canine. The dam material is secured on the distal of this tooth with a double loop of floss, a corner cut of the dental dam material, or stabilizing cord (Figure 28-16).

15. Place the dental napkin around the patient's mouth (Figure 28-17).

16. Place the frame or holder to stretch the dam to cover the oral cavity. The frame can be placed either under or over the dental dam material, depending on the type of frame and the preference of the operator (Figure 28-18).

17. Isolate the remaining teeth. The dental dam is worked gently between the contacts. Dental floss is used to assist in placing the dental dam and exposing the teeth. When using the floss, catch the edge of the hole with the floss and pull it over the tooth, into and through the contact (Figure 28-19). Using the air syringe to dry the teeth at this time facilitates the placement of the dam material.

FIGURE 28-18 Frame stretching the dam.

FIGURE 28-16 Clamp with dental dam material positioned on the tooth and the dam secured to the opposite cuspid.

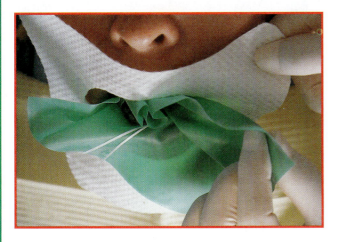

FIGURE 28-17 Dental napkin being placed around the patient's mouth.

FIGURE 28-19 Dental assistant placing the dam between the contacts with floss.

(continued)

P R O C E D U R E   **2 8 - 1** *continued*

18. Invert or tuck the dam material. (The edge of the dam that surrounds the tooth must be inverted or tucked into the sulcus of the gingiva to seal the tooth and prevent leakage. There are several ways this is accomplished. Carefully pull the dental dam material slightly apically, and the dam will often invert when the dam is releases. When using the floss to place the dam interproximally, the dam may be inverted. Or, use a T-ball burnisher, a plastic instrument, or a spoon excavator to tuck the buccal and lingual surfaces (Figure 28-20). Use the instrument with the air from the air-water syringe to dry the surface and then invert the edge of the dam. Continue until all edges of the dam are sealed.

19. Coat all tooth-colored restorations with lubricant.

20. Place and position a saliva ejector and/or a bite-block under the dam for patient comfort, if needed.

21. Double-check dam placement and patient comfort (Figure 28-21).

FIGURE 28-21 Patient with dental dam on and ready for the dentist.

Alternate Technique for Placing the Dental Dam

Some operators prefer to carry the clamp, dental dam material, and, in some placements, even the frame to the tooth when applying the clamp. This technique requires practice and confidence when placing the clamp but does take less time (Figure 28-22). The clamp is selected (usually a winged clamp), and the ligature is secured on the bow of the clamp. The bow of the clamp and the forcep holes on the jaws are exposed through the dental dam material. The clamp forceps are placed in the forcep holes and secured. The operator holds the rest of the dam material up and out of the way while placing the clamp and dam on the anchor tooth. After the clamp is secured on the tooth, the wings of the clamp are exposed and placement is completed following the procedure steps.

FIGURE 28-20 Dam is in place and the dental assistant is tucking the dam with an instrument.

FIGURE 28-22 Dental dam clamp secured in the forceps with the dental dam material in position for placement.

(continued)

Removal of the Dental Dam

When the operator is ready to remove the dental dam, the area is rinsed and dried using the evacuator and the three-way syringe.

1. Explain to the patient the procedure to remove the dental dam and caution him or her not to bite down when the dam is removed.

2. Free the interseptal dam with scissors. To protect the patient, slip the index or middle finger underneath the dam material and stretch it facially, away from the tooth. Slant the scissors toward the occlusal surface, and clip each septum with the scissors (Figure 28-23). Pulling the dam material toward the facial, the operator cuts the interseptal dam.

3. Remove the dental dam clamp. Place the forceps in the clamp holes and squeeze the handles to open the clamp jaws. Usually, the clamp can be lifted straight off the tooth, but if this is not possible, rotate the clamp facially so the jaws clear the lingual and then rotate the clamp lingually to clear the buccal (Figure 28-24).

4. Remove the frame or holder and the dam material.

5. Remove the napkin, wiping the area around the mouth.

6. Examine the dam material by spreading the dental dam material out flat and examining to make certain that all the interseptal material is present (Figure 28-25). If there are any pieces missing,

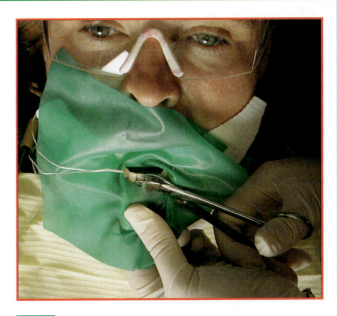

FIGURE 28-23 Pulling the dental dam material toward the facial, the operator cuts the interseptal dam.

floss between the teeth. This should dislodge any small segment of remaining dam.

7. Massage the gingiva around the anchor tooth to increase circulation of the area.

8. Rinse the patient's mouth thoroughly.

FIGURE 28-24 Clamp forceps remove the clamp from the anchor tooth.

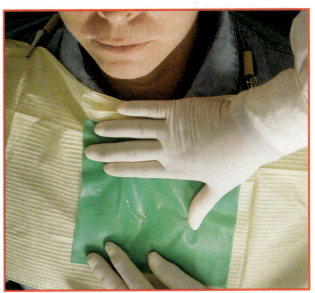

FIGURE 28-25 Dental dam material is placed on the patient's bib for the operator to examine.

DENTAL DAM FOR THE CHILD PATIENT

Dental dam is used on children as routinely as it is on adults. The key advantages become even more important when trying to control the busy tongue and lips of a child. The basic technique is the same for both adults and children. There are, however, several modifications.

It is important to explain to the child the parts of the dental dam and the procedure. Use terminology and explanations that are appropriate for the maturity of the child. Words that are commonly used to describe the dental dam include "raincoat" or "umbrella," the clamp might be the "button" or the "tooth raincoat holder," and the frame is the "coat hanger." Explain to the child how to swallow and breathe with the dental dam in place. Let him or her help by holding the saliva ejector during the procedure and establish a way for him or her to communicate, for example, raising a finger on the dental assistant's side. When people try to talk with the dental dam in place, it is amazing how well the dentist and the dental assistant understand "dental dam talk."

Look at the patient's dentition and determine whether all primary teeth are present, there are missing teeth, partially erupted teeth, and/or if the patient is in mixed dentition. The holes are punched according to these conditions. Generally, the holes are punched closer together and no holes are punched where teeth are missing or just barely erupted.

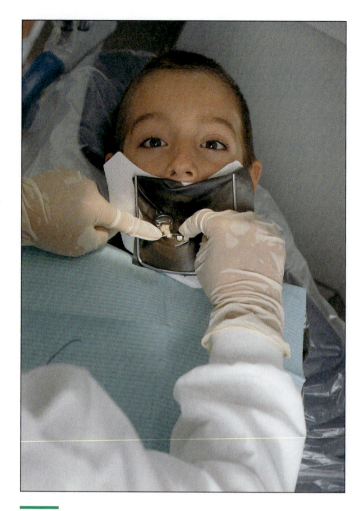

FIGURE 28-26 Dental dam is placed on child patient.

Placing the Dental Dam for the Pediatric Patient

When placing the dental dam for the pediatric patient (Figure 28-26), punch the holes in the same manner as for adult patients, with the anchor hole the same but the holes for the individual teeth smaller. The arch is still punched following the pattern of the child's arch, going to the opposite cuspid. In some cases, the holes are punched only for the teeth that are directly involved. Dental dam clamps with projections are used on "short teeth" or teeth that are partially erupted. Ligatures on the primary first molars or cuspids aid to retain the dam on the tooth. Wooden wedges are also used interproximally to depress the gingiva and the dental dam.

ALTERNATIVES FOR FULL DENTAL DAM PLACEMENT

An alternative to the full dental dam placement is an oval piece of dental dam that has a border of flexible plastic. This dental dam comes with its own template to mark each tooth. The **Quickdam** is punched using a regular punch and the same size holes. After the holes have been punched, the dam frame is folded and inserted into the patient's mouth, lying in the vestibular area. The dam must be fitted around the teeth to be isolated; sometimes, a ligature or dental dam clamp is used to secure the dam.

PROCEDURE

28-2 Rubber Dam Application for the Child Patient

The procedure is performed by the dentist or the dental assistant. The dental dam is quickly placed on the teeth. The patient's dentition must be evaluated to determine which teeth can be included in the isolation. Look for partially erupted teeth and teeth that are loose.

EQUIPMENT AND SUPPLIES

▶ Basic setup: mouth mirror, explorer, and cotton pliers

▶ Dental dam material (5x5)

▶ Dental dam napkin

▶ Dental dam punch

▶ Assortment of pedodontic clamps

▶ Dental dam clamp forceps

▶ Dental dam frame

▶ Dental floss

▶ Lubricant

▶ Cotton tip applicator

▶ Tucking instrument (plastic instrument, T-ball burnisher, or spoon excavator)

▶ Scissors

PROCEDURE STEPS *(Follow aseptic procedures)*

1. Prepare the child for the dental dam placement by explaining the materials and the procedure at a level the child can understand.

2. Determine the number of teeth to be isolated and the size and shape of the arch.

3. Using the five-inch, square, heavyweight dental dam, punch the predetermined pattern. The holes are punched closer together than they would be for adults.

4. Select the clamp. Winged clamps are often selected because they retract the heavyweight rubber dam for better vision. The wings are also used to position the clamp below the height of contour of teeth that are partially erupted. Tie a piece of floss to the bow of the clamp for security.

5. The clamp is positioned on the tooth with the clamp forceps. Often, the clamp, dental dam, and frame are carried all in one to be applied to the tooth.

6. Check to see whether the clamp is securely positioned. Slide the dam over the wings of the clamp to expose the wings.

7. Place the dental dam over the remaining teeth.

8. A ligature of widget is placed to secure the dental dam (Figure 28-27).

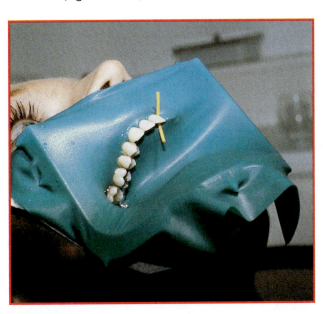

FIGURE 28-27 Patient with widgets securing the dental dam in place. *(Courtesy of Coltène/Whaledent, Inc.)*

P R O C E D U R E

28-3 Quickdam Placement

This procedure is performed by the dentist or the dental assistant. The patient is anesthetized and the Quickdam is placed.

EQUIPMENT AND SUPPLIES

▶ Quickdam

▶ Quickdam template

▶ Dental dam punch

▶ Dental dam clamps

▶ Dental dam clamp forceps

▶ Dental floss

▶ Tucking instrument

PROCEDURE STEPS (Follow aseptic procedures)

1. Examine the patient's dentition to determine the punch pattern. Note any malpositioned teeth and the curve of the arch.

2. Use the Quickdam template to mark each tooth to be punched and allow for any deviations. Mark with a felt-tip pen.

3. Punch the marked teeth according to the corresponding hole size for each tooth.

4. The Quickdam can be used with or without a dental dam clamp. Without a clamp, fold the ends of the Quickdam toward each other and press the sides together. Insert the Quickdam into the patient's mouth and release the sides. The Quickdam fits into the patient's vestibule. Slide the dam over the teeth to be isolated. Use dental floss to tuck the dental dam, and secure the dam with floss ligatures on the distal of the last isolated teeth.

5. With a clamp, select a clamp and attach a ligature to the bow of the clamp. To place the clamp and dam in one step, secure the clamp in the hole punched for the tooth to be clamped. Apply the clamp forceps, and place the clamp over the tooth. Once the clamp is securely on the tooth, remove the clamp forceps. Place the dam over the teeth to be isolated and tuck the dam.

MATRIX AND WEDGE

OBJECTIVES

The student should strive to meet the following objectives and demonstrate an understanding of the facts and principles presented in this chapter:

1. Define matrix and wedge. List the uses and types of matrices.

2. Describe the functions, parts, placement, and removal of the Tofflemire matrix.

3. Explain and demonstrate placement and removal of the strip matrix.

KEY TERMS

band (p. 645)

burnish (p. 648)

circumference (p. 646)

contra-angle (p. 646)

guide channels (p. 646)

matrix (p. 645)

retainer (p. 645)

spindle (p. 646)

vise (p. 646)

wedge (p. 645)

INTRODUCTION

During the preparation of a tooth for an amalgam or a composite restoration, often one or more axial surfaces are removed. Once these surfaces are removed, the only way to restore the tooth is to have an artificial wall in place of the missing wall or surface. This wall holds the restorative materials in the preparation during the filling of the cavity. A matrix replaces the surface and acts as the artificial wall.

The **matrix** is a collective term used to refer to the matrix **band** and the **retainer**. The matrix band forms the missing surface or wall and reestablishes the normal contour of the prepared tooth while the tooth is being filled with the restorative material. The matrix band is inserted into the retainer and then placed on the tooth. The retainer is the device which holds the band. It is tightened on the tooth and secures the band in place.

In addition to replacing the missing tooth surface of the cavity preparation, the matrix restores the natural contours of the tooth and the proximal contact with the adjacent tooth. A matrix also contains the restorative material within the walls, thereby preventing any excess material from getting near the gingiva. In addition, the matrix must be stable enough to withstand the pressure of the restorative material being placed in the cavity preparation.

Types of Matrices

There are several different matrices available, and the type of matrix selected depends on the type of restorative materials being used. For amalgam restorations, the **Tofflemire matrix** or the **Automatrix** is used. With the composite material, a **plastic strip matrix** or **shell matrix** is used.

WEDGES

Once the matrix is in place, a wedge (small, triangular piece of wood or plastic) is inserted interproximally against the matrix band or strip near the gingival margin of the preparation. This **wedge** holds the band securely in place and also prevents excess filling material from escaping between the tooth and the matrix band. This excess is called an **overhang**. An overhang can be damaging to the gingival tissues if left in place, so the correct positioning of the wedge is important in order to prevent this from occurring. The wedge also separates the teeth slightly to compensate for the thickness of the band. This ensures good contact with the adjacent tooth after the band has been removed.

Types of Wedges

Wedges come in different sizes that are either natural, clear, or colored. They usually come in an assortment kit with various sizes, with the colors marking the different sizes (Figure 28-28). The wedges can be altered in shape with a knife, if needed. Once the procedure is complete, the wedges are discarded.

Placement of Wedges

Wedges are only used when the preparation includes a proximal surface(s). For example, if the tooth had a mesiocclusal (MO) cavity preparation, only one wedge would be needed on the mesial. On the posterior teeth, either the wooden or plastic wedges can be used. On the anterior teeth, when light-cured materials are used, the plastic wedges are best.

The wedges are usually placed from the lingual on the posterior teeth. This makes placement easier and prevents interference with the retainer. Cotton pliers or a hemostat are used to place and remove the wedges. When placing the wedge, the smallest of the three sides is placed toward the gingiva. The wedge should fill the space and fit snugly (Figure 28-29A).

TOFFLEMIRE MATRIX

The Tofflemire matrix is the most common matrix used for amalgam restorations. It has two parts: the retainer and the band (Figure 28-29B). The retainer can be sterilized and reused, but the bands are disposed of in the sharps container after the procedure.

FIGURE 28-28 Assortment of wedges.

(A)

Occlusal aspect

(B)

Guide channels

2. Gingival aspect

FIGURE 28-29 (A) Matrix and wedge in place. (B) Parts of the straight Tofflemire retainer: Guide channels, vise, diagonal slot, spindle, inner knob, outer knob, and frame. 1. Occlusal view. 2. Gingival view.

Parts of the Tofflemire Matrix Retainer

Table 28-1 identifies the parts and functions of the Tofflemire matrix retainer.

The Tofflemire matrix retainer has a top (occlusal) side and a bottom (gingival) side. The occlusal side is directed toward the occlusal surface and is the smooth side of the guide channels and the vise. The gingival side is directed toward the gingival tissues and has the diagonal slot on the vise and the open ends of the guide channels (Figure 28-31).

Tofflemire Retainer Styles. The Tofflemire retainer is available in several styles so it can be positioned from either the lingual or the facial. The straight Tofflemire retainer is the most commonly used, and it is placed on the buccal or facial side, while the **contra-angle** Tofflemire retainer is placed on the lingual surface. It is angled slightly to accommodate clearance of the anterior teeth (Figure 28-30).

Matrix Bands

Matrix bands are made of stainless steel and are approximately all the same length. They differ in the shape of one edge and their widths (Figure 28-31). The size and shape of the cavity prep indicate which band is used. The more the prep extends toward the gingiva, the wider the matrix band needs to be. The matrix band is slightly curved and when looped over so both ends meet, the small **circumference** edge faces toward the gingiva and the larger circumference edge faces toward the occlusal.

> ▶ Hold the retainer with the guide channels and diagonal slot on the vise facing the operator.
> ▶ Keep the guide channels and the vise within one-quarter inch of each other.
> ▶ The looped matrix band correlates to the shape of the tooth, with the smaller circumference at the gingiva and the larger circumference at the occlusal.

TABLE 28-1 COMPONENTS OF THE TOFFLEMIRE MATRIX RETAINER

Part	Function
Frame	The main body of the retainer.
Guide channels	The slots in the end of the retainer that hold the matrix band. The slots direct the band to the right or left of the retainer.
Vise (locking)	Holds the ends of the matrix band in place in the diagonal slot.
Spindle	A screw-like rod used to secure the band in the vise.
Inner knob (adjusting knob)	Used to adjust the size of the matrix band loop by moving the vise along the frame of the retainer.
Outer knob (locking knob)	Used to tighten and loosen the spindle against the band in the vise.

FIGURE 28-30 Contra-angle Tofflemire retainer (note the angle of the guide channel section).

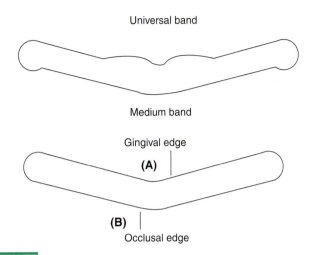

Universal band

Medium band

Gingival edge

(A)

(B)

Occlusal edge

FIGURE 28-31 Examples of matrix bands. Width of band selected is determined by the extension of the cavity preparation. (A) Occlusal edge. (B) Gingival edge.

P R O C E D U R E

28-4 Assembly of the Tofflemire Matrix

This procedure is performed by the dentist or dental assistant. The assembly is completed before the procedure begins.

EQUIPMENT AND SUPPLIES

▶ Tofflemire retainer

▶ Assortment of matrix bands

PROCEDURE STEPS (*Follow aseptic procedures*)

1. Hold the retainer so the guide channels and the diagonal slot on the vise are facing the operator.

2. Holding the frame of the retainer, rotate the inner knob (adjustment knob) until the vise is within one-quarter inch of the guide channels.

3. Turn the outer knob (locking knob) until the pointed end of the spindle is clear (below) of the slot in the vise.

4. Prepare the matrix band for placement in the retainer by holding the band to look like a smile, with the gingival edge on the top and the occlusal edge on the bottom.

5. Bring the ends together to form a teardrop-shaped loop (Figure 28-32). Be careful not to crease the band at any time. The larger circumfer-

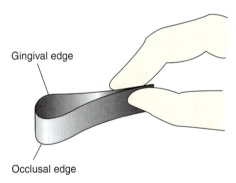

Gingival edge

Occlusal edge

FIGURE 28-32 Hold the matrix band in a smile and loop the ends of the band together. The gingival edge will be on the top and the occlusal edge on the bottom.

ence of the band, the occlusal, will be on the bottom and the smaller, the gingival, will be on the top.

6. With the gingival edge still on the top, place the occlusal edge of the band in the diagonal slot of the vise. The loop is extended toward the guide channels.

7. Place the matrix band in the appropriate guide channels. The direction of the matrix band depends on the tooth being restored (Figure 28-33).

(continued)

P R O C E D U R E **2 8 - 4** *continued*

FIGURE 28-33 Hold the Tofflemire retainer with the guide channels and the slot facing up, and insert the matrix band into the vise slot and the guide channels.

Hold the matrix retainer with the guide channel up, facing the operator, and the matrix band looped. Then:

▶ If the matrix is to be applied to the maxillary right or mandibular left quadrant, place the matrix band in the guide channels toward the operator's right (Figure 28-34A).

▶ If the matrix is to be applied to the maxillary left or mandibular right quadrant, place the matrix band in the guide channels toward the operator's left (Figure 28-34B).

(A)   (B)

FIGURE 28-34 The matrix band is positioned in the guide channels for the different quadrants. (A) Maxillary right/mandibular left. (B) Maxillary left/mandibular right.

8. Once the band is placed in the vise slot with the guide channels, turn the outer knob until the tip of the spindle is tight against the band in the vise slot.

9. Move the inner knob to increase or decrease the size of the loop to match the diameter of the tooth (Figure 28-35).

10. If the band becomes creased or bent during the assembly, it can be smoothed out by inserting the handle of the mouth mirror into the loop and running it around the inside of the loop (similar to curling ribbon when wrapping a gift) (Figure 28-36).

FIGURE 28-35 By turning the inner knob of the Tofflemire retainer, the matrix band loop increases and decreases in size.

FIGURE 28-36 Smoothing the loop of the matrix band.

The AutoMatrix

The AutoMatrix is a matrix without a retainer. The stainless steel bands are conical shaped and come in four sizes. The conical shape makes the band easy to **burnish** (smooth) for better contact in proximal areas. The

bands are circles with autolock loops that lock the matrices on the teeth. The tightening coil on the outside of the band is where the matrix is adapted to the tooth. There is no retainer to obstruct the operator's access or vision. The AutoMatrix comes in a kit that contains the clipping

P R O C E D U R E

28-5 Placement of the Tofflemire Matrix

This procedure is performed by the dentist or dental assistant. After the Tofflemire matrix is assembled, it is ready for positioning on the prepared tooth.

EQUIPMENT AND SUPPLIES

▶ Assembled Tofflemire retainer and matrix band

▶ Cotton pliers or hemostat

▶ Ball burnisher

▶ 2 × 2 gauze sponges

▶ Assortment of wedges

PROCEDURE STEPS *(Follow aseptic procedures)*

1. Place the matrix band over the prepared tooth with the smaller edge of the band toward the gingiva. The slot on the vise is directed toward the gingiva. Keep the retainer parallel to the buccal surface as the loop is placed around the tooth.

2. Move the loop through the interproximal surface. Place one finger over the loop to stabilize the loop and the retainer.

3. Once the matrix band is around the tooth, adjust the guide channel to center the retainer on the buccal surface of the tooth (Figure 28-37).

4. Turn the inner knob to tighten the band around the tooth. The band should be securely around the tooth and the retainer should be snug to the

FIGURE 28-37 Placing the Tofflemire retainer with the matrix band on the tooth and centering the retainer on the buccal surface of the tooth.

tooth. If the band is too tight or too loose, the contour of the restoration may change the contours of the tooth and the proximal contact.

5. Check the margins of the matrix band. The band should extend no more than 1 to 1.5 mm beyond the gingival margin of the cavity preparation on the gingival edge, and the occlusal edge should extend no more than 2 mm above the highest cusp (Figure 28-38).

6. To ensure contact with the adjacent teeth, the band needs to be contoured. To accomplish this, use a

(A) Band should be tight near the gingival margin

1.0–1.5mm

(B) Band should extend 1.0 to 1.5mm beyond cavity preparation near the gingiva

(C) Band should fit the circumference of the tooth near the occlusal surface

2.0 mm

(D) Band should extend no more than 2mm above the cusp of the tooth and occlusal ridge

FIGURE 28-38 Criteria for correct placement of the matrix band.

(continued)

P R O C E D U R E   **2 8 - 5** *continued*

ball burnisher. Place the burnisher on the inner surface of the band and apply pressure until the band becomes slightly concave at the contact area.

7. Once the matrix band has been placed on the tooth, a wedge(s) is (are) placed to stabilize the

band at the gingival margin of the preparation. (Refer to Wedges for placement suggestions.)

8. Check the seal at the gingival margin of the preparation with an explorer. There should be no gap between the band and the preparation.

P R O C E D U R E

28-6 Removal of the Wedge and the Tofflemire Matrix

This procedure is performed by the dentist with the assistance of the dental assistant. Once the tooth has been filled with restorative material, the matrix and wedge are removed to finish carving the anatomy of the tooth.

EQUIPMENT AND SUPPLIES

▶ Cotton pliers or hemostat

▶ 2 × 2 gauze

PROCEDURE STEPS *(Follow aseptic procedures)*

1. To remove the wedge, use cotton pliers or a hemostat. Grasp the wedge at the base and pull in the opposite direction of the insertion.

2. To remove the retainer, hold the matrix in place with a finger on the occlusal surface, then turn the outer knob of the retainer to loosen the spindle in the vise.

3. Separate the retainer from the band by lifting the retainer toward the occlusal surface.

4. Using cotton pliers, gently free the band from around the tooth, then lift one end of the band in a lingual occlusal direction.

5. Lift the band from the proximal surface and repeat with the other end of the band. The tooth is ready for the final carving.

pliers, the tightening device, and bands in assorted sizes (Figure 28-39).

To place the AutoMatrix, position the matrix on the tooth following the same criteria as with the Tofflemire. Place the tightening device in the coil and rotate the handle to tighten the band around the tooth. Once the matrix is securely on the tooth, place the wedges as needed. To remove the AutoMatrix, remove the wedges and then, using the removal pliers, clip the end of the auto-lock loop. The pliers clip the loop and then have a plastic cover to catch the ends of the loop as they fall after being cut. Open the matrix and slide toward the buccal or lingual while pulling it occlusally.

PLASTIC STRIP MATRIX

The thin, transparent, strip matrix is used with composite, glass ionomer, or compomer restorative materials on anterior teeth. The strip can be made of nylon, acetate, celluloid, or resin and is approximately three

FIGURE 28-39 AutoMatrix kit: assortment of bands and tightening device. *(Courtesy of Dentsply)*

inches long and three-eighths inch wide. The functions of the strip matrix are to:

▶ Provide anatomical contour and proximal contact relation

▶ Prevent excess material at the gingival margin

▶ Confine the restorative material under pressure while the material is being cured

▶ Protect the restorative material from losing or gaining moisture during the setting time

▶ Allow the polymerizing light to reach the composite restorative material

P R O C E D U R E

28-7 Placement of the Strip Matrix

This procedure is performed by the dentist or the dental assistant. After the tooth has been prepared, the strip matrix is placed.

EQUIPMENT AND SUPPLIES

▶ Strip matrix
▶ Cotton pliers
▶ Mouth mirror
▶ Assortment of clear wedges

PROCEDURE STEPS *(Follow aseptic procedures)*

1. Contour the strip by drawing the strip over the rounded edge of the handle of the mouth mirror. The procedure is the same here as it is with the Tofflemire matrix band.

2. Place the strip matrix between the teeth. Hold the strip tightly and slide toward the gingiva.

3. Adjust the position of the strip so that the entire preparation is covered by the strip.

4. Seat the wedge to secure the strip in place.

5. Restorative materials are placed and the strip matrix is pulled tightly around the tooth to adapt the material to the convex surface of the tooth.

6. The strip matrix is held in place by hand or with a clip retainer until the material has been cured (Figure 28-40).

FIGURE 28-40 Strip matrix and wedges on tooth.

P R O C E D U R E

28-8 Removal of the Strip Matrix

This procedure is performed by the dentist once the restorative material is placed and cured.

EQUIPMENT AND SUPPLIES

▶ Cotton pliers or hemostat
▶ 2 × 2 gauze sponges

PROCEDURE STEPS *(Follow aseptic procedures)*

1. Once the material has been cured and is completely hardened, remove the clip retainer, if one was used. Then, remove the wedges with cotton pliers.

2. The strip matrix is gently pulled away from the restorative material.

3. Remove the strip by pulling the matrix strip in a lingual incisal or facial incisal direction.

Crown Matrix Form. The **crown matrix form** is a thin, plastic form that is shaped like the crown. On anterior teeth when the incisal edge is involved, Class IV, a crown form is often used to restore the tooth. The crown forms come preformed in various designs and sizes. The restorative material is placed in the cavity preparation and in the crown form. The crown form is then placed on the tooth. These crown forms are clear and can be used with light-cured materials. Once the restorative material is set, the crown form is removed and the tooth is ready for final contouring and finishing.

CORONAL POLISH

OBJECTIVES

The student should strive to meet the following objectives and demonstrate an understanding of the facts and principles presented in this chapter:

1. Define coronal polish.
2. Explain the indications and contraindication for a coronal polish.
3. Describe and identify dental deposits and stains.
4. List the types of abrasives and explain the characteristics of each type.
5. List and explain the types of equipment and materials used to perform a coronal polish.
6. Explain how to maintain the oral cavity during the coronal polish.
7. List auxiliary polishing aids and explain their functions.
8. Describe the steps in the coronal polish procedure.

KEY TERMS

abrasives (p. 656)
auxiliary polishing aids (p. 664)
black line stain (p. 656)
calculus (p. 655)
clinical crown (p. 653)
dental fluorosis (p. 655)
endogenous (p. 655)
exogenous (p. 655)
extrinsic stains (p. 653)
flour of pumice (p. 657)
fulcrum (p. 654)
green stain (p. 656)
hard deposits (p. 653)
humectant (p. 657)
interproximal brushes (p. 664)
intrinsic (p. 655)
materia alba (p. 655)
metallic stains (p. 655)
oral prophylaxis (p. 653)
pellicle (p. 655)
polishing (p. 656)
proximal (p. 663)
soft deposits (p. 653)
subgingival (p. 655)
supragingival (p. 655)
tetracycline stain (p. 655)
tobacco stains (p. 655)
yellow stains (p. 655)
zirconium silicate (p. 657)

INTRODUCTION

The **oral prophylaxis** procedure is actually twofold. First, the **hard deposits** (scaling) are removed by the dentist or dental hygienist. Second, the teeth are polished with a rubber cup. In some states, a registered or an expanded-function dental assistant can do this part of the prophylaxis, in addition to the dentist and the hygienist.

Coronal Polish Defined

The **coronal polish** procedure involves removing **soft deposits** and **extrinsic stains** (stains removed from tooth surface by polishing) from the surfaces of the teeth and restorations. This is accomplished with an abrasive, a dental handpiece, a rubber cup (sometimes this procedure is called a "rubber cup" polish), a brush, dental tape, and floss. The coronal polish is the polishing of the **clinical crown**, which may involve both enamel and exposed dentin that is visible in the mouth (Figure 28-41). Often, exposed dentin is not polished because of the possibility of increased sensitivity. Composite restorations, acrylic veneers, and porcelain-filled surfaces are also not polished because of the possibility of removing the finish and decreasing surface hardness. Different abrasives are used on each surface.

RATIONALE FOR PERFORMING THE CORONAL POLISH

After the teeth have been scaled to remove the hard deposits, the polish is done to provide a smooth, polished surface. Additional benefits and indications include:

▶ A polish makes it easier for the patient to keep the teeth clean.

▶ The tooth surface absorbs fluoride better.

▶ The process of accumulation of new deposits is slowed.

▶ A clean tooth surface motivates the patient to maintain good oral hygiene habits.

▶ The tooth is prepared for placement of enamel sealant.

▶ The teeth are prepared for orthodontic bracket and band placement.

CONTRAINDICATIONS AND MODIFICATIONS

The conditions that contraindicate a coronal polish involve the gingival tissues. The abrasive agents used in the coronal polish may cause problems, and the actual technique of the polish could traumatize the already irritated tissues. Whether the cause of the gingival irritation is systemic or local, whenever the gingival tissues are irritated, inflamed, sensitive, or hemorrhage easily, it is best to evaluate the necessity of the coronal polish. For some patients, the polish should be postponed until the condition of the tissue improves. For other patients, the polish removes the source of irritation. The dentist makes the decision on an individual basis.

The following conditions may require that coronal polish techniques be modified:

▶ **Orthodontic appliances**—Use of a small rubber cup and a pointed or tapered brush, especially around the brackets.

▶ **Hypersensitive teeth**—Use a very wet abrasive agent with a light, intermittent stroke. Use a cotton roll or cotton swab to dry the area.

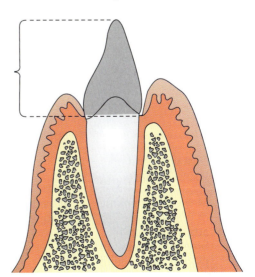

Clinical crown length

FIGURE 28-41 Clinical crown of a tooth.

▶ **Green chromogenic bacterial stain**—Before beginning the coronal polish, use a solution of equal parts of 3 percent hydrogen peroxide and water. Apply to the stained areas with a cotton tip applicator for a few seconds and then rinse.

▶ **Minor oral irritations, such as cold sores**—Avoid the areas when polishing and retracting the tissues or establishing a fulcrum (position of stabilization). Apply a protective coating of lubricant.

 In states where the dental assistant can perform a coronal polish, legal and ethical issues must be considered. The following are guidelines when performing a coronal polish:

▶ Consistently meet the high standards of the profession in performing a coronal polish.

▶ Follow aseptic techniques and OSHA guidelines.

▶ Request assistance when needed to best serve the patient.

▶ Refer all diagnosing to the dentist.

▍DENTAL DEPOSITS

Dental deposits is a collective term referring to a variety of deposits and/or stains, intrinsic and extrinsic, that accumulate on the teeth and on appliances in the mouth. The dental assistant must be able to recognize these deposits and know how to remove them. Dental deposits are often classified as soft deposits, hard deposits, and stains (refer to Table 28-2).

TABLE 28-2 SOFT DEPOSITS

	Pellicle	Materia Alba	Food Debris	Plaque
Appearance	Thin, clear film, sometimes stained.	Soft, bulky mass, cottage cheese-like, white to yellow	Small particles of food.	Soft, dense, furry-like deposit.
Composition	Acellular. Insoluble proteins, fats, and other materials.	Unstructured, living and dead micro-organism. Food debris, desquamated epithelial cells, disintegrating leukocytes, and proteins.	Food particles.	Organized mass of many types of micro-organisms in a sticky matrix. Approximately 80 percent water and 20 percent organic and inorganic solids, with most of the solids being microorganisms.
Source	Saliva and sulcular fluids.	Accumulation of materials and bacterial growth.	Diet.	Microorganisms.
Formation	Forms within minutes of removal.	Time varies.	Forms while eating.	Forms within 12-24 hours of removal.
Attachment	Tooth surface, restorations, and appliances.	Loosely attached, collects in grooves and spaces on and between teeth, gingiva, and. appliances.	Loosely attached, collects in spaces and grooves in and around teeth and appliances.	Gingival areas in difficult areas to clean and lingual and occlusal grooves.
Classification	Unstained and stained surface.	None.	None.	Location on the tooth and pathogenic effect.
Significance	May protect enamel or may provide attachment and breeding ground for plaque and calculus.	Provides source for plaque development.	Provides nutrients.	Dental caries, gingivitis, and periodontal disease.
Methods of removal	Polishing with an abrasive.	Rinsing, toothbrushing, and flossing.	Rinsing, toothbrushing, and flossing.	Toothbrushing, flossing, and coronal polish.

Soft Deposits

Soft deposits include the acquired dental **pellicle**, **materia alba**, food debris, and plaque. The dental assistant can remove these soft deposits while performing a coronal polish.

Calculus

Dental **calculus** is a hard, calcified deposit that forms on the teeth, restorations, and dental appliances. Another name for calculus is "tartar," which many people use. Calculus is mineralized plaque with few, if any, living organisms in its structure. It is often covered with a layer of plaque and is attached firmly to the tooth. The dental assistant should recognize both **supragingival** (above the gingiva) and **subgingival** (below the gingiva) calculus, even though the dental assistant is not legally allowed to remove it. Calculus may be present on a patient scheduled for a coronal polish (refer to Table 28-3 for characteristics of calculus).

Dental Stains

Stains are discolorations of the teeth and are caused by a variety of things, including foods, bacteria, tobacco, metals, drugs, imperfect tooth development, and excess fluoride. Stains adhere to the tooth structure, plaque, and calculus or may be part of the internal structure of the tooth. They are classified according to location, as either **intrinsic** or **extrinsic**, and by their origin, either **exogenous** or **endogenous**. Intrinsic stains are inside the tooth structure and are mostly permanent (in some cases, bleaching is successful). The origin of intrinsic stains can be both endogenous (originating from inside the tooth) and exogenous (originating from outside the tooth). Extrinsic stains are on the outside of the tooth structure and can be removed by scaling and polishing. Extrinsic stains are only exogenous in origin.

The significance of dental stains is their unattractive appearance. They also may provide rough surfaces for deposits to adhere to. They may indicate past or present physical habits or conditions of the patient, which aids the dental assistant in determining the oral hygiene information and instructions to be given to the patient.

Intrinsic Stains. Intrinsic stains have several categorizations.

Dental Fluorosis. **Dental fluorosis** occurs as a result of high concentrations of fluoride received systemically during tooth development. The color of the stain varies from white to yellow-brown or gray-brown. The outer surface may be pitted and rough depending on the severity. The stain is distributed relative to the stage of development of the teeth. Other names include brown stain and mottled enamel.

Pulp Damaged or Non-Vital Tooth Stain. This type of intrinsic stain occurs when the pulp is damaged or removed. This stain can vary in color from light yellow to black to green to magenta and is caused by blood and pulp tissues seeping into the dentin tubules.

Tetracycline Stain. **Tetracycline stain** is the result of high concentrations of tetracycline antibiotics taken during the time the tooth was developing. The stain varies in color from light green or yellow to dark gray-brown.

Metallic Stain. **Metallic stains** can be intrinsic and/or extrinsic. The metals and metallic salts may be inhaled in industrial settings, taken orally in certain drugs, or be part of the materials used to restore teeth. The metals adhere to the pellicle and other soft deposits, or they penetrate the tooth surface to become part of the tooth structure. Several of the metals that can cause permanent stains are copper dust, which causes green to greenish blue stain amalgam; which causes a gray to black or bluish black stain; iron dust, which causes a brown stain; and iron drugs, which cause a black stain.

Extrinsic Stains. Extrinsic stains also have several classifications.

Yellow and Brown Stains. **Yellow stains** and brown stains are usually associated with poor oral hygiene and are dull yellow to a light brownish color. They are generally associated with plaque and most commonly found on the buccal surface of the maxillary molars and the lingual surface of the mandibular incisors.

Tobacco Stain. **Tobacco stains** are the result of coal tar combustion in cigarettes and pigments from chewing

---

TABLE 28-3 CALCULUS

	Supragingival Calculus	Subgingival Calculus
Appearance	Chalky white, yellow, gray, or stained by food.	Black, brown, or dark green.
Formation	Surfaces above the gingival margin. Most common on lingual of mandibular incisors and buccal of maxillary molars.	Surfaces below the gingival margin.
Removal	Mechanical methods.	Mechanical methods.
Age of patient	Uncommon in children under age nine.	Very rare in children under age nine.

tobacco penetrating the pits and fissures on the enamel and dentin surfaces. The stain is light brown to black in color, and the amount of stain depends on the individual's oral hygiene habits and how often the person smokes.

Green Stain. Green stain varies in color from light to dark green or a yellowish green and is found most frequently in children. It is found on the facial surface of the maxillary anterior teeth at the cervical third and contains chromogenic bacteria and fungi.

Black Line Stain. Black line stain forms a thin black to dark-brown line slightly above the gingiva and follows the contour of the gingival margin. It is found primarily in women and often where there is excellent oral hygiene. The black line stain forms on the facial and lingual surfaces of the teeth and tends to reform after removal.

Orange Stain. This extrinsic stain is believed to be caused by chromogenic bacteria often related to drug therapy, such as antibiotics. It is uncommon, but if it does occur, it can be found on the lingual and facial surfaces of the anterior teeth near the gingival margin.

Chlorhexidine Stain. This stain occurs with prolonged use of chlorhexidine, which is found in chewing gum and mouth rinse. It is yellowish to brown in color and appears on restorations, the tongue, in plaque, and in the cervical and interproximal surfaces of the teeth. This is not a permanent stain and can be removed with toothbrushing and/or a coronal polish.

▮ ABRASIVES AND POLISHING AGENTS

There are abrasives and polishing agents available to remove deposits and stains. **Abrasives** are materials that cut or grind the surface, leaving grooves and a rough surface, while **polishing** produces a smooth, glossy surface with fine abrasive materials. It is impor-

tant to understand abrasives, their characteristics, and their actions in order to select the best materials for the patient without damaging the tooth. Abrasives remove small amounts of enamel during the polishing procedure; therefore, it is best to follow the coronal polish procedure with a fluoride treatment and/or to use a fluoride prophy agent.

Abrasives

Abrasives are materials composed of particles that come in powders or pastes. They are selected according to the amount of stain and soft deposits that are to be removed. Abrasives should always be as moist as possible yet easy to use without dripping or spattering. These particles have characteristics that affect their abrasiveness (refer to Table 28-4).

Rate of Abrasion. The rate of abrasion is the time it takes to remove stains and deposits from a surface. This depends on several factors:

▶ By *increasing the speed of the handpiece*, the rate of abrasion is increased accordingly. This also increases the heat production.

▶ The *pressure* can control the rate of abrasion. The firmer the pressure, the more abrasive. Also, the rate of frictional heat increases.

▶ The *amount of abrasive* material used affects the rate of abrasion. The more material that is used, the faster the abrasive works.

▶ The *type of abrasive* used determines the rate of abrasion. The larger and harder the particles, the faster the abrasion. Also, the rate of heat production increases.

▶ The *dryer the abrasive* materials, the more abrasive they are.

TABLE 28-4 CHARACTERISTICS OF ABRASIVES

Characteristic	Effect on Abrasive
Particle shape	Sharp-edged particles are more abrasive than dull, rounded particles.
Hardness of particle	Harder particles abrade faster. Particles must be harder than the surfaces they are used on.
Strength of particles	The strength of the particles not to break up during the polish; therefore less material is used.
Size of particles	The larger the particle, the more abrasive it is.
Grit or grade of abrasive particles	Materials are sifted through standardized sieves to grade the fineness of the materials. Fine abrasives are called powders or flours and are graded F, FF, and FFF for increasing fineness.
Attrition resistance of particles	Particles that do not dull or become imbedded in the surface being polished are the most effective.

Select an abrasive material that is coarse enough to cut through the deposits and stains and polish until the surfaces are as smooth as possible. Then, select a finer material, if needed, to polish the surface until it is smooth and free of deposits and stains. Usually, one abrasive is enough to complete the task, but if the patient has a lot of stain, a more coarse abrasive should be used. In the case of gingival recession, a finer abrasive is used on these areas after finishing all other areas with a more coarse abrasive. When using two types of abrasives, completely finish with one abrasive, then rinse the patient's mouth thoroughly before beginning with another abrasive. Also, use separate dappen dishes, rubber cups, and brushes for each abrasive.

Types of Abrasives

There are many abrasives available that are used for the coronal polish procedure. The abrasives come in powders and pastes and in bulk form or individually packaged. Besides the abrasive, most commercial preparations contain water, a binder, **humectant** (retains moisture), color, and a flavoring.

▶ **Zirconium silicate**—Used for stain removal and polishing. This material may be used on gold restorations, exposed dentin, and tooth-colored restorations, as well as enamel.

▶ **Tin oxide**—A very fine polishing agent used on enamel and metallic restorations. To use in a paste form, mix with water, alcohol, or glycerin.

▶ **Flour of pumice**—Used to remove stains from the enamel. It is relatively coarse and should be followed by a fine polishing agent. It is not used on exposed dentin, tooth-colored restorations, or gold restorations because of its abrasiveness.

▶ **Chalk** (also known as whiting)—A mild abrasive. It is used in some prophylactic pastes.

▶ **Fluoride prophylaxis pastes**—Are available and are very popular. Fluoride is added to commercially prepared prophylaxis pastes to replace the fluoride lost in the enamel surface during the polishing procedure due to abrasion. Fluoride prophylaxis pastes should not be used if the teeth are to receive enamel sealants after the coronal polish.

▌ EQUIPMENT AND SUPPLIES

The tray setup for the coronal polish includes patient safety glasses, hand mirror, mouth mirror, explorer, cotton pliers, cotton swabs (Q-tips), 2 × 2 gauze, cotton rolls, saliva ejector, evacuator, air-water syringe tip, low-speed handpiece, rubber cups, brushes, prophy paste, tongue depressor, dental floss, dental tape, disclosing solution, and dappen dish for disclosing solution (Figure 28-42). Barriers are placed on the dental unit, and

the dental assistant follows OSHA guidelines and wears PPE.

Use of the Dental Handpiece for the Coronal Polish

For the coronal polish procedure, a low-speed dental handpiece is used with a prophy angle attachment (right angle). The handpiece is held in a modified pen grasp. The fingers should close up on the prophy angle attachment, and the body of the handpiece should rest in the "v" of the hand. This gives the operator control and prevents fatigue (Figure 28-43).

When the correct grasp is used, the procedure is performed efficiently and effectively. The speed of the handpiece is controlled by steady foot pressure on the rheostat. Keeping the speed even takes practice. An even, slow speed is desired, with just enough pressure to keep the cups and brushes rotating. Apply the handpiece to the tooth with light to moderate pressure. The handpiece should be started when it is in the mouth, near the tooth to be polished. This establishes the speed of the handpiece before placing the cup/brush on the tooth. When the handpiece is removed from the tooth for more than a moment, release the pressure on the rheostat so that the handpiece stops before being removed from the mouth. This prevents debris from splattering.

When the modified pen grasp is used, the ring finger is the fulcrum finger. The little finger is also used to supplement the ring finger as a fulcrum. During the procedure, tooth structure provides the most stable fulcrum. However, the soft tissue is used as a fulcrum. Cover the tissue with a 2 × 2 gauze first to prevent slipping. Using a fulcrum provides stability and control of the handpiece, provides for patient comfort, and helps reduce fatigue of the dental assistant.

FIGURE 28-42 Tray setup for the coronal polish procedure.

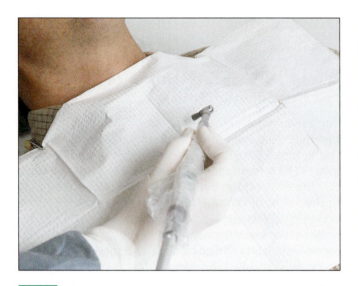

FIGURE 28-43 Modified pen grasp and the dental handpiece.

Points for Using the Dental Handpiece

▶ Use a slow, even speed.
▶ Use a light to moderate pressure.
▶ Always use a fulcrum.
▶ Start and stop the handpiece inside the patient's mouth.

Use of the Rubber Prophy Cup

The **rubber prophy cup** is used with abrasive agent to polish the teeth and dental appliances. Rubber prophy cups are available in several designs to fit the prophy angles. On the back of the prophy cup there may be a small metal-screw attachment that is screwed into the corresponding prophy angle or a small hole that slips over a knob on the prophy angle. Disposable prophy angles with attached prophy cups and brushes are also available (Figures 28-44A through J).

The rubber prophy cups are made of either natural or synthetic rubber. The natural rubber cups are resilient and will not stain the teeth. The synthetic rubber cups are stiffer than the natural rubber, and the black cups may stain the teeth during the polish.

The rubber cup should be soft and flexible to adapt to the contours of the teeth. Edges should not be rough or frayed—This could irritate the tissues. The number of cups needed for the polishing depends on the number of abrasives used. One cup is used for each polishing agent. The edge of the cup is the part that actually does the polishing. The center of the cup holds and transports the abrasive agent. The cup is flexed to adapt to the tooth surface by applying slight pressure to one edge (Figure 28-45). The cup is most efficient on the facial and lingual surfaces of the teeth and fixed appliances, along the gingival margin, and 1 to 2 mm into the sulcus.

The hand and wrist are used to move the handpiece to adapt the cup to the tooth surface. When working on the

FIGURE 28-44 (A) Contra-angle with latch prophy cup. (B) Disposable prophy angle cup. (C) Right angle with snap on prophy cup. (D) Right angle (prophy angle) for screw cup or brush. (E) Snap-on prophy brush. (F) Screw-on prophy cup. (G) Rubber point. (H) Screw-on prophy brush. (I) Latch brush. (J) Assortment of cups, brushes, and points.

lingual or facial surfaces, move the edge of the rubber cup as far as possible into the proximal and manipulate the cup into the sulcus, *not on* the gingival margin. The next step in learning to use the prophy cup is to learn the stroke. A short, intermittent, overlapping stroke is used with a slow-revolving rubber cup. This stroke covers the tooth, leaves no unpolished surfaces, and minimizes the frictional heat produced (Figure 28-46).

FIGURE 28-45 Adapting the rubber cup to the tooth surface.

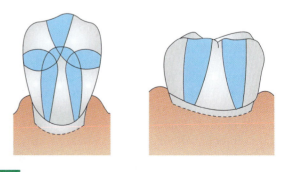

FIGURE 28-46 Examples of the polishing stroke.

PROCEDURE

28-9 Polishing with the Rubber Cup

This procedure is performed by the dental assistant, hygienist, or dentist. The following procedure for polishing with the rubber cup explains the positioning techniques and the action of the rubber cup. Examine the rubber cup placement on both arches and each quadrant on the facial and lingual surfaces.

EQUIPMENT AND SUPPLIES

▶ Basic setup: mouth mirror, explorer/periodontal probe, cotton pliers

▶ Saliva ejector, HVE tip, air-water syringe tip

▶ 2 × 2 gauze sponges, cotton tip applicator

▶ Dappen dish

▶ Lip lubricant

▶ Disclosing solution (optional)

▶ Low-speed handpiece

▶ Prophy angle attachment

▶ Assortment of rubber cups and brushes

▶ Prophy paste in different grits

▶ Finger rings to hold prophy paste cup

▶ Dental tape and dental floss

PROCEDURE STEPS *(Follow aseptic procedures)*

1. The patient is seated and prepared for the coronal polish procedure. Sometimes, lip lubricant is offered for the patient's comfort. The dental assistant reviews the patient's medical history and inspects the oral cavity. The amount of extrinsic stain determines the grit of the abrasive to be used.

2. The dental assistant may dry the teeth and place disclosing solution on the teeth for easier detection of plaque.

3. After the teeth are dry, a cotton tip applicator is used to place the solution on all surfaces of the teeth. This is accomplished one quadrant, one arch, or one side at a time.

4. After placing abrasive polishing agent in the cup, place the cup near the gingival sulcus and as far into the mesial or distal surface as possible. Establish a fulcrum as close to the tooth being polished as possible.

5. Apply light pressure to flex the cup and flare it into the sulcus 1 to 2 mm.

6. Sweep the rubber cup toward the incisal or occlusal edge. If the crown of the tooth is long, lift the cup halfway up the tooth and make a second stroke toward the occlusal.

7. At the incisal or occlusal edge, lift the cup slightly off the tooth and re-place it near the gingiva to repeat the stroke, moving toward the opposite side of the tooth.

8. Repeat the stroke, overlapping each time, until the entire tooth surface is polished.

9. When finished with one tooth, move to the adjacent tooth using the same steps until the surfaces of all teeth have been polished.

10. For the patient's comfort, rinse the mouth frequently, at least after polishing each quadrant.

11. When all the teeth have been polished, rinse and evacuate the patient's mouth thoroughly, removing all debris (Figures 28-47A through F).

(A1)

FIGURE 28-47 Correct cup placement and fulcrum for: A Maxillary right posterior: Buccal surface, lingual surface.
  A1. Cheek is retracted to position cup on tooth. Fulcrum on same arch. *(continued)*

(continued)

(A2)

(C1)

(B1)

(C2)

(B2)

(D1)

FIGURE 28-47 *(continued)*
  A2. Use indirect vision and fulcrum on same arch.
B Maxillary anteriors: Facial surface, lingual surface.
  B1. Retract lip and fulcrum on incisal edge.
  B2. Use indirect vision.
C Maxillary left posterior: Buccal surfaces, lingual surface.

C1. Retract cheek to position prophy angle and have
    patient close slightly. Fulcrum on same arch.
C2. Adapt cup to lingual surface.
D Mandibular right posterior: Buccal surface, lingual
 surface.
  D1. Retract tissue to place prophy angle and have patient
    close slightly.

(continued)

P R O C E D U R E   **2 8 - 9** *continued*

(D2)

(F1)

(E1)

(F2)

(E2)

FIGURE 28-47 *(continued)*
D2. Retract tongue with mouth mirror.
E   Mandibular anteriors: Facial surface, lingual surface.
E1. Retract lip with finger.
E2. Use mouth mirror for indirect vision and retraction.
F   Mandibular left posterior: Buccal surfaces, lingual surface.
F1. Retract cheek and position prophy cup.
F2. Retract tongue with mouth mirror to position prophy cup.

Systematic Procedure

Follow a systematic procedure when polishing the entire mouth by developing a sequence that is always followed. For example, always start in the same quadrant. Or, begin on the buccal surface of the most posterior tooth in the mandibular right quadrant and polish each tooth, moving around the entire arch; then, make a loop around the most posterior tooth on the mandibular left quadrant and polish the lingual surface, ending up on the right side.

The Prophy Brush

The **prophy brushes** used for the coronal polish procedure come in several styles. Like the rubber cup, they are either "snap on" or "screw on," depending on which prophy angle they are used on (Figure 28-44). Brushes are available with either nylon or natural bristles. Some brushes are tapered, while others are flat on the end. For the coronal polishes, a soft and flexible brush is used. The softening can be accomplished by soaking the brush in hot water before using it.

The prophy brushes are used on the occlusal surfaces to effectively clean the deep pits and fissures and also on the lingual of the anteriors, but the bristles should *never* contact the gingival tissues and should be positioned only above the gingival third of the tooth. The prophy brush is used only on the enamel surface. The brush is used in the same manner as the cup: flexed in the central fossa with a light, intermittent, and overlapping stroke. With the lingual surfaces, the brush is placed in the lingual pit and moved toward the incisal edge.

P R O C E D U R E

28-10 Using the Prophy Brush

This procedure is performed by the dental assistant, hygienist, or dentist. The prophy brush procedure follows the rubber cup polish. It includes the techniques used to manipulate and position the brush (Figure 28-48).

EQUIPMENT AND SUPPLIES

▶ Refer to Procedure 28-9, Polishing with the Rubber Cup.

PROCEDURE STEPS *(Follow aseptic procedures)*

1. Place the softened brush on the prophy angle and apply prophy paste to the brush.

2. Establish a fulcrum close to the posterior tooth to be polished.

3. Move the brush bristles toward the mesial buccal cusp tip and continue until the brush comes off the occlusal surface.

4. Replace the brush bristles in the central fossa.

5. Apply slight pressure again, and move the brush up toward the distal buccal cusp until the brush comes off the occlusal surface.

6. Repeat this procedure on the occlusal surface of each posterior tooth until all of the occlusal surfaces are cleaned.

7. Repeat this process on the occlusal surfaces of all teeth.

8. For the lingual surfaces of the anterior teeth, place the prophy brush in the lingual pit, above the cingulum.

9. Apply light pressure to flex and spread the bristles of the brush.

10. Move the brush toward the incisal edge to polish the lingual surface.

11. Repeat on all lingual surfaces that have deep pits and grooves.

12. When finished with the brush, rinse and evacuate the oral cavity thoroughly.

FIGURE 28-48 Prophy brush positioned on occlusal surface.

Dental Tape and Dental Floss

Dental tape is used on the interproximal surfaces of the teeth with an abrasive agent. Care must be used not to damage the interdental papilla and free gingival margins when using the tape. After all the interproximal surfaces have been polished with dental tape and abrasive, the teeth must be flossed to remove any particles of abrasive that were left after rinsing. The **dental floss** is placed interproximally, wrapped around the tooth, and moved in an up-and-down motion.

> **NOTE:** If fluoride is going to be applied as the next step of this procedure, unwaxed floss should be used instead of waxed floss. Waxed floss coats the teeth, preventing the fluoride from being absorbed by the teeth.

MAINTAINING THE OPERATING FIELD

During the coronal polish, it is important to keep the mouth free of excess saliva and debris, direct the dental

light for maximum light for the operator (dental assistant), keep the patient comfortable, and maintain correct positioning for the dental assistant and the patient.

Dental Assistant

The dental assistant should follow the guidelines for positioning found in previous chapters. When the dental assistant becomes the operator, he or she should sit on the side of the patient where he or she is the most comfortable. For example, a right-handed dental assistant usually finds being on the right side of the patient more convenient to work from. The dental assistant should adjust the operator's chair so that his or her feet are flat on the floor and movement around the patient's head is unrestricted. The dental assistant usually sits between the 8 and 9 o'clock positions when performing the polish if right handed and between 3 and 4 o'clock if left handed.

Patient

The patient is seated and reclined to the correct height for the dental assistant. During the coronal polish

PROCEDURE

28-11 Polishing with Dental Tape and Dental Floss

This procedure is part of the coronal polish. After the rubber cup and brush have been used, the interproximal surfaces of the teeth are cleaned with dental tape and then dental floss is used.

EQUIPMENT AND SUPPLIES

▶ Refer to Procedure 28-9, Polishing with the Rubber Cup.

PROCEDURE STEPS (*Follow aseptic procedures*)

1. Cut off a piece of dental tape twelve to eighteen inches long.

2. Wipe some abrasive agent into the interproximal contact areas of the teeth in a quadrant, with a cotton tip or finger.

3. Wrap the tape around the middle fingers of both hands, leaving a length of tape just long enough to wrap around the tooth while maintaining control.

4. Take the tape through the contact at an oblique angle (\ ) in a back-and-forth motion, using gentle pressure and holding the tape against the tooth.

This assists in preventing the tape from snapping through the contact and damaging the gingiva.

5. Wrap the tape around the tooth to cover the line angles of the tooth on both the buccal and the lingual.

6. When the **proximal** surface of one tooth is complete, lift the tape up and over the interdental papilla without removing the tape through the contact and readapt the tape on the proximal surface of the adjacent tooth.

7. Polish this surface with the tape and abrasive and then remove the tape up through the contact. If the tape is pulled through the embrasure area, be careful not to injure the gingival tissues.

8. Continue around each tooth in both arches until all proximal surfaces have been polished, including the most distal surface of each quadrant. Use different areas of the tape as needed, and rinse areas thoroughly and evacuate all debris.

9. Follow the taping by using dental floss to remove any debris left. Floss all areas and rinse thoroughly.

procedure, the patient's head may be positioned up and down and left and right depending on the arch and the quadrant the dental assistant is working on.

Dental Light

The dental light needs to be adjusted for good direct and indirect vision. The dental assistant can maintain good illumination of the mouth by remembering to adjust the light whenever the patient's head position is changed.

Oral Cavity

The oral cavity should be rinsed frequently during the polish using the air-water syringe and the evacuator. The saliva ejector helps to keep the saliva to a minimum if placed in the patient's mouth during the use of the prophy cup and brush. This also reduces splattering of the polishing agent. Another way to reduce splattering is to wipe the debris from the cup and the brush with a 2 × 2 gauze when removing the cup and brush from the mouth.

▌ AUXILIARY POLISHING AIDS

There are several **auxiliary polishing aids** that may be needed during a coronal polish. These aids include bridge threaders, abrasive polishing strips, soft wooden points, and small interproximal brushes (Figure 28-49).

Bridge Threaders

The **bridge threaders** are used to pull the dental tape and floss under fixed appliances, around orthodontic appliances, and around splints so that all proximal surfaces can be cleaned and polished. There are several types of bridge threaders. Usually, they are made of plastic with loops or eyes for the tape or floss to slide through and pointed ends (Figure 28-50). After the floss or tape is threaded through the eye of the threader on the facial side, slip the pointed end through the gingival embrasure. Once the bridge threader is through the embrasure, take hold of the floss or tape and proceed as described in the previous section on using the dental tape and floss.

Abrasive Polishing Strips

Abrasive polishing strips are used occasionally when a small stain is difficult to remove. Polishing strips or "finishing strips" are used only on enamel surfaces. They come in different grits and widths. The polishing strip is worked interproximally, pulled tight against the proximal surface of the tooth, and then moved in a back-and-forth motion until the stain is gone. Care must be taken not to cut the surrounding soft tissues, because the edges of the strip are sharp.

Soft Wood Points

Soft wood points are sometimes used with polishing agents to polish occlusal grooves and pits, proximal surfaces of sensitive teeth, and areas other polishing instruments cannot reach. Soft wood points are made of balsa wood; orangewood sticks; round, wooden toothpicks; and several other types of soft wood. The soft wood points can be used alone or with handles. The points are narrow and come in either wedge shapes for the proximal surfaces or cone shapes for the pits and grooves.

Interproximal Brushes

Interproximal brushes are small, soft-bristled brushes that come in a variety of shapes and sizes. The brushes

FIGURE 28-49 Various auxiliary polishing aids, such as bridge threaders, abrasive polishing strips, soft wooden points, and small interproximal brushes.

FIGURE 28-50 Bridge threader going under a fixed bridge near abutment tooth.

come in packages of three or four and are used by attaching them to metal or plastic handles. After selecting the best shape of brush to clean a specific area, attach the brush to the handle and insert the brush with light pressure. Use a back-and-forth motion to work the brush.

Interproximal brushes are useful in the following conditions:

▶ Open contact areas

▶ Around orthodontic braces and wires

▶ Around exposed bifurcation or trifurcation of the roots

▶ On abutment teeth of a hygienic bridge

P R O C E D U R E

28-12 Coronal Polish

This procedure is performed routinely by the dental assistant and the dental hygienist. This procedure describes the protocol for performing a coronal polish, including preparation of materials and the patient, positioning of the operator and the patient, sequence of procedure, and evaluating the procedure.

EQUIPMENT AND SUPPLIES

▶ Basic three setup: mouth mirror, explorer, cotton pliers

▶ Saliva ejector, HVE tip, air-water syringe tip

▶ 2 × 2 gauze sponges, cotton tip applicators, tongue blade, and cotton rolls

▶ Lip lubricant and disclosing solution in dappen dish

▶ Low-speed handpiece with prophy angle attachment

▶ Prophy cups and brushes (dappen dish with warm water to soak brushes in)

▶ Prophy pastes, with a variety of grits and finger ring holder

▶ Dental tape and dental floss

▶ Auxiliary aids as needed

The following items are needed off the tray:

▶ Patient's chart

▶ Red/blue pencil, lead pencil, and pen

▶ Barriers for the dental unit

▶ Patient napkin and napkin chain

▶ Patient safety glasses

▶ Patient hand mirror

PROCEDURE STEPS *(Follow aseptic procedures)*

1. After gathering the preceding equipment and materials, prepare the operatory for the patient.

2. Prepare the patient.

▶ Following the established procedure, seat the patient and review and update the patient's records.

▶ Explain the procedure to the patient.

▶ Follow aseptic procedures to prepare the patient for the coronal polish.

▶ Evaluate the patient's condition by performing an oral inspection.

▶ Select abrasive agents to be used after examining the teeth. Depending on the amount and type of stain, abrasives are selected.

▶ Lubricate the patient's lips, dry the teeth, and apply the disclosing agent with the cotton tip applicator.

▶ Adjust the dental unit light for good vision.

3. Position the operator and the patient. When the operator is polishing the maxillary and mandibular right facial and the maxillary and mandibular left lingual, the patient's head is turned away from the operator (Figure 28-51). When the operator is

FIGURE 28-51 Positioning patient's head away from the dental assistant.

(continued)

polishing the maxillary and mandibular right lingual and the maxillary and mandibular left facial, the patient's head is turned toward the operator (Figure 28-52).

4. Begin the sequence of the procedure.

   ▶ Begin the polish on the quadrant or arch according to the predetermined, established routine.

   ▶ Follow criteria previously discussed regarding the use of abrasives and the rubber cup, prophy brush, tape, and floss.

   ▶ Rinse the patient's mouth after each quadrant is polished, or as needed.

5. Evaluate the coronal polish.

   ▶ Once all steps of the coronal polish have been completed, rinse the patient's mouth thoroughly with the spray from the air-water syringe and the evacuator.

   ▶ Apply disclosing solution to detect any areas of plaque or stain that were missed.

   ▶ Using the mouth mirror and the air syringe, inspect each surface for any remaining soft deposits and/or stains. Note these areas on the patient's chart or paper for future reference.

   ▶ Polish the areas missed with a prophy cup and/or brush.

   ▶ Rinse the patient's mouth to remove all the abrasive agent.

FIGURE 28-52 Positioning patient's head toward the dental assistant.

   ▶ Inspect the teeth for a lustrous shine showing no debris or extrinsic stains. The soft tissues should be free of abrasion or trauma. The patient is ready for a fluoride treatment. The dentist may want to see the patient before he or she is dismissed.

6. Chart the coronal polish. It is the dental assistant's responsibility to record the coronal polish completely and accurately on the patient's dental chart. The entry is recorded in ink, dated, and signed or entered into the computer system. Include any comments about the condition of the patient's mouth and the type(s) of material(s) used.

PLACING CAVITY LINERS, CAVITY VARNISH, AND CEMENT BASES

OBJECTIVES

The student should strive to meet the following objectives and demonstrate an understanding of the facts and principles presented in this chapter:

1. Classify cavity preparations according to their relationships with the pulp.

2. Explain the different options for protecting the pulp with cavity liners, cavity varnish, and cement bases.

3. Describe the purpose of using cavity liners. List types of materials that can be used and explain the placement procedure.

4. Describe the purpose of using cavity varnish and explain the placement procedure.

5. Describe the purpose of using cement bases. List types of materials that can be used and explain the placement procedure.

INTRODUCTION

The dental assistant should be familiar with and knowledgeable about the properties and preparation of cavity liners, varnishes, and cement bases (refer to Chapter 26, Chairside Restorative Materials). Cavity preparation and terminology also should be familiar so that the dental assistant can plan ahead and be ready to prepare and place the materials the dentist asks for. Not all states allow dental assistants to place bases, liners, and cavity varnish, but the dental assistant can assist the dentist during this step of restorative procedures.

CAVITY PREPARATION/ PULPAL INVOLVEMENT

The **cavity preparation** for a restoration depends on the amount of decay, the location of the decay, and the type of materials used to restore the tooth. If the dental assistant is placing the liners, base, or varnish, he or she should examine the cavity preparation to assess pulpal involvement (see Table 28-5).

TREATMENT OF CAVITY PREPARATIONS

The treatment of the cavity preparations varies with the amount of enamel and dentin removed and how near the prep is to the pulp. Using the categories from Table 28-5, possible treatments are as follows:

1. Treatment of the ideal cavity preparation:
   ▶ A base is not required because only a minimal amount of enamel and dentin has been removed. Some dentists place only the restoration, while others prefer to place a fluoride-releasing liner. If an amalgam restoration is going to be placed, two thin layers of cavity varnish are often placed over the dentin.
   ▶ If a composite restoration is going to be used, a glass ionomer liner or calcium hydroxide is placed over the exposed dentin.

2. Treatment of the beyond-ideal cavity preparation:
   ▶ With a beyond-ideal preparation, the level of the dentin is restored with a cement base.

   ▶ With an amalgam restoration, there are several options. One option is to place two thin layers of varnish to seal the dentin tubules and then place a layer of a cement base, such as zinc phosphate.
   ▶ Another option is a reinforced ZOE base, which has a soothing effect on the pulp. Varnish is not used with this material.
   ▶ Other options include polycarboxylate or glass ionomer base, which also do not require varnish.
   ▶ Under composite restorative materials, use a glass ionomer base or calcium hydroxide.

3. Treatment of the near-exposure cavity preparation:
   ▶ The closer the cavity preparation comes to the pulp, the more precautions that are needed. There are also several options of treatment of the near-exposure preparation.
   ▶ With preparations that are going to be restored with amalgam, a liner of calcium hydroxide, glass ionomer, or ZOE is placed first over the deepest portion of the prep in the dentin. Once this layer is placed, two thin layers of varnish are inserted over the exposed dentin. Then, a layer of cement base is applied. Zinc phosphate, polycarboxylate, or glass ionomer cements can be used for this layer.
   ▶ Another option for amalgam restorations is to place a liner over the deepest portion of the preparation, then a layer of reinforced ZOE, polycarboxylate, or glass ionomer cement. This is then sealed with cavity varnish.
   ▶ With some preparations, the dentist may choose not to place cavity varnish.
   ▶ When composite materials are going to be used to restore the tooth, a liner is placed first, then a layer of either polycarboxylate or glass ionomer cement. Varnish is not placed and a ZOE base liner is not used because they inhibit the setting of the composite.
   ▶ When a cavity liner is placed on a near exposure, the procedure is often referred to as an **indirect pulp capping**.

4. Treatment of the exposed-pulp cavity preparation:
   ▶ In an exposed pulp, the dentist must decide whether endodontic treatment is indicated or attempt to save the vitality of the tooth. If the

TABLE 28-5   DEPTH OF CAVITY PREPARATIONS AND PULPAL RELATION

Pulpal Involvement	Illustration
1. Ideal Level This preparation does not involve the pulp but is through the enamel and just in the dentin. It is large enough to retain a restoration.	
2. Beyond Ideal More enamel and dentin are removed, but the preparation is not close to the pulp.	
3. Near Exposure This cavity preparation involves a large amount of enamel and dentin being removed, but the pulp is not exposed. The floor of the preparation may be slightly pink in color.	
4. Pulp Exposure Enough enamel and dentin have been removed to expose a portion of the pulp. There will be blood in the cavity preparation.	

treatment of choice is to save the pulp, a procedure called a **direct pulp capping** is performed.

▶ One treatment involves the placement of calcium hydroxide or glass ionomer liner and then reinforced ZOE as a temporary restoration. This gives the dentist time to see whether the pulp is going to heal.

▶ Another treatment involves the placement of a liner, followed by a layer of ZOE cement, two thin layers of varnish, and a cement base.

▶ Some dentists prefer to place a liner and then a layer of polycarboxylate or glass ionomer cement base.

CAVITY LINERS

Cavity liners are placed in the deepest portion of the cavity preparation on the **axial walls** or pulpal walls. After the liners are hardened, they form a cement layer with minimum strength. They are placed on the dentin or on an exposed pulp and protect the pulp from chemical irritations and also provide a therapeutic effect to the tooth. Examples of cavity liners are calcium hydroxide, zinc oxide eugenol, and glass ionomer. Liners also are often called **low-strength bases**.

CAVITY VARNISH

Cavity varnish is used to seal the dentin tubules to prevent acids, saliva, and debris from reaching the pulp. Cavity varnish is used under amalgam restorations to prevent microleakage and under zinc phosphate cements to prevent penetration of acids to the pulp. If cavity liners or medicated bases are used, varnish is placed after or on top of these materials.

CEMENT BASES

Cement bases are mixed to a thick putty consistency and placed in the cavity preparation to protect the pulp and provide mechanical support for the restoration. These cement bases are placed on the floor of the cavity preparation to raise the level of the floor of the preparation to the ideal height. There are several different types of cements that can be used for bases. These include glass ionomers, hybrid ionomers, reinforced zinc oxide

P R O C E D U R E

28-13 Placing Cavity Liners

This procedure is performed by the dentist or an expanded-function dental assistant. The preparation of the cavity has been completed, and this procedure begins the restorative process.

EQUIPMENT AND SUPPLIES

▶ Cavity liner (calcium hydroxide, glass ionomer, zinc oxide eugenol)

▶ Application instrument—small, ball-shaped instrument or explorer

▶ Gauze sponges and cotton rolls

▶ Mixing pad and spatula, if material is mixed

▶ Curing light (if material is light cured)

PROCEDURE STEPS *(Follow aseptic procedures)*

1. Examine the cavity preparation. Determine the deepest portion of the cavity preparation and access to that area.

2. Clean and dry the cavity preparation. Remove any debris from the cavity preparation. Wash and dry the area with the air-water syringe.

3. Prepare the liner to be used. Dispense and mix according to directions. NOTE: Usually, light-cured materials do not have to be mixed but are placed directly in the preparation.

4. Place the liner in the cavity preparation. Using a small, ball-ended instrument, place the material in the deepest portion of the cavity preparation in a thin layer. Be careful not to touch the instrument to the sides of the preparation. The material will flow into the area and can be spread by pushing the liner in the direction desired with the small ball of the instrument.

5. Complete the placement. Remove the instrument, wipe it clean with a gauze, and repeat this procedure until the liner covers the deepest portion of the cavity preparation (Figure 28-53).

6. If the liner is self-curing, the mix must be allowed to harden. If the liner is light curing, the light is held over the tooth and activated to cure the material for the appropriate time (usually ten to twenty seconds).

7. Examine the cavity preparation. After the liner has cured, examine the preparation. If any material is on the enamel walls, remove it with an explorer.

FIGURE 28-53 Placement of cavity liner in preparation.

P R O C E D U R E

28-14 Placing Cavity Varnish

This procedure is performed by the dentist or the expanded-function dental assistant. The preparation of the cavity has been completed, and this procedure is part of preparing the tooth for the restoration.

EQUIPMENT AND SUPPLIES

▶ Cavity varnish (varnish and solvent)

▶ Cotton pliers

▶ Application instruments (cotton balls or cotton pellets, sponge applicators, brush applicators)

▶ Gauze sponges

PROCEDURE STEPS *(Follow aseptic procedures)*

1. Prepare two very small cotton balls or pellets about 2 mm in size to look like small footballs.

(continued)

ᵃᵃᵃ

P R O C E D U R E   **2 8 - 1 4** *continued*

2. Evaluate the cavity preparation to determine access, visibility, and placement of liners or bases.

3. If the tooth has not been washed and dried, do so at this time with the air-water syringe.

4. To prevent contamination of the varnish, pick up both cotton pellets or balls with the sterile cotton pliers and place in the varnish. Then, place the cotton on gauze to remove excess varnish.

5. Using the cotton pliers, pick up one cotton ball or pellet and paint a thin layer of varnish on the dentin in the cavity preparation. A sterile disposable brush or sponge may also be used (Figure 28-54).

6. Allow the cavity to dry for thirty seconds. Place a second coat of varnish. Using the cotton pliers, pick up the second cotton pellet or ball from the gauze and apply a second layer of varnish (this prevents any voids). To prevent contamination,

FIGURE 28-54 Placement of cavity varnish in preparation.

never place an applicator that has been used in the mouth back in the bottle of varnish.

7. Clean up after the procedure. If any excess varnish was placed on the enamel surface, remove it with varnish solvent and a small applicator.

eugenol, zinc phosphate, and polycarboxylate. The preparation, sensitivity of the pulp, and type of restoration indicate which cement to use (Refer to Chapter 26, Restorative Materials, for specific uses of each material mentioned). These materials are often referred to as **high-strength bases**.

P R O C E D U R E

28-15 Placement of Cement Bases

This procedure is performed by the dentist or the expanded-function dental assistant. The preparation of the cavity has been completed, and this procedure is part of preparing the tooth for the restoration.

EQUIPMENT AND SUPPLIES

▶ Cement base materials, usually powder/liquid
▶ Mixing pad
▶ Cement spatula
▶ Gauze sponges
▶ Plastic filling instrument
▶ Explorer or spoon excavator

PROCEDURE STEPS (*Follow aseptic procedures*)

1. Determine the previous treatments and decide where to place the base and the size of area. Evaluate access and visibility.

2. Prepare the preparation area. Remove any debris with the air-water syringe and HVE.

3. Prepare the cement base materials according to manufacturer's instructions. Mix the cement base to a thick putty consistency and gather into a small ball.

4. Collect the base on the blade of the plastic filling instrument. Place the base in the cavity preparation.

5. Using the small condensing end of the plastic filling instrument, condense the base into place on the floor of the cavity prep (Figure 28-55). If the material is sticky, place a small amount of powder on the mixing pad and dip the end of the condenser as needed. Continue until a sufficient base layer is placed.

(continued)

P R O C E D U R E **28-15** *continued*

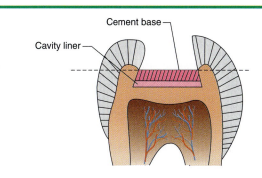

FIGURE 28-55 Placement of cement base in cavity preparation.

6. Evaluate the placement. The base should cover the floor of the cavity preparation, leave enough room for the restorative materials, and should not be on pins or in retentive grooves.

7. Remove any excess materials with a spoon excavator or an explorer.

8. Clean up the mixing materials. Remove cement from the spatula as soon as possible and remove the paper from the pad.

SUTURE REMOVAL

OBJECTIVES

The student should strive to meet the following objectives and demonstrate an understanding of the facts and principles presented in this chapter:

1. Explain the function of sutures and when they are placed.

2. List the equipment and supplies needed for suture removal.

3. Determine and identify the location and number of sutures and how to evaluate the healing process.

4. Identify the following suture patterns: simple, continuous simple, sling, continuous sling, horizontal, and vertical mattress.

5. List the basic criteria for suture removal.

6. Explain the steps of removal for identified suture patterns.

7. Explain postoperative patient care.

KEY TERMS

continuous simple suture (p. 673)
continuous sling suture (p. 673)
debride (p. 672)
horizontal mattress suture (p. 673)
simple suture (p. 673)
sling suture (p. 673)
vertical mattress suture (p. 674)

INTRODUCTION

Sutures hold displaced or incised tissue in its original position (refer to Chapter 19, Oral and Maxillofacial Surgery). Sutures close the wound to promote healing and limit contamination by bacteria and food debris. The dental assistant assists the dentist in the placement of sutures and observes the type and number of sutures, then records this information on the patient's chart for later reference. In five to seven days, the patient returns to the office for the sutures to be removed. In some states, qualified dental assistants are allowed to remove the sutures under the supervision of the dentist. It is the responsibility of the dental assistant to gain the knowledge and the experience necessary to perform this task to the highest standard. The dentist must be aware of the patient's status and be notified immediately if diagnostic decisions are required.

PROCEDURES PRIOR TO REMOVAL OF SUTURES

Prior to the suture removal, several steps and considerations are necessary to ensure patient comfort and safety. Included are reviewing the patient's chart, preparing the equipment and supplies, evaluating the suture site, and consulting with the dentist.

A. Suture Removal Equipment and Supplies

Before the patient's appointment, the tray is set up with the following items: mouth mirror, explorer, cotton pliers, suture scissors, gauze sponges, air-water syringe tip, and evacuator. This is a sterile procedure, so all aseptic guidelines are followed.

B. Review the Patient's Chart

After the patient has been seated and before the procedure has begun, check the patient's chart for information concerning the sutures. Ask the patient if any problems had occurred with the sutures since the last appointment.

C. Examine the Suture Site

Check the suture site for the following information:

1. Location of the sutures
2. Number of sutures

3. Type or pattern of the sutures
4. Healing of the tissues in the wound area

Healing of the Tissues

The healing of the tissues depends on a number of factors, including the extent of the wound, the healing capabilities of the patient, whether a periodontal dressing was applied, and the amount of healing time. To evaluate the healing process, the dental assistant should **debride** (remove debris from) the suture site. Once the tissues have been cleaned, the suture site is evaluated for progress of healing and signs of infection. See Table 28-6 for descriptions of what to look for in the suture area.

> **Ways to Debride the Suture Site**
>
> 1. Use light air and a warm water spray.
> 2. Use a cotton tip applicator moistened with warm water or diluted hydrogen peroxide.
> 3. Use a moist cotton gauze and gently dab the suture site.

D. Consult with the Dentist

The dental assistant should always consult with the dentist when removing sutures. After the patient has been seated, the dental assistant should check the healing of the suture site and identify the correct number of sutures to be removed. Consult with the dentist prior to suture removal for instructions, especially if there is anything unusual in the healing process or sutures cannot be located.

TYPES OF SUTURE PATTERNS

To remove sutures, it is necessary to understand how the sutures are placed. There are several different basic patterns, although each dentist may vary his or her suturing techniques depending on the procedure

TABLE 28-6 SUTURE SITE HEALING SIGNS

Size of Wound	Appearance
Large area for flap or multiple extractions without a periodontal dressing	Area is slightly red with granulation tissue present, but no infection.
Large area for flap or multiple extractions with a periodontal dressing	Area appears slightly red with granulation tissue present. A milky film is seen where the dressing was placed.
Small area for minor surgery without a periodontal dressing placed	Area appears almost healed, with dark pink granulation tissue and no inflammation.
Any size wound that is red and inflamed, tender, and has some bleeding	This wound is infected or irritated or has not had enough time to heal.

and the patient. Detailed charting when the sutures are placed will help the dental assistant during the sutures' removal. Most sutures are tied with simple, square knots, referred to as surgeon's knots. The dental assistant should ask the dentist to place a variety of sutures in a tissue simulation, such as cotton rolls rolled into 2×2 gauze or dental dam material, to practice the sutures' removal.

The Simple Suture

The **simple suture** is the most widely used suture stitch, it is very versatile, and is used in may areas of the mouth (see Figure 28-56 for steps the dentist follows to place the simple suture). Once the suture is placed, it is tied with a surgeon's knot.

The Continuous Simple Suture

The **continuous simple suture** is placed when there have been multiple extractions (Figure 28-57). This series of sutures looks like hem stitching, with a surgeon's knot at either end. The number of stitches depends on the wound site.

The Sling Suture

The **sling suture** is used for interproximal suturing (Figure 28-58). When a flap has been necessary, the sling suture is especially useful. An example of when a sling suture would be used is on the facial surface of the tissue. The suture needle and thread are inserted through the tissue on the facial surface (distal-facial of the tooth) and then the thread is wrapped around the lingual of the tooth, where the needle and thread are placed through the facial tissue on the opposite side of the tooth (mesial-facial). The thread is then wrapped back around the lingual of the tooth and a surgeon's knot is used to secure the suture.

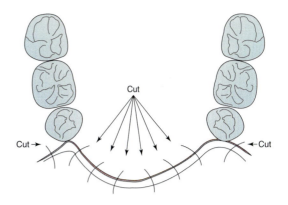

FIGURE 28-57 Continuous simple suture pattern with removable cuts.

The Continuous Sling Suture

The **continuous sling suture** is placed where a large flap involving several teeth has been used (Figure 28-59). This suture involves the same steps as with the single sling, except the suture thread is wrapped around to the next tooth instead of back to the beginning side. When the tissue has been secured interproximally of each tooth involved, the suture is tied off (see Figure 28-59 for a continuous sling suture securing the facial tissue of several teeth).

Mattress Sutures

Mattress sutures also are used when a flap is to be sutured. The difference between the simple and the mattress sutures is that the simple suture goes into the facial surface and then emerges from the lingual surface, while the mattress sutures go in and out of the tissue on the same surface. For example, on the facial surface, the suture goes into and comes back out of the tissue on the same surface. If the stitch, or bite, is taken horizontally, it is a **horizontal mattress suture** (Figure 28-60A). If the

Step 1   Step 2   Step 3   Step 4

FIGURE 28-56 Simple suture pattern.

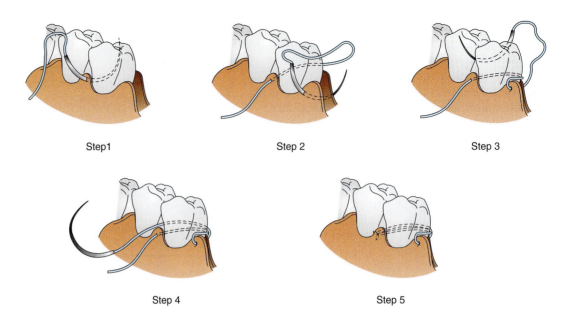

Step1   Step 2   Step 3

Step 4   Step 5

FIGURE 28-58 Sling suture pattern.

stitch is taken vertically, it is a **vertical mattress suture** (Figure 28-60B). With the mattress sutures, the same stitch is taken on the facial and lingual. The mattress sutures are tied with one surgeon's knot on the surface where the suture procedure began.

FIGURE 28-59 Continuous sling suture pattern.

SUTURE REMOVAL CRITERIA

The following are basic criteria to guide the dental assistant when removing sutures:

▶ Explain the procedure to the patient.

▶ The healing process should not be disturbed when removing the sutures.

▶ The suture is removed with the least amount of trauma to the tissues.

▶ All sutures are removed from the suture site.

▶ The knot is not cut.

▶ The suture is cut as closely to the tissue as possible.

▶ A suture that has been exposed in the mouth is not pulled through the tissue. (This suture is contaminated with saliva, food, and bacteria.)

▶ The knot is not pulled through the tissue.

▶ The hemorrhage is controlled following established procedures.

▶ The sutures are placed on a gauze so they can be counted.

SUTURE REMOVAL

Each type of suture is placed in a specific pattern. To remove the sutures, identify the pattern and determine where the cuts are to be made. Then, follow the basic criteria and remove the sutures from the suture site.

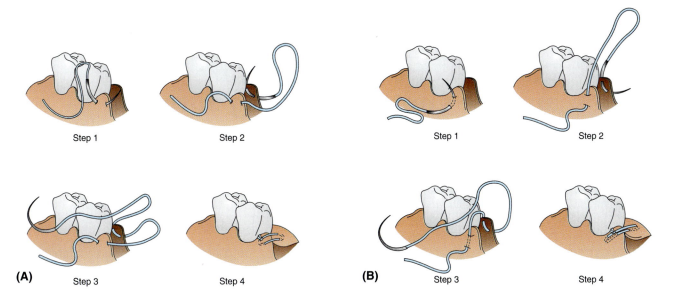

FIGURE 28-60 (A) Horizontal mattress suture pattern. (B) Vertical mattress suture pattern.

28-16 Removal of the Simple Suture and Continuous Simple Sutures

This procedure is performed by the dentist or the expanded-function dental assistant. The patient returns to the office for suture removal. The dental assistant prepares the materials needed and the patient before beginning the procedure.

EQUIPMENT AND SUPPLIES

▶ Basic setup: mouth mirror, explorer, cotton pliers
▶ Suture scissors
▶ Hemostat
▶ Gauze sponges
▶ Air-water syringe tip, HVE tip

PROCEDURE STEPS *(Follow aseptic procedures)*

1. Using cotton pliers, gently lift the suture away from the tissues.

2. Take the suture scissors and cut the thread below the knot, close to the tissue.

3. Secure the knot with the cotton pliers and gently pull, lifting the suture out of the tissues.

4. Place the suture on a gauze sponge.

5. For continuous simple sutures, cut each suture and remove individually. Begin with one end and then proceed with each suture stitch.

6. Loosen the suture with the cotton pliers and, while still holding the suture thread with the cotton pliers, cut the thread close to the tissue (Figure 28-61).

7. As each suture is removed, place it on a gauze sponge so it can be counted when finished with the procedure.

Always carefully evaluate the sutures before cutting them to be sure sutures exposed in the oral cavity are not pulled through the tissue during removal.

FIGURE 28-61 Removal of simple and continuous simple sutures.

PROCEDURE

28-17 Removal of the Sling Suture and the Continuous Sling Sutures

This procedure is performed by the dentist or the expanded-function dental assistant. The patient returns to the office for suture removal. The dental assistant prepares the materials needed and the patient before beginning the procedure.

PROCEDURE STEPS *(Follow aseptic procedures)*

1. The sling suture is cut in two places. With cotton pliers, lift the suture gently on each side of the tooth to loosen the suture from the tissue (Figures 28-62A and B).

2. Lift the knot gently and cut below the knot, near the tissue.

3. Lift the suture thread on the other side of the tooth, near the tissue, and cut it as close to the tissue as possible without cutting the tissue.

NOTE: When removing a continuous sling suture, this process is repeated, cutting on each side of the tooth until all sutures have been removed.

4. Using cotton pliers, remove each thread carefully, pulling toward the opposite surface, away from the flap. For example, if the suture is taken on the facial and wrapped around the lingual, pull toward the lingual to remove the sutures.

5. Place each thread of the suture on a gauze sponge to be counted.

6. Examine the suture site.

(A)

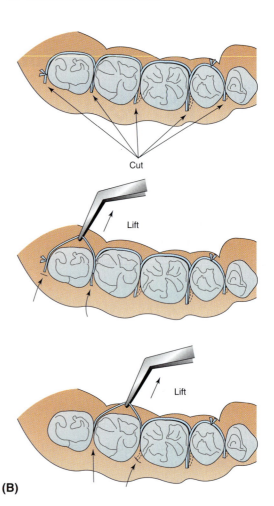

(B)

FIGURE 28-62 Removal of (A) sling and (B) continuous sling sutures.

28-18 Removal of the Horizontal and Vertical Mattress Sutures

This procedure is performed by the dentist or the expanded-function dental assistant. The patient returns to the office for suture removal. The dental assistant prepares the materials needed and the patient before beginning the procedure.

PROCEDURE STEPS *(Follow aseptic procedures)*

Although the horizontal and vertical mattress sutures are placed differently, the basic steps are the same. This holds true for their removal, also. Two cuts are made with each mattress suture, one on each side of the suture stitch (see Figure 28-63A for the horizontal mattress and Figure 28-63B for the vertical mattress).

1. Gently lift the knot with cotton pliers.

2. Cut the suture below the knot, close to the tissue.

3. Make the second cut on the opposite surface, close to the tissue.

4. Remove one piece of the suture by holding the knot with the cotton pliers and lifting gently. Place it on a gauze sponge.

5. Remove the remaining suture thread.

6. Count pieces of the suture.

7. Examine the suture site.

(A)

(B)

FIGURE 28-63 Removal of (A) horizontal mattress suture and (B) vertical mattress suture.

POST SUTURE REMOVAL

If there was bleeding when the sutures were removed, apply pressure with gauze sponge for a few minutes until the bleeding stops. Check the patient's mouth for any debris, and wipe around the outside of the patient's mouth if necessary. After the sutures are removed, the dental assistant should instruct the patient to continue with a soft diet and rinse with warm saltwater for several days. Before the patient is dismissed, the dental assistant should document the procedure on the patient's chart. The chart entry should include any complications encountered and the degree of healing of the suture site.

Summary of Steps of Suture Removal

1. Review patient's chart and medical history.
2. Prepare armamentarium.
3. Seat the patient.
4. Explain the procedure and ask whether the patient has had any problems or has any questions.
5. Examine the suture site for healing.
6. Check the number and type of sutures.
7. Consult with the dentist.
8. Debride the suture site to prepare for suture removal.
9. Evaluate the sutures to determine where to make the cuts.
10. Gently secure and lift the sutures to position for cutting.
11. Using suture scissors or sharp, pointed surgical scissors, cut the sutures.
12. Remove the sutures and place on a gauze.
13. Blot the suture area if there is blood.
14. Count the sutures on the gauze.
15. Instruct the patient regarding care of the suture area.
16. Document the procedure on the patient's chart
17. Call the dentist to check the patient.
18. Dismiss the patient.

GINGIVAL RETRACTION

OBJECTIVES

The student should strive to meet the following objectives and demonstrate an understanding of the facts and principles presented in this chapter:

1. Explain the function of gingival retraction.

2. Describe the different types of gingival retraction.

3. Explain the steps of placing and removing gingival retraction cord.

KEY TERMS

electrosurgery unit (p. 680)

ischemia (p. 680)

gingival retraction (p. 678)

INTRODUCTION

After a tooth is prepared for a crown, **gingival retraction** is done to ensure that an impression with clear margins can be obtained. During this process, all hemorrage must be arrested and all the hard and soft tissue the operator wants to reproduced must be clean and dry. The margins ideally are supragingival, or above the gingiva, but many may be subgingival, or below the gingiva. The tissue must be retracted horizontally to allow room for sufficient impression material and displaced vertically to expose the margin completely. Retraction may be done chemically, mechanically, surgically, or a combination of these.

Retraction cord is available in a variety of sizes, configurations, and chemical treatments (Figure 28-64). The cord comes in a dispensing package for easy use. The cord may be twisted, braided, or woven to hold its shape.

(A)

(B)

FIGURE 28-64 (A) Various types of retraction cord. (B) Tissue management gel kit. *(Courtesy of Pascal, Co., Inc.)*

TYPES OF GINGIVAL RETRACTION

Mechanical Retraction

Mechanical retraction can be accomplished in a number of ways. Without the use of drugs, tissue shrinkage or hemostasis will not be accomplished; however, the tissue can be displaced to allow access to the margin. Retraction cord is placed in the sulcus of healthy and inflamed free gingiva. The cotton cord is left in place for ten to fifteen minutes (instead of the five minutes as it would be with the chemical retraction cord).

If any of the cords is placed too deep, the crevice opens at the bottom but is narrow at the top (Figure 28-65A). The operator may be able to get the impression material into the crevice after the cord is removed, but the material has a tendency to fracture near the edge of the preparation. If the cord is placed too shallow in the crevice, the space is inadequate to allow an accurate

reproduction of the margin of the preparation (Figure 28-65B). The proper position of the tucked cord is 1 to 3 mm into the V-shaped crevice (Figure 28-65C). The dentist may want two cords placed to retract the gingival tissues. The crevice is V shaped, and this dictates the size of cords to use. The smaller cords are placed at the depth of the crevice, and the larger cord is placed on top (Figure 28-65D).

Another means of mechanical retraction is accomplished by lengthening a temporary crown form to cause tissue displacement and taking the impression at a later date. Another method uses a dental dam clamp and rubber dam to displace the tissue. The clamp and rubber dam are placed and then removed just prior to

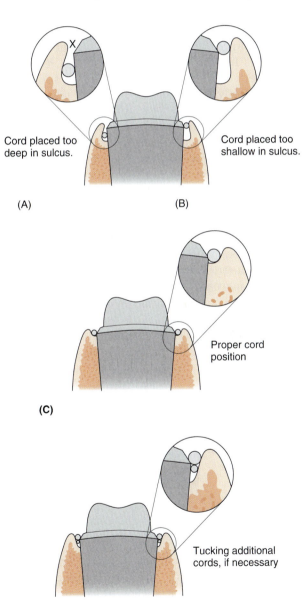

Cord placed too deep in sulcus.

Cord placed too shallow in sulcus.

(A)

(B)

Proper cord position

(C)

Tucking additional cords, if necessary

(D)

FIGURE 28-65 (A) Retraction cord placed too deep. (B) Retraction cord placed too shallow. (C) Retraction cord placed properly. (D) Double retraction cords placed properly.

taking the final impression. Both of these techniques may cause the tissue to bleed and the impression to be distorted.

Chemical Retraction

Chemical retraction may be done prior to the placement of the cord or by impregnating the cord and then placing it, or both ways. One of the newer ways is to use a topical hemostatic solution, astringent with dento-infusion tubes, and a plastic lure lock syringe. The solution is placed using a disposable metal tip bent to the desired area. As the solution is placed, the blood and the solution merge together and are washed away with the air-water syringe. What is left in the tissue is a temporary coagulum seal that does not allow any seepage. The tissue may appear slightly darkened, but this technique allows hemorrhage to be arrested. A retraction cord of interwoven cotton with or without solution is packed vertically to expose the prepared margin. This packing of the cord allows for horizontal retraction to allow for sufficient bulk of impression material to flow around the margin.

The retraction cord could also be impregnated with aluminum chloride or astringent of aluminum salts for chemical retraction. This technique causes a shrinking of the tissues, or **ischemia**, to obtain clear access to the margin of the preparation. A substance used to obtain this result is epinephrine, which is an astringent and a vasoconstrictor. It provides hemostasis and shrinks the tissues by constricting the blood vessels. Epinephrine brings on an increase in the heart beat, or **tachycardia**, for the patient. The epinephrine definitely is contraindicated for a patient with heart disease, diabetes, or hyperthyroidism or a patient taking certain drugs.

NOTE: The dental assistant should watch for patients who exhibit hypertension, knowing that most hyperthyroid and diabetic patients are usually hypertensive. Normally, the dentist prefers to use chemical retraction cord, so the patient's medical history should be reviewed carefully.

Surgical Retraction

Instead of retraction, the dentist may choose to remove the tissue around the preparation. This approach is accomplished by using a surgical knife or by performing electrosurgery. With the surgical knife, the dentist excises the tissue and exposes the margin of the preparation. The area where the tissue has been removed may bleed and cause additional treatment in order to get a good impression of the area.

The dentist may decide to use an **electrosurgery unit**, which cauterizes the tissues as it removes them. Therefore, the tissue is removed without bleeding. The unit passes high-frequency current to a small electrode passing through the tissue. The tip of the unit appears as a metal wire or loop. As the tip touches the tissue, the unit is activated to remove the tissue. It is especially important with this treatment that soft tissue anesthesia is maintained. Electrosurgery is not used with patients who are receiving radiation therapy, have cardiac pacemakers, or have any diseases that slow healing.

Constant use of a non-metal HVE tip during the surgery is important due to the odor given off as the tissues are cauterized. The evacuator reduces the odor if it is placed near the surgical site. After the tissue is removed, the sulcus is cleaned with a hydrogen rinse. Immediately following the procedure, the final impression is taken.

PROCEDURE

28-19 Placing and Removing the Retraction Cord

This procedure is performed by the dentist or the expanded-function dental assistant. After the tooth has been prepared, the retraction cord is placed. The equipment and supplies are included as part of the crown/bridge tray setup. The specific items needed to place and remove the retraction cord are listed.

EQUIPMENT

▶ Basic setup: Mouth mirror, explorer, cotton pliers

▶ HVE tip and air-water syringe tip

▶ Scissors

(continued)

PROCEDURE 28-19 *continued*

- ▶ Hemostat
- ▶ Retraction cord(s)
- ▶ Retraction cord placement instrument or plastic instrument
- ▶ Cotton rolls, 2 × 2 gauze sponges

PROCEDURE STEPS *(Follow aseptic procedures)*

1. The dentist prepares the tooth for the crown.

2. Rinse and dry the area in preparation for placement of the retraction cord.

3. Cotton rolls are placed on the facial and, if mandibular, on the lingual surface. The area is carefully dried.

4. The dentist selects the retraction cord(s) to be placed around the tooth.

5. The length of the cord needed is determined by the circumference of the prepared tooth. NOTE: The desired length is determined by wrapping the cord around the small finger for an anterior tooth and around a larger finger for a molar.

6. The cord is cut to the appropriate length.

7. Twist the cord ends to compress the fibers together.

8. The cord is looped and placed in a hemostat or cotton pliers.

9. The cord is looped around the margin of the prepared tooth and tightened slightly (Figure 28-66). This aids in slipping the cord into the sulcus area. Normally, the ends of the cord are toward the buccal surface for easy access.

10. The hemostat or cotton pliers is/are released, leaving the cord in the sulcus.

11. The retraction cord is packed into position with a packing instrument or a plastic instrument.

12. The cord is gently packed around the cervical area, apical to the preparation.

13. The cord is packed around the tooth and overlaps, usually on the facial surface.

14. A tip of the cord is left showing out of the sulcus in order for easy removal just prior to taking the impression (Figure 28-67).

15. The retraction cord is left in place for five minutes when chemical retraction cord is used and for ten to fifteen minutes for mechanical retraction.

16. The end of the retraction cord is grasped and removed in a circular motion just prior to the impression material being placed.

FIGURE 28-66 Retraction cord looped around the prepared tooth for placement in the gingival sulcus.

FIGURE 28-67 Retraction cord in place around the prepared tooth with a tag left out for easy removal.

ENAMEL SEALANTS

OBJECTIVES

The student should strive to meet the following objectives and demonstrate an understanding of the facts and principles presented in this chapter:

1. Explain the purpose of using enamel sealants and where they are placed.
2. List the indications and contraindications of placing sealants.
3. Discuss the role of the dental assistant in the placement of enamel sealants.
4. Describe the types of sealant materials.
5. List and describe the steps of the application procedure.

KEY TERMS

acid etched
    (p. 683)
chemically cured
    (p. 683)
coalesced (p. 682)
**dental composites
    (BIS-GMA)** (p. 683)
light cured (p. 683)
mechanical bond
    (p. 683)
occlusal (p. 682)
polymerization
    (p. 683)

INTRODUCTION

Enamel sealants are hard resin materials that are applied to caries-free **occlusal** surfaces of premolars and molars. These pit and fissure teeth are particularly susceptible to caries because of the deep pits and fissures in the enamel on the occlusal surface. Tooth-brushing is not always an adequate means of removing the bacteria and debris that are lodged in the pits and fissures. Fluoride is very effective in preventing decay on the smooth enamel surfaces but less effective in the pits and fissures. Sealants bond to the tooth to "seal" the pits and fissures, thereby preventing the decay process from starting. The barrier costs less than a restoration but does not last as long. On the average, sealants remain in place for five to seven years. The combined use of pit and fissure sealants and fluoride has proven to be an effective measure that greatly reduces dental caries in patients through age sixteen.

INDICATIONS AND CONTRAINDICATIONS FOR SEALANTS

Enamel sealants are indicated and would be most beneficial if applied:

▶ On occlusal pits and fissures of non-carious primary and permanent teeth

▶ On recently erupted teeth

▶ On patients with a high number of occlusal caries and deep fissures

▶ Along with preventive treatment

Contraindications to placing enamel sealants include:

▶ Teeth that have been caries free for four or more years (the chances are minimal that occlusal decay will occur)

▶ Teeth with shallow open grooves. Usually, these teeth are easy to keep clean, making them more resistant to decay. Also, sealants are not well retained in these areas

▶ Teeth with well-**coalesced** (blended) pits and fissures

▶ Patients with occlusal decay or who have occlusal restorations

ROLE OF THE DENTAL ASSISTANT

Applying enamel sealants is an expanded duty delegated to the dental hygienist or the dental assistant in some states. The laws governing the dental assistant's responsibilities vary greatly with each state, so become familiar with state practice acts. In some states, the dental assistant can assist the dentist in this procedure, in which help is always needed to isolate the teeth and keep them dry and free of debris until the sealant is placed. In other states, with education and training the dental assistant can place the sealants. The dental assistant can then follow through with the total preventive program and apply both the fluoride and the pit and fissure sealants.

It is important for the dental assistant to stay informed and current on enamel sealants. Research on sealants' effectiveness, chemical properties, and potential is ongoing, so reading articles and attending seminars keeps the dental assistant well informed.

ENAMEL SEALANT MATERIALS

Several materials have been used as sealants for occlusal pits and fissures, but the most commonly used are **dental composites (BIS-GMA)** that have been diluted to be less viscous to enhance the flow characteristic needed with sealants. These materials come in clear, opaque, or lightly tinted colors. The advantage to the opaque and tinted is visibility, which makes placement less difficult and identification of the sealants at follow-up exams easier; however, patients prefer the clear sealants because of esthetic appeal.

The main difference in the types of sealant materials is in the curing or hardening process. The two methods of **polymerization** (hardening) are:

1. **Chemically cured**, also known as self-cure or autopolymerization

2. **Light cured**, the use of curing light to harden materials

The chemically cured materials come with a two-component system with a catalyst and a base. When mixed together, they react chemically to polymerize in about one minute. The light-cured sealants are packaged as one-component systems that are activated by a curing light. The advantages of the light-cured sealants are that the operator has control of the setting time and there is no mixing required.

Acid Etching/ Conditioning Material

Enamel sealants bond mechanically to the tooth surface, not chemically. The **mechanical bond** is accomplished by the sealant flowing into the irregularities of the treated enamel and locking into place. The enamel surface is **acid etched**, or **conditioned**, by a phosphoric acid solution that is applied to a clean tooth with a brush, syringe, or cotton pledget. The etchant comes in a gel or a liquid and is applied for thirty to ninety seconds. During that time, the etchant is "dabbed" or flowed over the area, but never rubbed. When the time is complete, the tooth is rinsed thoroughly for the specified amount of time. The tooth surface looks frosted or chalky and appears dull. If the enamel does not appear chalky and white, the procedure must be repeated. If the tooth is contaminated with saliva before the sealant is placed, the etching procedure must be redone (Figure 28-68). The acid etchant/conditioner is applied on the occlusal surface 2 to 3 mm beyond the area to be sealed. The tooth must be etched beyond the sealant to prevent fracture of the sealant and possible microleakage.

PLACEMENT OF ENAMEL SEALANTS

The dentist diagnoses which teeth need enamel sealants after a thorough examination, including radiographs. Children with newly erupted molars and premolars that are caries free benefit the most from sealants. Partially erupted teeth may be sealed provided there is not a flap over the occlusal surface that interferes with the sealant application. It is the operator's preference when to isolate the teeth, before or after the polish. Usually, sealants are placed on one or two quadrants at a time to ensure adequate isolation of the teeth.

The sealant kits are usually supplied with everything needed for applying the sealants. The sealant kits often vary according to how the material is cured and application methods.

FIGURE 28-68 View of where the acid etchant was placed.

P R O C E D U R E

28-20 Procedure for Placing Enamel Sealants

This procedure is performed by the dental assistant, hygienist, or dentist depending on the state dental practice act. Before the sealant is placed, the tooth/teeth is/are polished with a rubber cup. Equipment for the preparation of the tooth/teeth and the sealant procedure are listed.

EQUIPMENT AND SUPPLIES (Figure 28-69)

FIGURE 28-69 Equipment for placing enamel sealants.

▶ Basic setup: mouth mirror, explorer, cotton pliers

▶ Air-water syringe tip, HVE tips, and saliva ejector

▶ Rubber cup

▶ Low-speed handpiece with right angle attachment

▶ Flour of pumice or prophy paste without fluoride

▶ Dental dam setup or Garmer cotton roll holders and short and long cotton rolls

▶ Etchant/conditioner

▶ Sealant material: base material and catalyst (for self-cure) or base material (for light cure)

▶ Applicators (brush, small cotton pellets, or syringe) for etchant and sealant

▶ Sealant dappen dish

▶ Light-curing unit

▶ Articulating paper and forceps

▶ Assorted burs and/or stones

▶ Floss

PROCEDURE STEPS (*Follow aseptic procedures*)

1. Polish the occlusal surface of the teeth to receive sealants. Use flour of pumice or a non-fluoride prophy paste with a rubber cup or bristle brush to clean the occlusal surfaces. Once polished, rinse the teeth and dry thoroughly. If the pits and fissures are deep, check them with an explorer and then rinse and dry again.

2. Dental dam isolation is ideal because it keeps the teeth dry and protects the tissues from the etchant. Depending on the skill of the operator, the dental dam may be placed on more than one quadrant at a time. (Refer to information on dental dams in this chapter.) Cotton roll isolation is commonly used, but care must be given to ensure that the teeth are kept isolated. Garmer clamps used with long and short cotton rolls are very effective.

3. After the tooth is isolated, completely dry the tooth. Following manufacturer's directions, apply the acid etchant. Using an applicator, apply etchant to the occlusal surface, into the pits and fissures and two-thirds up the cuspid incline. Use a gentle dabbing motion while applying the sealant for the designated amount of time (usually sixty seconds).

4. Rinse the tooth with water, and use the evacuator tip to remove the remaining acid and water. Rinse for twenty to thirty seconds. Reisolate with dry cotton rolls if this method was used.

5. Dry the tooth with the air for twenty to thirty seconds. Examine the etched surface. It should appear dull and chalky white. If the tooth does not have this appearance, etch again for fifteen to thirty seconds (Figure 28-70).

6. Follow manufacturer's directions to prepare and apply the sealant material. With the applicator

(continued)

FIGURE 28-70 Isolated tooth with enamel etched. Appearance is white and chalky where etchant was placed.

FIGURE 28-71 Tooth with sealant in place.

selected, place the sealant so that it flows into the pits and fissures and reaches the desired thickness. The applicator tip or an explorer can be used to move the sealant and prevent air bubbles.

7. Allow the self-curing sealants to set (polymerize) for the time recommended by the manufacturer. For light-cured sealants, hold the curing light 2 mm directly above the occlusal surface and expose for the appropriate time (materials differ, so the curing time can range from twenty to sixty seconds).

NOTE: Use tinted protective eyewear during the curing process.

8. Evaluate the sealant (Figure 28-71). With an explorer, check to see whether the sealant is hardened and smooth. If there are irregularities or voids, repeat the process to properly seal those areas. If the surface has been free of saliva, then additional sealant can be added without etching the tooth first. However, if saliva has contacted the tooth, then the process must be repeated.

9. After the sealant has set, rinse or wipe the surface with a moist cotton roll/pellet to remove the air-inhibited layer.

10. Remove cotton rolls or the dental dam. Check the contacts with dental floss, and look for any excess materials. Dry the teeth and, with articulating paper, evaluate for any high spots (Figure 28-72). If the markings are dark, use a bur or stone to reduce them. It does not take much to reduce the sealant,

and areas just a little high will wear down in two to three days with very little patient awareness.

11. Apply fluoride to the sealed tooth to cover any areas that were etched but not sealed. Sealants are recorded on the patient's chart. Instruct the patient to check the sealants every six months to a year to ensure that they have been completely retained.

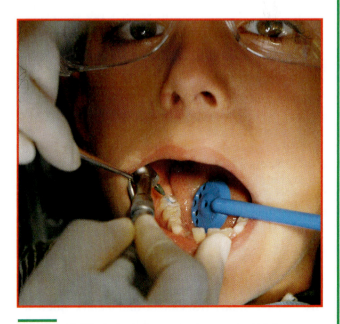

FIGURE 28-72 Articulating paper has marked high spots on the sealant. The sealant is reduced with assorted burs and stones before the patient is dismissed.

BLEACHING TECHNIQUES

OBJECTIVES

The student should strive to meet the following objectives and demonstrate an understanding of the facts and principles presented in this chapter:

1. Explain the benefits of the bleaching process used in dentistry.

2. List and describe the types of bleaching techniques and describe the procedures for dental office bleaching for vital and non-vital teeth and for home bleaching.

3. Explain information given to the patient concerning outcomes, procedures, responsibilities, and precautions related to bleaching.

KEY TERMS

assisted bleaching (p. 689)

carbamide peroxide (p. 686)

hydrogen peroxide (p. 686)

power bleaching (p. 688)

sodium perborate (p. 686)

walking bleach technique (p. 687)

INTRODUCTION

Many attempts have been made to esthetically improve the shade of one's teeth. Today, the most commonly used materials are **sodium perborate**, **hydrogen peroxide**, and **carbamide peroxide**. These bleaching agents are sometimes used with a light or a heat source.

Bleaching has become one of the most requested services provided by the dental profession and is often delegated to a dental assistant. Specific training and clinical experience are required for this person to become confident and competent. Although the bleaching procedures have been proven safe and effective through the ADA and the Federal Drug Administration, research is continually being done and the office must keep up-to-date on new information.

Types of Stains

Teeth are stained by a variety of causes, and the source may be intrinsic or extrinsic. Examples of **extrinsic stains** include stains from diets and habits, such as tobacco, tea, and coffee. These leave yellow to brown stains, and the success of the bleaching process depends on the amount of stain. **Intrinsic stains** include tetracycline stains, dental fluorosis, discoloration due to injury, and non-vital endodontically treated teeth.

(See Coronal Polish in this chapter for more information on dental stains.) Sometimes, the shade of the teeth is naturally toward the yellow or gray shades, and these patients can esthetically enhance the color of their teeth with bleaching.

BLEACHING TECHNIQUES

There are two methods of bleaching: One method is done in the dental office, and the other method is done at home. Patients can have one or the other or a combination of both services to meet their needs. Both vital and non-vital teeth are bleached in the office. There are advantages and disadvantages with each method, so the options should be presented to the patient. Considerations include the amount of stain and its origin, the number of visits to the office versus the amount of time the bleaching trays are worn at home, the expense of the in-office bleaching (which is higher than in-home bleaching), and the amount of instruction and guidance the patient requires.

Non-Vital Bleaching

Endodontically treated teeth sometimes turn dark due to blood, pulpal debris, and restorative materials that are used to fill the canal. These teeth can be lightened by both internal and external bleaching. One of the most common bleaching techniques is the **walking bleach technique**. This technique calls for a thick paste of hydrogen peroxide, sodium perborate, or a combination of the two to be placed in the coronal portion of the non-vital tooth. With the bleach mixture temporarily sealed in place, the patient can leave the office and return for evaluation and another possible treatment as instructed by the dentist. Sometimes, heat is applied with a heated instrument/unit in order to achieve the results desired.

P R O C E D U R E

28-21 Non-Vital Bleaching

This procedure is performed by the dentist. The patient has received information on the procedure and the possible outcome before the procedure begins. More than one treatment may be necessary.

EQUIPMENT AND SUPPLIES

▶ Basic setup: mouth mirror, explorer, cotton pliers

▶ Cotton rolls, gauze sponges, cotton pellets

▶ HVE tip, air-water syringe tip, saliva ejector

▶ Dental dam setup

▶ Protective gel

▶ Waxed dental floss

▶ High-speed handpiece and assorted burs

▶ Low-speed handpiece

▶ Prophy brush

▶ Cement base materials

▶ Bleaching materials

▶ Heat source

▶ Temporary coverage and cement

▶ Finishing burs

PROCEDURE STEPS (*Follow aseptic procedures*)

1. The dentist examines and evaluates the root canal treated tooth.

2. Place the dental dam and ligature of waxed dental floss on the designated tooth or teeth. Once the dam is in place, apply more protective gel to further seal the dam.

3. Remove the access restoration and any debris in the crown. With the crown of the tooth open, some dentists scrub the chamber with a soap solution and a prophy brush or cotton pellet.

4. The root canal is sealed with 2 to 3 mm of a thick base cement or with a light-cured resin ionomer or bonded composite. This is a critical step, because the tooth must be sealed in order to prevent the bleaching from penetrating the root. This can be done using the gel bleach in the office or the walking technique, or a combination of both techniques. If bleaching results are not achieved, heat may be also used with the office bleaching gel technique. Stains caused by endodontic procedure and drugs often need the application of heat with the bleaching agents.

   ▶ Gel bleaching in the office involves the chamber being filled for thirty minutes. Change the bleaching gel every ten minutes. Then, place a cotton pellet and temporary in the crown. The patient should be reappointed in three to seven days for evaluation.

   ▶ With walking bleaching, a thick mixture of bleaching agent is placed in the crown and covered with temporary cement. Reappoint the patient in two to five days to remove the cotton pellet.

5. Desired results should be achieved in three appointments, but if the tooth remains darker than the patient prefers, a veneer should be considered. The shade can be altered slightly with the shade of the restorative materials. The temporary filling is removed, and the chamber is rinsed and evacuated. Etching is applied to the inside of the crown. Rinse. Apply the dental adhesive and then fill the chamber with restorative material and light cure.

6. Polish the restoration with finishing burs and polish.

7. Reappoint the patient in a few days to evaluate the color and whether there is the possible need of a veneer.

Vital Bleaching In-Office

Bleaching vital teeth in the office involves the application of bleaching liquids or gels, often with the application of heat and a curing light. This is sometimes called **power bleaching**. The patient's teeth are isolated tightly to prevent irritation to the gingiva by any chemicals, and then they are polished with a pumice or prophy paste. The actual bleaching steps depend on the type of materials used, but, for most, a fresh mix is applied every ten to fifteen minutes for three to four applications. The bleaching materials are evacuated between applications and then completely when the procedure is finished. Then,

rinse thoroughly, remove isolation, and polish with a fluoride prophy paste.

The patient is scheduled for his or her next appointment within one to two weeks. The patient should be told that the teeth may be sensitive. This process usually takes three appointments.

Home Bleaching Techniques

For home bleaching, the patient applies a bleaching agent, usually carbamide peroxide or diluted hydrogen peroxide, in a custom-fit tray for specific amounts of

P R O C E D U R E

28-22 In-Office Bleaching for Vital Teeth

This procedure is performed by the dentist in the dental office. The procedure is explained to the patient with the possible outcomes.

EQUIPMENT AND SUPPLIES

▶ Protective gel

▶ Waxed dental floss

▶ High-speed handpiece and assorted burs

▶ Low-speed handpiece

▶ Prophy brush

▶ Cement base materials

▶ Bleaching materials

▶ Heat source

▶ Temporary coverage and cement

▶ Finishing burs

PROCEDURE STEPS (*Follow aseptic procedures*)

1. The procedure is explained and videos, photos, and pamphlets may be available for the patient. The teeth and surrounding tissues are examined. Before photos may be taken of the patient.

2. Cover all surrounding tissues with protective gel. Isolating with the dental dam is the safest method to protect the tissues. Place the dental dam, punching the holes as close as possible to match the tooth. With the dental dam on, place a ligature of

waxed floss around each tooth, and pull the floss toward the cervix and secure.

3. Polish the crowns of the teeth to remove plaque and debris that may interfere with the bleaching process. Prophy paste or flour of pumice may be used.

4. Follow the manufacturer's instructions for the specific steps of the materials being used. Materials are mixed to a thick consistency and placed on the facial and lingual surfaces of the tooth or in a tray. Some materials require the use of a bleaching heat and/or light source and are used for approximately thirty minutes. The no-heat materials are applied every ten minutes, with fresh materials mixed each time for three to four applications. Rinse and evacuate between each application to remove the bulk of the bleaching gel.

5. After thoroughly rinsing the area, cut the ligatures and interseptal dental dam and remove these from the patient's mouth. Rinse again, and remove any protective gel with floss and wet gauze.

6. Polish the teeth with a composite resin polishing cup or a fluoride prophy paste. (This step may vary with different types of materials.)

7. Although the bleaching process may take some time before the shade can be evaluated, the patient's tissues are examined and the patient is instructed to avoid substances that may stain the teeth. The patient should also be warned that the teeth may be sensitive following the bleaching procedure. Usually, three appointments one to two weeks apart are required to reach the desired shade.

time. There are multiple materials, and the techniques vary greatly. The dental staff must become familiar with materials being prescribed for their patients. The advantages of the home bleaching techniques include fewer visits to the dental office, less expense, and patients can apply the bleach when it is convenient. The disadvantages of these techniques are that the patients must be motivated to following the routine, the time involved for the bleaching process can take several weeks, the bleaching materials can cause nausea and sensitivity to the gingiva, and there is lack of direct monitoring by the dentist. Home bleaching is very popular with patients because of the lower cost and the positive results when done properly. As an alternative, patients can come to the office for a startup, or **assisted bleaching**, appoint-

ment and then complete the process with home bleaching. Usually, the two appointments are needed to set up the patient for home bleaching. At the first appointment, the impressions for the custom trays are made. The second appointment is for delivery of the bleaching trays; instructions are also given to the patient (Figure 28-73).

PATIENT INFORMATION

With all bleaching procedures, the patient needs to understand the procedure steps and the outcome possibilities. The bleaching process will "lighten" most teeth, but some teeth will never be the whitest or the brightest—but they will be improved. The patient's dedication

PROCEDURE

28-23 Home Bleaching

This procedure is performed by the patient at home after an examination by the dentist. The patient is given a bleaching kit and step-by-step instructions from the dentist. This procedure is divided into appointments and steps that occur between appointments.

EQUIPMENT AND SUPPLIES

▶ Basic setup: mouth mirror, explorer, cotton pliers

▶ Alginate

▶ Rubber mixing bowl and spatula

▶ Impression trays

▶ Camera

▶ Custom-fit, vacuum-formed tray

▶ Home bleaching kit

PROCEDURE STEPS (*Follow aseptic procedures*)

First Appointment

1. The dentist examines the teeth, considering the shade of the teeth, sensitivity, restorations, and areas of abrasion and erosion. General procedures are completed before the bleaching process begins. The bleaching techniques are explained, and the procedure that best meets the patient's needs is selected.

2. Alginate impressions are taken of the arches being bleached. Before photographs are taken.

Between Appointments

1. The alginate impressions are poured in stone and prepared.

2. A custom-fit, vacuum-formed tray is made. This may be done in the office lab or at a commercial lab.

Second Appointment

1. With the home technique, the patient tries on the trays to ensure a good fit.

2. Instructions are given, including when and for how long to wear the trays, how to prepare the materials, how to place the custom-fit trays, what to do in case the gingiva becomes irritated, and how to handle other side effects.

3. In some cases, the patient receives one bleaching in the office, before beginning the home bleaching. The teeth are polished, and then the bleaching agent is prepared and placed in the trays. The trays are inserted into the patient's mouth for thirty to sixty minutes, then removed. The teeth are suctioned off and rinsed thoroughly.

4. Some offices schedule an appointment to follow-up with the patient's progress and to examine the tissues. This appointment is usually within two weeks of the second appointment.

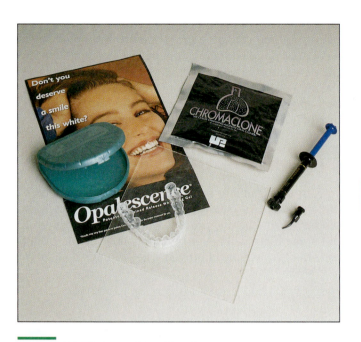

FIGURE 28-73 Home bleaching kit.

to following procedures and limiting foods and habits that stain the teeth will enhance the process and bleach the teeth faster. The health of the gingiva and surrounding tissues must be protected by adhering to technique suggestions. Ingestion of the solutions should be kept to a minimum. The patient must realize that bleaching may be an ongoing treatment, with repeated bleaching necessary every few years.

CHAPTER SUMMARY

Expanded functions, such as, dental dam; matrix and wedge; coronal polish; placing cavity liners, cavity varnish, and cement bases; suture removal; gingival retraction; placing enamel sealants; and bleaching techniques; are specific advanced tasks that require increased skill and responsibility. These functions are delegated by the dentist according to the Dental Practice Act within the state. Some states require additional education, certification, or registration to perform these functions.

CASE STUDY

Tina Jerrod, a blind patient, had been a patient for several years but has not had any work done other than routine examinations and cleanings. Tina was scheduled for a restoration today. Nitrous oxide sedation, local anesthetic, and the dental dam were to be part of the preparation for the procedure. Tina did fine until the assistant stretched the dam over the dental dam frame, which gave Tina the feeling that she could not breathe. She panicked and began grabbing at the dental dam and the nitrous hose.

Case Study Review

1. Should the dental assistant have anticipated Tina's reaction?

2. What steps might have been taken to prevent Tina from going through this experience?

3. Should the dentist proceed with the appointment or reappoint Tina on another day?

 To complete your study of this chapter, work the review activities that follow. Also, refer to the software that accompanies this text.

REVIEW QUESTIONS

Multiple Choice

1. Dental dam clamps have the letter "W" imprinted on the bow if
   a. they are winged.
   b. they are wingless.
   c. they have jaws that are bent sharply downward.
   d. they are for use on children only.

2. The smallest circumference of the matrix band when looped is placed
   a. toward the gingival tissue.
   b. toward the occlusal surface of the tooth.
   c. toward the mesial surface of the tooth.
   d. toward the distal surface of the tooth.

3. When cleaning deep pits and fissures while polishing the occlusal surfaces, which aid is most effective?
   a. Rubber cup.
   b. Prophy brush.
   c. Dental tape.
   d. Dental floss.

4. Treatment of the beyond ideal cavity preparation includes all of the following *except*
   a. a base is not required.
   b. a cement base is required.
   c. varnish is placed first, then a cement base.
   d. reinforced ZOE base is placed.

5. When removing sutures, follow all of these statements *except*
   a. do not cut the suture knot.
   b. do not pull the suture thread that was exposed in the oral cavity through the tissues.
   c. cut the suture thread away from the tissues as far as possible.
   d. place all sutures removed on a gauze following removal.

6. To constrict the blood vessels, retraction cord may be impregnated with
   a. aluminum chloride.
   b. sodium hypochlorite.
   c. gluteraldehyde.
   d. epinephrine.

7. Enamel sealants are indicated for all of the following *except*
   a. recently erupted teeth.
   b. teeth that have been caries free for four or more years.
   c. on occlusal pits and fissures of non-carious primary teeth.
   d. on deep occlusal fissures.

8. Bleaching can remove both intrinsic and extrinsic stains to varying degrees.
   a. True
   b. False

Critical Thinking

1. Once the dental dam is placed, the patient is unable to speak. Can you suggest two ways in which the patient might let the dentist know something is hurting him or her?

2. If tooth #20 was to be restored, which tooth would be the anchor tooth if tooth #19 was missing? On what tooth would the last punch on the opposite end of the arch be? Why?

3. Describe how you would punch a dental dam for the following patient: Tooth #4 needs an MOD amalgam, tooth #3 is missing, and teeth #7 and #10 are inclined toward the facial.

4. What classes of cavity preparations would need wedges?

5. Which class of restoration is the strip matrix used for?

6. Explain where cavity varnish is used and why. Which material is cavity varnish not compatible with?

7. If the patient's tooth was sensitive, describe two possible treatments. Include materials and sequence of placement.

8. When a patient comes in for a six-month recall appointment and the sealant on tooth #30 is missing, can the sealant be replaced without etching the tooth first? If so, why?

Dental Practice Management

Dental Office Management

OBJECTIVES

The student should strive to meet the following objectives and demonstrate an understanding of the facts and principles presented in this chapter:

1. Identify the dental office staff and their areas of responsibility.
2. Identify marketing ideas for dentistry.
3. Outline the proper procedure for answering an incoming call.
4. Describe the information every message should contain.
5. Describe telephone and business office technology and its uses.
6. Give examples of the ways in which computers are used in the dental office.
7. Explain how database management concepts can be used in the dental office.
8. Explain why ergonomics is important at a computer workstation.
9. Explain ways in which effective patient scheduling can be accomplished in the dental office.
10. Identify the equipment needed for record management.
11. Define key terms related to accounts receivable.
12. Identify computerized and manual systems for management of patient accounts.
13. Identify accounts payable expenses that the dental practice is responsible for.

KEY TERMS

accounts payable (p. 697)
accounts receivable (p. 697)
Americans with Disabilities Act (p. 696)
check register (p. 724)
computerized systems (p. 701)
down time (p. 706)
ergonomics (p. 703)
etiquette (p. 698)
expendable (p. 720)
facsimile (p. 700)
file folder (p. 707)
gross income (p. 718)
hardware (p. 701)
net income (p. 718)
non-expendable (p. 720)
packing slip (p. 721)
personal computers (PCs) (p. 701)
petty cash (p. 724)
overlap of time (p. 706)
overtime (p. 706)
software (p. 701)
tickler file (p. 708)
usual, reasonable, and customary fee (p. 709)

INTRODUCTION

The dental reception area needs to be an environment in which all patients feel welcome and comfortable. Dentists have worked long and hard to overcome the negative image of dentistry performed years ago. Today, dentistry can be a positive experience, and the dental treatment can be pain free. That image is developed when the patient first steps into the reception area. Many dentists have hired interior design consultants and space-planning advisors to aid the practice in developing an area that is inviting and pleasant for the patients. Some offices have themes while others are designed to be like warm, comfortable, home atmospheres. The creation of this area takes not only appealing colors, but a staff that greets patients with smiles and makes them feel welcome.

The Reception Area

The reception area is a place where patients are received (Figure 29-1). Calling it a waiting room gives it a negative connotation—Patients are busy and their time is important and they do not want to wait. The colors, design, and artwork should be relaxing and adequate, comfortable seating should be available so that each patient can have his or her own space. Keep in mind that individuals from different cultures require different spatial needs. The seating should be arranged in a way that allows people to cluster together or remain distant from others.

Have magazines containing short stories so that the patients can read while they are waiting. The magazines should be current issues. An office that has out-of-date magazines shows indifference to the patient, and it reflects negatively on the overall care. Many dentists

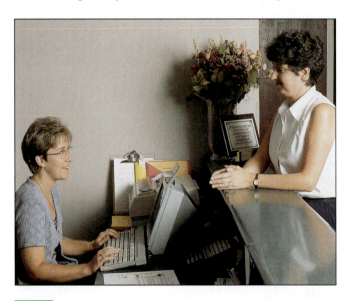

FIGURE 29-1 The reception area is where the patient is first received. It should portray a welcome environment.

have brochures and pamphlets related to the procedures being done in the office. This is also an area in which to display marketing procedures. Some offices also have photo albums showing each staff member and his or her family. Patients like to feel that they can get to know the staff who are taking care of them. Some dental offices have areas for coffee and juice for patients.

The needs of the reception area may change as the practice grows. In 1990, the **Americans with Disabilities Act** was passed by Congress. It mandated that individuals with disabilities have accessibility to health-care facilities having more than fifteen employees. Even though most dental offices have fewer than fifteen employees, it is still the goal to have access for all patients. All doors and hallways should be wide enough for wheelchair access, and a ramp should be available in areas where stairs are present and no elevator is available.

The overall appearance and initial feeling that is obtained from the reception area should give the patients a feeling of well-being and confidence. The patients may not realize consciously the message that is being received, but the dental office should present an atmosphere that relieves the feelings of anxiety.

DENTAL RECEPTIONIST AND BUSINESS OFFICE STAFF

The front office staff has changed dramatically in recent years. One person used to provide the greetings and do all the bookwork for the office. That no longer is the case due to the increased demand for skills the front office personnel are required to perform.

Dental Receptionist

The receptionist in a dental office needs to be able to organize time efficiently and handle multiple tasks concurrently. While being interrupted numerous times, the dental receptionist must be able to complete all tasks on time, paying close attention to details. The dental receptionist must be able to communicate effectively, listen and observe patients, and serve as a liaison between the patient and the office staff. This mature individual must be able to respond to patients who may be upset in a calm, tactful, and appropriate manner.

The receptionist is normally responsible for, but not limited to, the following tasks:

▶ Greeting the patients

▶ Assisting the patients in filling out the initial paperwork required for treatment

▶ Answering the telephone and taking messages as necessary

▶ Scheduling the appointments

▶ Maintaining the patient chart system and records

Dental Office Bookkeeper

The dental office bookkeeper might be the same person as the dental office receptionist or another individual, depending on the size of the office. This person must pay close attention to detail. All the office finances are handled by this person. This includes **accounts receivable**, the money owed to the practice, and **accounts payable**, the money the office owes to others. These finances are normally handled in two separate bookkeeping systems. This individual may also handle the patient dental insurance and make financial arrangements with the patients for payment of the dental service. The inventory and supply system may also be handled by this individual. This person must be organized, have a knowledge of dental treatments, and exhibit good communication and problem-solving skills. These tasks may be shared with other individuals, such as the dental receptionist, depending on the size of the practice. All the individuals in the front office need to be knowledgeable using business machines, such as computers, faxes, and copy machines.

DENTISTRY MARKETING

Marketing tips, which are used throughout this text, are an important part of the dental profession. Even though the first priority of the office team is to care for the patients' dental needs, it cannot be done if there are no patients. A dental office is a business as well as a health-care facility. If there are no patients, employees are not needed. Marketing is a means of attracting and retaining patients who are satisfied with the practice. Dental assistants, along with all the members of the dental team, need to be involved in marketing the practice. It can be rewarding for members of the dental team to use effective efforts in attracting patients to the practice, either through external or internal methods.

Even in off hours, a dental assistant is still associated with the dentist with whom he or she is employed. When people ask what your occupation is, it provides an opportunity to do external marketing for the practice. Other planned external activities can be done, such as dental health education in the community, schools, and centers. The professional manner and enthusiasm that is projected enhances any marketing attempts.

Internal marketing can be accomplished in a number of ways. One person or the whole staff can participate. The ideas are limitless, but the following are suggestions:

▶ Monthly newsletters with tips for dental health

▶ Timed giveaways, such as teddy bears for children and gift certificates for teens (CDs) and adults (dinners)

▶ Flowers given out at each appointment or sent to patients for referral thank-yous

▶ Birthday greetings or cards for special occasions, such as new baby, anniversary, and graduation

▶ Bulletin board with patient pictures on it (for example, the good hygiene club)

▶ Map of the world with postcards from patients

▶ Special dental services coupons

▶ Bulletin board showing photos of patients flossing while on vacation and in different locations throughout the world

▶ Refrigerator magnets noting the dental office and phone number

Keep in mind that the goal of marketing is to attract new patients to the practice and retain the ones who are there. The positive attitude and professional approach in providing dental care to each patient is one of the most productive marketing approaches. Go that "extra mile" to make patients comfortable. Treat them with dignity every time they are in the office.

TELEPHONE TECHNIQUE

The telephone may be the first contact the patient has with the office, and it sets the stage for the kind of care the person can expect to receive. The first impression tends to be a lasting impression. Make sure that the tone of voice and the message substance is informational and welcoming to the caller. Handle the call in the same manner that would be done if meeting the patient face to face. Posture and the way the body is carried, along with attitude through facial expressions, are carried through the telephone lines to the patient. If the telephone is answered by an individual who is slumped over, leaving the diaphragm constricted, it may be interpreted on the other end as being tired or frustrated. Correct posture allows an individual to sound alert and more professional. Attitude is "heard" by the patients over the phone. Never forget that the patients who are calling are not an interruption of work but the reason for the job. Some reception areas have mirrors placed in front of the phone so that anyone answering can look at the expression on his or her face and be reminded of the importance of communicating a good attitude to the caller.

Answer the telephone in a manner that depicts pleasure that the individual called the office. Speak clearly and distinctly, identify the dental practice and yourself, and ask, "How can I help you?" Then, listen carefully. Personality and attitude sparkle through the telephone or come out flat and drab.

Basic Telephone Techniques

▶ No food or drink while on the telephone.

▶ Answer within two or three telephone rings.

▶ Smile because "the patient can hear your smile."

▶ Speak directly into the mouthpiece with it not more than one and one-half inches away.

▶ Use the same volume you would use if speaking to the person directly.

▶ **Enunciate**, speak clearly, and articulate carefully.

▶ Speak at a normal rate of speed.

▶ Pronounce the words correctly.

▶ Always use telephone **etiquette** (good manners).

▶ Get the caller's name and use it during the conversation.

▶ Listen carefully.

▶ Allow the caller to end the call.

Types of Calls

Several types of calls come into the dental office. They all should be handled in a professional manner. Some of the calls are more critical for patient care than others.

Answering Incoming Calls

A receptionist must be prepared to answer the incoming calls, at any time, while juggling the other responsibilities of the front desk. It is crucial that the caller feel that he or she has the total attention of the receptionist. Good listening and communication skills help portray an image of an organized, efficient, and courteous dental office. The receptionist must be able to listen carefully to the caller and make judgments after gathering information that will aid in the patient's care. It may be necessary to **screen** the calls in order to get the caller in touch with the right person to solve the problem. Patients may ask to speak to the dentist. The receptionist must first try to help, identify the patient's concern, and take a telephone number where the doctor can call back. Give the caller an idea of when to expect the call from the dentist. The dental receptionist must ensure that the dentist's time is managed efficiently. Most dentists prefer not to be interrupted at chairside while caring for another patient. With the infection control concerns, the chance of being inconsiderate to the current patient, and the delay in patient treatment and a day's schedule, it is important not to disrupt the dentist with a telephone call. Some dentists will take calls from another dentist, the dental laboratory technician needing an answer to further a case, and/or family members. Know your doctor's policies in regard to taking incoming phone calls. Handle the calls with tact by saying something such as, "The doctor is with a patient. Can I help you?"

Placing the Caller on Hold

If it becomes necessary to place the caller on hold and handle emergent situations or answer another phone line, ask the patient if he or she would mind holding for a minute and then listen to the answer. One of the rud-est ways to handle patients on the telephone is by asking, "Can you hold?," then, without waiting, push the hold button and cut the patient off.

The caller should never have to wait any longer than one minute on hold. If necessary, check in and ask whether the caller would like to continue to hold or whether it be more convenient to receive a call back. Handle on-hold calls in this manner and the patients will know that their time is being respected and their needs facilitated as soon as possible. Some offices have one-minute timers by the telephone to remind the receptionist of the person waiting and how long he or she has been on the other line. Do what is necessary to get back to the person on hold or that patient may be lost from the practice.

Taking Messages

When taking messages, be thorough. It is advisable to use standard telephone message pads with carbon so that the office can retain copies of all messages. Record and ask the caller the following information:

▶ Date and time the call was received

▶ Name and telephone number of the caller

▶ Who the message is for

▶ Message and urgency of the telephone call

▶ What action is required

▶ A good time to return the call

▶ The receptionist's initials or name in case the person receiving the messages has questions

After the message is written, repeat it to the caller to verify that it was written correctly. Give the caller an approximate time when to expect the return call to be placed.

Outgoing Calls

When telephone calls are made from the office, the same professional, positive approach should be followed. Be prepared and know the information that needs to be conveyed or sought. Most offices call the next day's patients to confirm their appointments. Doing this tedious task requires attention. More than one receptionist has called a patient to confirm the appointment and totally forgotten which individual was dialed. Use some type of indication system to keep track of which patients have been called. If calling an insurance company, have all the information, including the patient's chart and forms, handy so that any questions that come up can be answered readily.

If calling and leaving a message, take care with any information recorded on the answering machine. Remember that all health-care issues are confidential and should be discussed only with the patient. Try not to leave the information with small children, because the information can become confusing and get passed on to the adult inaccurately.

It is best if no personal telephone calls are made at the office. If the need arises, make them during the lunch hour, if possible. The telephone is for dental office business, and personal matters belong outside of employment.

Long-Distance Telephone Calls

Dental office assistants normally use direct-dialing telephone calling for long-distance calls. This means that the number is dialed directly into the telephone and not placed through the operator. Most of the long-distance calls are made to insurance carriers to verify patient coverage or to follow up on payments. It is important to be aware of the location of the call and plan ahead according to the time zone (Pacific, Mountain, Central, and Eastern) (Figure 29-2). Keep in mind that there is a three hour difference from one zone on the Pacific coast to the other time zone on the Atlantic coast.

English as a Second Language

 It is probable in the dental office to encounter many patients whose primary languages are not English. The dentist is responsible for providing an interpreter, if necessary, for communication. Some patients bring family members who speak English to translate. It is important that communication on the telephone and in the office be handled in a manner that provides the patient with the pertinent information. Things to remember when speaking to patients who have English as their second language are:

▶ Be patient.

▶ Speak at a normal volume. Raising the voice does not increase the other person's ability to understand the words.

▶ Speak more slowly, if necessary, and avoid complicated words.

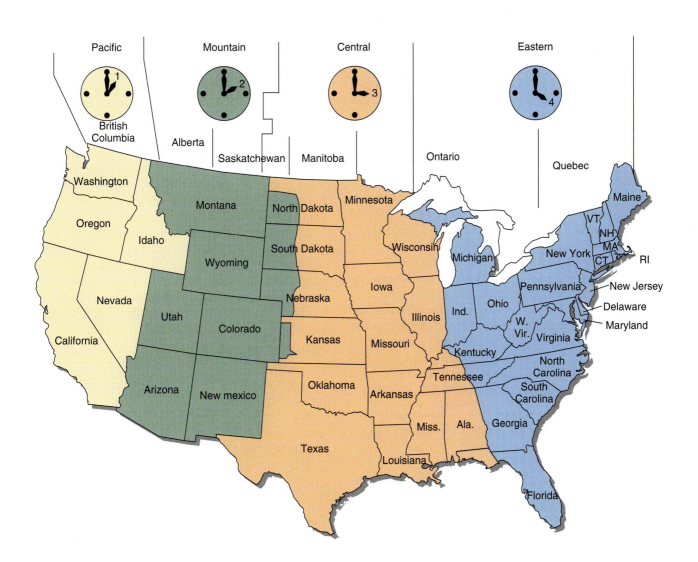

FIGURE 29-2 Pacific, Mountain, Central, and Eastern time zones.

▶ A patient who does not speak English may be able to understand English well. Do not assume that the patient does not comprehend what is being said.

▶ Ask the patient if clarification is needed.

▶ Repeat the information, if necessary, until understood.

Telephone and Business Office Technology

Most offices have telephones that are multi-functional. Normally, the telephones have a minimum of three lines and hold buttons. Spend time understanding the functions of the telephone so that if transfers are done, the patient is not lost. Spend time thoroughly learning the entire system. All the telephone calls become a great expense to the dental office. Do research into the best service available at the most economical price. Check the statements and identify the highest cost items, then contact the telephone services and tell them the office's needs. The services are happy to discuss the current packages available. The advances in telecommunications have a tremendous impact on dental office communication, so stay informed.

Answering Systems.
Dental offices need to provide a way for patients to contact them in the event of an emergency. Answering machines are commonplace today, and patients have grown to accept them. They are not replacements for a live person answering but can be utilized to give patients emergency telephone numbers and information. Many offices use answering systems that are turned on each evening when the dentist and staff leave for the day and during lunch hour, staff meetings, and seminars. These systems are checked promptly each morning for messages and turned off during the day.

It is the responsibility of the receptionist to record the message on the answering machine and check frequently for messages. With heavy usage, the taped message may become poor and difficult to understand. The receptionist should call it occasionally to check that the message being received by the patients is acceptable. The phone message reflects the dental office and, like all other aspects, it is important that the recording is clear and of good quality.

Answering Services.
Many offices have opted for answering services that are staffed by live operators. Having a person at the other end of the line is more reassuring to patients and other callers. These services also can provide flexibility in screening and routing calls. Most of the fees for the answering services are by the month or by the number of calls placed. This service is more expensive than that of an in-office answering machine.

Voice Mail.
If working at a large group practice, a voice-mail or automated routing unit may be used. This system answers the call, and a recorded voice identifies choices for the caller to pick by pressing a specific number on a touch-tone telephone. Some of the automated routing systems have mailboxes for the caller to leave a message for the person being called. All the messages are done by a recorded voice. Some patients who are not familiar with a system like this can become frustrated by it, especially elderly patients who may have more difficulty hearing the directions. Some offices provide information sheets to patients to clarify the telephone options available with this type of system.

Fax Machines.
Fax machines are becoming more common in the dental office. A **fax** is a facsimile transmission used to send and receive written messages through the telephone lines. It can contain typed or written data, pictures, and line art. It is important that it be sent to the correct address, taking care that confidential information be handled conscientiously. The fax is used to relay information to and from patients and insurance companies and to order dental supplies, among other things.

Electronic Mail (E-Mail).
Electronic mail (E-mail) is another form of communication done through the telephone lines via a computer. It is for sending, receiving, storing, and forwarding messages in digital form. It can be very convenient and saves time. A person can send a message to an electronic mailbox and the receiver reads it at a convenient time and responds, if necessary, by pushing the respond notation, typing the reply, and pushing send. Many of the new systems identify whether the person received and read the message that was sent. It is a great way to send inter-office memos to personnel in other areas. It also can be programmed to send the same message to a group of people.

It is possible to subscribe to on-line services that allow information to be transmitted around the world through the World Wide Web. These services also feature bulletin boards that are an electronic method of exchanging information publicly. Information regarding medical research and new treatment techniques can be found on the Internet.

Cellular Phones and Services.
Patients, dentists, and staff members may use cellular phones routinely for communication. The person who owns the cellular phone pays for the time the call takes, even if that individual did not place the call. Cellular phone usage is more expensive than using traditional telephone lines. If a patient gives a cell phone number to the office, verify that he or she does not mind receiving a call on that phone and be mindful to keep the messages brief and to the point.

Paging Systems.
Another telecommunication option available is a pager, or "beeper." Medical personnel have used the paging systems for years, and now they are available to individuals at a reasonable cost. The pagers are not as convenient as a cellular telephone,

because they are one-way communication systems. The pager does have several options available:

▶ A beep or vibration to notify the person to call one designated phone number

▶ Voice alert in which the person hears the message from the caller along with a number

▶ Digital message display in which the receiver scrolls it out and reads it

BUSINESS OFFICE SYSTEMS

Historically, the business office systems were manual, but today most of the offices have **computerized systems** (units of computer parts that function together to perform a particular task) of some sort. The office staff may choose to do only one or more aspects of the office business on a manual system. In today's fast-paced dental office, time and efficiency are important. The computer reduces the time involved in many routine office procedures. Once the dental assistant becomes familiar with the computer, its software, and its applications, he or she will find more and more uses for the computer. The responsibility of picking the correct **hardware** (computer physical equipment) and **software** (computer program or set of instructions that tells the hardware what to do) for the office may fall on the dental office manager or receptionist. Research the options available and know what is needed from the system. Talk to other office personnel about the systems they are using and the pros and cons of each system. Work with a trusted and knowledgeable vendor who understands the needs of the practice before purchasing a system.

After the research is completed, bring it to the staff members for their input. It is important that all the staff members be familiar with the system. It takes a great deal of time to convert all the information to the new system and staff training will be necessary, so it is best if everyone is involved in the process. Make sure the system that is purchased allows for expansion. Most dental offices purchase the microcomputers in the format of desktop **personal computers (PCs)** (Figure 29-3).

Common Software Applications in the Dental Office

A variety of software applications are available for use in the dental office. Choose the software that meets the office's needs. It should have general-purpose software that includes word processing, graphics, spreadsheets, database, and on-line communication programs.

Word Processing. Word processing has largely replaced typing. It allows the user to type memos, letters and reports and to make corrections easily. Word processing software allows for spelling checks, deletions,

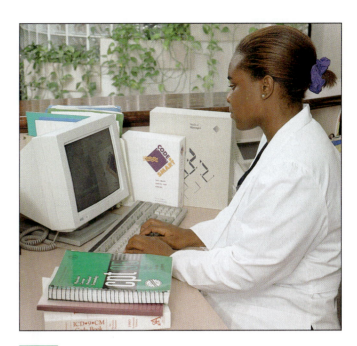

FIGURE 29-3 The traditional desktop personal computer comes in a variety of sizes and types.

cut and paste information, and much more. The documents can be stored for use at a later time and changed slightly for a different application. Typing a letter has been made much easier via the computer and word processing software.

Graphics. With the use of graphic software, numeric information can be transformed into graphs, pie charts, and bar graphs (Figures 29-4A through C). This allows the information to be summarized in a graphic format for easy visualization. Popular integrated packages of graphic software are Microsoft Works and Lotus Works. The dental software may allow usage with one of these possible systems.

Spreadsheets. Spreadsheets are the computerized format of the worksheets with calculations preprogrammed. Spreadsheets take numbers and electronically calculate the data to be analyzed. This calculation and recalculation that used to take hours is completed in seconds with spreadsheet software. Spreadsheets are used in the dental office to prepare monthly and yearly financial statements and accounts payable, along with other uses. The data from a spreadsheet can be converted to a graph or chart, therefore presenting information that can be interpreted at a glance.

Computer Database Management

To organize large quantities of related data into useful forms, computer database management software is used. The office can design the basic database that

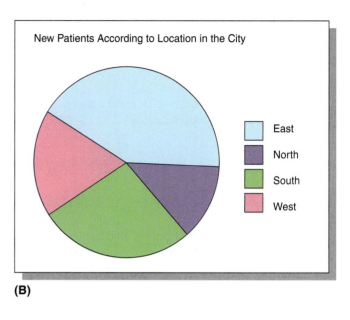

New Patients According to Location in the City

East

North

South

West

(B)

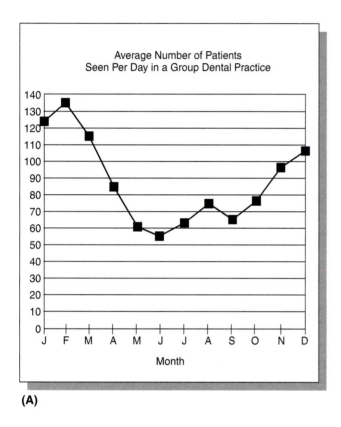

Average Number of Patients
Seen Per Day in a Group Dental Practice

Month

(A)

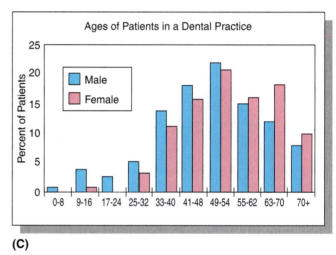

Ages of Patients in a Dental Practice

Male
Female

Percent of Patients

0-8 9-16 17-24 25-32 33-40 41-48 49-54 55-62 63-70 70+

(C)

FIGURE 29-4 Information can be presented in graphs and charts to make it easier to interpret. (A) Line graph. (B) Pie chart. (C) Bar graph.

would be beneficial to the practice. The general identifying information that is minimally required includes:

▶ Patient's name

▶ Spouse's name and/or other family members

▶ Patient's address

▶ Patient's home phone number

▶ Patient's work phone number

▶ Patient's insurance

Most office database systems have information about the patient and spouse, the patient's insurer, Social Security number, patient's date of birth, primary care physician, phone number, type of insurance, identification of the insurance carrier or carriers, place of employment,

and occupation. The patient's recall date can be placed in the computer with the other information.

Once the information is in the computer database, the information can be used with the word processor, graphs, or spreadsheets. This information can be grouped in a number of ways. For example, an office could identify all the patients who have birthdays in the current month and send birthday cards to them, or all the new patients could be identified so that welcome letters could go out to them. A large number of applications are beneficial to the dental practices both in marketing and collecting data.

Computer Safety

Use computer virus protection to protect the office system if there is any chance that the office downloads information from the internet or accepts files from other computer systems. Everything could be lost if unprotected. Most offices download the files daily to make sure that a backup document is available if the system "crashes." Even if the possibility of loosing the data is remote, it takes a great deal of time to reconstruct the system if this happens. Always have a backup document or file or disk.

Computer Ergonomics and Eye Care. For those individuals who spend a great deal of time on the computer, it is important to practice recommended computer **ergonomics** (human factors that affect the design and operation of tools and the work environment). For instance, posture is critical in preventing injury. A recommended sitting posture for computer users was developed by Gary Karp, Ergonomics Consultant of Onsight Technology Education Services of San Francisco, California (Figure 29-5).

Other recommended aids include the ergonomic keyboard, which allows the wrists to remain in a flat posi-

tion. A wrist rest for the mouse is used to keep the wrist in the level position. Screen glare protectors are utilized to deflect and reduce monitor glare. Eye care professionals advise that, for every hour of computer use, the user should relax the eyes by looking at a distance for ten minutes to reduce eye fatigue.

PATIENT SCHEDULING

Effective patient scheduling is the key to any dental office. Maintaining a smooth patient flow throughout the day determines the success and profitability of the dentist and the practice. Scheduling may seem to be a mundane task, but in reality it takes an organized person with good interpersonal and communication skills to schedule properly. If this task is done well, this job can be very challenging and satisfying. In this position, the receptionist acts as coordinator to help all the team members work together, keep their timing perfect, and reach goals. One of the first steps in the process is to

• Top of monitor just below eye level. This supports keeping the head over the shoulders. Comfortable viewing is generally 5 to 30° below horizontal. Place in front of the body to prevent sitting in a twisted posture or turning the head.

• Head over the shoulders to allow the skeleton to carry the weight of the head, relieving overuse of neck, shoulder, and back muscles.

• Monitor distance so that chin does not jut forward while the trunk is against the chair back.

• Seat back should support lower (lumbar) spine. High seat backs are recommended torelieve spinal pressures. A backward angle is preferred to allow the chair to take some pressure off the spine. Allow the chair to carry a share of the body weight.

• Keyboard should allow for relaxed shoulders, flat wrists, and at least 90° at the inside of elbow. Sit directly in front, close enough not to have to reach forward. Rest palms on rest only when fingers can remain relaxed.

• Armrests, if used, should be soft and wide. There should be no contact during keying. Close enough to not force extension of elbow and low enough for shoulder to be relaxed without slumping or leaning.

• Thighs level with or just above knees to promote a neutral spine.

• Feet in firm contact with the floor to distribute load through the whole body. Use a footrest only if necessary. Leave space under desk free of any obstruction to legs.

• Seat pan not so deep that comfortable contact with chair back is prevented. Contact behind the knees must be avoided. Optimal contact with thighs provides greatest degree of effortless support.

FIGURE 29-5 Recommended computer operator position. (*Courtesy of Gary Karp, Ergonomics Consultant, Onsight Technology Education Services, San Francisco, CA.*)

acquire the proper materials for scheduling effectively. Analyze the needs of the practice and plan accordingly. Understand that the needs may change and adjustments will have to be made.

Appointment Books

Appointment books are available in several options. To choose the correct one for the office situation, evaluate the qualities of each. Manual appointment books come in ringed or bound copies. The ringed appointment book allows for the addition or deletion of additional pages. It lays open and flat on the counter during use. A bound appointment book needs to be replaced when the current one is filled. This leaves a time frame in which two books are utilized, making it more difficult for the scheduling to be completed.

Another consideration is the number of appointment columns required. This is dependent on the unique needs of the physical facilities and the staff. Solo practitioners have two or three columns for scheduling patients. Larger practices need six or more columns if multiple dentists practice together. Some practices have a separate column for each expanded-duty dental assistant or dental hygienist. Dental practices also may have separate appointment books for the dental hygienist's patient schedule.

Appointment book pages may have day headings printed in them. The blank headings can be filled in by the receptionist so only the days worked are used in the appointment book and a minimum number of pages are wasted. Some appointment books have the days of the week across the top of the schedule and the correct day can be circled or underlined. Identify the appointment book that works the best for the practice.

Many of the appointment books are set up so that the pages show a week at a glance. The days not worked can be crossed out, still allowing the user to see the entire week at one time.

The time intervals in an appointment book are normally ten- or fifteen-minute intervals and are described as units of time (Figure 29-6A). There are six units in an hour if using the ten-minute intervals and four units in an hour if using the fifteen-minute intervals. Most dental offices use the ten-minute unit because it allows for more effective patient scheduling. The treatment procedures are broken down into units, and the doctor may request five units for a crown preparation. This equals fifty minutes of time in the appointment book.

Receptionists who are advanced and production conscious can color code the scheduling of appointments. The appointment book indicates whether the dentist or expanded-duty dental assistant is performing treatment for the patient. For example, if using the crown preparation appointment, the schedule would reflect that the first five minutes of the fifty minute allotted time are for the dental assistant to set up and take the preliminary impressions; the next thirty minutes are

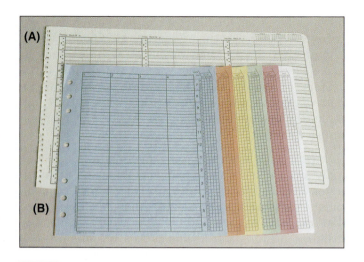

FIGURE 29-6 (A) Appointment book pages showing fifteen-minute units for patient scheduling. (B) Color-coded appointment book for efficient use of the dentist's and dental assistant's time. Both allow for a week at a glance.

for the dentist to anesthetize the patient, prepare the tooth for the crown preparation, and take the final impression; the final fifteen minutes are for the dental assistant to make the temporary (provisional) restoration and dismiss the patient. Therefore, the dentist's time can be scheduled for other patient care after the initial thirty-five minutes with the crown preparation patient. This method is utilized in a practice in which patients can be attended to by other staff members. This approach, called **double booking**, utilizes the dentist's time in the most productive manner. If patients are waiting for the staff or the dentist to attend to them, then the double-booking approach is not working effectively. Double booking can be done in a manual appointment book or on the computer.

Appointment Book Matrix. After the appointment book is selected with the appropriate days, columns, and units, the receptionist can begin establishing the appointment book matrix. This is where the whole year (if possible) can be mapped out to avoid scheduling patients when the dentist has other commitments or when the office is closed. It is advisable to use pencil, because even the best laid out plans may change. First, mark an X through the days when the office is closed. Identify all the continuing education seminars and meetings that the dentist and staff will be attending, along with the holidays when the office is closed.

In many offices, specific periods of time are set aside for emergencies. This time is referred to as buffer time. Each dental office identifies which time is best for buffer time. The most common buffer time is late morning, right before lunch, and late afternoon, right before closing. Buffer time is not previously scheduled but is reserved for emergency patients only.

Lunch time is marked out in the appointment book with an X or a diagonal line. The columns are identified for operatories or for specific dental team members, such as the dental hygienist. Color coding can be used in defining the appointment book matrix (Figure 29-6B).

When scheduling the dental appointments for patients, it is important to know the specific time intervals needed between appointments. For instance, after a crown is prepared and a provisional is placed, the dental laboratory needs time to process the case and return the finished product to the dental office before the next appointment. This interim time may be from two to seven days. Each dental laboratory varies in the amount of time needed to process the case. Whatever the time required by the laboratory, allow a couple of additional days to ensure that the case is complete prior to the patient's appointment. At times, multiple appointments are required in a series. The receptionist may have to consider healing time as well as laboratory production time when scheduling the advanced appointments.

Special Patient Appointment Times. All practices have patients who require special scheduling of appointment times due to health concerns, age, or just nervousness. If young children are to be scheduled for dental appointments, it is best to care for them in the morning or after nap times. Treating a child prior to nap time when he or she is cranky and unhappy may make it difficult for everyone. Children of school age normally require appointments after school or during vacation days. Call the local schools to become aware of the academic calendar year so the appointment book can be scheduled according to the children's needs.

Elderly patients should be scheduled at a time when they are not fatigued or tired. They may have concerns about transportation, bus routes, and the weather. Arrange times for their appointments that are convenient for them. Morning appointments often work well.

It is well documented that patients who are extremely anxious about dentistry have a greater cancellation rate for their appointments. If a patient expresses fear, the assistant can reassure him or her and make a notation for the receptionist. This alerts the receptionist that a short, easy appointment should be scheduled the first time to build the patient's confidence and lessen the risk of cancellation. Calls may be made prior to the appointment to confirm the time, and follow-up calls may be made after the appointment to ensure that everything went well for the patient.

Health concerns impact patient appointment scheduling. If a patient has diabetes or hypoglycemia, schedule the patient after a mealtime. Confirm that the patient has eaten and verify that the diabetes patient has taken the needed medication. A patient with heart problems may require shorter appointments so that the patient does not become overfatigued.

Other Scheduling Concerns. Discuss the appointment book scheduling with the dentist and the staff. The dentist may have the highest energy level in the morning. Scheduling a difficult, tedious treatment at the

end of the day may be overtaxing. Also, scheduling the same procedure repeatedly may make it difficult on the dental team members. Staggering the types of treatment allows the dental team to be prepared for the procedures and makes the day go smoother and faster. Also, scheduling the same procedure several times in a row may make it difficult to accomplish the sterilization procedures when only a limited number of specific instruments are available for the specific procedure. During staff meetings, talk over appointment scheduling that works well and define the best approach policy.

Computer Scheduling

When using computer scheduling, the program searches through the database for open appointment time frames. After finding a time and date that are convenient for the patient, the data is keyed into the computer schedule and the appointment is automatically scheduled. Software programs are available to develop any matrix the practice desires for any specific database. The scheduling can be designed to highlight open appointment times with very few directions.

Appointment Book Entries

When making appointment book entries using the manual system, it is important to write in pencil. First, establish an appointment time with the patient, noting any special considerations, such as laboratory work that might affect the appointment. Record the entry in the schedule. The entry should include the patient's name, phone number, procedure to be completed (abbreviated), length of procedure identified by an arrow, and age, if the patient is a child. Write out the information on an appointment card for the patient, including the day, date, and time (Figure 29-7). Clearly repeat the

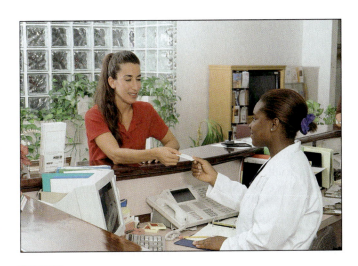

FIGURE 29-7 Patients are given appointment cards that have the next appointment and any preoperative instructions neatly printed on them.

information to the patient as the card is given to him or her, to verify it once again.

The receptionist must know the time units for each procedure in order to schedule patient treatment times. The more productive treatment procedures are called primary procedures. They tend to be the longer appointments dealing with crown and bridge preparations, amalgam and composite fillings, surgery, and endodontic treatment. With the increased time spent placing and removing barriers and sterilization, it is much more productive to take care of several teeth at the same appointment. Around the primary procedures, the dental receptionist can schedule a dovetail or conjunctive procedure that does not require the same concentrated attention by the dentist. These conjunctive procedures include routine examinations, consultations, or denture adjustments.

The receptionist's goal is to fill the appointment book with patient care so that the scheduling problems such as down time, overtime, and overlap time are nonexistent for the dentist and dental assistants.

▶ **Down time** is time in the appointment book that is not scheduled. If an appointment time using ten-minute units is open from 2:00 to 2:30, it is referred to as three units of down time.

▶ **Overtime** is where the patient treatment time went beyond the estimated time frame. This can affect the entire schedule. It can cause other patients to wait for their appointments, therefore making them unhappy.

▶ **Overlap of time** occurs when the dentist or dental assistant is required to be in two places at the same time or when two patients need to be seated in the same operatory at the same time.

All three of the scheduling problems occur, and care should be taken to eliminate them. Careful estimation of accurate time units reduces or eliminates some of these problems. If this is an ongoing concern, scheduling adjustments should be made accordingly. The office team should meet and discuss ideas to eliminate scheduling problems.

Recall Patients

Established dental offices consider the recall system the backbone of the dental practice. A recall system ensures that patients return for continued care and maintenance of their dental needs. Bringing patients back into the office at regular intervals allows the dentist to assess their teeth and tissues and keep them in optimum condition. This preventive measure prevents serious discomfort for the patient. During the continued-care appointment (recall appointment), the dental team reinforces oral hygiene techniques and educates the patient concerning any new dentifrices or other dental aids on the market that will aid the patient in overall oral care. Questions may arise about bleaching techniques, types of toothbrushes, and mouth rinses. It also allows the dentist to assess any other pathological concerns at an early stage.

Computer Recall. Recalling patients for their ongoing care can be accomplished with a number of methods. With the increase of computer use in the dental offices, most current recall is done from a computer-generated printout. Information is placed in the computer after the regular appointment is completed. The program allows a date for the recall or continued-care appointment to be indicated. At the end of the month, an alphabetical list of patients needing recall the following month, along with their addresses and phone numbers, can be generated. This list can be used to contact the patients by telephone or though the mail. The patients who schedule appointments can be removed from the list, while the others stay on the printout automatically.

Advanced Appointment Scheduling. The appointment book allows for advanced scheduling of continued-care appointments immediately after regular dental care is complete. This allows an appointment to be scheduled for the patient six months to a year in advance. The appointment book in this system is used as the primary listing. The patients need to reaffirm their appointments two weeks in advance as well as the day prior. The advantage to this system is that the task is completed immediately for the patient as well as the dental office. The disadvantage of this system is obvious: The patient does not always know what will be happening in his or her life that far in advance and may need to cancel or reschedule the appointment.

Chronological Card File. A minimum amount of time is invested in the chronological card file system. In this system, the patient fills out a postcard so that the next recall date will be mailed directly to him or her. The cards are filed according to the month the patient is to be recalled. The card is mailed to the patient two weeks before the given recall date. If this system is used alone, the card is sent to the patient and then all references for the patient recall are lost, unless someone goes through all the charts and makes a list of patients needing recall appointments. It is better to make a list and note the patients who do not schedule appointments and follow up with telephone calls to schedule the appointment.

Color Tagged Card File. Another type of recall system is the color-tagged card file. In this system, every patient has an index card with name, address, telephone number, and any other special notations printed on it. The cards are filed alphabetically, and a colored tag is clipped to each card indicating in which month the patient requires a recall appointment. For example, a yellow tag is clipped to a card if the patient needs a recall appointment in January. The tagged file cards are reviewed each month, and calls are made to schedule the patients needing continued care. If they do not schedule, they can be moved up to the next month or later, if requested. After the patient is scheduled, the card is attached to the chart and updated at the time of the patient's appointment. A new color-coded tag is then attached to the card and filed in the index system. The advantage of this system is that the cards are available with information on them about prior appointments. The disadvantages are the time it takes to complete a card for each patient and the possibility of the tag falling off.

Regardless of which system is used, the goal is to make sure that every patient in the dental office is either under regular treatment or on a recall system.

DENTAL RECORDS MANAGEMENT

Accurate dental records management is essential for quality patient care at any dental office. It is also necessary because of the legal issues that every dental office must face today. The records must be filled out completely, reflecting all pertinent information.

Equipment and Supplies Needed for Record Management

The dentist decides on the type of **file folder** to use in the office, normally with the advisement of the receptionist and staff. File folders are designed in many different ways to meet office needs. They should provide easy accessibility and yet enclose the information and protect it during storing. A patient folder may be like an envelope or have a book-type opening. The envelope folder may have preprinted data on the outside and all the information sheets, x-rays, and so on placed inside. The book type normally keeps the patient information in constant order. The book type normally is more costly because it requires added pockets and fasteners to hold the information sheets secure.

File cabinets are also available in several primary types, such as vertical, open-shelf lateral, and movable. The vertical file cabinet is widely used in home filing (Figure 29-8A). The files are retrieved by lifting the appropriate file upward and outward. The open-shelf file cabinets seem to be the most widely used in the dental office, normally with a color-coding system that allows for easy chart identification (Figure 29-8B). The records from the open-shelf lateral files are retrieved by pulling them out laterally from the shelf. Some large offices may have the movable file units that are powered electrically or physically by easy handles. Patient names are typed on the labels and attached to the file for quick identification.

Patient Chart Filing

Make sure that the filing system used is organized alphabetically. Most systems index the individual

(A)

(B)

FIGURE 29-8 (A) Vertical file cabinet. *(Courtesy HON® Company)*. (B) Open-shelf lateral file cabinet.

names. The patient name is divided into three units: the last name, first name, and middle name or initial. File all the charts according to the last name; if two patients have the same last name, such as Smith, then use the first name. Therefore, if the office has a John Smith and a Jim Smith, Jim is filed before John in the file cabinet. Occasionally, two patients with the same first and last names become patients. Use their middle names or initials to file properly. Alphabetical filing requires accuracy during the removal and replacement of the chart. These tasks must be done correctly or a lot of time can be wasted trying to find the chart.

Most dental offices use some form of color coding in regards to their patient filing (Figure 29-9). The file

FIGURE 29-9 Patient files color coded. Yellow file selected for "Carl," "F" side tab selected for "Friend." *(Courtesy of KARDEX System, Inc., Marietta, OH)*

folder may be color coded so that all the patients with a last name beginning in A or S have yellow charts and all the patients with B or T have blue charts. Following this system reduces the lost charts because they will stand out if not in the proper color section. Other charts may have colored tabs that are placed on either plain or colored charts to make the filing and retrieval of files more efficient. The larger the practice, the more tabs required to break down the total charts into small groupings. However, this makes filing easier and reduces the number of errors that may occur, because any visible color differences are quickly identified.

Tickler File. A well-organized office has a **tickler file** that serves as a reminder of any action that needs to be taken in the future. Most offices use sticky notes (reminder notes that have adhesive strips on one side) to remind office personnel of things that need to be taken care of immediately. A tickler file normally is index cards in an index box with approximate dates in which to complete the task (Figure 29-10). Many of the computer software programs have tickler files available so that the information can be stored and retrieved when necessary.

Record Confidentiality

The patient has the right to confidential treatment and records. The clinical record contains private information that must be kept confidential within the dental office. With the usage of computers and fax machines, great care must be used when placing anything on-line where others can access it. When sending a fax, attach a cover sheet that advises the receiver of the confidential nature of the material, and make sure that the fax machine that is receiving the material is located in an area where only the appropriate individuals can access it.

FIGURE 29-10 Tickler file for daily review and follow-up actions in patient management.

Archival Storage. Most dentists keep records for the entirety of their careers. This creates a storage concern for the practice. There is a process similar to microfiche and microfilm by which the records are copied with a laser beam and compressed onto an optical disc. These small discs can store a great deal of information, and this information can be easily retrieved and viewed, if needed.

Daily Schedule

The daily schedule is a form developed directly from the information in the appointment book for that day (Figure 29-11). It shows the time each patient is scheduled and the treatment that is to be provided. Normally, several daily schedules are generated so that one can be placed in each operatory and one in the sterilization area. This schedule allows the clinical staff to plan ahead and set up for the upcoming patients. Any changes throughout the day are changed on each daily schedule. If a computer monitor is in each operatory, the daily schedule can be available through the network and changed more readily from the main computer at the front desk.

ACCOUNTS RECEIVABLE

The primary concern of the dental office is patient care, but without sound financial management, the office will not thrive and the patients will ultimately suffer.

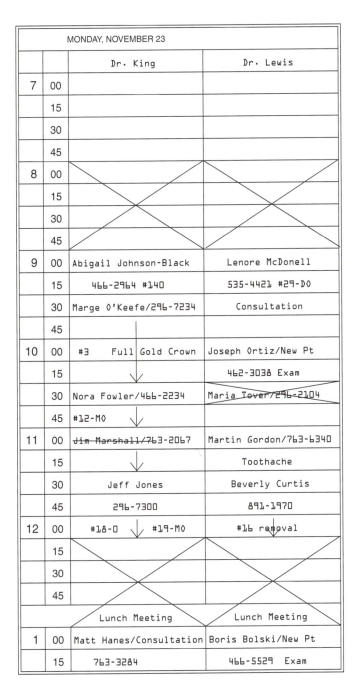

FIGURE 29-11 Computer-generated daily patient schedule.

for any theft. Insurance fraud also brings with it prosecution and possible imprisonment.

Patient Fees

In the dental office, a fee schedule is used to define what patients are charged for each service. It is referred to as the **usual, reasonable, and customary fee**. The usual fee refers to the fee typically charged by the dentist for a specific procedure. The reasonable fee is the midrange of fees charged for this same procedure; therefore, if it is a difficult case, then the usual fee may be raised to reflect the difficulty of the case. The customary fee is the average up to the 90th percent that the dentists in the area charge for the same procedure. The impact that the fee schedule has on the dental practice is that if a dentist feels that he or she would like to charge a greater amount for one service, the insurance companies will not pay above the usual, reasonable, and customary fee schedule. The patient will be billed for the overage. Patients may question the additional charge and become upset with the practice if this has not been discussed previously in the treatment plan or at the consultation appointment. Most dentists stay within the fee range. This range can be adjusted yearly, raising by 5 percent, by area dentists, but seldom does it raise that much.

The dentists have the right to adjust the fees by means of a **professional courtesy**. This professional courtesy, a discounted amount, may be offered to other dentists for dental work or to employees, family, and friends. The dentist has the discretion to make any adjustments desired. Another area in which dentists may make adjustments is insurance. Dentists who accept assignments in specific programs agree to accept a payment in full by the provider. For instance, a patient is covered on a program and the dentist does a restoration on this patient for a fee of $75. The provider only pays $55 for this particular service. The dentist has to adjust, or "waive," the remaining $20 of the fee and the patient will not be responsible for it.

Dental team members must be aware that the practice cannot survive if constant adjustments to the fees are made. Production must be balanced by other cases that meet the regular fee schedule to maintain a viable practice.

MANAGEMENT OF PATIENT ACCOUNTS

Patient accounts can be managed either through a computerized bookkeeping system or a manual system, such as the pegboard system. Many dental offices have converted the manual bookkeeping system to the computer system because it offers great versatility and reduces the need to record entries more than once. Changing from the manual system is, initially, time consuming until all the data is entered into the computer.

With the high cost of materials and equipment, profit management is critical. The accounts receivable of the dental office encompasses the money owed to the practice. The bookkeeping in this area must be accurate and carries with it a great responsibility. This position may be occupied by the receptionist or the business assistant. Like the information on the patient's records, the financial information must remain confidential. All transactions, payments, adjustments, and charges must be handled in a safe and professional manner. Any employee engaging in unlawful activities may be prosecuted under the law and required to repay the employer

29-1 Preparing for the Day's Patients

This procedure is performed by the receptionist in preparation for the upcoming day.

EQUIPMENT

▶ File

▶ Patient charts

▶ Computer with word processor

▶ Telephone

The Day Prior

1. The dental receptionist pulls the charts for the patients for the next day.

2. All the patient appointments are confirmed with telephone calls.

3. The records are reviewed for any special concerns.

4. Patient account balances are reviewed and notations are made on the chart.

5. The needed laboratory work is checked to ensure that it is ready.

6. Any premedications are identified and noted.

7. A daily schedule is typed and the appropriate number of copies are made.

8. The daily schedule is posted in the appropriate areas after the current schedule is completed for the day.

The Day of the Appointment

1. The office staff meet in the morning to look over the daily schedule. This brief meeting (five minutes or fewer) allows the staff to dialogue any treatment or patient concerns that may transpire during the day.

2. The charts are ready for the dental assistants as they seat the patients.

3. The patients are greeted and seated in the dental treatment rooms by the dental team.

Pegboard System of Account Management

The pegboard system (Figure 29-12) is designed as a "write it once" system that uses no-carbon-required (NCR) paper, permitting the user to enter the data only once. The system consists of day sheets, charge slips, ledger cards, and receipt forms (Figure 29-13). The forms are designed to work together and are aligned on a pegboard with matching columns. The system is relatively inexpensive. Several companies have developed similar systems but their forms are incompatible. Therefore, it is important to use the forms from one company.

Day Sheets. The day sheets record each charge, payment, and adjustment for the day. All the transactions must be written legibly and accurately in order to maintain accurate records. The day sheets consist of five sections: the first three are for posting and the last two are for balancing (Figure 29-12).

▶ **Section 1** is where the patient transactions are posted. All charges, credits, and previous and current account balances are noted.

▶ **Section 2** is where all the deposits for the day are listed and transferred from section 1. This list includes the cash and check payments. Some companies have detachable portions or carbon overlays for use as deposit slips from this area.

▶ **Section 3** is where individual production can be recorded.

▶ **Section 4** is where all the daily transactions are totaled and balanced. For example, the total of D is added to the total of A and the total of B1 and B2 are subtracted to equal the total of column C. What this means is that the previous balance is added to the charges and then the credits are subtracted to equal the new balance.

▶ **Section 5** is where the total cumulative accounts receivable is balanced. This is the amount that all patients owe the practice.

End-of-Month Balancing. When the last day sheet of the month is complete, there will be a total accounts receivable balance noted on it. The patient ledger cards (one ledger per family) need to be totaled (using the amount owed to the practice) to compare with the one on the last day sheet. These totals should be exactly equal; if they are not, the mistake must be traced down before it grows into a major problem. The most likely error is that a ledger card is misplaced. The patients are billed from the ledger cards, so this error needs to be rectified.

Computer System of Account Management

Patients ledgers that are computerized contain all the information about each patient, including name, address, telephone number, insurance coverage, and person responsible for the account. The ledger also has the office visits and the services provided and procedure codes. Each time the patient is in the office, the information about the service is entered from the charge slips. The computer automatically updates the ledger, posts the charges, and calculates the balance and the practice accounts receivable balance.

The patient account can be viewed on the computer monitor or printed out if the patient desires a copy (Figure 29-14). Specialized information such as missed appointments or family discounts may be programmed into the computer.

Monthly Billing

Every patient owing the practice is billed monthly. If using the pegboard system, the ledger cards are copied and sent out for payment. The computer generates monthly bills from the ledgers on the database with an age analysis of the balance (Figure 29-15). Many offices include return envelopes to aid the patients in sending in payment. The patient statements are requests for payment and ask for the balance to be paid in full. Dental office may charge a finance charge for balances that are not paid within the first thirty days after treatment.

Payment Options. At the time of treatment, the business assistant may set up financial arrangements. Often, an initial down payment is requested. The balance is then divided and this fixed amount is paid over an arranged time frame. For instance, a patient may have $1,000 worth of dentistry to complete. The office may request that 20 percent be paid as a down payment and the other $800 dollars be paid in $100 increments over the next eight months. The date that the payment is due is determined together. The patient signs the determined payment plan along with the office personnel or dentist. The patient is given one copy of the payment plan and the original is kept in the patient's record. This information may also be noted on the ledger, to remind the patient of the arrangements when the statement is sent out.

FIGURE 29-12 Pegboard system, shown with section 1, the record of charges and receipts; section 2, the record of deposits; section 3, business analysis summaries; section 4, daily and monthly totals; and section 5, proof of posting, and the accounts receivable control.

P R O C E D U R E

29-2 Day Sheet Preparation for Posting

The dental receptionist or office business assistant performs this task and prepares the day sheet prior to the first patient arriving.

EQUIPMENT

▶ Pegboard

▶ New day sheet

▶ Block of new charge slips and receipt forms

▶ Ledger cards for all the patients scheduled that day (or ledger card file)

PROCEDURE STEPS

1. Place the day sheet on the pegboard.
2. Attach the charge and receipt slips on the first corresponding line (Figure 29-13).
3. At the top of the day sheet, fill in the date and the page number.
4. Transfer information from the previous page and fill in the previous day's totals from columns A through D and write in place at the bottom of the day sheet under "previous page."

5. Prepare ledger cards for the patients scheduled that day by pulling or tabbing them or have the storage file close by.

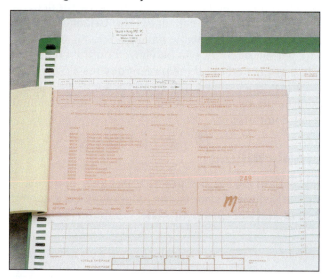

FIGURE 29-13 The pegboard accounting system with the day sheet, ledger card, and charge slip in place.

Financial Information

When a patient calls for an appointment, it is beneficial to gather all the information in regard to dental insurance. When the patient comes in, be sure to get a copy of his or her insurance identification and have the patient complete and sign the patient portion of the insurance form. With this information, the business assistant can gather information concerning the patient's dental coverage. Insurance coverage can have yearly limits and may have restrictions for specific services. By having knowledge about the most commonly used insurances, the business assistant can help the patients with making decisions concerning dental treatment.

Credit Reports. It may be necessary to obtain credit reports on patients who have large financial responsibilities for dental treatment. Essentially, the dental practice is loaning the patient the money to pay for this treatment. There are lab fees and overhead that must be paid, and the patient is requesting to be trusted to pay at a later date. Consumer credit reporting agencies provide financial profiles on individuals and verify whether they meet their obligations or are slow to meet their obligations through a rating system. The patient is to be informed prior to requesting a credit report. The

patient's Social Security number and birth date may be necessary to obtain the pertinent information. Any bankruptcies and lawsuits are identified on the credit report. After the report is received, the dentist or business assistant can determine whether the patient can pay in installments for dental treatment.

Dental Insurance

Dental insurance represents a large portion of the accounts receivable in most dental practices. By preparing the insurance forms accurately and submitting them in a timely fashion, payments come quickly to the dental office. Dental insurance seldom covers the entire fee, and the patient is responsible for the balance.

The individual who has dental insurance through employment is referred to as the **subscriber**. The patient who is entitled to benefits under any dental plan is referred to as the **beneficiary**. Some patients have dental insurance through their employment for themselves and have other coverage through their spouses. They would then be the subscribers for their primary insurance and the beneficiaries for the other dental insurance. This person is said to have dual coverage and may not have to pay for any additional

P R O C E D U R E

29-3 Posting Charges and Payments on the Pegboard

The dental receptionist or office business assistant performs this task during or at the end of each day.

EQUIPMENT

▶ Pegboard

▶ New day sheet

▶ Block of new charge slips and receipt forms

▶ Ledger cards for all the patients scheduled that day (or ledger card file placed close by)

PROCEDURE STEPS

When the Patient Enters the Dental Office for a Scheduled Appointment

1. Place the patient's ledger under the next charge sheet and on the corresponding line on the pegboard.

2. Write in the date, responsible party's name, the patient's name, and the previous balance, if any, in the spaces provided for each on the charge and receipt sheet. The information will automatically copy onto the ledger card and the pegboard day sheet.

3. Remove the charge sheet from the pegboard and clip it to the outside of the patient's chart. The chart is then ready for the dental assistant and the dentist to use during treatment.

4. The dentist or dental assistant completes the chart and the charge sheet prior to dismissing the patient. The chart is given to the patient to take to the reception area or is brought to the reception area by the dental assistant while dismissing the patient.

After the Patient Is Dismissed and Returned to the Reception Area

1. Replace the charge slip on the pegboard, align it with the patient's name, and insert the patient's ledger card back into place under the charge slip on the pegboard. Enter the charges and payments in the designated spaces in section 1 (Figure 29-12).

2. The final balance for the patient is totaled by adding the previous balance with the new charges and subtracting any payment the patient has made. Place the final charge in column C. Note that column D is the previous balance, column A is charges, column B1 is payments, and column B2 is adjustments. The proof of posting at the bottom on the day sheet indicates the procedure to be used for each entry as well as the entire day sheet.

Column D total + Column A total =

Subtotal – (Column B1 + B2) = Column C

3. When posting is completed, the first copy of the charge slip is filed in the patient's chart and the second copy is given to the patient for the purpose of payment and the patient's records. The final copy is used for submission for insurance expenses for dental treatment. If two coverages are used, the primary pays the normal fees and the secondary covers up to the amount owed. Together they pay the entire bill. Children are normally covered under dental insurance until they are of age eighteen or until they complete their full-time education. They are referred to as dependents under the dental insurance carrier. The carrier is the dental insurance company that pays the agreed benefits for the patient treatment. Patients who have benefits are normally given benefit booklets that state the coverage that the patients are eligible for. The coverage normally is negotiated with the employer for the employees. Limitations for benefits may be noted in the booklets along with the benefit plan.

Many of the insurance plans have an identified deductible amount. This means that a specified amount is deducted from the benefit amount before any benefits are paid. For example, if the policy has a $100 deductible each year, the individual must pay this amount before becoming eligible for payment of any benefits.

Some insurance plans have maximum amounts that can be paid out for the year. This means that no matter what the dental treatment is, the plan will not pay over a specified amount. So, if an insurance plan pays a

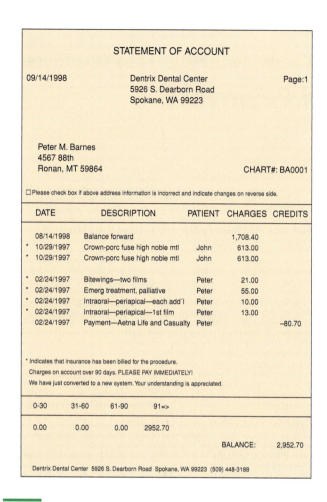

STATEMENT OF ACCOUNT

09/14/1998   Dentrix Dental Center   Page:1
                   5926 S. Dearborn Road
                   Spokane, WA 99223

Peter M. Barnes
4567 88th
Ronan, MT 59864   CHART#: BA0001

☐ Please check box if above address information is incorrect and indicate changes on reverse side.

DATE	DESCRIPTION	PATIENT	CHARGES	CREDITS
08/14/1998	Balance forward		1,708.40	
* 10/29/1997	Crown-porc fuse high noble mtl	John	613.00	
* 10/29/1997	Crown-porc fuse high noble mtl	John	613.00	
* 02/24/1997	Bitewings—two films	Peter	21.00	
* 02/24/1997	Emerg treatment, palliative	Peter	55.00	
* 02/24/1997	Intraoral—periapical—each add'l	Peter	10.00	
* 02/24/1997	Intraoral—periapical—1st film	Peter	13.00	
02/24/1997	Payment—Aetna Life and Casualty	Peter		−80.70

* Indicates that insurance has been billed for the procedure.
Charges on account over 90 days. PLEASE PAY IMMEDIATELY!
We have just converted to a new system. Your understanding is appreciated.

0-30	31-60	61-90	91=>
0.00	0.00	0.00	2952.70

BALANCE: 2,952.70

Dentrix Dental Center 5926 S. Dearborn Road Spokane, WA 99223 (509) 448-3188

FIGURE 29-14 Computer-generated dental patient account showing services rendered and insurance and patient payments. *(Courtesy of Dentrix Dental Systems, Inc. ©1989-1999)*

maximum annual amount of $2,000 per year and a patient has ten crowns costing $400 each, the insurance will only pay $2,000 of the bill. The patient would be responsible for the remaining $2,000 balance. So, for this patient, it would be beneficial to have five crowns completed each year for two years in order to utilize maximum benefits from the dental insurance.

If the dental coverage is difficult to determine, send the planned treatment to the insurance company to get a predetermination of benefits. This predetermination is often referred to as a pretreatment estimate. The insurance carrier may request dental radiographs before the predetermination can be made. After receiving the predetermination, both the dentist and the patient will know the *exact* amount of benefits available toward the cost of the entire dental treatment.

Submitting Dental Insurance Claims

As a courtesy to patients, most dental offices submit the insurance claims. The entire claim must be filled out. The patient fills in the patient and subscriber information and the dental office fills in the dentist's identification and the description of services. The American Dental Association developed a **Code on Dental Procedures and Nomenclature** to simplify the reporting of the confidential information regarding the patient's dental treatment. It is advisable for the patient to sign the area regarding assignment of benefits, as well as the area permitting payment from the insurance company directly to the dentist who provided the service. If this area is not signed, the dental office assumes that the patient is responsible for the entire fee. The business assistant must pay attention to and have the patients sign both areas in order to protect the practice.

L&K **LEWIS & KING, DDS**
     2501 CENTER STREET
     NORTHBOROUGH, OH 12345

STATEMENT DATE	08/29/--
PATIENT NUMBER	113
PREVIOUS BALANCE	$0.00

OFFICE PHONE: (404) 555-0078

DATE	CODE	DESCRIPTION	AMOUNT
02/12/--	00000	BALANCE FORWARD	23.00
02/16/--	00110	INITIAL ORAL EXAMINATION	40.00
03/14/--	01120	PROPHYLAXIS, CHILD	20.00
04/22/--	01220	TOPICAL FLUORIDE	12.50
06/13/--	02331	MI 2 SURFACE RESIN RESTORATION #7	75.00
07/05/--	08200	LOCAL ANESTHETIC	17.00
07/26/--	02140	0 1 SURFACE AMAL RESTORATION #3	35.00
08/29/--	PMT	PERSONAL CHECK	-93.65 CR
		BALANCE DUE	$128.85

STATEMENT DATE 08/29/--

CURRENT	0.00
OVER 30-DAYS:	52.00
OVER 60-DAYS:	75.00
OVER 90-DAYS:	1.85
BALANCE DUE	$128.85

THANK YOU FOR YOUR PAYMENT.

113

OFFICE CLOSED SEPTEMBER 5TH.
NEW CHARGES HAVE BEEN SENT
TO YOUR INSURANCE CARRIER(S).

MARTIN GORDON
107 KNOWLEDGE DRIVE
NORTHBOROUGH, OH 12345

FIGURE 29-15 Patient account showing age analysis.

PROCEDURE

29-4 Balancing the Day Sheets and the End-of-the-Month Figures

The dental receptionist or office business assistant balances the day sheets daily and totals the day sheets at the end of the month or prior to patient statements being sent out.

EQUIPMENT

▶ Pegboard

▶ Day sheets totaled for the month

▶ Ledger cards for all the patients in the storage file

▶ Calculator with tape that records the entries

PROCEDURE STEPS

1. Total each column and place that total in the spaces provided at the bottom of the page in "Totals this page." (This section is identified as section 4 of Figure 29-12.)

2. The column totals are added to the "Previous page" totals and these numbers are placed in the "Month to Date" total spaces.

3. The totals are verified in the "Proof of Posting" box in section 5 of Figure 29-12. This is where the total of column D is added to column A and subtotaled. The total of columns B1 and B2 are subtracted from the subtotaled amount of A + D. The final amount must equal column C. For example:

Column	D		A		Subtotal	B1–B2		C
	12	+	21	=	33	– 2	=	31
	10	+	14	=	24	– 9	=	15
	5	+	9	=	14	– 4	=	10
Column Totals	27	+	44	=	71	– 15	=	56

4. Once the proof of posting is complete, the accounts receivable control is totaled. This is accomplished by adding the total of column A to the previous day's total and subtracting the columns B1 and B2 from the subtotal. The amount owed to the practice is the accounts receivable total. By adding column A to this, the additional charges are added to the total (or additional money owed to the practice). The payments and adjustments (columns B1 and B2) are subtracted from the total, leaving a true balance of accounts receivable or a true amount that is owed to the practice.

5. The next step in balancing month-end figures is to total the amounts owed on the ledger cards. Use a tape to do this. The cards' totals can be verified on the tape to ensure that nothing was missed.

6. If the total of the ledger cards balances with the total on the day sheet, the accounts receivable is balanced. If it does not balance, recheck the figures and find the missing amount to balance the accounts receivable. Statements are sent out after the accounts receivable is balanced.

After the patient treatment is complete, the insurance is sent in for payment. The codes for service and their descriptions are completed, along with the fee and the date the service was performed. The form is submitted to the carrier through the mail or via electronic claims processing (Figure 29-16). Many software applications allow for the transmission of insurance claims through the modem. The claims are either transmitted to a national clearinghouse and then on to the carrier or directly to the carrier.

The business assistant is responsible for tracking the insurance claims and making certain that payment is received. A copy of each insurance claim submitted is essential for tracking. It is essential to follow up on claims that are not paid promptly in order to identify the problem so that it can be corrected.

The benefit checks received from the carrier are accompanied by an explanation of benefits. The benefit check is posted to the bookkeeping system on the patient ledger with information explaining the services covered. The check is then deposited along with other checks and cash in the daily deposit.

Insurance Schedule of Benefits. Insurance companies may list their schedules of benefits. This is a list of specified amounts that the carrier will pay for the service. This schedule is not in any way related to the dentist's actual fees. The schedule of benefits also identifies the services that are covered under the plan. For instance, some carriers (insurance companies) will not pay for orthodontic benefits. They may only cover two surface restorations at a $40 fee or a percentage of this

Attending Dentist's Statement

Check one:
☐ **Dentist's pretreatment estimate**
☒ **Dentist's statement of actual services**

Carrier name and address
Dental Care Insurance Company
1500 Western Avenue
Middleton, CA 98765

PATIENT SECTION

1. Patient name	2. Relationship to employee	3. Sex	4. Patient birth date	5. If full-time student
first m.i. last	☒ self ☐ child	m f	MM DD YYYY	school city
Jason P. Rangers	☐ spouse ☐ other—	x	11 24 1950	– –

6. Employee/subscriber name and mailing address	7. Employee/ suscriber soc. sec. number	8. Employee/ subscriber birthdate	9. Employer (company) name and address	10. Group number
Self 2356 Harmony Avenue Prospect, CA 98766	111-222-3333	MM DD YYYY 11 24 1950	Sanders Refuse 14th&Main Sts. Prospect, CA	4590

11. Is patient covered by another plan of benefits?	12-a. Name and address of carrier(s)	12-b. Group no(s)	13. Name and address of employer
Dental none Medical health	Maxima Health Ins.	2847B	none

14-a. Employee/subscriber name (if different than patient's)	14-b. Employee/subscriber Soc. Sec. number	14-c. Employee/subscriber birth date	15. Relationship to patient
– – –	same	MM DD YYYY – – – – – –	☒ self ☐ parent ☐ spouse ☐ other _____

I have reviewed the following treatment plan, I authorize release of any information relating to this claim. I understand that I am responsibile for all costs of dental treatment.

▶ *Jason P. Rangers* 8-15-XX
Signed (Patient, or parent, if minor) Date

I hereby authorize payent directly to the below named dentist of the group insurance benefits otherwise payable to me.

▶ *Jason P. Rangers* 8/15/XX
Signed (Insured person) Date

DENTIST SECTION

16. Dentist's name		24. Is treatment result of occupational illnesss or injury?	No	Yes	If yes, enter brief description and dates.
Jay V. School			x		
17. Mailing address		25. Is treatment result of auto accident?	x		
5600 Professional Building Suite D		26. Other accident?	x		
City, State, Zip		27. Are any services covered by another plan?			
Prospect, CA 98766			x		

18. Dentist Soc. Sec. or T.I.N.	19. Dentist license no.	20. Dentist phone no.	28. If prothesis, is this initial placement?	(If no, reason for replacement)	29. Date of prior placement
999-88-7777	CA8476	302-555-1111			

21. First visit date current series	22. Place of treatmet Office Hosp. ECF Other	23. Radiographs or models enclosed?	No	Yes	How many?	28. Is treatment for othodontics?	If services already commenced enter:	Date appliances placed	Mos. treatment remaining
8/1/xx	x		x			x			

Identify missing teeth with "x"

Tooth # or letter	Surface	31. Examination and treatment plan—List in order from tooth no. 1 through tooth no. 32—Use charting system shown. Description of service (including x-rays, prophylaxis, materials used, etc.) Line No.	Date service performed Mo. Day Year	Procedure number	Fee	For administrative use only
		1 oral examination	08 01 xx	0 0120	24 00	
		2 Bite wing radiographs(2)	08 01 xx	0 2720	16 00	
		3 Prophylaxis	08 01 xx	0 1110	32 00	
8	M	4 Composite restoration 1 sur	08 15 xx	0 2330	44 00	
18	MO	5 Amalgam restoration 2 sur	08 15 xx	0 2150	48 00	
		6				
		7				
		8				
		9				
		10				
		11				
		12				
		13				
		14				
		15				

32. Remarks for unusual services

I hereby certify that the procedures as indicated by date have been completed and that the fees submitted are the actual fees I have charged and intend to collect for those procedures.

▶ _____ Date 8/16/xx
Signed (Dentst)

Total Fee Charged	164 00
Max. Allowable	
Deductible	
Carrier %	
Carrier pays	
Patient pays	

Form approved by the
American Dental Association
ADS 851
029375 - Medical Arts Press 1-800-328-2179

FIGURE 29-16 The American Dental Association standard insurance claim form. *(Courtesy of Medical Arts Press 1-800-328-2179)* established fee. The patient is responsible for the balance of uncovered fees. Medicaid, a government program, requires that the dentist accept the reduced amount as payment in full without being able to bill the patient for the balance.

Payment for Dental Services

Ideally, every patient pays in full for the dental treatment he or she receives. Normally, however, the accounts receivable balance does not equal over three months of production. Offering several payment options helps the practice remain healthy and productive.

Cash Payments. Few patients pay for their dental treatment in cash. However, it is important to keep enough cash in the office to make change if the need arises. Some dental offices offer a discount to patients who pay cash in advance (checks included) for the entire treatment the patient is to receive. If a patient pays in cash, it is customary to give a written receipt showing payment on the account.

Check Payments. The majority of patients pay for their dental services with personal checks. Some offices require that the patient use a driver's license number on the check and/or another form of identification for the check. Some regular patients may take offense to this requirement, so be sure to identify how the dentist would like this to be handled. Other checks that may be received in the dental office are cashier's checks. A **cashier's check** is guaranteed by the bank for the amount in which it is written. It is actually the bank's own check that the patient has paid for. Traveler's checks may be used by out-of-town patients. They are safer than cash for the user. They are written in specific denominations ($20, $50, and so on) and require a signature from the user that matches the one on the check, when used. A certified check could be used by a patient as well. A **certified check** is one that the bank has verified as "good" for the amount indicated.

Credit Cards. Patients may use credit cards to pay for the services. The office takes the card and uses it with a credit card charge form. The totals are entered on the charge form and the patient signs it and is given a receipt. The dental office may call the credit card number in order to verify that the patient has not exceeded the limit available on the credit card. Credit card payments, accepted by the office, are assessed a service fee by the banks for handling the transaction. This service fee is actual funds collected. When credit card collections are used, they are documented on the ledger card as a payment. The bank charge is taken from the office checkbook as a fee and not added to the patient's account. The office may post the paid amount on the patient's account and post the bank charge as an adjustment. The patient is still given credit for the entire amount of the credit card transaction.

Collection Management

Collection on some accounts is necessary no matter how effective the billing process. The best business assistant still has to collect from individuals who have past due accounts. There are individuals who have financial difficulties. Work with these patients so that they can to continue paying small amounts on the accounts until they are in better financial states. There are also patients who are negligent in meeting their financial obligations. The longer the dental office puts off contacting these people, the less chance there is in receiving the delinquent amounts.

The dentist will give guidelines for patient collections. They must be handled carefully and tactfully. The best way to address this issue with a patient is in a manner of aiding the patient in finding a way to pay the account balance. The **Fair Debt Collection Practice Act** makes it illegal to telephone a debtor at inconvenient hours. It also prevents collection calls from being made to the debtor's employer, except to verify employment. It prevents anyone seeking collection from getting information through false pretense or by threatening violence.

The telephone is a more effective way to contact the debtor. First, identify that the person is the individual who is sought and then discuss methods for resolving the problem. Always set a date when the payment can be expected. If it does not arrive as promised, then contact the patient immediately to let the patient know that the dental office is not letting the debt slide.

Collection Letters. If unable to reach the debtor by telephone, a collection letter is necessary. The letters are sent to encourage patients to pay their overdue balances. Collection letters can be sent through certified mail (Figure 29-17). Any letters received via certified mail are signed by the people receiving them. This receipt is sent back to the sender to verify that the letter was received. The receipt should be kept in the patient's chart, along with a copy of the letter.

Occasionally, dental offices have to turn highly delinquent accounts over to an outside collection agency. The agency will normally charge one-third of the balance collected as its fee. All accounts that reach collection are reported to the credit bureau. After the money is collected, the fees are subtracted and the balance is sent to the office.

Special Collection Situations

▶ If the patient has declared bankruptcy, the dental office is notified. The dental office is no longer able to send statements or attempt to collect the amount owed. The patient's debt is written off as a loss for the dental office.

▶ If the patient has died and the finances are tied up, a person is designated to execute the deceased individual's estate and oversee the payment of outstanding

Tamara Riegel, D.D.S.
909 Central
Rockford, LA 20011

December 1, 19-

Mr. John Cooper
41 Santiford Drive
Locust, LA 22011

Dear Mr. Cooper:

Your account with our office
is three months past due, and
you have not responded to our
previous requests for payment.
Please pay your balance of
$152 at this time, or contact
us with an explanation of why
you cannot pay.

Please call me at 555-7823 if
you have a question about your
account. Otherwise, we expect
your payment immediately.

Sincerely,

Natalie Short
Accounts Manager

Tamara Riegel, D.D.S.
909 Central
Rockford, LA 20011

December 29, 19-

Mr. John Cooper
41 Santiford Drive
Locust, LA 22011

Dear Mr. Cooper:

Your son, Royce, had a
seriously infected tooth in
March when he came to Dr.
Riegel for treatment. Dr.
Riegel was pleased to use her
experience and education to
treat Royce, and it was in
this same spirit of
cooperation that we expected
you to pay your account within
a reasonable amount of time.

Four months have passed and
you have still not remitted
the $152 outstanding balance
on your account. We cannot
continue to keep your unpaid
account on our books. If you
are experiencing financial
difficulties, please call the
office so we can arrange a
payment schedule that is
agreeable to both of us.

Sincerely,

Natalie Short
Accounts Manager

Tamara Riegel, D.D.S.
909 Central
Rockford, LA 20011

February 1, 19-

Mr. John Cooper
41 Santiford Drive
Locust, LA 22011

Dear Mr. Cooper:

You have not replied to our
previous notices regarding
your unpaid balance of $152.
Unless we hear from you
personally within 14 days,
your account will be given to
the Rockford Medical and
Dental Collection Service.

Do not wait any longer to
contact me at 555-7823 if you
wish to maintain your previous
good credit record with Dr.
Riegel. As previously
suggested, we will cooperate
in arranging a suitable
payment schedule, if needed.

Sincerely,

Natalie Short
Accounts Manager

FIGURE 29-17 Collection letters sent to patients who have accounts that are delinquent. They are drafted to encourage patients to pay their bills.

bills. The statements should be addressed to the "Estate of" from that time forward until paid.

▶ There may be patients who "skip" town and leave no forwarding addresses. The statement will be returned with "no forwarding address" on the unopened envelope. Verify that the address was correct. If it is, the office needs to decide whether to pursue the unpaid debt or turn it over to a collection agency.

Recording Payments

All payments are written promptly onto the ledgers and into the bookkeeping system. The totals are deposited into the bank daily. The cash is noted separately and all the checks are endorsed with the office rubber endorsement stamp, which indicates the specific bank that is utilized. Most of the offices have restrictive endorsement stamps that state "for deposit only." This protects

the office if the check is stolen or lost. A **deposit slip** with the date, practice name, account number, currency and checks listed, and total amount of the deposit identified on it is written for each deposit. Most offices keep carbon copies of these slips along with the bank's deposit receipt, as records of these transactions.

ACCOUNTS PAYABLE

The accounts payable is the amount that the practice owes others. It includes the necessary expenses. The expenses that are required to run the dental practice are called **overhead**. The total accounts receivable is calculated as the **gross income**. Subtract the accounts payable from the gross income to identify the **net income**. The net income is the true profit the practice makes. The practice cannot remain vital if there is no

29-5 Preparing a Deposit Slip

The dental receptionist or office business assistant creates the deposit slip and either takes it to the bank or the dentist takes it to the bank to be deposited. Deposits normally are made in person or placed in the night deposit box.

EQUIPMENT

▶ Deposit slip (Figure 29-18)

▶ Cash and checks received for that day

▶ Office stamp for endorsing the check

▶ Envelope in which to place the deposit slip, checks, and cash

PROCEDURE STEPS

1. Place the date on the deposit slip.

2. Separate the currency (coin and paper money) from the checks.

3. Tally the coins and place the total sum in the designated space on the deposit slip.

4. Tally the paper money and place the total sum in the designated space on the deposit slip.

5. On the back of the deposit slip, list each check separately, listing the patient's last name and the amount of the check in the space provided in the right-hand column.

6. Total the list amounts from the checks on the back of the deposit slip and place this sum in the area on the front of the check slip in the space identified as checks.

7. Total the currency (both coins and paper money) and the check amount and place this sum at the bottom of the deposit slip under total. This amount should total the total identified on the payments column on the day sheet. One way to further check that the total is accurate is to add up the coins, paper money, and each check. This verifies that the sum is correct.

8. Enter the date and the amount of the deposit into the checkbook stub.

FIGURE 29-18 Sample deposit slip.

net income for the dentist. It is not advisable to operate a business in a non-profitable manner for long.

Some of the expenses are **fixed** (remain the same) each month. These include the mortgage, the full-time salaries, and some utilities. Other expenses are **variable,** meaning they fluctuate (do not remain constant), and are dependent on the needs for the month. Variable overhead expenses include dental supplies, dental laboratory costs, and equipment repairs. The business assistant, along with the dentist, can document the monthly overhead and evaluate whether costs can be cut without decreasing patient service. One of the highest monthly variable overhead costs is in the area of dental supplies.

Inventory Supply Systems

There are different types of supplies utilized in the dental office. Some of these supplies are disposable and used up quickly. They are referred to as **expendable**. Examples of expendable supplies are cotton rolls and stationery. Other supplies are retained in the office for long periods of time and are referred to as **non-expendable** supplies. Examples of non-expendable supplies are an autoclave and a light-curing unit.

A number of things must be taken into account when developing an efficient inventory supply system. Products need to be looked at according to the following factors:

▶ **Shelf life**—The length of time the product can be stored until it begins to deteriorate.

▶ **Item price**—The cost of one item.

▶ **Unit price**—The cost of a commonly grouped package of an item (for example, a dozen toothbrushes).

▶ **Bulk price**—The reduced price for a minimum of units (for example, twelve dozen units of toothbrushes).

▶ **Price break**—The minimum quantity of a supply at which the per unit or per item cost is reduced.

▶ **Lead time**—The time between when an order is placed and the time it is received.

▶ **Rate of use**—How much of a product is used in a specific time period. For example, twenty toothbrushes per week are given out to patients.

▶ **Reorder point**—The point that ensures that an adequate supply is available, taking into consideration the lead time and the rate of use for the product.

There are several inventory records systems that can be utilized in the dental office to keep track of the supplies. The goal of any system is that the supplies are available when they are needed. Maintenance of an adequate supply of materials and supplies is essential. Placing the supplies in a central location makes it easier to manage and restock. In most offices, one person is assigned to oversee the inventory system. The system should be simple, easy to use, and accurate. The computer has made an inventory list system easier to maintain. The system can be further designed to meet the needs of the practice. Another system that is routinely used in dental offices is the tag system. The tag system makes use of a reorder tag that is attached to the item in the inventory and represents the reorder point for that particular supply. Tags

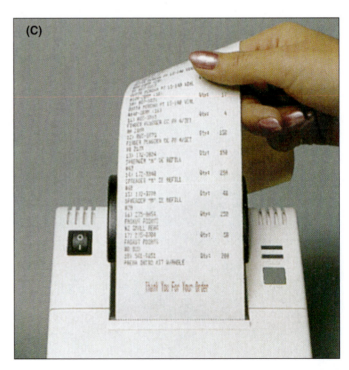

FIGURE 29-19 Electronic ordering system. (A) Scanner. (B) Assistant ordering supplies. (C) Receipt printout. *(Courtesy of Patterson Dental Supply, Inc.)*

P R O C E D U R E

29-6 Reordering Supplies

The dental assistant may be assigned specifically to order supplies or this task may be shared by several auxiliaries.

EQUIPMENT

Red Flag Reorder Tag System
▶ Red flag reorder tags that have surfaced for reordering

▶ Telephone

▶ Index card with order information

Electronic Bar Code System (Figure 29-20)
▶ Bar code wand

▶ Telephone

PROCEDURE STEPS

Red Flag Reorder Tag System
1. Gather the red flags indicating the items that require reordering.

2. Check the index card to obtain the ordering information for each item.

3. Place an indicator in the upper-right corner to indicate that this item is to be ordered immediately.

4. After the item is ordered, place the indicator in the upper-left corner until the product arrives.

5. When the item arrives, remove the indicator from the tag, place the most recently received items to the back of the supply (using the older materials first), and place the red flag ordering tag on the minimum quantity needed in stock before reordering must be accomplished again.

Electronic Bar Code System
1. Identify the items that require reordering. (This system is used for the commonly ordered items.)

2. Obtain the book that has product information and bar codes identified.

3. Use the bar code wand to input the items needed. Run the wand over the bar codes of the items needing ordering. Indicate on the transmitter the number of items needed. The order is then transmitted directly to the dental supply company for ordering.

4. Place a date on the listed items and indicate the number that have been ordered.

FIGURE 29-20 Electronic bar code ordering system. Assistant enters I.D. card using a portable bar code reader. *(Courtesy of Patterson Dental Supply, Inc.)*

---

can be attached with rubber bands. The information on the tag may include only the name of the item. Some dental supply companies come into the dental offices and set up this system by placing the initial tags on the inventory.

When supplies get down to the tagged item, the tagged item is placed in an area to be ordered from the dental supply representative or mail-order supply company.

NOTE: Mail-order supply companies require a slight increase in lead time.

Another supply inventory system that has become more popular is the bar code system. This system allows dental assistants to use a bar code wand that reads the bar code information and electronically transmits this data to the dental supplier to be ordered (Figure 29-19). This system cuts down on the dental assistant's time spent ordering supplies.

Receiving Supplies. When the supplies are delivered, check them for damage. If there is damage, immediately notify the manufacturer or distributor. A **packing slip** listing everything that was shipped is enclosed with the

P R O C E D U R E

29-7 Reconciling a Bank Statement

The dental receptionist or business assistant reconciles the bank statement each month.

EQUIPMENT

▶ Bank statement (Figure 29-21)

▶ Checkbook

▶ Calculator

PROCEDURE STEPS

1. Make sure that all checks and deposits have been added to or subtracted from the checkbook.

2. Subtract any bank service charge from the last balance listed in the checkbook.

3. Check off each listed check in the bank statement against the checkbook and verify the amount listed.

4. Check off each deposit listed in the bank statement against the checkbook and verify the amount listed.

5. On the back of the bank statement, place the ending balance from the front of the statement in the ending balance space on the worksheet.

6. List all checks from the checkbook that have not cleared the bank in the section provided on the back worksheet.

7. List all deposits from the checkbook that have not been received by the bank on the space provided on the worksheet on the back of the statement.

8. Total the checks not cleared and the deposits not received. Subtract the checks not received from the ending balance on the bank statement and add the deposits not received to the ending balance on the bank statement. This balance should agree with the checkbook balance. (If there are any bank charges on the statement, make the corresponding adjustments to the checkbook balance.)

Summary of Account Balance				Closing Date 1/15/99	
Account # 1257-164013				Ending Balance $8,347.62	
Beginning Balance	$7,152.18				
Total Deposits and Additions	$8,643.86				
Total Withdrawals	$7,433.21				
Service Charge	$ 15.24				
Number	Date	Amount	Number	Date	Amount
201	12/18/98	173.82	234	1/4/99	96.31
223*	12/18/98	44.12	235	1/4/99	73.48
224	12/20/98	586.00	236	1/6/99	325.40
225	12/21/98	24.15	237	1/7/99	40.00
226	12/22/98	33.90	238	1/8/99	66.77
228*	12/23/98	1250.00	241*	1/9/99	15.55
229	12/24/98	11.75	242	1/10/99	12.45
230	12/24/98	19.02	243	1/10/99	4441.64
231	1/2/99	43.80	244	1/10/99	64.55
232	1/3/99	39.00			
233	1/4/99	71.50			

*Denotes gap in check sequence

Date	Deposit Amount	Date	Deposit Amount
18-Dec	361.75	4-Jan	825.00
19-Dec	586.00	5-Jan	1286.71
20-Dec	918.21	7-Jan	608.00
21-Dec	201.00	8-Jan	811.15
2-Jan	475.00	9-Jan	1092.68
3-Dec	1478.36		

Front

1. Enter ending balance from the front of this statement
$ 8,347.62

2. Enter deposits not shown on this statement.
$ 3,162.50

3. Subtotal (add 1 and 2)
$ 11,510.12

4. List outstanding checks or other withdrawals here

Check #	Amount
222	37.89
227	161.15
239	11.50
240	92.12
245	835.17
246	21.75
247	586.00

5. Total outstanding checks.
$ 1,745.58

Balance (subtract 5 from 3)
$ 9,764.54
This should equal your checkbook balance

Back

FIGURE 29-21 Sample bank statement.

P R O C E D U R E

29-8 Writing a Business Check

The dental receptionist or business assistant writes out the office accounts payable for the dentist to review and sign.

EQUIPMENT

▶ Checkbook with check and stub (Figure 29-22)

▶ Calculator

PROCEDURE STEPS

1. Write or type in the date. Make sure the date is current.

2. Write or type in the name of the payee. Verify that this is the correct payee.

3. Write in the correct numbers for the correct amount and write out the amount in the designated area. Check that the numerical and written amounts agree and are correct.

4. Fill out the memo, indicating what the check is for.

5. Fill out the date, payee, memo information, and amount on the check stub.

6. Verify that everything is accurate, including spelling.

7. Have the dentist sign on the signature line after reviewing the account payable.

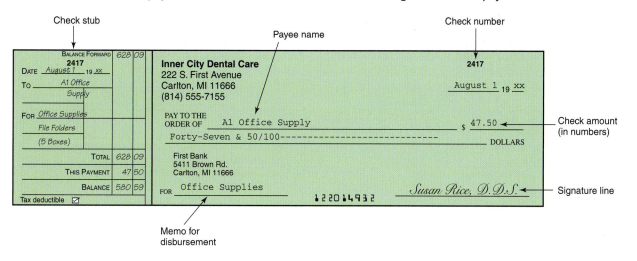

FIGURE 29-22 Sample of practice checkbook and check stub.

supplies. Check the items received against the packing slip list; if there are any discrepancies, contact the manufacturer.

NOTE: The packing slip does not have the price information. That is sent separately on the **statement**, a monthly summary with charges of all supplies.

If any items are returned for any reason to a supplier, a **credit slip** is issued. The credit slip assures the office that they will not be charged for the returned item. If the supplier cannot supply an item on the order, a **back order slip** is issued. This slip lists the items the supplier could not ship immediately and gives an estimated date when the items will be available.

Storing Supplies. After supplies are received and checked, the dental assistant places them in the storage area. The supplies should be rotated so that the older supply items are used before the more recently purchased items. The older supplies are placed directly in the front, ready for use. Some of the supplies require special storage. For example, some of the dental medications and restorative materials require refrigeration, while others require dry, dark areas. Read the manufacturer's instructions for special storage concerns.

Payment of Accounts

The accounts payable for a dental office are paid monthly or bimonthly by the dentist. The dentist reviews the accounts payable and approves payment and then the business assistant prepares the checks for the dentist to sign. All statements are checked for accuracy prior to being paid.

The checks, which are orders for the identified banks to pay the specific amounts indicated to the payee, should be dated. The name of the **payee** must be clearly indicated following the preprinted "Pay to the Order of." The amount of the payment must be entered in both figures and in words. It is advisable to complete the check stub information needed for tax purposes. The **check register** is a record of all the deposits and checks made from the account. It provides a running balance of the funds within the account.

Each month, the bank sends a statement showing any transactions that took place within the account during the month. It lists all checks that have cleared the bank, any deposits received by the bank, and any service charges that were deducted from the account. It should be reconciled against the entries made in the dental office check register.

Non-Sufficient Funds. If any check is written in excess of the amount in the account, it is returned to the payee and marked NSF for non-sufficient funds. The bank charges the account for returned, or "bounced," checks. Most offices require the payer to pay an additional charge to the office for the returned check.

Stop Payment. If a check is written and has not cleared the bank, the payer can stop payment of the check. The bank may charge for stopping payment of a check. Normally, if the payee deposits the check in the bank immediately, it clears within a day of issue.

Petty Cash

The **petty cash** is the money kept in the office for minor expenses, such as for coffee supplies or postage-due letters. Most offices keep less than $100 in this account. The receptionist oversees this cash account. Each time it is used, a voucher or receipt is placed in the cash box until the money gets low. Then, the fund is replenished by writing another check to the cash fund, bringing it up to the original amount. The check is noted as petty cash and the receipts total the amount replenished to the account.

Payroll

The business assistant may complete the employee payroll. Each employee fills out a W-4 form, or the Employee's

a Control number	22222	Void ☐	For Official Use Only OMB No. 1545-0008	
3203				

b Employer's identification number	1 Wages, tips, other compensation	2 Federal income tax withheld
317 600 23	18,500.00	2,950.00

c Employer's name, address, and ZIP code	3 Social security wages	4 Social security taxes withheld
Lewis & King, D.D.S. 2501 Center Street, Suite 23 Northborough, OH 12345	18,500.00	1200.00
	5 Medicare wages and tips 18,500.00	6 Medicare tax withheld 220.00
	7 Social security tips	8 Allocated tips

d Employee's social security number	9 Advance EIC payment	10 Dependent care benefits
263-58-5296		

e Employee's name (first, middle initial, last)	11 Nonqualified plans	12 Benefits included in box 1
Ellen L. Armstrong		
498 Menaul Road Northborough, OH 12345	13 See Instrs. for box 13	14 Other 360.00 Dental Care

	19 Statutory employee ☐	Deceased ☐	Pension plan ☐	Legal rep. ☐	Hshld. emp. ☐	Subtotal ☐	Deferred compensation ☐
f Employee's address and ZIP code							

16 State	Employer's state I.D. No.	17 State wages, tips, etc.	18 State income tax	19 Locality name	20 Local wages, tips, etc.	21 Local income tax
OH	24	18,500.00	750.00	OH	18,500.00	63.50

Cat. No. 10134D   Department of Treasury—Internal Revenue Service

Form **W-2** **Wage and Tax Statement** **19--**

Copy A For Social Security Administration

For Paperwork Reduction Act Notice, see separate instructions

FIGURE 29-23 W-2 form, summarizing all earnings and deductions for the year. A W-2 form is prepared for each employee by the employer by January 31.

Withholding Allowance Certificate, when he or she begins employment, which includes his or her name, address, Social Security number, and the total number of allowances to be claimed. With this information, the payroll is calculated using charts provided by the Internal Revenue Service. Federal tax is based on the amount earned, marital status, the number of allowances (exemptions) claimed, and the length of the pay period. Most of the state and local taxes are figured on the total gross earnings of the employee. A required deduction under the Federal Insurance Contributions Act (FICA), commonly called Social Security, is figured on the amount of gross pay. The employer is required to match this deducted amount and send both contributions to the federal government quarterly. Other deductions that may be taken from the employee's paycheck are health and life insurance payments, along with retirement or savings that are put in another account.

At the end of the year, the employer is required to give each employee a W-2 wage and tax statement (Figure 29-23). This statement is used by the employee to submit his or her federal income tax. The statement includes total wages earned and tax deductions made for the year by that employee.

CHAPTER SUMMARY

The dental reception area needs to be an environment in which all patients feel welcome and comfortable. Today, dentistry can be a positve experience, and the dental treatment can be pain free. That image is developed when the patient first steps into the reception area. The patients may not realize consciously the message that is being received, but the dental office should present an atmosphere that relieves feelings of anxiety.

The front office staff has changed dramatically in recent years. All of the individuals in the front office need knowledge of business machines such as computers, fax machines, and copy machines. These individuals must be organized, have a knowledge of dental treatments, and have good communication and problem-solving skills.

Marketing is also an important part of the dental profession. A dental office is a business as well as a health-care facility. Dental assistants, along with all the members of the dental team, need to be involved in marketing the practice and the dentistry that can be provided.

CASE STUDY

Melissa Jones is a new graduate of an accredited dental assisting program and has received her dental assisting national certification. She will be the dental receptionist in the office of Dr. Ward. Dr. Ward is using a computer-based patient management system and would like to expand on patient marketing ideas.

Case Study Review

1. What types of effective marketing and practice management functions can be done from a computer-based practice management system?

2. What types of reports can be generated by a computer-based patient management system?

3. Identify the background knowledge that Melissa received in her dental assisting program that will aid her in this task.

 To complete your study of this chapter, work the review activities that follow. Also, refer to the software that accompanies this text.

REVIEW QUESTIONS

Multiple Choice

1. When moving from a manual to a computerized bookkeeping system, the office can expect

   a. a week or so turnaround time to input the patient information.

   b. that the manual and computer systems may need to run concurrently for several weeks.

   c. the computer system to require a great deal of time until all patient information is entered into the system.

   d. all of the above.

2. A check guaranteed by the bank is called a
   a. certified check.
   b. cashier's check.
   c. voucher check.
   d. money order.

3. One of the primary reasons that dental patients do not pay their dental bills is
   a. patients consider the cost of dental care to be too high.
   b. patients think that the insurance company should pay the entire dental bill.
   c. patients become unable to pay their dental bills because of financial hardship.
   d. the treatment plan was not discussed and sound financial arrangements were not made at the time of the dental services.

4. An example of a fixed cost is
   a. cost of supplies.
   b. cost of treating dental patients.
   c. salaries.
   d. cost of dental materials.

5. The Employee's Withholding Allowance Certificate, which is completed by all employees, is the
   a. W-2.
   b. W-4.
   c. accounts payable.
   d. accounts receivable.

Critical Thinking

1. Why is it critical to the success of the dental office to bill patients promptly and accurately?

2. List the five sections of the pegboard day sheet and describe the functions of each.

3. Explain why a color-coding system is used for filing charts.

Employment Strategies

OBJECTIVES

The student should strive to meet the following objectives and demonstrate an understanding of the facts and principles presented in this chapter:

1. Identify four pathways to obtain DANB certification.

2. Explain how to obtain employment and identify different types of practices.

3. Set goals and identify sources to obtain employment in the dental field.

4. Identify the steps of preparing a cover letter and a résumé.

5. Define how to prepare for the interview.

6. Explain the interview process and identify skills and preparation techniques that will aid in obtaining the job.

7. Identify the skills that a successful dental assistant possesses. Explain how to terminate employment.

KEY TERMS

American Dental Assistants Association (ADAA) (p. 728)

American Dental Association (ADA) (p. 728)

Dental Assisting National Board, Inc. (DANB) (p. 728)

dental associate (p. 729)

partnership (p. 729)

INTRODUCTION

As the required formal training necessary to become a dental assistant nears completion, the student must switch his or her goals toward becoming an employed dental assistant. The first step in this process is obtaining national certification. Then, the employment search begins.

When conducting the search for suitable employment, it is necessary to be well prepared and goal oriented. Being knowledgeable about how to write a cover letter and prepare a résumé is very important. Effective cover letters and résumés lead to job interviews. Understanding the interview process and possessing the skills necessary to interview successfully lead to job offers.

OBTAINING NATIONAL CERTIFICATION

National certification for dental assistants is not mandatory in every state. Once obtained, however, the patients and the dentist can be assured that the assistant has the basic knowledge and background necessary to perform as a professional on the dental team. The **Dental Assisting National Board, Inc. (DANB)**, assumes the responsibility for credentialing dental assistants. This board is independent of the **American Dental Association (ADA)** and the **American Dental Assistants Association (ADAA)**. Upon completing and passing the chairside dental assisting examination of DANB, the dental assistant can display the certificate that verifies successful completion of the DANB test (Figure 30-1). The assistant can also wear the official certified dental assistant (CDA) pin acknowledging that he or she is a certified dental assistant and can use that title (Figure 30-2). The DANB examination is divided into three major categories: radiology, infection control, and general chairside. An assistant must pass all three sections in order to become a certified dental assistant. Maintenance of the CDA credential is through yearly continuing education hours and a renewal fee.

A dental assistant is eligible to take the dental assisting examination and can obtain national certification by DANB through four pathways:

1. **Pathway I**
   - ▶ Is a graduate of an accredited dental assistant or dental hygiene program
   - ▶ Has a current cardiopulmonary resuscitation (CPR) card, health-care provider level
   - ▶ Has completed the application and paid the fee

2. **Pathway II**
   - ▶ Is a high school graduate or equivalent
   - ▶ Has a current CPR card
   - ▶ Has two years of full-time employment or 3,500 hours
   - ▶ Has verification of dentist employer
   - ▶ Has completed the application and paid the fee

3. **Pathway III**
   - ▶ Status as a current or previous DANB CDA or graduation from a DDS or DMD program accredited by the American Dental Association
   - ▶ Has a current CPR card
   - ▶ Has completed the application and paid the fee

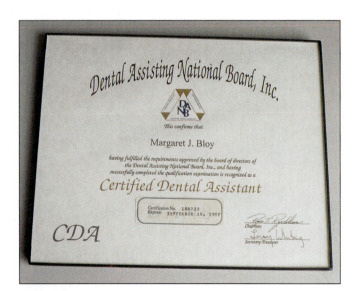

FIGURE 30-1 Dental Assisting National Board (DANB) certificate.

FIGURE 30-2 The official Certified Dental Assistant (CDA) pin of the Dental Assisting National Board.

4. **Pathway IV**
   ▶ Is a high school graduate or equivalent
   ▶ Has four years of part-time work experience (at least 3,500 hours accumulated over a forty-eight-month period) as a dental assistant
   ▶ Has verification of dentist employer
   ▶ Has completed the application and paid the fee

Reprinted with permission of the Dental Assisting National Board, Inc. (DANBI)]

Every dental assistant should obtain national certification to ensure that his or her patients receive the best care possible and to build the self-esteem of each dental assistant employed in the field.

EMPLOYMENT

Whether graduating from an accredited program or just trying to obtain a position in the dental office, there are several important steps that must be accomplished first. It is important that a dental assistant plans future employment before proceeding forward. It may be essential to obtain dental assisting national certification for the state in which that employment is sought. If that is the case, reflect on the pathways available and seek the one that suits the individual's needs best.

After obtaining the necessary credentials, the next goal is to prepare to obtain successful employment. Research should be done to identify the type of practice that will be the most interesting, stimulating, and enjoyable. When choosing an employer, find one who has a good reputation and whose philosophy is similar to the individual's own. A dental assistant needs to feel that he or she is working together with the dentist and the other team members in order to care for the patients in the best manner possible. Do research and talk to employees who work for the dentist to make sure that a good match for employment will be accomplished prior to obtaining the position. The other aspect of the employment is working well with the other employees. Are they team players and is compatibility possible?

It is important to find employment that best suits the individual's needs and allows for the best possible situation for the dental assistant, the employer, and the patients. Before taking the first position offered, consider the following:

▶ What qualities are desired in an employer?

▶ What areas of growth are available in this situation?

▶ From an employee's position, what strengths can be brought to this position?

▶ What individual areas can be improved upon?

▶ Overall, what type of dentistry is interesting?

Solo or Partnership Practice

The majority of dentists practice in solo practices where there are single dentists. A dentist may hire another dentist under a contractual agreement; this hired dentist is a **dental associate**. An associate relationship may turn into a **partnership**, in which each dentist has equal rights and duties. A partnership is developed through a legal agreement and makes both dentists responsible for any accounts payable. Partners are not held responsible for any malpractice suits against the other partner.

There is an increase in partnerships in dental practices. This is due to the tremendous startup costs a dentist faces upon graduation from dental school. Therefore, a newly graduated dentist may work in an established practice as a dental associate for some time and then, after an allotted time frame, become a partner. Another way dentists are dealing with the costs of a practice is to share a building and/or front office employees while still maintaining solo practices.

Group Practice

Another type of dental office is the group practice. In a group practice, any number of dentists (both general and specialty) can share a building and still remain independent. The positive aspects of this type of practice is the opportunity to talk over cases with each other. In addition, the total number of employees in the group practice may lend itself to offering more complete and extensive benefit packages. The more employees under the same insurance plan, the better the rates for the employer.

Dental Specialty Practice

There are a number of dental practices that are specialty practices. If a dental assistant likes to assist primarily in oral surgery, endodontics, periodontics, orthodontics, prosthodontics, pathology, pediatric dentistry, or dental public health, there are specialty offices available. However, fewer employment opportunities are available in the areas of pathology and dental public health. The dental specialties work with the general dentists to care for specific cases. The general dentist refers the patient to a specialty office to obtain a special service and then the patient returns to the general dental office for routine care.

Other Employment Choices

Dental assistants can gain employment in government clinics that care for patients who are eligible to receive dental care at a reduced rate. Often, federal or state grants set up programs to meet the specific needs of people who cannot afford dental care. These programs may also collect data on specific diseases this group of people may have. Usually, the guidelines of the programs change or have to be renewed annually. A dental assistant is an employee hired by the overseer of the grant. This dental assistant may receive great satisfaction treating patients in this type of program.

School Clinics and Laboratories. Dental schools and dental assisting schools also employ dental assistants to either work in the clinic with students, teach, and/or be administrators for the program. In dental schools, the dental assistants work with student dentists to simulate four-handed dentistry or in dental laboratories to help the students perfect their skills.

Veterans' Hospitals. Veterans' hospitals hire dental assistants to assist the dentists on staff in the clinics. Employment in this area must be obtained through the civil service office. Points are given to individuals who have worked in the service or been employed in veterans' programs before. A list of qualifications can be obtained from the civil service office that advertises the employment position.

Dental Supply Companies. Dental supply companies hire dental assistants as sales representatives for goods and supplies. Normally, a dental assistant in this position does not utilize his or her chairside skills but does become knowledgeable about the products and travels from dental office to dental office giving product knowledge and ordering supplies.

Insurance Companies. Dental assistants are also hired by insurance companies to process dental insurance claims. Having knowledge and background in dental terminology and procedures is an asset in understanding situations and processing the dental insurance claims.

EMPLOYMENT SEARCH

After a decision is made about the type of dental practice employment is desired in, locating open positions is the next step. Many dentists advertise in the daily paper in the classified section. Other areas where employment opportunities are posted include the local dental and dental assistant societies. Most local societies have newsletters or employment people who list the job openings. If graduating from a dental assisting program, career placement services may be available at the school. Some employment agencies have listings for dental assistant jobs, and most of the dental supply houses know of dentists who are hiring. Leaving a cover letter and résumé with some of these agencies may be a consideration.

PREPARING A COVER LETTER AND A RÉSUMÉ

The next step in the employment search is to prepare a cover letter and a résumé. These documents introduce the prospective employee and present the individual's educational background, training, and previous employment experiences. The cover letter states reasons why the individual is right for the position and when he or she is available for employment.

The cover letter and the résumé should be printed on quality rag-bond paper (normally white, light gray, or off-white) and follow a professional format. It is crucial that the cover letter and résumé be prepared on a word processor, printed on a laser printer or high-quality dot matrix printer, and contain correct spelling, punctuation, and grammar. Every cover letter and résumé must be proofread several times before being submitted to a prospective employer.

Cover Letter

A cover letter is an introduction to a prospective employer (Figure 30-3). It communicates to the employer or hiring personnel the individual's potential value and any specific personal attributes that can be called attention to. A cover letter should accompany every résumé. A standard format can be used to develop a cover letter.

▶ **Return address**—Include a street address, city, state, and zip code.

▶ **Date**—Month, day, and year.

▶ **Inside address**—Addressee's name and title; company name, if different; street address; city; state; and zip code.

▶ **Salutation**—Make every effort to use the correct name. If unknown and as a last resort, use "To Whom It May Concern:" At the end of every salutation, a colon (:) is used.

▶ **First paragraph**—Tell why the letter is being written and indicate where the information about the employment opportunity was obtained and which position is desired.

▶ **Second paragraph**—Identify the reasons for interest in the position (such as the dental office has a good reputation for providing quality dental care). List the qualifications that would be assets to the employer and dental team members (for example, a graduate of an accredited dental assisting program and an explanation of how the academic background makes for a qualified dental assistant). Make mention of any relevant work experience. Refer the employer to the résumé, which lists individual qualifications, education, training, and experience.

▶ **Third paragraph**—Ask for a personal interview, indicate flexible available times to be reached, and list a phone number with area code, if applicable, and an e-mail address, if available. Close with a statement that encourages a speedy response: "I am available for an interview at your convenience and will be calling within the next five days to confirm an interview time with you," or "I am looking forward to meeting with you and your dental team in the near future."

625 "B" Street
Spokane, WA 99228

January 12, 1999

Dr. Conrad Jones
312 33rd
Spokane, WA 99205

Dear Dr. Jones:

I am writing in response to your advertisement in the April 25th edition of the *Spokesman Review* for an expanded-function dental assistant.

I believe that I am the "gentle, caring, enthusiastic" dental assistant that you are looking for. I am flexible and capable of working individually or as a team member. I am a recent graduate of the Spokane Community College Dental Assisting program, and I am currently awaiting the results of my Dental Assisting National Board examination. With the combination of my training, my desire to work, and my love of helping people, I will be a valuable asset to your office.

Looking at my enclosed résumé, you will see that I have worked in several offices during my training. I have also assisted several dentists in the volunteer clinic, provided dental education in the area schools, and worked with patients in my other health-related employment. I have obtained computer proficiency during my other employment opportunities.

I would like to request an opportunity for a personal interview to further discuss the position and to answer any questions you may have. My schedule is flexible so feel free to call me at (509) 555-1857 as soon as is convenient so an appointment can be arranged.

I look forward to meeting you and your staff and to getting the opportunity to demonstrate my abilities as a valuable member of your office team.

Sincerely,

Jean Lucas
Dental Assistant

Enclosure: résumé

FIGURE 30-3 A cover letter for employment as a dental assistant in a dental office.

▸ **Closing**—Close the letter with "Sincerely" and a comma. Then, type four returns and the name. The four spaces provide room for a signature, written in black ink. (Using other colors may detract from the professionalism that has been established in the cover letter.)

▸ **Enclosures**—After the typed name, type two returns and then type the words "Enclosure: Résumé" (any other enclosures can be listed beneath the word "Résumé," such as letters of recommendation).

Résumé

A résumé should fit on one page (Figure 30-4). It should be attractive and professional. Present specific information. Stress achievements and skills related to employment. Include personal data, a career objective, education, employment history (including qualifications, skills, and abilities), and references.

▶ **Personal data**—Include the name, address, phone number, and e-mail address, if available, where the individual can be reached. Marital status and birth date are no longer appropriate for a résumé.

▶ **Career objective**—Identify the desired goal (for example, "To gain a position in a dental office as a dental assistant who will utilize the skills and abilities obtained in dental assisting school").

▶ **Education**—List certificates, registration, degrees, and continuing education courses that have been completed. Do not include grade point average unless it is in some way pertinent to the position. Also, list any academic awards received, such as scholarships. List the most recent education first

---

625 "B" Street
Spokane, WA 99228

Phone: 509-555-1857
Fax: 599-555-3038
E-mail:
Jlucas@spokane.wa.us.com

Jean Lucas

Career Objective	To obtain a dental assisting position in which my education and skills can be utilized, in an office that uses the team approach to providing quality dental care.		
Education	1991–1993	Spokane Community College	Spokane, WA

AAS Degree, Dental Assisting
♣ Vice President's Honor Roll for academic achievement

Employment History   1993–1995   Community Clinic   Palouse, WA
Chairside Dental Assistant
♣ Assisted in a variety of dental procedures
♣ Developed and taught a program in oral hygiene to elementary children
♣ Provided patient care and service
♣ Maintained inventory and supplies
♣ Volunteered in community clinic care programs

1990–1991   Ice Cream Delight   Seattle, WA
Senior Assistant Manager
♣ Supervised employees while providing customer service
♣ Created and decorated cakes
♣ Managed telephones
♣ Maintained accounts payable and receivable
♣ Organized employee work schedule

References	Dr. Michael Smiley	Ms. Elaine Garcia	Ms. Jean Norman
	Dentist	Director of Clinic	Instructor, Dental Assisting
	(523) 555-5436	(569) 555-7895	(589) 555-6547

FIGURE 30-4 A résumé for employment as a dental assistant in a dental office.

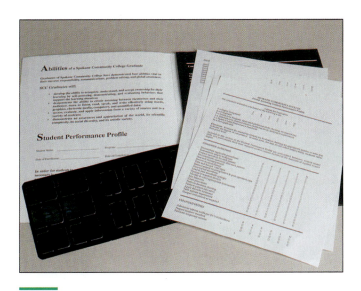

FIGURE 30-5 A personal portfolio is a nice way to share with the dental office your certificates and letters of recommendation.

FIGURE 30-6 During the interview, be prepared and listen carefully to the interviewer prior to answering the questions.

with corresponding dates. High school graduation information is not necessary.

▶ **Employment history**—Employment history should be listed with an idea of what was accomplished in each position. Use action words to explain what was done. For instance, instead of writing, "I worked as a cashier," it would be better to write, "I was responsible for maintaining cash payables while resolving daily problems, projecting a positive attitude, and developing good customer relations." Present the abilities in the best manner, but always be honest about the job description.

▶ **References**—It is appropriate to use the sentence "References are available upon request." In many areas of the country, it is beneficial to list three references using name, title, and phone number. It is likely that a dentist will call a fellow dentist to inquire about an individual's skills and abilities. Make sure that the references listed have been checked first to ensure that they will give positive references and that they are aware that they are listed as references. It is important to have references who relate specifically to the desired characteristics and who pertain to the employment that is sought.

SETTING UP AN INTERVIEW

Follow through on what was said in the cover letter. For example, if the letter mentions making a follow-up call in five days, be sure to call back on the fifth day. When making a follow-up call, make sure the background noises are not distracting. If an individual is nervous using the telephone to set up the interview, visit the dental office or practice in person or with a friend and identify a script that is comfortable to use while making the contacts. When setting up an interview, the individual should make sure that his or her schedule can accommodate the appointment time. It is also important to make sure that it is scheduled at a convenient time for the dentist and staff.

INTERVIEW PROCESS

When preparing for the interview, there are several things to consider. It is important to be at least five minutes early for the interview, so allow additional time to get there. It is important that some research has been done regarding the dental office. The additional interest in the dental office will have a positive effect on the prospective employer. Know yourself and know your strengths and abilities in order to be prepared for the question that is most often asked: "Why should we hire you for this position?"

Develop questions that can be asked of the dentist and staff. Salary questions should not be the only thing that is brought up in the interview. Ask questions related to team work, prevention programs, or continuing education.

Prepare a portfolio with letters of recommendation, copies of certificates, radiographs you have taken, or any additional items that attest to your abilities and skills (Figure 30-5). Place them in a folder to present to the dentist and staff.

Practice the interview before actually going to one. Ask a friend or family member to do a mock interview and to give feedback on any areas that can be improved. A firm handshake, eye contact, and a smile are still important in the interview process. Sit up straight and speak distinctly. Try to relax and enjoy it. How is the situation

Jean Lucas

625 "B" Street
Spokane, WA 99228
Fax: 599-555-3038
E-mail: Jlucas@spokane.wa.us.com

April 24, 1999

874 Jefferson Street
Chicago, Ill 60891

Dear Dr. Jones and Staff:

I wanted to thank you for your time and interest in interviewing me for the position of chairside dental assistant. I am extremely interested in working with you and your office in this position.

Your office reputation is one that above all provides quality dental care. My personal professional philosophy has always been that patient care is the number one priority and that teamwork is essential to the success of any dental office.

Dr. Jones, thank you again for taking time out of your schedule to interview me. Please review my résumé for my qualifications for the chairside position. I will look forward to hearing from you in the near future. I am available at (509) 555-1857.

Sincerely,

Jean Lucas

Certified Dental Assistant

FIGURE 30-7 Sending a follow-up letter is advisable after an interview.

going to be handled if the office staff ask you if you would like a cup of coffee? Identify the possible situations and plan ahead.

Appearance is crucial. Wear something that feels comfortable, but a rule of thumb is to dress like an individual who cares about being hired. Many individuals feel comfortable in jeans, but jeans are not appropriate attire for an interview. Dress appropriately and demonstrate good hygiene. Make sure that the clothes are clean and pressed. Do not wear clothes that appear to be flamboyant or dowdy; instead, err on the side of conservatism. Think about the small details, such as where the car keys or purse are going to be placed during the interview. Is a pen available if asked to fill out an application? If necessary, are references with addresses and phone numbers available? If asked to write a paragraph

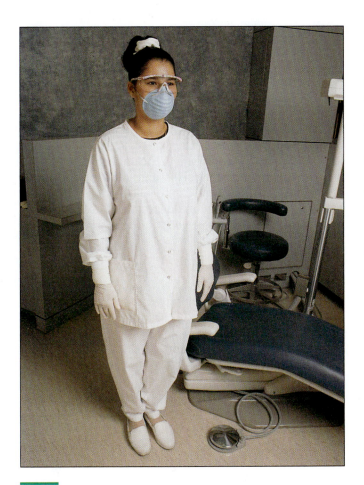

FIGURE 30-8 Maintaining a professional appearance on the job is important for the dental assistant.

about yourself, can this be accomplished with the correct spellings of the words needed to express yourself properly? Are the questions available to ask the dental team members? Many of these items may not be necessary, but it is important to be prepared.

Be yourself and, if nervous, say so, then continue on. Make sure that the dentist's name is pronounced correctly and always address the dentist as Dr. __ unless asked otherwise. The dentist may request that a working interview be done. If that is the case, ask about time, uniform, and parking in order to be ready for the identified day. Stay calm and do the best work possible. The interviewer usually closes the session by asking if the interviewee has any further questions (Figure 30-6). This is the time to ask the prepared questions. If all areas have been covered, say, "The specific questions I had prepared to ask have been answered. Can I clarify anything in regard to my background and experience?"

Leaving the Interview and Following Up

Be sure to thank the interviewers for their time and shake their hands. It is good to close by stating that you are interested in the position and look forward to hearing from them. If they have not stated it during the interview, ask when they anticipate making a decision on the open position. Dentists look for dental assistants who have positive attitudes, good interpersonal skills, good clinical skills, good dental educational foundations, flexibility, team player attitudes, and the willingness to learn.

If, after the interview, the interviewee confirms that he or she would like to obtain the position in that dental office, send a follow-up letter referring the office to the résumé and restate an interest in becoming part of the dental team (Figure 30-7).

Receiving an Offer of Employment

Before accepting an employment offer, it is important to ask a few more questions. If it was not mentioned during the interview, now is an appropriate time to discuss salary. Also, ask about benefits and find out the office's policies on sick days, holidays, and vacation time. Know what the dental assistant's specific responsibilities are and what the office hours will be. Find out when performance evaluations are conducted and what performance objectives lead to a raise in pay.

PROFESSIONAL CONDUCT DURING EMPLOYMENT

Once the job is obtained, the dental assistant's goal becomes keeping the job. Basic requirements for keeping the job are to always be on time, be ready to accomplish the necessary skills, plan ahead, and prepare for success. Take care of all outside practical matters so that attention can be placed on fulfilling employment responsibilities. Make sure child care is arranged (if applicable) and that backup care is available in case the primary caregiver has an emergency. Arrange for reliable transportation.

Maintain high standards of personal hygiene (Figure 30-8). As an employee in a health profession, it is important to present good health standards. Uniforms should be clean and well pressed; shoes should be clean and in good condition. Unfortunately, an employer's perception of an employee's abilities may be influenced by the employee's appearance. Therefore, dental assistants should always look and act like professionals and be well prepared for the job.

Make sure that expectations of the job are identified and then try to go above and beyond those expectations, especially if planning to advance. If expectations are unclear, talk with the office manager or employer to clarify areas of concern. A positive attitude is key to becoming an ideal employee. The dental office can be stressful, especially when a patient procedure changes and the schedule is off course, so tackling each challenge with a positive attitude and flexibility makes the office environment better for everyone. It is a well-known fact that the majority of patients who leave one dental office for another do so because of the poor attitude of one employee. Each dental assistant is responsible for maintaining a positive attitude at work.

Set goals to learn new skills, and stay current with the changes in technology and materials. One way to continue education is through the dental assistant association, other professional courses, and seminars. Other courses in the nearby community or four-year colleges may be of benefit to an individual's professional growth. Seek them out. Occasionally, do a self-evaluation. Be honest and look at overall individual attitude, skill, and professionalism. Try not to look at others to correct these behaviors, because the only person an individual can change is himself or herself.

Terminating Employment

If an individual continues to dread going to work, determine where employment could be obtained that would correct the problem. Evaluate the career goals, the qualifications pertaining to these goals, and the new path that is desired. If it is determined that employment in a different office is the plan of action, submit a letter of termination or verbally notify the employer and allow him or her two weeks' notice so that a replacement can be found. Do everything possible to leave a position on good terms with the employer. Then, if the new career does not proceed as planned, returning to the job if an opening is available is a possibility.

Continued Success

The career of dental assisting is a very rewarding one, both professionally and personally. The work environment is a pleasant one that usually does not require evenings or night shifts. The goal of dental offices is to provide the best care possible for the patients. The patients are appreciative of the dental assistants who care for their needs. The dental assistant who provides a pleasant smile while providing care makes everything go better for the patient. Most days, dental assistants go home feeling good about the skills and knowledge used to provide quality dental care to the patients. Continue to improve dental assisting skills and knowledge through continuing education, and stay challenged to stay knowledgeable about new techniques and materials. Be the best dental assistant possible. Good luck in your career!

Chapter Summary

It is important to find employment that will best suit individual needs and that allows for the best possible situation for the dental assistant, employer, and the patients. Before taking the first position available, plan ahead. It may be essential to obtain dental assisting national certification for the state in which employment is sought. National certification for dental assistants is not mandatory in every state, but it assures the patients and the dentist that the assistant has the basic knowledge and background to perform as a professional on the dental team. Make sure that expectations of the job are identified and then try to meet and exceed those if planning to advance. Each dental assistant is responsible for maintaining a positive attitude at work. Set goals to learn new skills and stay abreast of changes in technology and materials. A dental assisting career is very rewarding, both professionally and personally. Be the best dental assistant possible.

Case Study

Drs. Bryan and Lucas are hiring a dental assistant to replace Phong Ho, a dental assistant who is leaving at the end of the month. Phong has been a chairside dental assistant for seven years for Drs. Bryan and Lucas. Svetlana Maklavic has applied for the position and will be the first dental assistant applicant to be interviewed.

Case Study Review

1. What paper work should Svetlana bring to the interview?

2. How should Svetlana prepare for the interview?

3. What clothes should Svetlana wear for an interview with Drs. Bryan and Lucas?

4. Why should Svetlana arrive ten minutes early for the interview?

 To complete your study of this chapter, work the review activities that follow. Also, refer to the software that accompanies this text.

REVIEW QUESTIONS

Multiple Choice

1. A cover letter is:
   a. a listing of personal data for the employer.
   b. a listing of education.
   c. an introduction to your employer.
   d. a career objective for the position that is being sought.

2. The interview:
   a. does not require follow-up.
   b. is a time for questions and answers about salary and benefits.
   c. requires very little preparation.
   d. requires that you prepare, listen carefully, and think before answering questions asked.

3. If an individual is a graduate of an accredited dental assisting program, what would not be required in order to be eligible to take the Dental Assisting National Board?
   a. Current cardiopulmonary resuscitation care, health-care provider level.
   b. Verification of dentist employer of work experience.
   c. Completed application.
   d. Application fee.

4. A _____ practice is one in which any number of dentists can share a building and still remain independent.
   a. Group.
   b. Specialty.
   c. General.
   d. Partnership.

5. The key to becoming an ideal employee is
   a. high standard of personal hygiene.
   b. skill.
   c. knowledge.
   d. positive attitude.

Critical Thinking

1. Discuss methods of researching a prospective employer.

2. Identify the differences in a solo, partnership, group, or specialty dental practice.

3. Identify areas in which a dental assistant can obtain employment.

Ethics and Jurisprudence

OBJECTIVES

The student should strive to meet the following objectives and demonstrate an understanding of the facts and principles presented in this chapter:

1. Identify the difference between civil and criminal law.

2. Define the Dental Practice Act and what it covers.

3. Identify who oversees the Dental Practice Act and how licenses for the dental field are obtained.

4. Define expanded functions.

5. Identify the components of a contract.

6. Identify due care and give examples of malpractice and torts.

7. Identify fraud and the service that can be given under the Good Samaritan Law.

8. Identify the four areas of the Americans with Disabilities Act.

9. Identify the responsibilities of the dental team in regard to dental records, implied and informed consent, subpoenas, and the statute of limitations.

10. Define ethics and give examples of the American Dental Association and American Dental Assistants Association principles of ethics.

11. State how dentistry follows ethical principles in regard to advertising, professional fees and charges, and professional responsibilities and rights.

KEY TERMS

abandonment (p. 742)

Americans with Disabilities Act (p. 743)

assault (p. 742)

battery (p. 742)

breach of contract (p. 741)

civil law (p. 740)

contract (p. 741)

contract law (p. 740)

criminal law (p. 740)

defamation of character (p. 743)

dental jurisprudence (p. 740)

Dental Practice Act (p. 740)

Doctrine of Respondeat Superior (p. 741)

ethics (p. 740)

expanded functions (p. 740)

expressed contract (p. 741)

Good Samaritan Law (p. 743)

implied consent (p. 744)

implied contract (p. 741)

informed consent (p. 743)

malpractice (p. 742)

reciprocity (p. 740)

statutes (p. 740)

tort (p. 740)

INTRODUCTION

Each dental team member is faced with daily decisions that require judgments regarding legal and ethical principles. Maintaining professional ethical standards at all times is essential. The area of **dental jurisprudence**, the law(s) that governs dentistry, is more clearly defined than dental **ethics**, moral judgment(s). The consequences of not doing what should be legally done or doing what should not be done can be imposed on an individual in the form of fines or imprisonment.

THE LAW

The U.S. Constitution is the supreme law in the United States of America. If a question of how to read, or interpret, this law occurs, a decision is made in a court of law. The first case that relates to that particular question is referred to as the precedent. From that time on, all cases relating to that same situation are based on the primary decision, the principle of *stare decisis*, meaning "let the decision stand." All future cases are determined in the same manner. Following these guidelines, everyone is treated fairly under the same circumstances. These laws and rules are known as **common laws** and are to be followed by everyone.

Civil and Criminal Law

Law, the set of rules established and enforced by local, state, and federal governments, can be divided into two primary classifications: **civil law** and **criminal law**. The most frequent law exercised in the dental care setting is civil law, which can be further broken into two subclassifications: **contract law** and **tort** law.

If a civil charge is brought against a dentist, he or she becomes the **defendant**. The **plaintiff**, the person who is bringing the charges against the defendant, must prove that a civil wrong was committed. If able to prove wrongdoing, restitution is awarded to the plaintiff in a monetary amount for any pain, suffering, and loss of wages the dentist or dental treatment has caused.

Criminal law addresses wrongs committed against the welfare and safety of society as a whole. Criminal charges are brought against the defendant by the state to prevent any further harm to the society and its members. If a case is proven against a defendant in criminal law, the defendant faces fines and/or imprisonment. A dentist would also face disciplinary action from the board of dentistry in his or her practicing state.

Dental Practice Act

In each state, **statutes** are enacted by each legislative body to make rules and regulations. The state board of dentistry is an administrative agency in each state that enforces these statutes and rules in regard to performance of specific functions. Each state has a **Dental Practice Act** that describes the legal restrictions and controls on the dentist, the hygienist, and the other dental assistants. The Dental Practice Act describes the dental team members as licensed or non-licensed and lists what are allowed or disallowed duties for each, including the **expanded functions** (delegated functions that require increased responsibility and skill) that may be performed by each dental team member. Even if the job classification or title is unused in the state Dental Practice Act, any employee working in a dental office is covered in the law. The Dental Practice Act of each state gives guidelines for eligibility for licensing and identifies the grounds by which this license can be suspended or repealed. Changing the content of the Dental Practice Act can be done by an amendment of the dental law, by an entirely new law and regulations being enacted to replace the old law, or by a combination of the two.

State Board of Dentistry

The practice act includes the name of the administrative board that supervises the dental practice act, such as The State Board of Dental Examiners or Dental Quality Assurance Board of the state. This board has the basic responsibility of enforcing adherence to the Dental Practice Act of that specific state. The members of this board are appointed by the governor of that state, normally from a list of recommendations from the state dental association. The membership usually has one lay member from the state, and the rest of the board members are normally licensed dentists. Another function of this board is to examine applicants for dental licenses and grant licenses if the criteria are met.

License to Practice. A license is granted to a dentist if he or she has met all the minimum requirements. The license is to protect the public from unqualified individuals providing dental treatment. Each state requires that the dental hygienist become licensed, as well. Some of the states require dental assistants to become licensed in order to perform specific dental tasks.

To obtain a license, an individual must meet the educational and moral requirements and pass a written theory examination and a clinical practice examination as specified by the administrative board of that state or region. The requirements may vary from state to state, so if the individual wants to practice in another state, an additional license may be required. In some states, an individual who has passed the requirements for one state may apply for a **reciprocity** agreement in another state and be allowed to perform dental skills without taking a written or clinical examination again. Reciprocity is an agreement between two or more states that allows an individual licensed in one state to receive, without further examination and testing, a similar license in the other state(s) identified in the reciprocity agreement. The reciprocity agreement normally takes place in states with adjoining borders and similar testing requirements.

The factors for revoking, suspending, or denying renewal of a license vary from state to state. Most states take action if the licensed person has a felony conviction and/or misdemeanors of drug addiction, moral corruptness, incompetence, or mental/physical disability that may cause harm to patients under his or her dental care.

Expanded Functions.
Expanded functions are specific advanced tasks that require increased skill and responsibility. These functions are delegated by the dentist according to the Dental Practice Act within the state. Some states require additional education, certification, or registration to perform these functions. Like all functions the dental assistant performs, the expanded functions fall under the **Doctrine of Respondeat Superior**. Translated this means, "Let the master answer." So, if wrongdoing took place under the guidelines of employment, the dentist is liable for the negligent act. However, this does not mean that the dental assistant is not held responsible and cannot be sued. It merely means that a suit can be filed against either the employee and the dentist or both. Often, the dentist is sued because the plaintiff anticipates greater recovery in financial damages from the dentist. The doctrine is based on the assumption that the dentist has the right to direct and control the employees; therefore, along with the duty comes the responsibility of the consequences. In addition, if the patient is damaged, it is due to the employer exposing the patient to his or her employee. Therefore, the dentist is required to compensate the patient for any harm that was caused.

The expanded functions are most often specified in the dental practice acts according to how they are to be delegated. They may be stipulated for general supervision, which means that the procedure authorized in the dental practice act can be performed legally on a patient of record by the dental assistant under the general supervision of the dentist. If it is specified to be delegated under direct supervision, the dentist must be in the treatment facility to authorize this function and he or she must evaluate the performance of the procedure.

Certification, Licensure, and Registration.
Dental assistants can become nationally certified by the Dental Assisting National Board, Inc. (DANB) (see Chapter 30, Employment Strategies). Some states require dental assistants to be certified, licensed, or registered to perform specific functions in the dental office. The first state to grant licensure to dental assistants was Minnesota. Certification from DANB is granted after education or work requirements have been met and a written test covering general chairside, radiology, and infection control has been passed. Continuing education is required to maintain current certification from DANB, and many states require continuing education to maintain registration or licensure.

THE DENTIST, THE DENTAL ASSISTANT, AND THE LAW

 The dental assistant must thoroughly understand the law in order to protect the patient, the dentist, and the profession. Dental health care continues to change, and the dental assistant must understand how these changes are impacted by the law.

Contracts

A **contract** is a binding agreement between two or more people. This agreement must be between two competent people, to do or not to do something lawful, in exchange for a payment ("competent" eliminates the mentally incompetent, individuals under the influence of drugs or alcohol, infants, and minors). The dentist has a legal obligation to care for a patient under the principles of contract law after a patient arrives for dental care and the dentist accepts him or her by providing dental care.

A contract can be expressed or implied. An **expressed contract** is written or verbally agreed upon. It describes specifically what each party in the contract will do. An **implied contract** is implemented by actions, not words. Most of the dentist/patient contracts are implied. If a patient comes to the dentist with a toothache and the dentist checks the area and requests that a radiograph be taken, this is an implied contract because it exists due to the circumstances. The law says that the dentist does what is necessary and what the patient would have requested had there been an expressed contract.

Dental assistants are **agents** of the dentist. What a dental assistant says and does can be used in a court of law against the dentist. For instance, if a dental assistant said the dentist can cure a problem but the dentist does not cure it, the dentist—not the dental assistant—is at fault. This is considered an admission by an employee and under the doctrine of Respondeat Superior would be the legal equivalent of the dentist saying that this can be accomplished even if it cannot be done. The dental assistant should be cautious because his or her actions and words at work may become binding on the employer, the dentist. Any statements either pro or con made spontaneously at the time of an alleged act can be admissible as evidence in a court of law. This is true because of the principle of *res gestae*, which translates to "part of the action," at the time of the offense and becomes admissible evidence in a case.

Termination of a Contract.
A contract can be terminated when one of the parties does not meet contractual obligation. Until the contract is broken, or a **breach of contract** occurs, the dentist is legally bound to treat the patient. The contact can be terminated if:

▶ The patient discharges the dentist or fails to return to the office

▶ The patient fails to follow instructions given by the dentist

▶ The dentist formally withdraws from patient care

▶ The patient no longer needs treatment/all requirements agreed upon have been met

Patient Discharges the Dentist.

The patient often discharges the dentist by not continuing to return to the office to complete services or continued care appointments. Legally, the dentist should send a letter to the patient to confirm and document the termination of the contract. This is normally done with a recall notification, documentation on the chart, and follow-up notification. Ideally, it should be done through certified mail, requesting a return receipt, so that a copy is in the patient's chart.

Patient Fails to Follow Instructions from the Dentist.

The patient may fail to follow the instructions of the dentist in regard to the dental treatment. For instance, a patient has dental implants and is told by the dentist that ongoing cleaning appointments are necessary in order to maintain the health of the area. The patient is warned that failing to undergo ongoing cleaning may cause the implants to fail. The dental office repeatedly contacts the patient to have the prophy (cleaning) appointments, yet the patient does not return. Further, the dentist writes a letter telling the patient again that the implants may fail without the ongoing cleaning appointments and asks the patient to schedule necessary appointments. If the patient chooses not to follow the instructions from the dentist and fails to schedule the needed appointments, the contract would be broken. Any time the patient fails to respond to or follow instructions of the dentist, the contract between the dentist and the patient is broken.

Dentist Formally Withdraws from the Case.

To avoid any charges of abandonment (desertion), the dentist should send the patient a certified letter, with return receipt requested, to formally withdraw from a dental case. This would happen if the dentist feels that he or she can no longer provide service to the patient or if the patient becomes **noncompliant** and the dentist can no longer work with the patient.

Patient No Longer Needs Treatment.

The dentist is responsible for providing treatment until the patient no longer needs treatment or the dentist has formally withdrawn from the case. For example, if an oral surgeon has seen a patient to remove four wisdom teeth and this service has been completed and the patient has healed accordingly, therefore no longer needing this treatment, the contract would be terminated.

STANDARD OF CARE

The dentist and the dental team members have the responsibility and duty to perform due care in treating all patients. **Due care** is what any reasonable and prudent dental care professional in the same circumstances would do. The dental professional must provide sufficient care, within his or her scope of training, in all dental procedures, not excluding prescribing, dispensing, or administering drugs.

Malpractice

Malpractice is failure to use due care in dental treatment, which is considered negligence. **Negligence** is the failure to exercise the standard of care that a reasonable person would exercise in similar circumstances. Negligence is the primary cause of malpractice suits. Negligence comes about when an individual suffers injury because of another person's failure to live up to the normal standard of care. Malpractice is professional negligence. There are normally four elements of negligence (sometimes called the four "Ds"): duty, derelict, direct cause, and damage. Dental professionals are held to a high standard of care by virtue of their knowledge, intelligence, and skills. It is their duty to provide high performance, and they are expected not to be derelict (careless) in their skills. If they directly cause injury due to deviation from the normal standard of care and damage or harm occurs, they are negligent. At times, in a court of law, **expert witnesses** will testify in regard to the standard of care that is to be expected.

Torts

A tort is a wrongful act that results in injury to one person by another. For example, a dental assistant breaks the aseptic chain and causes the patient to be exposed to infection. If this infection causes the patient damage or harm, then the case may result in litigation. If the dental assistant broke the aseptic chain and the patient care resulted in no infection, damage, or harm, then a tort did not result. A tort must have a wrongful act that is a breach in due care that causes injury because of this action. Some wrongful areas of negligence may result in torts when the standard of care is not followed. Practicing good risk management protects the dentist and dental assistant from litigation.

Assault and Battery

Assault is the threat of touching a person without consent, and battery is the actual touching. The basis of the tort of assault and battery is the threat of or unprivileged touching of one person by another without consent. For example, an assault would be to insinuate that a desired touch is indicated. If dental personnel touch any areas other than the oral cavity or perioral region (palpation of neck, TMJ, lymph nodes, and so on), this could be considered battery. An unwanted hug without consent is battery. If a child was refusing treatment and the dental assistant threatened and restrained him or her without parental consent, assault and battery charges could be brought against the dental assistant according to the tort law.

Defamation of Character

Another tort law protects an individual(s) from causing injury to another person's reputation, name, or character. This injury, called **defamation of character**, can come from written or spoken words. Defamation of character can come from either libel or slander. **Libel** is false and malicious written comments. In the dental office, untrue comments on the patient's chart may be libel. For instance, if the dental assistant wrote on the chart that he or she suspected the patient's grinding of the teeth was a result of a bad marriage, it would be libel if someone else read the chart and took it as truth. **Slander** is false or maliciously spoken words. For example, a patient said, "Dr. Smith removes teeth even if they do not need to be removed." If the statement was overheard by another individual, it would be considered slander if untrue. A third party must hear or see it and understand what was said in order for defamation of character to exist.

Invasion of Privacy

Another kind of tort is the invasion of privacy. It includes unwanted publicity and exposure to public view and unauthorized publicity of patient information or anything in the patient's records.

> **NOTE:** In the dental office, unwanted exposure to public view is not a problem; this occurs in the medical field where body parts are exposed for treatment.

The dental office must take great care to protect the disclosure of any patient information, spoken or written, on patient records. A dental assistant cannot use any information about the patient, medical or personal, that was obtained as a course of treatment without the person's approval or permission.

Fraud

Fraud is deliberate deception that is practiced to secure unfair or unlawful gain. The most common area of fraud in the dental office is in the area of insurance fraud. Dental personnel who send information that is incorrect to the insurance companies for payment are committing fraud.

Good Samaritan Law

The **Good Samaritan Law** is for those individuals who are not seeking payment but are rendering medical assistance to the injured. This care is usually given because of an accident and the law protects people or grants immunity for acts performed while providing emergency care. If this care is given without the intent to do bodily harm and without being compensated for this care, the Good Samaritan Law provides protection.

Americans with Disabilities Act

The **Americans with Disabilities Act** nationally mandates that individuals will not be discriminated against because of their disabilities. The four areas noted in the act refer to:

▶ Employment discrimination due to disabilities.

▶ The disabled are provided access to public services.

▶ Public accommodations and access to equal goods and services are open to the disabled.

▶ Telecommunication services to the hearing and speech impaired are extended.

In the dental offices, ramps must be provided to allow individuals with disabilities access. The doorways and treatment rooms should allow for care to be provided for individuals with disabilities. One dental operatory needs to have access for those patients confined to wheelchairs.

▌ DENTAL RECORDS

The dentist and the dental team members must be responsible to maintain accurate, up-to-date patient records. In litigation, the accuracy of the dental record directly relates to the credibility of the professionals. All actual care and charges must be reflected in the patients' dental records. Charts must be written in ink and be legible and all necessary corrections should be made by drawing a line through the initial content and then making the correction, initialing it, and dating the new data (Figure 31-1).

Informed Consent

 One important area of documentation is the **informed consent** form. Each patient has the right to know and understand any procedure that is to be performed. The patient is informed in words that can be understood. The patient should be told of the procedure, risks involved, expected outcome, other optional methods to treat the same problem, and the risk of denying the treatment. The health-care worker must make certain that the patient understands the treatment. In today's world, a large number of patients speak English as a second language or not at all. An interpreter must be used to explain the procedure to the patient, if necessary.

If surgical procedures are to be performed, it is advisable to receive a consent form. The dental assistant may sign as a witness on the consent form. One copy is kept in the patient's chart and one is given to the patient for his or her records.

Chart No. ———————

HEALTH HISTORY COMMENTS:

Patient's Name _Bradley Plummley_

Date _4/9/99   #2 MOD Amal_

#3 DO Amal dycal

#4 O Amal

2 anes.   KJM

5/2/99   #15 Full cold Crown prep

acrylic temp cemented w/tempbond KJM

5/13/99   #15 Full Gold Crown

cemented with zinc phosphate   KJM

R 250 mg. V-cillin K ~~20 tabs~~ 10 tabs KJM

FIGURE 31-1 When changes are made on the dental chart, a red line must be drawn through the initial content and then the correction made with the person initiating the change notating it by initialing the chart.

Implied Consent

Implied consent may happen in a number of subtle ways. When a dentist sits down and the patient opens his or her mouth, the patient is implying consent for the dentist to begin treatment. Patients rolling up their sleeves prior to blood pressure being taken are implying that the action for the blood pressure procedure can be taken.

Subpoenas

Subpoenas are court orders mandating that an individual shows up at a specific time and date and with a specific reason to testify. Dental records can also be subpoenaed by the court and must be released to the court. Any records that provide documentation about sensitive material, such as sexually transmitted diseases including AIDS, substance abuse, and so on, may require an additional court order. **Confidentiality** must be maintained, because the information the patient shares with the dentist is always held in confidence.

Statue of Limitations

The statute of limitations is different in every jurisdiction (state, county). The statute of limitations defines the period of time in which legal action can take place. Some time limits run from the beginning of treatment, some from the time the accused neglect took place, and others from the time the treatment was completed. Most time frames run for three to six years. With the confusion about the time limits, most dentists keep their records for indefinite time periods.

ETHICS

Ethics is defined in terms of what is right or wrong, or moral judgment of these two. In dentistry, it is defined by a code as The American Dental Association Principles of Ethics. Unlike the law, which rarely changes, ethics constantly change and evolve just as personal values and morals change and evolve.

Advertising. Traditionally, dentists as professionals did not advertise. Advertising was not illegal if the advertising was truthful and not misleading, but many thought it to be unethical. Currently, it is not thought to be unethical, and there is a trend to advertise in a number of ways, such as telephone books, television, radio, media, Internet, and dental service coupons. Advertising is becoming more popular in the dental profession. Patients who are satisfied with their dental care are still the best advertising source.

Professional Fees and Charges. Professional fees are based on what is customary to the locale and should represent the difficulty of the dental procedure and the quality of the service rendered. The services documented on the patient's chart are the ones that are charged. The office can also charge the patient for insurance processing and missed appointments if the patient has been reminded of the appointment (see Chapter 29, Dental Office Management, for further information).

Professional Responsibilities and Rights. The dentist has professional responsibilities and rights when treating patients. Dentists cannot refuse to serve a patient on the basis of race, color, religion, national origin, sexual origin, or because he or she is an HIV-infected individual. If the dentist takes a dental patient for treatment, the dentist must provide the care in a timely manner unless that patient was given official written notice of possible delays.

If a dentist is HIV infected, the dentist should refrain from performing procedures that may risk transmission of the virus to the other health-care providers or patients.

A dentist is not to be influenced by financial interests. For instance, if the dentist owns a large amount of stock in a company that sells specific dental medications, the dentist should not only prescribe that medication in order to enhance personal gain.

The American Dental Assistants Association Principles of Ethics and Professional Conduct

Each individual involved in the practice of dentistry assumes the obligation of maintaining and enriching the profession. Each member shall choose to meet this obligation according to the dictates of personal conscience based on the needs of the general public the profession of dentistry is committed to serve.

The member shall refrain from performing any professional service which is prohibited by state law and has the obligation to constantly strive to upgrade and expand technical skills for the benefit of the employer and consumer public. The member should additionally seek to sustain and improve the local organization, state association, and the American Dental Assistants Association through active participation and personal commitment.

Code of Professional Conduct

As a member of the American Dental Assistants Association, I pledge to:

▶ Abide by the Bylaws of the Association

▶ Maintain loyalty to the Association

▶ Pursue the objectives of the Association

▶ Hold in confidence the information entrusted to me by the Association

▶ Maintain respect for the members and employees of the Association

▶ Serve all members of the Association in an impartial manner.

▶ Recognize and follow all laws and regulations relating to activities of the Association

▶ Exercise and insist on sound business principles in the conduct of the affairs of the Association

▶ Use legal and ethical means to influence legislation or regulation affecting members of the Association

▶ Issue no false or misleading statements to fellow members or to the public

▶ Refrain from disseminating malicious information concerning the Association or any member or employee of the Association

▶ Maintain high standards of personal conduct and integrity

▶ To not imply Association endorsement of personal opinions or positions

▶ Cooperate in a reasonable and proper manner with staff and members

▶ Accept no personal compensation from fellow members, except as approved by the Association

▶ Promote and maintain the highest standards of performance in service to the Association

▶ Assure public confidence in the integrity and service of the Association

Dental Assistants Following Ethics and Jurisprudence

The profession of dentistry will continue to advance, and dental assistants will have more decisions to make in the arena of ethics and jurisprudence. The necessity to stay abreast of the changes and to make decisions that are educated and concrete are essential. The dental assistant should always strive to stay within the law, handle patients in a professional manner, maintain a high standard of care, obtain patient consent, preserve confidentiality, maintain legible accurate records, and not judge others who have belief systems that are different.

CHAPTER SUMMARY

Each dental team member is faced with daily decisions that require judgments regarding legal and ethical principles. Maintaining professional ethical standards at all times is essential. The consequences for not doing what should be legally done or doing what should not be done can include fines or imprisonment. A license is granted to protect the public from unqualified individuals providing dental treatment. Some states require dental assistants to become licensed to perform specific dental tasks. The expanded functions are most often specified in the Dental Practice Act according to how they are to be delegated. They may be stipulated for general supervision, which means that the procedure authorized in the Dental Practice Act can be legally performed on a patient of record by the dental assistant under the general supervision of the dentist, or they may be specified to be delegated under direct supervision. The dental assistant must thoroughly understand the law in order

CASE STUDY

Two weeks ago, Dr. Greenwood treated a new patient, Desiree Jordan, for a fractured tooth. Peggy Jones assisted Dr. Greenwood during the examination and the restoration of the tooth. Today, both Dr. Greenwood and Peggy Jones were served with subpoenas by Desiree's attorney. Desiree is alleging that unsafe conditions took place at a local restaurant and she bit down on a rock in her hamburger. Dr. Greenwood and Peggy Jones are called as expert witnesses in a civil hearing. Peggy is nervous about going to court and being on the witness stand. Peggy does not know what to expect.

Case Study Review

1. How will Desiree's dental record help Peggy answer questions at the hearing?

2. As an expert witness, what is Peggy expected to testify about in this case?

3. What should Peggy do to prepare for the testimony?

 To complete your study of this chapter, work the review activities that follow. Also, refer to the software that accompanies this text.

REVIEW QUESTIONS

to protect the patient, the dentist, and the profession. Dental health care continues to change and the assistant must understand how the law affects these changes.

Multiple Choice

1. Occasionally, a dentist is sued for the negligence of a dental assistant employee, even though the dentist is not guilty of the negligent act himself or herself. This is done on the basis of the doctrine of
   a. contract law.
   b. expressed law.
   c. respondeat superior.
   d. civil law.

2. The contract that most often exists between the dentist and the patient is
   a. civil.
   b. implied.
   c. expressed.
   d. proximate.

3. The legal restrictions and controls that governs dentistry in each state are the
   a. statutes.
   b. expanded functions.
   c. Dental Practice Acts.
   d. reciprocities.

4. A binding agreement between two or more people is a(n)
   a. agent.
   b. reciprocity.
   c. contract.
   d. breach.

5. A wrongful act that results in injury to one person by another is a(n)
   a. tort.
   b. contract.
   c. assault.
   d. libel.

Critical Thinking

1. Explain the standard of care as it applies to dental assistants. Give an example.

2. What is the Good Samaritan Law? What must the dental assistant remember when giving first aid during an accident?

3. Define the difference between ethics and jurisprudence.

DENTAL AND DENTAL RELATED ORGANIZATIONS RESOURCE LIST

American Dental Association (ADA)
211 E. Chicago Avenue
Chicago, IL 60611
(312) 440-2500
(800) 621-8091
online: *http://www.ada.org*

American Dental Assistants Association (ADAA)
203 N. LaSalle Street, Suite 1320
Chicago, IL 60601
(312) 541-1550
online: *http://members/aol/com/adaa1/index.html*

Dental Assisting National Board, Inc. (DANB)
676 N. St. Clair, Suite 1880
Chicago, IL 60611
(312) 642-3368
(800) FOR-DANB

Centers for Disease Control and Prevention (CDC)
Atlanta, GA 30333
(404) 488-4450

Environmental Protection Agency (EPA)
401 M Street SW
Washington, DC
Waste Hotline: (800) 424-4372
                     (202) 260-2090

Food and Drug Administration (FDA)
5600 Fishers Lane
Rockville, MD 20857
Devices and Radiological Health (800) 638-2041
Drug Evaluation Research (301) 295-8000

Occupation Safety and Health Administration (OSHA)
Department of Labor
200 Constitution Avenue
Washington, DC 20210
(800) 321-6742
online: *http://www.osha.gov*

STAGES OF TOOTH ERUPTION

Development of Human Dentition

Prenatal	Infancy	Early Childhood

4 months in utero

Birth

18-30 months

6 months in utero

4-8 months

2-3 years

Primary Dentition

Permanent Dentition

8-12 months

3-4 years

9-15 months

4-5 years

15-21 months

5-6 years

Late Childhood

6-7 years

7-8 years

8-9 years

9-10 years

Adolescence and Adulthood

10-11 years

11-12 years

14-15 years

21 years

Copyright by the American Dental Association. Reprinted with permission, 1999.

GLOSSARY

abandonment desertion, refusal to treat a patient without prior notice (Ch. 31)

abrasive rotary instruments non-bladed instruments used to finish and polish restorations and appliances (Ch. 15)

abrasives materials that cut or grind the surface leaving grooves and a rough surface, in the form of either powder or paste (Chs. 15 & 28)

abscess local area of pus and infection (Chs. 7, 18 & 20)

abscessed tooth an infected tooth that causes the patient pain (Ch. 13)

absorption the process of transferring digested food into the bloodstream (Ch. 3)

abutment a tooth, root, or implant used for the retention of a fixed or removable prosthesis; the teeth adjacent to a pontic in a bridge (Chs. 24 & 25)

accelerates starts the process of (Ch. 27)

accounts payable amount that the business or office owes for goods or services (Ch. 29)

accounts receivable amount that the business or office is owed for goods or services (Ch. 29)

acid etchant process of applying phosphoric acid solution to a tooth (to alter the surface of the tooth enamel by creating microscopic undercuts between the enamel rod) to allow for adhesion of dental materials to the enamel by brush, syringe, or cotton pledget (Chs. 26 & 28)

acquired immunodeficiency syndrome (AIDS) disorder of the immune system caused by the human immunodeficiency virus (HIV) that ultimately destroys the body's ability to fight infection. There is no known cure for AIDS. (Ch. 8)

actinomycosis an infection caused by bacteria, characterized by painful swelling followed by discharge of pus and yellow granules (Ch. 20)

activator orthopedic appliance that expands the width of the maxillary arch (Ch. 21)

activity zones the division into four zones of the area around the patient: operating, assisting, static, and transfer (Ch. 14)

ADA Seal of Acceptance classification given by the ADA Council on Dental Therapeutics that notes product is safe and effective for use (Ch. 2)

addiction physical or psychological dependency (Ch. 12)

adhesive materials used to improve retention between two objects; also known as bonding agent (Ch. 26)

adjacent next to, as in, the teeth are adjacent to each other (Ch. 6)

air abrasion a technique used for specific dental procedures, to remove micro amounts of tooth structure in the cavity preparation (Ch. 15)

air compressor provides compressed air for handpieces and air/water syringes (Ch. 14)

air-water syringe device used by the dentist that provides air or water, or a combination spray of air and water (Ch. 14)

ALARA the principle of keeping radiation exposure "As Low As Reasonably Possible"; it involves combining radiation protection procedures with common sense practices (Ch. 17)

alimentary canal forms a tube from the mouth to the anus as part of the digestive system (Ch. 3)

alkalosis an increase in blood alkalinity (Ch. 13)

allergens substances that produce allergic reactions (Ch. 13)

allergic reactions the overreaction of the body to particular allergens; itching, redness of the skin, and hives are symptoms (Ch. 13)

allergy an overreaction of the body to a particular allergen (Ch. 13)

alloy combination of two or more metals (Ch. 26)

alveolar crest where two cortical bone plates come together between each tooth (Ch. 5)

alveolar mucosa thin, loosely attached mucosa covering the alveolar bone; alveolar process forms the bone that supports the maxillary and mandibular teeth (Chs. 4 & 5)

alveoli part of the alveolar sacs in the lungs where the exchange of gases takes place (Ch. 3)

alveolitis complication following tooth extraction involving the loss of the blood clot, leaving a "dry socket" that can be very painful (Chs. 13 & 19)

alveolus the bone that surrounds the root of the tooth, the socket (Ch. 5)

alveoplasty a surgical contouring of the alvelar bone (Ch. 19)

amalgam an effective, long lasting, and comparatively inexpensive material (an alloy with mercury) used for tooth restoration (Ch. 26)

amalgamator a small machine that mixes dental amalgam and other dental materials (Ch. 14)

ameloblasts enamel-forming cells (Ch. 5)

American Dental Assistants' Association (ADAA) the national professional organization for dental assistants; local and state branches exist with a national office in Chicago (Chs. 1 & 30)

American Dental Association (ADA) the national professional organization for dentists (Chs. 1, 9 & 30)

American Dental Hygienists' Association (ADHA) the national professional organization for dental hygienists (Ch. 1)

Americans with Disabilities Act passed by Congress in 1990, this act was intended to end discrimination against disabled people (Chs. 29 & 30)

analgesic a drug that relieves pain; for example aspirin and morphine (Ch. 12)

anaphylactic shock an immediate, severe, sometimes fatal reaction by an individual to specific allergens (Chs. 8 & 13)

anatomical term for describing posterior denture teeth; anatomical teeth resemble natural teeth with cusps and developmental grooves (Ch. 25)

anatomical crown portion of the tooth covered with enamel (Chs. 6 & 28)

anchor tooth tooth that the dental dam clamp is placed on, usually one or two teeth distal to the tooth or teeth being restored (Ch. 28)

anesthesia drugs that cause a loss of pain but not a loss of all sensation; usually used before surgeries (Ch. 12)

angina pectoris pain in the chest that may radiate into the jaw, neck, or arm (Ch. 13)

angioedema Large urticaria (hives) brought on by an allergic reaction (Ch. 13)

Angle's classification system used to classify malocclusion (Ch. 21)

angular cheilitis inflammation of the corners of the mouth (Ch. 20)

ankylosis a condition in which the tooth, cementum, or dentin fuses with the alveolar bone, restricting movement of the tooth (Ch. 20)

anode the positive terminal of an electrolytic cell (Ch. 17)

anodontia the congenital absence of teeth (Ch. 20)

antibodies a disease-fighting protein developed by the body in response to the presence of a specific antigen (Chs. 8 & 13)

antigen pathogens that stimulate the production of antibodies (Chs. 8 & 13)

antihistamine a drug that counteracts the body's production of histamine (Ch. 13)

antimicrobial a microorganism growth inhibitor; antimicrobial soap, for example (Ch. 9)

antipyretic an agent that reduces fever (Ch. 11)

antitoxins antibodies produced in response to and capable of neutralizing a specific biologic toxin (Ch. 8)

apexogenesis pulpotomy of permanent tooth whereby pulp vitality is maintained, allowing time for the root end to develop and close (Ch. 22)

aaphthous ulcers painful ulcers that appear in the oral cavity; a circular lesion appears with a yellow center and red "halo" surrounding the lesion; sometimes referred to as a canker sore (Ch. 20)

apical foramen an opening in the end of the tooth through which nerve and blood vessels enter (Ch. 6)

apical periodontitis pulpal inflammation that extends into the periapical tissues (Ch. 18)

apicoectomy removal of the apex of the root and infection surrounding the area (Ch. 18)

arch wire wire used to apply force to either move or hold teeth in the desired position (Ch. 21)

Aristotle (384-322 BC) wrote early oral hygiene instructions (Ch. 1)

arteriosclerosis hardening of the arteries (Ch. 13)

articulation joints where two or more bones meet or form a junction (Ch. 3)

articulator a frame which holds models of the patient's teeth in order to maintain the patient's occlusion, representing his or her jaws; a mechanical device that represents the temporomandibular joints to which upper and lower casts of the dental arches may be attached to simulate mouth functions (Chs. 25 & 27)

asepsis/aseptic technique steps necessary to ensure an environment free from pathogens; handwashing, for example (Ch. 9)

assault/battery assault is the threat of touching a person without their consent; battery is the actual touching (Ch. 31)

assisted bleaching initial in-office stages of home bleaching process; patient makes dental impressions, then returns to the office to obtain custom bleaching trays and instructions for home bleaching (Ch. 28)

asymmetric shape, size, and relative position of body parts on opposite sides are not equal; for example, if the face were divided into halves, the halves would not be equal (Ch. 11)

atrium (auricles) upper chambers of the heart (Ch. 3)

attached gingiva extends from the mucogingival junction to the gingival groove. It is stippled and attached tightly to the alveolar bone (Ch. 5)

attrition the wearing away of the incisal or occlusal surfaces of the tooth during normal function. The final stage of the life cycle of the tooth (Ch. 5)

automatic processing processing of dental X-rays using automated equipment (Ch. 17)

auxillary polishing aids aids used during coronal polishing procedures, including bridge threaders, abrasive polishing strips, soft wooden points, and small interproximal brushes (Ch. 28)

avulsed tooth a tooth that has been completely removed from the mouth; avulsed teeth should be replanted immediately (if possible) or transported to the dentist in milk, saliva, saline, or water (Ch. 22)

axial wall wall that is parallel to the long-axis of the tooth (Ch. 28)

band part of the matrix that forms the missing surface or wall of a tooth (Ch. 28)

barbed broaches endontic instruments used for the removal of soft tissue from the pulp canal (Ch. 18)

basal cells one of the deepest cells in the dermis (Ch. 17)

basal metabolic rate (BMR) energy used when a person is at rest (Ch. 2)

base material applied in a putty or thick layer between the tooth and restoration to protect the pulp from chemical, electrical, mechanical, or thermal irritation (Ch. 26)

baseline vital signs the initial reading of basic signs of life, including body temperature, pulse, blood pressure, and respiration rate (Ch. 11)

baseplates a preformed semi-rigid acrylic resin material that temporarily represents the denture base (Ch. 25)

behavior management plan to modify or maintain the desired behavior of a person or group of persons (Ch. 22)

bevel the slanted edge or side on the working-end of an instrument (Ch. 15)

bifurcated one tooth with two roots (Ch. 6)

binangle a dental instrument where the shank has two angles (Ch. 15)

biopsy surgical removal of a small amount of tissue (Chs. 19 & 20)

bisecting technique X-ray technique that applies the geometric principle in which the central ray bisects the angle formed by the dental film and the long axis of the tooth (Ch. 17)

bite registration an occlusal record of the relationship between the upper and lower teeth (Ch. 24)

bite rim the several layers of baseplate wax that are attached to the baseplate that represent the space provided by teeth in normal occlusion, registering the vertical dimension for the denture and establishing the occlusal relationship of the mandibular and maxillary arches (Ch. 25)

bite-wing radiograph intraoral radiographs that show the maxillary and mandibular crowns in occlusion (Ch. 17)

black line stain formation of a thin black to dark brown line slightly above the gingiva and following the contour of the gingival margin; found primarily in women and often in cases of excellent oral hygiene (Ch. 28)

Black, G.V. (1836-1915) the grand old man of dentistry, he authored numerous articles and books and invented numerous machines and instruments for cavity preparation (Ch. 1)

Black's formula formula developed by G.V. Black to standardize the exact size and angulation of an instrument. See pg. 276 for more information (Ch. 15)

blade the flat working end on a dental instrument (Ch. 15)

blister a raised, fluid-filled area, usually oval or circular in shape (Ch. 20)

Bloodborne Pathogens Standard effective in 1992, this federal standard came about in the hope of reducing the occupational-related cases of HIV and hepatitis B infection among health-care workers (Ch. 9)

blurred image image on X-ray film that is out of focus (Ch. 17)

bonding agents materials, usually low viscosity resins, used to improve retention between two objects (in dentistry, between the tooth structure [enamel and dentin] and the restoration) also known as adhesives, bonding resins; mainly light- or dull-cured (Ch. 26)

bone restoration surgery to correct defects and/or deformities by reshaping the bone or removing parts of the bone (Ch. 23)

bone resorption bone loss caused during periodontal disease (may be horizontal or vertical)

border molding when receiving a final impression, the impression compound is heated and placed along the borders of the custom tray. The tray is cooled and placed in the patient's mouth, and the lips, cheeks, and tongue are moved to establish accurate length for the periphery and adjacent tissues to be included in the final impression (Ch. 25)

brachial artery the main artery of the arm (Ch. 11)

bracket a device attached to the teeth that holds the arch wire in place and transmits the force of the arch wire to move the tooth (Ch. 21)

bradycardia abnormally slow heart rate (Ch. 11)

bradypnea abnormally slow respiratory rate at rest (Ch. 11)

brand names drug names assigned by the manufacturer that are trademarked; for example, Tylenol® is a brand name, aspirin is a generic name (Ch. 12)

breach of contract breaking of a contract (Ch. 31)

bridge a fixed prosthetic device placed in the mouth to replace missing teeth (Ch. 7)

broad spectrum refers to drugs, specifically antibiotics, that are effective against a wide range of bacteria, not just one specific bacteria (Ch. 12)

bronchioles a smaller branch of the bronchiole tubes that divide into alveolar sacs (Chs. 3 & 13)

bruxism grinding of the teeth (Ch. 23)

buccal nerve branch nerves that pass through the buccinator muscle to the cheek where it innervates the buccal mucosa, buccal gingiva, and the buccal of the mandibular molars (Ch. 4)

buccal the surface of the posterior tooth that is toward the cheeks (Chs. 6 & 7)

buccal tubes small cylinders of metal welded to the molar bands providing a means of attachment for the arch wire to the band in the posterior area (Ch. 21)

buccinator a muscle of facial expression (Ch. 4)

buccoversion a tooth that is tipped toward the lip or cheek (Ch. 21)

bulla a large, fluid-filled blister; greater than ½ inch in diameter (Ch. 20)

burnish to smooth (Ch. 28)

burs one of the dental rotary instruments, burs are used for cavity preparation, finish and polish restorations, surgical procedures, and for adjusting dental appliances (Ch. 15)

calcification the process of depositing calcium salts and other materials in the formed tooth, it takes place in the apposition stage of tooth development (Ch. 5)

calcination the process of driving a specific amount of water out of gypsum to create specific plasters, stones, or investment die stones (Ch. 27)

calcium hydroxide type of cementation used as a low-strength base under any restoration (Ch. 26)

calculus hard, calcified deposit of mineralized plaque that forms on teeth, restorations, and dental appliances; also known as tartar (Chs. 23 & 28)

calorie unit of heat. The large Calorie (which is always capitalized) is the amount of heat needed to change the temperature of l gm. of water from 14.5° C to 15.5° C.; one thousand kilo calories make up l calorie. (Ch. 2)

cancellous tissue sponge-like appearing tissue (Ch. 3)

candida albicans yeast-like fungus (Ch. 20)

canker sores painful ulcers that appear in the oral cavity; the circular lesion appears with a yellow center and red "halo" surrounding the lesion; sometimes referred to as aphthous ulcers (Ch. 20)

carbamide peroxide popular bleaching agent used to whiten teeth (Ch. 28)

cardiopulmonary resuscitation (CPR) rescue breathing and chest compressions performed on a patient experiencing cardiac arrest (Ch. 13)

caries also known as dental cavities; tooth decay (Ch. 2)

cariogenic foods foods that breakdown into simple sugars and are used by bacteria to cause dental caries (Ch. 2)

carpules (cartridges) glass containers of anesthetic solution (Ch. 16)

cartilage a tough nonvascular, resilient, specialized connective tissue (Ch. 3)

cartridges (carpules) glass containers of anesthetic solution (Ch. 16)

cassette a container for extra oral radiographic film containing intensifying screens; available in hard or soft light-proof containers (Ch. 17)

catalyst an ingredient that starts or accelerates a process (Ch. 27)

cathode the negative terminal of an X-ray tube (Ch. 17)

cavities also known as dental caries, tooth decay (Ch. 2)

cavity liner low-strength bases placed in the deepest portion of the cavity preparation, on the dentin or exposed pulp, which harden to form a cement layer to protect the pulp from chemical irritations and provide a therapeutic effect on the tooth (Ch. 28)

cavity preparation preparation for a restoration; technique depends on the amount and location of decay, degree of pulpal involvement, and type of materials used to restore the tooth (Ch. 28)

cavity varnish used to seal the dentin tubules to prevent acids, saliva, and debris from reaching the pulp; when used with cavity liner or medicated base, it is placed on top of these materials (Ch. 28)

cavosurface margin the angle that is formed by the junction of the wall of a cavity preparation and the untouched surface of the tooth; sealing of this margin is critical to prevent marginal leakage (Chs. 26 & 28)

cellulitis swelling and discomfort of facial tissues caused by an abscess (Ch. 18)

Celsius the centigrade measure of temperature; the freezing point is 0 degrees and the boiling point is 100 degrees (Ch. 11)

cement base high-strength bases of thick putty-like consistency placed on the floor of a cavity preparation to protect the pulp and provide mechanical support for the restoration; preparation, pulp sensitivity, and type of restoration indicate which cement to use (Ch. 28)

cementoblasts cementum-forming cells (Ch. 5)

cementum the tooth structure that is located around the root covering the dentin on the root portion of the tooth (Ch. 5)

Centers for Disease Control and Prevention (CDC) the organization that investigates, reports, and tracks specific diseases and public health concerns for the United States (Ch. 9)

central beam the primary ray emitting from the x-ray tube head (Ch. 17)

central vacuum system provides suction for saliva ejectors and oral evacuators (Ch. 14)

centric occlusion closing of the jaws in a position that produces maximal contact between the occluding surfaces of the maxillary and mandibular arch (Ch. 25)

cephalometric radiograph an extraoral radiograph showing a profile of the patient, including bones and tissues (Ch. 17)

cerebral embolism a blood clot that blocks the normal flow of blood to the brain (Ch. 13)

cerebral hemorrhage rupture of a blood vessel in the brain (Ch. 13)

cerebral infarction an interruption of the flow of blood to the brain (Ch. 13)

Certified Dental Assistant (CDA) a dental assistant who has obtained national certification through the Dental Assisting National Board (Ch. 1)

Certified Dental Technician (CDT) an individual who has successfully passed an examination in dental laboratory skills (Ch. 1)

cervical clamp double-bowed clamps used for Class V restorations on anterior teeth that assist in gingival retraction; often must be stabilized with stick impression compound after the teeth have been exposed (Ch. 28)

cervical line where the anatomical crown and root join together (Ch. 6)

Chauliac, Guy de (1300-1368) influential author on surgery who wrote rules for dental hygiene (Ch. 1)

check register a record of all checking account transactions; deposits to and checks made from the account are included (Ch. 29)

chemical retention attachment of materials to a surface achieved through a chemical reaction (Ch. 26)

chemically cured type of sealant material that is hardened by use of a catalyst and a base; also known as self-cure or autopolymerization (Ch. 28)

chuck a small metal cylinder in the head of the handpiece that holds rotary instruments (Ch. 15)

chyme mixture of food and gastric juices (Ch. 3)

cingulum a convex area found on the lingual surface of the anterior teeth near the gingiva (Ch. 6)

circumference the distance around (Ch. 28)

civil law law related to actions and circumstances between individuals; civil law can be broken down into contract law and tort law (Ch. 31)

classifications of motion the five classifications that show the amount of motion the dental team is involved with (Ch. 14)

cleft lip cleft in or separation of the upper lip; also known as harelip; failure of the maxillary processes to fuse with the medial nasal process (Chs. 5 & 20)

cleft palate a fissure in the roof of the mouth that forms a passage between the nasal cavities and the mouth; failure of the palatal shelves to fuse with the primary palate or with each other (Chs. 5 & 20)

cleft uvula the uvula is separated slightly (Ch. 5)

clinical crown exposed coronal portion of the crowns (Ch. 28)

coalesced fused together (Ch. 28)

collimator a device used to eliminate peripheral radiation (Ch. 17)

commissures corners of the mouth where the upper lip meets the lower lip (Chs. 4 & 11)

common carotid artery artery suppling blood to most of the head and the neck, divided into internal and external branches (Ch. 4)

composite direct, tooth-colored restorative material (Ch. 26)

Comprehensive Drug Abuse Prevention and Control Act of 1970 identifies drug according to five schedules of potential abuse. See pg. 208 in the text for the complete rundown of the schedule (Ch. 12)

compules single-application cartridges (Ch. 26)

computed tomography (CT) computer-produced image; also known as CT scanning (Ch. 17)

computerized system a unit of computer parts that function together to perform a particular task (Ch. 29)

cone cutting partial image created when the central beam misses the x-ray film (Ch. 17)

congestive heart failure a condition that occurs as the heart weakens, rendering it unable to achieve the level of cardiac output that meets the body's needs (Ch. 13)

connectors unite the various parts of the partial into one unit, holding working parts in the proper position (Ch. 25)

contamination the presence of an infectious agent (Ch. 9)

continuous simple sutures series of stitches that look like hem stitching, placed in areas of multiple extractions, and tied with a surgeon's knot at either end (Ch. 28)

continuous sling sutures series of sling stitches placed in areas where a large flap involving several teeth is used (Ch. 28)

contra-angle attachment head for the low-speed handpiece; contra-angles hold burs, discs, stones, rubber cups, and brushes for intraoral and extraoral procedures; type of Tofflemire retainer, placed on the lingual side, angled slightly to accommodate clearance of the anterior teeth (Chs. 15 & 28)

contract a binding agreement between two or more persons (Ch. 31)

coronal polish procedure whereby coronal surfaces of the teeth are polished with rubber cups, brushes, an abrasive, polishers, and dental tape (also known as prophylaxis) (Chs. 23 & 28)

corrective orthodontics the improvement of existing orthodontic problems (Ch. 21)

corrosion the result of chemical or electrochemical attacks (Ch. 26)

Council on Dental Therapeutics part of the ADA, this body gathers and releases to dentists information about drugs being used in dentistry (Ch. 12)

criminal law related to wrongs committed against the welfare and safety of society as a whole (Ch. 31)

cross-section technique technique used to expose occlusal radiographs (see procedure 17-3) (Ch. 17)

crown top or highest part of a tooth; often called a cap by the patient (Ch. 6)

curettes hand instruments used for removing subgingival calculus, smoothing the root surface, and removing the soft tissue lining of the periodontal pocket (Ch. 23)

curing light a high-intensity light that hardens or sets many dental materials (Ch. 14)

cusp a pointed or rounded mound on the crown of the tooth (Ch. 6)

Cusp of Carabelli a fifth cusp located on the mesial lingual surface of most maxillary first molars (Ch. 6)

cutting edge on a dental instrument, the sharpened edge used for refining the cavity preparation (Ch. 15)

cyst fluid-filled or semi-solid fluid-filled sac (Ch. 20)

daVinci, Leonardo (1452-1519) defined morphology of teeth (Ch. 1)

DDS doctor of dental surgery (Ch. 1)

debride to remove debris (dead tissue) (Ch. 28)

defamation of character causing injury to another's reputation, name, or character; this injury can be verbal or written (Ch. 31)

delivery systems types of dental units that are at various positions—such as front delivery, side delivery, and rear delivery—to accommodate dental team members (Ch. 14)

demineralization when the minerals calcium and phosphorus are lost from the enamel surface (Ch. 2)

dental (BIS-GMA) composites most commonly used as a sealant for occlusal pits and fissures; available in clear, opaque, and lightly-tinted colors (Ch. 28)

dental assistant an auxiliary to the dentist, he or she provides comfort to the patient and performs independent skills depending on the State Dental Practice Act; for example, exposing dental radiographs (Ch. 1)

Dental Assisting National Board, Inc. (DANB) the independent organization that administers the credentialing examinations for dental assistants (Ch. 30)

dental associate a hired dentist that works under contractual agreement, usually for a dentist that has a solo practice (Ch. 30)

dental casting alloy combination of metals (gold, iron, tin, zinc) used in crowns (Ch. 24)

dental dam latex material used to isolate teeth that are to be restored (Ch. 28)

dental dam clamp used to stabilize and secure the dental dam material in place; comes in numerous designs and sizes to fit around the teeth (Ch. 28)

dental dam forceps forceps with two beaks that fit in the holes of the jaws of the clamp; used to place and remove the dental dam clamp (Ch. 28)

dental dam frame holder designed to stretch and secure the dam in place across the patient's face; keeps the operating area open (Ch. 28)

dental dam napkin soft, pre-cut, disposable, absorbent fabric used for patient comfort and for absorbing saliva, water, and perspiration (Ch. 28)

dental dam punch similar in action to a paper punch, although much differently designed, with a sharp projection to punch through the dental dam to create holes for the teeth (Ch. 28)

dental fluorosis a condition caused by an excess intake of flourides during tooth development; enamel surface appears mottled and stained but is carie-free (Ch. 28)

dental hygienist a state licensed individual who specializes in the treatment of cleaning including plaque stain and calculus; also provides oral health education (Ch.1)

dental implants fixed prosthesis, attached to bone, used to replace missing teeth (Ch. 19)

dental jurisprudence the law(s) that govern dentistry (Ch. 31)

Dental Practice Act state regulations that describe legal restrictions and controls on the dentist, the hygienist, and other dental assistants (Ch. 31)

dental public health the specialty in dentistry that is concerned with dental disease; works with the community to promote dental health (Ch.1)

dental unit positioned according to the dentist, it consists of handpieces, air-water syringe, saliva ejector, oral evacuator (HVE), ultrasonic scaling unit, and numerous other options (Ch. 14)

dentifrice the toothpaste used with brushing and flossing for patient oral hygiene self-care (Ch. 2)

dentin makes up the bulk of the tooth structures located around the pulp cavity and under the enamel within the anatomical crown, and under the cementum within the root (Ch. 5)

dentinal tubules tubules that pass through the entire surface of the dentin and contain dentinal fluid (Ch. 5)

dentition natural teeth in position (Ch. 6)

denture a prosthesis that replaces missing teeth within the same arch; a full denture is used when all of the natural teeth are missing, a partial denture when some of the natural teeth are missing (Ch. 7)

denture base sometimes referred to as the saddle, denture teeth are held here (Ch. 25)

developer solution the first chemical solution used to process radiographs (Ch. 17)

developmental groove a groove formed by the uniting of lobes during development of the crown of the tooth (Ch. 6)

diabetes mellitus insufficient insulin production in the pancreas leading to high levels of glucose in the blood (Ch. 13)

diastolic blood pressure created as the arteries return to their original state when the heart relaxes between contractions (Ch. 11)

diet food an individual eats (Ch. 2)

digastric muscle muscle on the floor of the mouth that assists in the opening of the mouth (Ch. 4)

digital imaging technology imaging system that reduces x-rays received by the patient by over 90% (Ch. 17)

dimensional change change in length or volume of a material, usually from exposure to heat or cold (Ch. 26)

direct contact an individual has "direct contact" with a lesion or microorganism while performing intraoral dental procedures; acutal touching or first-hand contact (Ch. 9)

direct pulp capping (DPC) technique used to treat permanent tooth when pulp has been exposed due to mechanical or traumatic means but chance exists that pulp will still heal; involves placement of medicament directly over exposed pulp, followed by restoration of tooth (Chs. 22 & 28)

disinfection the process of killing pathogens by physical or chemical means; it does not destroy spores and resistant viruses (Ch. 9)

distal the surface of the tooth that is away from the midline (Chs. 6 & 7)

distortion a dimensional change in shape (Ch. 27)

distoversion a deviation in the positioning of a tooth; the tooth is distal to normal position (Ch. 21)

diuretics substances that cause the body to lose water (Ch. 2)

DMD doctor of medical dentistry (Ch. 1)

Doctrine of Respondeat Superior simply put, the dentist is responsible for the actions of the dental assistant, as well as any assistant; if there were a complaint or act of negligence on the assistants part, the dentist is liable for the act (Ch. 31)

dorsal surface on the back side of the body or organ (Ch. 3)

dorsal cavity posterior portion of the body, containing spinal canal and cranial cavity (Ch. 3)

double exposure a technique error where the film was exposed twice (Ch. 17)

down time time in the appointment book that is not being used for scheduled appointments (Ch. 29)

drifting movement of a tooth into the space created by a missing tooth (Ch. 7)

drug any substance that changes the body's life chemical processes (Ch. 12)

Drug Enforcement Agency (DEA) agency that regulates controlled substances; part of the Department of Justice (Ch. 12)

drug interaction the effect one drug can have on another when taken at the same time; intended results may be increased or decreased (Ch. 12)

dual-cured materials materials containing chemicals for self curing as well as materials that set by light curing (Ch. 26)

ductility the ability of a material to withstand forces of tensile stress without failing (Ch. 26)

duplication technique a technique whereby dental radiographs are reproduced on specialized film (Ch. 17)

ecchymosis the bruising of tissue (Ch. 20)

edema excessive amounts of fluid in body tissue; swelling (Ch. 13)

elastics rubber bands or elastic threads, often used between the upper and lower arches, providing force for movement (Ch. 21)

electronic pulp tester test, usually battery operated, that creates an electrical stimulus to the tooth indicating whether pulp is vital or non-vital (Ch. 18)

electromagnetic energy a form of energy that is the result of electric and magnetic disturbances in space (Ch. 17)

electrosurgery procedure that uses tiny electrical currents to incise gingival tissue and coagulate blood; setup consists of control box, foot-operated on-off controls, a termi-

nal plate that is placed behind patient's back or shoulders, and terminal probe with variety of cutting tips (Ch. 23)

electrosurgery unit tool which cauterizes tissues as it removes them in order to prevent bleeding (Ch. 28)

elevators instruments used to loosen and remove teeth, retained roots, and root fragments (Ch. 19)

elongation a technique error; the image of the teeth is lengthened (Ch. 17)

enamel hypocalcification soft and undercalcified tooth enamel (Ch. 2)

enamel hypoplasia incomplete development of tooth enamel (Ch. 2)

enamel tooth structure that covers the outside of the crown of the tooth; the hardest living tissue in the body (Ch. 5)

endocardium thin lining on the inside of the heart (Ch. 3)

endodontics the branch of dentistry that deals with the diagnosis and treatment of diseases of the pulp and the periapical tissues (Chs. 1 & 18)

endogenous originating from within the tooth (Ch. 28)

endosteal implant an implant placed into the bone surgically; these implants are used to replace a single tooth and for patients who are partially edentulous (Ch. 19)

Environmental Protection Agency (EPA) a regulatory agency involved in the safety and effectiveness of disinfecting and sterilizing solutions (Ch. 9)

epiglottis a leaf-shaped organ at the end of the larynx whose function is to close off the larynx during swallowing (Ch. 3)

epilepsy a recurrent disorder of cerebral function, due to excessive neuronal discharge (Ch. 13)

epithelial attachment the gingiva in the floor of the gingival sulcus that attaches to the enamel surface of the teeth just above the CEJ of the tooth (Ch. 5)

ergonomics study of work and space, including factors that affect worker's health, productivity, and mental well-being. (Ch. 29)

erythema redness or inflammation of the skin (Ch. 13)

essential amino acids (ten are needed) part of the protein molecule that the body cannot synthesize or produce; must be obtained through diet (Ch. 2)

ethics although different from person to person, ethics are what is morally right or wrong (Ch. 31)

ethmoid bone bone that forms part of the nose, orbits, and the floor of the cranium (Ch. 4)

etiologic agent a causative agent of a disease (Ch. 8)

etiology the cause of a disease (Ch. 20)

etiquette treating people/customers with respect; manners, politeness (Ch. 29)

excisional biopsy complete removal of a lesion along with a small border of the normal tissue surrounding it (Ch. 19)

exfoliative cytology removal of a layer of cells from the surface of a lesion (Ch. 19)

exhalation breathing out (Ch. 11)

exodontia the area of dental practice concerned with the extraction of teeth (Ch. 19)

exogenous originating from outside the tooth (Ch. 28)

exothermic reaction a chemical reaction that releases heat (Chs. 26 & 27)

expanded functions skills and functions beyond those normally associated with dental assisting that require increased skill and responsibility; expanded functions are delegated by the dentist according to the Dental Practice Act in their given state (Ch. 31)

expendable supplies that are used up or disposed of after use; for example, cotton balls and envelopes (Ch. 29)

expressed contract a contract, written or verbal, that specifically describes what each party in the contract will do (Ch. 31)

external jugular vein vein that drains the superficial veins of the face and neck into the subclavian vein (Ch. 4)

external oblique ridge extending from the mental foramen, follows the length of the body of the mandible past the last tooth and up to the ramus (Ch. 4)

external pterygoid muscles one of the muscles of mastication, opens jaw by depressing the mandible (Ch. 4)

extraction forceps instruments used to remove teeth from the alveolar bone (Ch. 19)

extraoral film film utilized outside the oral cavity (Ch. 17)

extrinsic stain discoloration on the outside of the tooth structure that can be removed by scaling and polishing; (Ch. 28)

exudate pus

facsimile (Fax) a communication system that sends and receives written messages through the telephone line (Ch. 29)

Farenheit system used to measure temperature; the freezing point is 32 degrees and the boiling point is 212 degrees (Ch. 11)

Fauchard, Pierre (1678-1761) founder of modern dentistry, organized all known information about dentistry and compiled it into a textbook (Ch.1)

Federation Dentaire Internationale (FDI) international system used for coding teeth and the oral cavity in charting (Ch. 7)

fever elevation of the body's temperature above the normal range (Ch. 11)

fiberoptic light source available with high-speed handpieces, fiberoptic systems greatly improve visibility of the treatment area for the operator (Ch. 15)

fibroblasts cells that form connective tissue (Ch. 5)

field block anesthesia an injection method that places the anesthetic solution near larger terminal nerve branches (Ch. 16)

file folders an envelope or book-type holder that stores patient information (Ch. 29)

files endontic instruments used to enlarge and smooth the canal (Ch. 18)

fissure a developmental groove that has an imperfect union where the lobes come together (Ch. 6)

fissured tongue a wrinkled, deeply grooved surface on the tongue (Ch. 20)

fistula a tube-like passage from an abscess to the external surface; used to drain the abscess (Ch. 18)

fixed appliance appiance attached to the teeth that cannot be removed by the patient; braces, for example (Ch. 21)

fixed prosthetic artificial part for missing tissue or tooth that becomes part of the natural dentition (Ch. 24)

fixer solution the second chemical solution used in processing radiographs (Ch. 17)

Flagg, Josiah a skilled surgeon for procedures in cleft lips, orthodontics, endodontics and operative dentistry; also designed the first dental chair (Ch.1)

flossing manual cleaning of the interproximal tooth surfaces (Ch. 2)

flour of pumice a relatively coarse (abrasive) material used to remove stains from enamel; should be followed by a fine polishing agent (Ch. 28)

flow continuing deformation of a solid; also referred to as creep and slump (Ch. 26)

fluoridation the process of adding fluoride to the water supply (Ch. 2)

fluoride a natural mineral nutrient that has been proven to make the tooth more resistant to tooth decay (Ch. 2)

fluoride systemic fluoride that is ingested and circulated through the body to the developing teeth, leaving the teeth more resistant to caries (Ch. 2)

fluoride topical fluoride that is applied to the outer layer of tooth enamel to make the tooth more resistant to caries (Ch. 2)

fluoropatite crystal new tooth structure formed when fluoride replaces the hydroxyl ion of the enamel (Ch.2)

fluorosis mottled enamel; results from excessive fluoride during tooth development; tooth enamel appears pitted and multicolored (Ch 2)

focal spot an area on the anode that electrons hit during the production of x-rays (Ch. 17)

focusing cup an area on the anode that directs the electrons to the focal spot during the production of x-rays (Ch. 17)

Food and Drug Administration a division of the United States Department of Health and Human Services that regulates the manufacturing and labeling of medical devices and solutions (Ch. 9)

Food and Drug Administration (FDA) a federal regulation agency (Chs. 9 & 12)

Fordyce spots sebaceous oil glands near the surface of the epithelium that appear in the oral cavity as round, yellow spots (Ch. 20)

foreign body airway obstruction (FBAO) obstruction of normal breathing; dental instruments, crowns, amalgams, composite, cotton rolls, and gauze are items that mat obstruct the airway (Ch. 13)

forensic dentistry an area of dentistry that deals with identification of an individual through tooth restorations and morphology utilizing dental records (Ch.1)

foreshortening a technique error whereby the image of the teeth is shortened (Ch. 17)

fossa a shallow rounded or angular depression (Ch. 6)

four-handed dentistry the dentist and dental assistant are working together at the dental chair (Ch. 14)

framework the skeleton of the removable partial to which rests, connectors, and retainers are attached (Ch. 25)

Frankfort plane the imaginary horizontal plane from the bottom of the eye socket to the top of the ear canal (Ch. 17)

free gingiva or marginal surrounds the teeeth and is attached only at the gingival groove, appears lighter in color (if healthy) and is about 1 mm in width (Ch. 5)

frenectomy complete surgical removal of the frenum, including the attachment to the underlying bone (Ch. 23)

frenum raised lines of mucosal tissue found in the vestibule areas of the oral cavity (Ch. 4)

frictional heat heat produced when a moving surface contacts another (Ch. 15)

fulcrum the support or point on which a level turns; for example, position of finger-rest for support when working in a patient's mouth (Chs. 14 & 28)

full-cast crown   full covering over a tooth that has extensive decay or damage (Ch. 24)

furcation   the dividing point of a multi-rooted tooth; division of the roots (Chs. 6 & 23)

galvanism   creation of electrical shock caused by two different metals coming together (Ch. 26)

gel   a solid (Ch. 27)

general anesthesia   anesthesia that causes the patient to become unconscious (Ch. 16)

generic names   drug names that are not protected by trademark, are less expensive than brand names, and may be used by any business (Ch. 12)

gingiva   composed of a mucosa that surrounds the necks of the teeth, and covers the alveolar processes (Ch. 5)

gingival grafting   procedure in which tissue is taken from one site and placed on another (Ch. 23)

gingival hyperplasia   an overgrowth of gingival tissue (Ch. 13)

gingival retraction   chemical, mechanical, surgical, or combination process used to ensure an impression with clear margins can be obtained when preparing a tooth for a crown (Ch. 28)

gingival sulcus   the space between the attached gingiva and the tooth (Ch. 5)

gingivectomy   surgical removal of diseased gingival tissue (Ch. 23)

gingivitis   inflammation of the ginigival tissues, marked by red, swollen, and/or bleeding gums; caused by buildup of plaque and calculus, poor fitting appliances, malocclusion, and may occur in association with certain systemic diseases, hormonal changes, or prolonged drug therapy (Ch. 23)

gingivoplasty   reshaping of the gingival tissue to remove deformities such as clefts, craters, and enlargements; performed only to recontour the gingiva (Ch. 23)

glass ionomer   permanent cementation with diverse types and applications: Type I is a finer grain that bonds chemically to teeth; Type II is coarser grain and is used in selected restorations; Type III is used as a liner and dentin bonding agent; Type IV is admixtures of glass ionomers used for build-ups (Ch. 26)

Glick #1   endontic instrument used to remove excess gutta percha (Ch. 18)

glutaraldehyde   solution used for high-level disinfection and sterilization (Ch. 9)

gold foil   a restoration created when several layers of pure gold are placed in the cavity preparation (Ch. 7)

Good Samaritan Law   protection for people that provide medical assistance to those in emergency situations that are not seeking payment for it; those providing the assistance are given immunity (Ch. 31)

grand mal seizure   seizure marked by person becoming unconscious, the body jerking, twitching, and stiffening; they usually last 2 to 5 minutes (Ch. 13)

granuloma   a neoplasm or tumor filled with granulation tissue (Ch. 20)

Gray (GY)   the Systeme Internationale unit of absorbed dose of ionizing radiation (Ch. 17)

green stain   discoloration most frequently found in children; found on the facial surface of the maxillary anterior teeth at the cervical third, containing chromogenic bacteria and fungi; varies from light to dark green or yellowish-green (Ch. 28)

gross income   the total accounts receivable (Ch. 29)

guide channels   slots in the end of a retainer that hold the matrix band and direct the band to the right or left of the retainer (Ch. 28)

gutta percha   filling material; usually thermoplastic in nature (Ch. 18)

gypsum   calcium sulfate dihydrate; used when pouring an impression to make a model; water-powder ratio dictates strength, accuracy, resistance, reproduction detail, and setting times (Ch. 27)

habit forming   drugs that lead to psychological or physical dependency (Ch. 12)

halitosis   bad breath (Ch. 2)

hallucinate   a drug reaction that causes the user to see images and hear sounds that do not actually exist (Ch. 12)

hand-over-mouth (HOM) technique   act by which a medical or dental professional places his or her hand over the patient's mouth and calmly explains behavior expectations; informed consent is required (Ch. 22)

handpieces   instrument used with rotary burs, discs, and stones; connected to power, air, and water sources (Ch. 14)

hard deposits   hard, calcified deposit (mineralized plaque) firmly attached to teeth, restorations, and dental appliances; also called calculus or tartar (Ch. 28)

hardware   physical equipment used by the computer system to process data (Ch. 29)

Harris, Chapin A. (1806-1860)   along with Horace Hayden, founded the first dental college in the world; the Baltimore College of Dental Surgery (Ch. 1)

Hayden, Horace (1769-1844)   along with Chapin A. Harris, founded the first dental college in the world; the Baltimore College of Dental Surgery (Ch.1)

headgear   orthodontic appliance comprised of a strap that goes behind the patient's head or neck, and a facebow that attaches to buccal tubes on molar bands, applying force to move teeth, restrain or alter facial bone growth, and reinforce stability of intraoral appliances (Ch. 21)

hematoma   appearing as a bruised area, it is a lesion caused by bleeding from a ruptured blood vessel (Ch. 20)

hemiplegia   weakness, numbness, or paralysis on one side of the body (Ch. 13)

hemisection   surgical removal of one root and the overlying crown (Ch. 18)

hemostasis   to stop bleeding (Ch. 3)

hemostats   a forceps instrument used during surgery to retract tissue, remove small root tips, clamp off blood vessels, and grasp loose objects (Ch. 19)

hepatitis   inflammation of the liver; usually caused by a virus, but sometimes originating from toxic agents (Ch. 8)

herpes labialis   a form of Herpes Simplex Type I; also known as fever blisters (Ch. 20)

herpes zoster   unilateral, painful lesions that can last up to five weeks; also known as shingles (Ch. 20)

herpetic gingivostomatitis   inflammation of the gingiva caused by a virus (Ch. 20)

herpetic whitlow   exposure to the Herpes virus that manifests itself as a crusting ulceration on the fingers or hands; may be very painful (Ch. 20)

herringbone pattern   a cross pattern that appears on film that has been placed backward in the mouth; caused by the pattern on the lead foil (Ch. 17)

high volume evacuation (HVE) a device used by the dental assistant to remove fluids from the patient's mouth; also called the oral evacuator (Ch. 14)

high-speed handpiece handpiece used for rapid cutting of tooth structure and finishing of restorations; rotates between 10,000 and 800,000 rpm (Ch. 15)

high-strength base cement bases including glass ionomers, hybrid ionomers, reinforced zinc oxide eugenol, zinc phosphate, and polycarboxylate (Ch. 28)

Hippocrates (460-377 BC) father of medicine; attempted to explain health and disease

histamine chemicals released by specialized cells as the body responds to disease and injury; brings about the inflammation process (Ch. 20)

hoe scalers instrument with sharp, beveled, 90-degree angled blade, which, when placed in the periodontal pocket to the base, and pulled toward the crown of the tooth with even pressure, planes and smooths the root surface (Ch. 23)

homeostasis cells, tissues, organs, and systems all functioning together to maintain harmony within the body (Ch. 3)

homogenous uniformly mixed (Ch. 27)

horizontal angulation the adjustment of angulation from left to right; improper angulation shows teeth overlapping (Ch. 17)

horizontal mattress suture used when suturing a flap, it goes in and out of the tissue on the same surface; identified by horizontal stitch or "bite"; tied with one surgeon's knot on surface where suture procedure began (Ch. 28)

human immunodeficiency virus (HIV) the AIDS virus; it ultimately destroys immune system cells (Chs. 8, 9 & 20)

humectant material or substance that retains moisture (Ch. 28)

hydrogen peroxide popular bleaching agent used to whiten teeth (Ch. 28)

hydroxyl ion located on the surface of the apatite crystal in the enamel (Ch. 2)

hyperkeratinized epithelium tissue that has built up a layer of keratin as a protective coating (Ch. 20)

hyperplasia excess tissue; in dentistry, resulting from ill-fitting dentures that initially cause small ulcers, which, after continued irritation, become folds of excess tissue (Ch. 20)

hyperventilation abnormally rapid and deep breathing, resulting in decreased levels of carbon dioxide (Ch. 13)

hypothermic having a body temperature below normal (Ch. 11)

imbibition enlargement due to the absorption of fluid or swelling (Ch. 27)

imbrication lines small curved lines running parallel to the CEJ located near the gingival area of the labial of the crown of a tooth (Ch. 6)

implied consent consent for a given procedure given by the patient's actions; for example, a patient that rolls up his or her sleeve for a blood pressure reading or to receive an injection (Ch. 31)

implied contract a contract implemented by actions, not words (Ch. 31)

impression compound thermoplastic impression material, rigid at mouth temperature (Ch. 28)

incipient beginning tooth decay that has not broken through the enamel into the dentin (Ch. 7)

incisal edge cutting or tearing edge of the anterior teeth (Ch. 6)

incisional biopsy removal of a small section of a lesion along with a small border of normal tissue (Ch. 19)

incisive nerve branch innervating the anterior teeth and the labial gingiva; it is a branch of the inferior alveolar nerve (Ch. 4)

incisive papilla a raised area of tissue lying behind the maxillary central incisors (Ch. 4)

indirect contact an individual has contact with a microorganism through means such as contaminated instruments, supplies, and equipment. (Ch. 9)

indirect pulp treatment (IPT) technique used when treating permanent teeth with potentially infectious tissue (due to caries or traumatic injury), when pulp is not exposed but when chance exists that pulp will be exposed during tissue removal; also known as indirect pulp capping (Chs. 22 & 28)

infection control methods to eliminate or reduce the transmission of infectious microorganisms (Ch. 9)

inferior alveolar nerve branch a main branch of the mandibular nerve (Ch. 4)

infiltration anesthesia an injection method that places anesthetic solution into the tissues, near the small terminal nerve branches for absorption (Ch. 16)

inflammation body's defense against infection or trauma; redness, pain, and swelling may occur (Ch. 20)

informed consent agreement by the patient to the procedure that is about to be performed after being told of the procedure, risks involved, expected outcome, and alternative treatments; patient acknowledges his or her understanding and acceptance by signing (Chs. 19 & 31)

inhalation breathing in, in the administration of drugs, the patient breathes in the gas or aerosol; an individual contacts a microorganism by "breathing it in"; (Chs. 9, 11 & 12)

inhaler a pressurized canister with a mouthpiece that administers antihistamines to a user (Ch. 13)

inlay a restoration replacement for missing tooth structure within the tooth; covered are the area between the cusps in the middle of the tooth and the proximal surfaces (Ch. 24)

innocuous causing no harm (Ch. 20)

inscription name of the drug prescribed and the dosage; the inscription appears within the prescription (Ch. 12)

intensifying screens screens used with extraoral films found in cassettes (Ch. 17)

interceptive treatment prevention and treatment of orthodontic problems (Ch. 21)

interdental aids aids used to clean the area between the teeth and stimulate the gingival tissue in that area (Ch. 2)

interdental knife periodontal knives used to remove soft tissue interproximally; spear-shaped with long narrow double-edged blades (Ch. 23)

internal jugular vein receives blood from the cranium, face, and neck and drains into the brachiocephalic vein, then into the superior vena cava, which drains into the heart (Ch. 4)

internal oblique ridge (mylohyoid ridge) follows the inside of the ramus and the body of the mandible (Ch. 4)

internal pterygoid muscles one of the muscles of mastication that elevates the mandible (Ch. 4)

interproximal radiographs, also known as bite-wing radiographs (Ch. 17)

interproximal brushes small, soft-bristled brushes attached to a metal or plastic handle for cleaning open contact areas, around orthodontic braces and wires, around exposed bifurcation or trifurcation of the roots, or on abutment teeth of hygienic bridge (Ch. 28)

intracanal instruments instruments used in endontics with precise diameters and lengths and which are made of stainless steel and nickel titanium alloy wire (Ch. 18)

intradermal administering drugs by injection under the epidermis (Ch. 12)

intramuscular administering drugs by injection into muscle tissue (Ch. 12)

intraoral camera a small camera attached to the intraoral wand that transmits images to a television monitor (Ch. 14)

intraoral film utilized inside the oral cavity (Ch. 17)

intravenous administering drugs by injecting directly into the vein (Ch. 12)

intrinsic stain discolorations, usually permanent, within the tooth structure (Ch. 28)

inverting tucking of the dental dam material around the teeth to prevent moisture leakage (Ch. 28)

iodophor solution used as an intermediate-level disinfection agent (Ch. 9)

irreversible hydrocolloid commonly called alginate, it is the material used in the formation of dental impressions; setting of the material is accomplished by a chemical reaction (Ch. 27)

irreversible pulpitis inflammation of the pulpal tissue to the point where it cannot recover; treatment includes root canal or extraction (Ch. 18)

ischemia shrinking of tissues (Ch. 28)

Jacksonian epilepsy characterized by a patient that remains conscious during their seizure, recalling details of the events (Ch. 13)

jugular vein vein that drains the blood from the cranium, face, and neck (Ch. 4)

Kaposi's sarcoma malignant neoplasm, normally flat, reddish purple to dark blue in appearance, most commonly occurring in AIDS patients and men over 60 (Ch. 20)

Kells, C. Edmond the first dentist to hire a female dental assistant (1885) (Ch.1)

key hole punch the largest hole punched in the dental dam; slides over the clamp and onto the anchor tooth; point from which next holes are punched (Ch. 28)

kilovoltage (kV) unit of electrical potential equal to 1,000 volts; dental kilovoltage is responsible for the quality of radiographs or penetrating power (Ch. 17)

labial the surface of the anterior tooth that is toward the lips (Chs. 6 & 7)

labial commissures the corners of the mouth, where the upper and lower lips meet (Ch. 4)

labio-mental grooves the groove just below the lower lip that separates the lip from the chin (Ch. 4)

laboratory area of the dental office where non-patient work is performed; for example, it may be used for finishing crowns, bridges, etc. (Ch. 14)

lacrimal bones small delicate bones forming part of the corner of the eye; anterior to the ethmoid bone (Ch. 4)

lamina dura radiopaque line that represents the thin compact alveolus bone lining the socket (Ch. 5)

laryngopharynx the lower section of the pharynx (Ch. 3)

latent period the time lapsed between the exposure and the response; for example, the time between exposure to the sun and production of a sunburn (Ch. 17)

lateral toward the outside or away from the midline (Ch. 3)

leakage radiation the radiation comes out in all directions from the tube or tube head due to a malfunction or leakage (Ch. 17)

lesions term used to describe tissue damage; in dentistry, term for all abnormal structures in the oral cavity (Ch. 20)

ligature a piece of floss or a cord that stabilizes the dental dam in different applications; used in fixed bridge isolation, bleaching procedures, and individual teeth isolation (Ch. 28)

ligature wire a thin, flexible wire that holds the arch wire to the brackets (Ch. 21)

light-cured type of sealant that is hardened by use of a single-component system activated by a curing light (Chs. 26 & 28)

light-cured materials materials that are set by means of a curing light (Ch. 26)

linea alba raised white line on the buccal mucosa that runs parallel to where the teeth meet (Ch. 4)

liner material placed in a thin layer on the walls and floor of the cavity preparaton (Ch. 26)

lingual the surface of the tooth that is toward the tongue (Chs. 6 & 7)

lingual nerve branch the nerve that innervates the floor of the mouth, ventral side of the tongue, tastebuds on the anterior two-thirds of the tongue, and the lingual gingiva (Ch. 4)

linguoversion a deviation in the positioning of a tooth; the tooth is lingual to normal position (Ch. 21)

lobe term often used to describe the separate divisions that come together to form a tooth. Often in the molars, the lobes become cusps (Ch. 6)

local anesthesia anesthesia that produces a deadened or pain-free area (Ch. 16)

long wavelengths in dental radiographs, wavelengths have low energy, low frequency, and are unsuitable for exposing dental radiographs (Ch. 17)

low-speed handpiece handpiece used to polish teeth and restorations, remove soft carious material, and define cavity margins and walls; rotates between 6,000 and 25,000 rpm (Ch. 15)

low-strength base also referred to as cavity liners, materials placed on dentin or on exposed pulp to protect the pulp from chemical irritation and provide therapeutic effect to the tooth; include calcium hydroxide, zinc oxide eugenol, and glass ionomer (Ch. 28)

lumbar lower region of the back (Ch. 14)

luting bonding or cementing together (Ch. 26)

luxate to move or dislocate; for example, the dentist uses forceps to luxate a loose tooth from the socket (Ch. 19)

macule a spot on the skin of abnormal texture or color (Ch. 20)

magnetic resonance imaging (MRI) technique used mainly in the diagnosis of TMJ disease; allows the dentist to look at soft tissues of TMJ with little risk to the patient (Ch. 17)

malleability the ability of a material to withstand compressive stresses without fracturing (Ch. 26)

malnutrition a disorder resulting from lack of correct nutrients for the body (Ch. 2)

malocclusion any deviation from normal occlusion; may be a missing tooth, group of teeth, or entire arch (Ch. 21)

malpractice   incorrect or negligent treatment given to a patient by their doctor, dentist, or health care provider (Ch. 31)

mamelons   three bulges on the incisal edge of the newly erupted central incisor (Ch. 6)

mandibular arch   lower arch in the dentition (Ch. 6)

mandrels   rods of various lengths used in low-speed hand-pieces; mandrels are available in three shanks—latch, friction grip, or straight (Ch. 15)

manual processing   processing of dental x-rays using a manual tank with developer, running water, and fixer (Ch. 17)

marginal ridge   elevated areas of enamel which form the mesial and distal borders of the lingual surface on the anterior teeth and the mesial and distal borders of the occlusal surface of the posterior teeth (Ch. 6)

Maryland bridge   a resin retained fixed bridge that replaces one tooth (Ch. 24)

masseter muscles   one of the four pairs of muscles of mastication (Ch. 4)

master cone   the primary cone, normally gutta percha, used in a root canal (Ch. 18)

materia alba   soft, bulky, cottage cheese-like mass of food debris and bacterial growth that collects in grooves and spaces on teeth, gingiva, and appliances, which provides the source for plaque development (Ch. 28)

Material Safety Data Sheets (MSDS)   health and safety information about each chemical, provided by the manufacturer (Ch. 10)

matrix   an essential artificial wall used to replace the missing or removed surfaces of a tooth during the filling of a cavity; comprised of a band and a retainer (Ch. 28)

maturation   growth to and learning on a certain level (Ch. 22)

maxillary arch   upper arch in the dentition (Ch. 6)

maxillofacial   branch of dentistry focusing on diagnosis and treatment of diseases, injuries, and malformations (Ch. 19)

Maximum Possible Dose (MPD)   the maximum dose of radiation that, in light of present knowledge, would not be expected to produce negative effects in a life

mechanical bond   bonding of sealant accomplished as sealant flows into the irregularities of the treated enamel and locks into place (Ch. 28)

mechanical retention   the attachment of materials to surfaces by means of grooves in the cavity preparation (Ch. 26)

medicine   drugs that are used to treat diseases (Ch. 12)

mentalis muscle   one of the major muscles of facial expression (Ch. 4)

mesial   the surface of the tooth that is toward the midline (Chs. 6 & 7)

metabolism rate   the physical and chemical changes that take place in relationship to the usage of energy (Ch. 20)

metallic stains   discoloration of the teeth due to metals and metallic salts inhaled (in industrial settings), taken orally in certain drugs, or as part of the materials used in tooth restoration; copper dust, amalgam, iron dust, and iron drugs can cause permanent stains (Ch. 28)

microleakage   the seepage of saliva and debris from the oral cavity between the tooth structure and restorative materials (Ch. 26)

midline or median line   imaginary line that divides the dental arches into two halves (Chs. 5 & 6)

milliamperage (mA)   a measurement unit for electrical current (Ch. 17)

minerals   inorganic element or compounds necessary to regulate body function; positive or negatively charged, referred to as electrolytes (Ch. 2)

mitosis   cell division in the sex cells in which the number of chromosomes in each is reduced by one-half (Ch. 17)

mobile carts   movable cart that contains dental equipment (Ch. 14)

mobility   tooth movement in the socket; may be due to periodontal disease or trauma (Ch. 7)

modeling technique   technique that aims to modify a patient's undesirable behavior by pairing the patient with another who demonstrates more desirable behavior (Ch. 22)

modified pen grasp   the grasping of an instrument as one would with a pen, except the pad of the middle finger is placed on the top of the instrument with the index finger (Ch. 14)

monangle   a dental instrument with a shank which has one angle (Ch. 15)

monomer   self-curing acrylic tray resin (liquid catalyst) (Ch. 27)

mottled enamel   fluorosis (Ch. 2)

mouth guards   protective device used to prevent premature loss or fracture of teeth (Ch. 22)

mouth props   a device used to prevent the patient from closing the mouth (Ch. 19)

mucogingival junction   the line of demarcation between the attached gingiva and the alveolar mucosa (Ch. 5)

mucogingival surgery   reconstructive surgery on the gingiva and/or mucosa tissues; involves covering exposed roots, increasing the width of gingival tissue, and reducing frenum or muscle attachments (Ch. 23)

mucoperiosteum   mucosa and periosteum surfaces that combine to form a membrane (Ch. 19)

muscle trimming   molding the borders of the custom tray to achieve margin adaption of the tray prior to final edentulous impression (Ch. 25)

myelin sheath   the protective and insulating covering of some nerves (Ch. 3)

myocardial infarction   a condition in which the coronary arteries are blocked or severely narrowed; also known as a heart attack (Ch. 13)

myocardium   a tough muscular wall (middle layer) of the heart (Ch. 3)

Nasmyth's membrane   a covering over the enamel of newly erupted primary teeth left over from the epithelium and the ameloblasts (Ch. 5)

nasopharynx   the first section of the pharynx, located behind the nasal cavity (Ch. 3)

National Fire Protection Association's color and number method   labeling system for hazardous chemicals using data from MSDS sheets (Ch. 10)

needle holders   hemostat-like instrument with a grooved beak used to hold the suture needle (Ch. 19)

neonatal teeth   those teeth present at birth or within the first month after birth (Ch. 20)

neoplasm   an abnormal growth that can be either malignant (cancerous) or benign (non-cancerous); a tumor (Ch. 20)

nerve block anesthesia   injection of anesthesia near a main nerve trunk (Ch. 16)

net income   the accounts payable subtracted from the gross income (Ch. 29)

nitrous oxide   an odor-free gas derived from nitrogen and oxygen, used as a sedative prior to anesthesia; relieves anxiety and fear (Ch. 16)

nodule(s)   small lump of tissue, either hard or soft, usually more than ¼ inch in diameter (Ch. 20)

non-anatomical   term for describing posterior denture teeth; non-anatomical lack detailed anatomy on the occlusal, usually a concave and flat surface (anatomical teeth have cusps and developmental grooves) (Ch. 25)

non-cutting   instruments not used for cutting tooth structure; for example, mouth mirrors and cotton pliers (Ch. 15)

non-expendable   supplies that are not used up or disposed of after use; for example, the dental chair or an autoclave (Ch. 29)

non-vital pulp   the pulp of the tooth that does not respond to sensory stimuli (Ch. 18)

normal occlusion   the term that describes the contact relationship of the mandibular arch with the maxillary arch (Ch. 21)

nursing bottle syndrome   extensive decay of the newly formed teeth due to the sweetened liquid frequently bathing the teeth (Ch. 2)

nutrients   any chemical substance present in food that provides the body tissues and structures with the elements that are necessary for growth, maintenance, and repair (Ch. 2)

nutrition   the manner in which foods are used to meet the body's needs (Ch. 2)

objective fears   fears based on a person's own experiences (Chs. 6 & 22)

oblique ridge   elevated areas of enamel which extend obliquely across the occlusal of the tooth (Ch. 6)

obturating   the process of filling the root canal (Ch. 18)

occlusal   chewing surface of the molars and pre-molar teeth (Chs. 6, 7 & 28)

occlusal equilibration   process of alleviating areas with an excessive force (Ch. 23)

occlusal radiographs   the radiograph that exposes either the maxillary or mandibular occlusal surface of the dental arch (Ch. 17)

Occupational Safety and Health Administration (OSHA)   regulating body that enforces the requirements established for employers to protect their employees (Chs. 9 & 10)

odontoblasts   dentin-forming cells (Ch. 5)

onlay   replacement for missing tooth structure within the tooth (Ch. 24)

open bay   treatment area designed with several dental chairs arranged in one open area; reassuring for patients to see others experiencing similar treatment (Ch. 22)

operating light   adjustable light used by the dentist during examinations and procedures (Ch. 14)

opportunistic infections   infections resulting from a weakened immune system (Ch. 20)

oral   the taking of medications by mouth; usually in tablet, capsule, pill, or liquid form (Ch. 12)

oral and maxillofacial surgery   the dental specialty concerned with the diagnosis and surgical treatment of the oral and maxillofacial region (Chs. 1 & 19)

oral hypoglycemics   drugs taken orally that lower blood sugar levels (Ch. 13)

oral pathology   a dental specialty concerned with the diagnosis and nature of the diseases that effect the oral cavity (Chs. 1 & 20)

oral prophylaxis   two-fold procedure involving removal of hard deposits and polishing of the teeth with a rubber cup (Ch. 28)

oral vestibule   the pocket formed by the soft tissue of the cheeks and gingiva (Ch. 4)

orifice   openings of the salivary glands (Ch. 20)

oropharynx   the middle section of the pharynx, located behind the mouth (Ch. 3)

orthodontic bands   stainless steel bands that are fitted around each tooth to hold and control tooth movement (Ch. 21)

orthodontics   the dental specialty concerned with the diagnosis and supervision and guidance and correction of the malocclusion in the dental facial structures (Chs. 1 & 21)

orthognathic surgery   surgery involving the face, maxilla, and mandible (Ch. 19)

osseointegration   compatible interface between the bone and the dental implant (Ch. 19)

osseous surgery   restoration of bone by removal of defects and deformities caused by periodontal disease and related conditions; can be either additive (augmentive) or subtractive (Ch. 23)

ostectomy   form of osseous surgery in which deformed bone is removed (Ch. 23)

osteoblasts   bone-forming cells (Chs. 3 & 5)

osteoclasts   dissolve and reabsorb the calcium salts of the bone matrix when bone is stressed or damaged (Ch. 3)

osteomyelitis   an advanced stage of periapical infection that spreads into and through the bone (Ch. 18)

osteoplasty   form of osseous surgery in which deformed bone is reshaped (Ch. 23)

other potentially infectious materials (OPIM)   any materials or bodily fluids other than blood; precautions should be taken to avoid contact (Chs. 9 & 10)

over-the-counter drugs (OTC)   drugs that can be purchased without a prescription (Ch. 12)

overbite   the projection of the upper teeth over the lower (Ch. 21)

overdenture   retained roots providing support to a complete or partial denture (Ch. 25)

overhang   excess restorative material projecting over the cavity margin (Ch. 7)

overlap of time   when a doctor/dentist is required to be in two different places at the same time, or when two patients are scheduled for treatment at the same time (Ch. 29)

overlapping   an x-ray technique error resulting from improper horizontal angulation (Ch. 17)

overtime   the patients estimated treatment time goes beyond what was scheduled (Ch. 29)

packing slip   a list included with supply shipments stating everything that was included; contents of the package should be checked against the packing slip to make sure there are no discrepancies (Ch. 29)

palm grasp   the holding of an instrument in the palm of the hand (Ch. 14)

Palmer System for numbering   system of teeth identification that numbers permanent teeth 1 through 8, divided into quadrants; the deciduous teeth are labeled A through E, also by quadrants. (Ch. 7)

palm-thumb grasp the grasping of an instrument that has the handle in the palm of the hand, four fingers wrapped around the handle, and the thumb extended upward from the palm (Ch. 14)

palpation examining the body with the hands or fingers for detection of abnormalities, checking pulse rate, etc. (Chs. 11 & 20)

panoramic technique rotation system used when taking radiographs that captured the entire dental arch on one film (Ch. 17)

papilla small, raised projection covering the dorsal side of the tongue (Ch. 4)

papule a small, solid, raised area of skin less than ½ inch in diameter (Ch. 20)

paralleling technique x-ray technique, also known as the right angle technique, whereby the film and tooth and PID are parallel (Ch. 17)

parenteral piercing of the mucous membranes of the skin through such events as needlesticks, cuts, and abrasions (Chs. 10 & 12)

parotid glands the largest of the salivary glands (Ch. 4)

partial denture prosthetic device containing artificial teeth supported on a metal framework and attached by clasps to natural teeth (Chs. 7 & 25)

partial seizure divided into two categories, they can be simple (patient remains conscious and remembers all of the event) or complex (patient is unconscious, remembers very little and experiences involuntary actions) (Ch. 13)

partnership a legal agreement that makes both doctors and dentists responsible for accounts payable; partners are not responsible for malpractice suits against the other (Ch. 30)

patch an area of the skin that is different in color or texture (Ch. 20)

pathogenic causing disease (Ch. 9)

pathogens disease-producing microorganisms (Chs. 8 & 9)

patient records a patient history; examined prior to procedures to see if there were any previous problems or concerns (Ch. 14)

pediatric dentistry the dental specialty concerned with prevention of oral disease, diagnosis, and treatment of oral care in children from birth to adolescence (Chs. 1 & 22)

pedodontics dental care for children (Ch. 22)

pellicle thin, clear film of insoluble proteins, fats and other materials from saliva that forms within minutes of removal; may protect enamel or provide breeding ground for plaque and calculus (Ch. 28)

pen grasp the grasping of an instrument in the same manner as one would with a pen or pencil (Ch. 14)

percussion examination of a tooth by tapping on the occlusal or incisal surface with fingers or instruments (Ch. 18)

periapical abscess a localized destruction of tissue and accumulation of exudate in the periapical region (Ch. 18)

periapical film x-ray showing the tooth and surrounding tissues (Ch. 17)

pericardial around the heart (Ch. 10)

pericardium a double-wall sac that forms the outer layer of the heart (Ch. 3)

periodontal dressing bandage-like material applied to protect a surgical site as it heals (Ch. 23)

periodontal flap surgery surgical separation of the gingiva from the underlying tissue (Ch. 23)

periodontal knives instruments used to remove gingival tissue during periodontal surgery; also known as gingivectomy knives (Ch. 23)

periodontal ligament connective tissue that secures the tooth into the socket with a number of organized fiber groups (Ch. 5)

periodontal pocket a space in the gingival sulcus (beyond the normal 1 - 3 mm) created by periodontal disease (Chs. 7 & 23)

periodontal probe calibrated instrument used to measure depth of periodontal pockets, areas of recession, bleeding, or exudate; primary instrument used in periodontal examinations (Ch. 23)

periodontal probing measuring of the depth of the periodontal pocket with a periodontal probe (Ch. 23)

periodontics the dental specialty concerned with the diagnosis and treatment of the diseases of the supporting and surrounding tissues of the tooth (Chs. 1 & 23)

periodontitis the formation of periodontal pockets, occurring when margins of the gingiva and periodontal fibers recede and the supporting bone becomes inflamed and destroyed (Ch. 23)

periodontium a collective term for the periodontal tissues (Chs. 5 & 23)

periosteal elevators used to reflect soft tissue away from the bone; usually double-ended, with one long-tapered end and one round-bladed end (Chs. 19 & 23)

periosteum a tough fibrous layer of tissue covering compact bone (Ch. 3)

peritoneal abdominal (Ch. 10)

personal computer (PC) a desktop computer; microcomputer (Ch. 29)

personal protective equipment (PPE) items that should be worn to protect against contact with all body fluids; protective eyewear, for example (Ch. 9)

petechiae small red or purple spots that appear on the skin or mucosa tissue (Ch. 20)

petit mal seizure seizure marked by a momentary loss of consciousness; usually lasts 5 to 10 seconds (Ch. 13)

petty cash small amount of money kept in the office for unexpected or emergency situations (Ch. 29)

pharmacology the study of all drugs (Ch. 12)

philtrum vertical groove on the midline of the upper lip (Ch. 5)

Physician's Desk Reference (PDR) published annually, the PDR is a comprehensive listing of drugs and drug information; drugs are listed by trade or product name, generic and chemical name, and category (Ch. 12)

pit area on occlusal surface of the teeth where the grooves come together or the fissures cross (Ch. 6)

plaque any raised or flat patch in the oral mucosa; common cause of inflammation of gingival tissues; is a sticky mass that contains bacteria and grows in colonies on the teeth. (Chs. 2, 20 & 23)

pleural pertaining to the pleura; the membrane surrounding the lungs (Ch. 10)

pocket marking pliers instrument with two "beaks" that when pinched together leave small pin-point perforations on the gingival tissue; used to transfer measurement of a pocket to the outside of the tissue so the operator can see the depth level of the pocket (Ch. 23)

polishing process of using fine abrasives to produce a smooth, glossy surface (Ch. 28)

polycarboxylate   type of permanent cementation for crowns, bridges, inlays, onlays, and orthodontic bands and brackets; sets in 3-5 minutes, does not exhibit exothermic heat (Ch. 26)

polymer   self-curing acrylic tray resin (powder) (Ch. 27)

polymerization   process by which a material changes from a plastic pliable state into a rigid state (Chs. 27 & 28)

polynitrile autoclavable gloves   sterilizable gloves used for disinfection and sterilization (Ch. 9)

polysulfide   material used in taking final impressions; comprised of a base and lead peroxide accelerator, resulting in good stability, accuracy, sharpness of detail, and a relatively long shelf-life (Ch. 27)

pontic   portion of a bridge that replaces the missing tooth (Ch. 24)

porcelain-fused-to-metal crown   crown that has a veneer (veneers are used to cover badly stained teeth and to reshape the anatomy of teeth) (Ch. 24)

posterior (teeth)   the molars in the primary dentition and the premolars and molars in the permanent dentition (Ch. 6)

post-retained cores   a metal post fitted into the pulp canal of an endodontically treated tooth for retention of a crown (Ch. 24)

power bleaching   multi-step application of bleaching liquids or gels, often with application of heat or curing light; patient's teeth are isolated to protect chemical irritation to the gingiva (Ch. 28)

prescriptions   an authorization written by a doctor, dentist, or other that makes specific drugs available to patients (Ch. 12)

primary radiation   the central beam that comes from the x-ray tube head (Ch. 17)

primer   conditioner used before a bonding material is placed (Ch. 26)

prophylaxis   procedure whereby soft and hard deposits are removed from teeth; includes scaling and polishing (Ch. 23)

prosthesis   a replacement for a missing body part; in dentistry, missing teeth and tissues are replaced with artificial structures (Chs. 24 & 25)

prosthodontics   the dental specialty concerned with the diagnosis and restoration and maintenance of oral function with replacement of missing teeth and supporting structures through artificial means (Chs. 1, 24 & 25)

proximal   nearest the point of attachment (Chs. 3 & 28)

psychological dependence   a person who develops an emotional need for taking a drug, even though there may no longer be a physical need to take it (Ch. 12)

pulp   vascular and nerve network of fleshy connective tissue that fills the center of the tooth in the cavity formed by the dentin (Ch. 5)

pulpal floor   the surface overlapping the pulp on the floor of the cavity preparation; also called a pulpal wall (Ch. 28)

pulpal necrosis   the death of pulpal cells; often results from irreversible pulpitis (Ch. 18)

pulpectomy   non-vital pulp therapy involving tooth extraction and complete removal of the pulp (Chs. 18 & 22)

pulpotomy   removal of pulp exclusively in the coronal portion of the tooth (Chs. 18 & 22)

purpura   small purplish or reddish-brown areas or spots caused by bleeding in underlying tissues (Ch. 20)

purulence   containing pus (Ch. 8)

pustule   small, pus-containing blister (Ch. 20)

radiation absorbed dose (rad)   amount of ionizing radiation absorbed in a substance

radiolucent   a black region on the x-ray indicating where radiation passed through the tissue (Ch. 17)

radiopaque   a white or light region on the x-ray indicating where radiation was blocked by tissue or a substance (Ch. 17)

radiosensitive   condition of being sensitized and effected by radiant energy (Ch. 17)

reamers   endodontic instrument with a tapered metal shaft used to clean and enlarge a root canal (Ch. 18)

reception room   the area that the patient initially enters in the dental office (Ch. 14)

recession   the movement of gingival tissue away from the tooth (Ch. 23)

reciprocity   one who has passed the medical/dental requirements for one state that applies for the same "rights" in another state, without taking another written or clinical examination (Ch. 31)

rectal   administration of drugs through the anus; enemas and suppositories may be used (Ch. 12)

relative biological effectiveness (REB)   measurement unit used to compare the biological effects of different tissues irradiated by different forms of radiation (Ch. 17)

reline   resurfacing of the under surface or tissue surface of a full or partial denture to improve the fit (Ch. 25)

removable appliances   devices that are inserted into the mouth and removed by the patient; retainers, for example (Ch. 21)

resin cements   type of permanent cementation for cast crowns, bridges, inlays, onlays, and endodontic posts (Ch. 26)

resorption   the body's process of removing existing bone (Ch. 21)

restoration   an agent used to replace missing tooth structure; known to most as "fillings" (Ch. 7)

rests   the part of the removable partial denture that contacts a tooth to provide vertical and horizontal support (Ch. 25)

retainers   used to tighten and support the matrix band on the tooth while the tooth is being restored; part of a partial denture that contacts the abutment teeth and prevents the partial from moving (Chs. 25 & 28)

retention pins   small metal pins placed for retention of a restoration (Ch. 24)

reticulation   a processing error that shows on the dental film when the film emulsion is exposed to extreme temperature variations; normally shows as pitting or wrinkling of the emulsion (Ch. 17)

retractors   oral surgery instrument that clears tissue from the surgical site (Ch. 19)

retrograde filling   a filling material placed in the apex of a tooth during an apicoectomy (Ch. 18)

reverse palm-thumb grasp   grasping with the evacuator tip held in the palm of the hand, thumb directed toward the assistant instead of toward the patient (Ch. 14)

reversible hydrocolloid   sometimes referred to as agar-agar; material used in formation of dental impressions that can be converted from a gel to a sol back to a gel due to thermal reaction; produces accurate impressions (Ch. 27)

reversible pulpitis inflammation of the pulp caused by an irritant; when irritant is removed, pulp will heal (Ch. 18)

revolutions per minute (rpm) used to determine speeds for dental handpieces (Ch. 15)

rheostat a foot pedal on a dental handpiece that controls the speed of the handpiece (Ch. 14)

ridge a linear elevation of enamel found on the tooth (Ch. 6)

Roentgen the amount of radiation that will ionize one cubic centimeter of air (Ch. 17)

roentgen equivalent man (rem) a radiation unit of measurement (Ch. 17)

Roentgen, Wilhelm Conrad (1845-1923) discovered x-rays in 1895 (Chs. 1 & 17)

rongeurs forceps with sharp-cutting edges used to trim and shape the alveolar bone following tooth extraction (Ch. 19)

root amputations surgical procedure to remove one or more roots of a multi-rooted tooth (Ch. 18)

root canal procedure where the pulp is removed and replaced with a filling material (Ch. 7)

root canal sealer cement used with gutta percha to seal the pulp canal (Ch. 18)

root planing process of smoothing the root surface with curettes and other periodontal instruments to leave a smooth root surface (Ch. 23)

root tip picks delicate instrument used to tweese the root tips or fragments from the bone socket (Ch. 19)

rotary instruments instruments that are mechanically driven (Ch. 15)

rubber stops pieces of rubber placed on files and reamers to mark the length of the root canal (Ch. 18)

saliva ejector a low-volume suction device that removes saliva and fluids from the patient's mouth (Ch. 14)

scaling technique to remove plaque, calculus, and stains from the surfaces of the teeth (Ch. 23)

scatter radiation radiation that is deflected from its path as it strikes matter (Ch. 17)

sealant enamel sealant is a resin material used to seal pits and fissures to prevent future decay (Ch. 7)

secondary radiation formed when the primary X-rays strike the patient or come in contact with any matter or substance (Ch. 17)

sedative palliative effect a soothing effect a material may have (Ch. 26)

self-curing materials that set by means of a chemical reaction (Ch. 26)

separators devices placed in the contact areas between teeth, forcing teeth to spread apart to accommodate the orthodontic bands; the separators are placed a few days before the patient is to have bands placed (Ch. 21)

septum amount of dental dam that slides between the teeth (Ch. 28)

shade guide samples of tooth shades used for tooth-colored restorations and denture teeth (Ch. 24)

shaft the handle of an instrument (Ch. 15)

shank the section of the instrument that connects the handle to the working end (Ch. 15)

Sharpey's fibers collagen fibers from the periodontal ligament, found within the outer part of the cementum (Ch. 5)

short wavelengths radiation wavelengths that have high frequency, high energy, and high-penetrating power; also known as hard radiation (Ch. 17)

sickle scalers sharp hand instruments used to remove hard deposits such as supragingival and subgingival calculus from the teeth (Ch. 23)

side effect an unintended result from the use of a drug (Ch. 12)

sievert a radiation unit of measurement (Ch. 17)

silicones material available in various forms used in taking final impressions; benefits include high rate of accuracy, no shrinkage, dimensional stability, high tear resistance, no taste and no odor (Ch. 27)

simple suture most versatile, widely used stitch; suture goes into the facial surface and emerges from the lingual surface, and is tied with a surgeon's knot (Ch. 28)

six-handed dentistry the dentist and two dental assistants are working together at the dental chair (Ch. 14)

sling suture used for interproximal suturing, stitch wraps around tooth to act like a sling; especially useful when a flap is necessary (Ch. 28)

smear layer layer of debris (created when the dentin is cut with a bur during cavity preparation) that lays on the cavity floor and walls and prevents contact between the intact dentin and the bonding agent/adhesive (Ch. 26)

smile line position of the lips when the patient smiles (Ch. 11)

sodium perborate popular bleaching agent used to whiten teeth (Ch. 28)

soft deposits acquired dental pellicle, materia alba, food debris, and plaque, removed during coronal polish (Ch. 28)

software the computers program (set of instructions) that tells the hardware what to do (Ch. 29)

sol a liquid (Ch. 27)

soluble the ability of a material to dissolve in a fluid (Ch. 26)

Southard, Juliette founded the American Dental Assistants' Association in 1924 (Ch. 1)

space maintainer a band and a wire loop that are soldered together providing a space for the permanent tooth to erupt after the premature loss of the primary tooth (Ch. 21)

space maintainers devices (either fixed or removable) designed to hold a space (left from the premature loss of a primary tooth) until the permanent tooth erupts (Chs. 21 & 22)

sphenoid one of the bones of the cranium, it is a wedge-shaped bone that goes across the skull anterior to the temporal bones (Ch. 4)

sphygmomanometer instrument used to measure blood pressure (Ch. 11)

spot-welded matrix bands custom-made bands constructed with the use of a spot-welding unit and used in class II restorations; does not require a retainer (Ch. 22)

spreaders endontic instrument used when sealing the root canal (Ch. 18)

springs specially bent or shaped wires attached to the main arch wire; used to exert pressure on teeth (Ch. 21)

stainless steel crown   used in the restoration of badly decayed teeth; usually used as a space maintainer in primary tooth replacement, or as temporary crown to be replaced by cast gold or porcelain (Ch. 22)

standard precautions   precautions developed in 1996 by the Centers for Disease Control (CDC) that augment universal precautions and body substance isolation practices (Ch. 9)

status epilepticus   the experience of continually having one seizure after another (Ch. 13)

statutes   a law enacted by a state (Ch. 31)

sterilizing area   area of the dental office where all sterilization procedures are performed (Ch. 14)

sternum   the breastbone (Ch. 13)

stethoscope   instrument used to listen to body sounds; for example, heartbeat and breathing (Ch. 11)

stomedeum   primitive mouth (Ch. 5)

strain   change or deformation of an object brought about by the object's resistance to a stress (Ch. 26)

stress   reaction of an object to resist an external force (Ch. 26)

stroke   a disruption of the blood flow to the brain because of a ruptured or blocked blood vessel (Ch. 13)

study models   diagnostic casts (Ch. 27)

subcutaneous   beneath the skin (Ch. 12)

subgingival   below the gingival margin (Ch. 28)

subjective fears   fears based on feelings, attitudes and concerns that have developed from suggestions by others (Ch. 22)

sublingual   in the administration of drugs, this method places the medication under the tongue and lets it dissolve (Ch. 12)

sublingually   placed under the tongue (Ch. 13)

subperiosteal implant   implanted beneath the periosteum, placed on top of the bone (Ch. 19)

subscription   part of the prescription, it is the area where the doctor writes the name and strength of the drug being prescribed, the doseage, and the form in which the drug is to be dispensed (Ch. 12)

subsupine position   the patient is in a reclined position with the head lower than the feet (Ch. 14)

succedaneous (teeth)   permanent teeth that replace primary teeth (Ch. 6)

supernumerary teeth   extra teeth, usually dwarfed in size or shape (Ch. 20)

superscription   part of the prescription directly below the heading used for filling in patient information; includes blank lines where the dentist can fill in the name and address of the patient, space for when the prescription was written, patient's phone number, age, gender, etc. (Ch. 12)

supine position   the patient is in a reclined position with the nose and knees on the same plane (Ch. 14)

supplemental groove   shallow linear grooves that radiate from the developmental groove (Ch. 6)

supragingival   above the gingival margin (Ch. 28)

surgical bone file   instrument used to trim and smooth the edges of the alveolar bone following tooth extraction (Ch. 19)

surgical chisels   instruments used to remove or shape the bone (Ch. 19)

surgical currettes   instrument used for debridement of the tooth socket or diseased tissue (Ch. 19)

surgical mallets   instrument (shaped like a small hammer and used with a chisel) used to remove bone (Ch. 19)

surgical scalpels   surgical knives used to incise or excise soft tissue in a precise manner with the least amount of trauma (Chs. 19 & 23)

surgical scissors   instrument, made of stainless steel and available in a variety of sizes, used to cut sutures and trim soft tissues (Ch. 19)

symmetric   shape, size, and relative position of body parts on opposite sides are equal; for example, when dividing the face into halves, both halves would be mirror images of each other (Ch. 11)

syncope   fainting (Ch. 13)

syneresis   shrinkage from a loss of water content due to heat, dryness, or exposure to air (Ch. 27)

synovial   pertaining to the lubricating fluid of the joints (Ch. 10)

systolic blood pressure   created when the heart contracts and forces blood through the arteries (Ch. 11)

tachycardia   abnormally rapid heart rate (Ch. 11)

tachypnea   abnormally rapid respiratory rate at rest (Ch. 11)

T-band matrix   restorative band made of brass strips that are crossed at one end; secured on primary teeth; adjustable, do not require a retainer (Ch. 22)

tell, show, and do technique   a technique for easing a patient's fears by introducing the patient to the instrument to be used, deomonstrating its use, then actually performing the technique (Ch. 22)

template   a guide showing either the adult or pediatric arches indicating where the holes for the teeth should be punched (Ch. 28)

temporal muscles   one of the four pairs of muscles of mastication (Ch. 4)

tetracycline stain   discoloration of the teeth resulting from high concentrations of tetracycline antibiotics taken during the time the tooth was developing; vary in color from light green or yellow to dark gray-brown (Ch. 28)

The Pure Food and Drug Act   passed in 1906 by the United States government, this act controlled and regulated the composition, sale, and distribution of drugs (Ch. 12)

The Pure Food, Drug, and Cosmetic Act   passed in 1938, this act made it mandatory for the FDA to have control of all food, cosmetics, and drugs sold, as well as their advertising (Ch. 12)

thermal properties   heat-related characteristics of a material (Ch. 26)

thermionic emission   the process of heating the current to an extremely high temperature to allow electrons to be given off (during radiation production) (Ch. 17)

thrush   fungal infection of candidiasis in children, appearing as a thick white covering over the oral mucous membrane (Ch. 20)

tickler file   a system that serves as a reminder that events are to take place on specific dates (Ch. 29)

tissue forceps   instruments used to hold and retract tissue during dental procedures (Ch. 19)

tobacco stain   discoloration (light brown to black) of the teeth caused by coal tar combustion in cigarettes and pigments from chewing tobacco penetrating the pits and fissures on the enamel and dentin surfaces (Ch. 28)

tongue thrust habit whereby a person's (usually a child's) tongue pushes against the anterior teeth during swallowing, causing an anterior open bite (Ch. 22)

tooth mobility movement of the tooth within the socket (Ch. 23)

topical anesthetic anesthesia that numbs the area about to be injected with local anesthesia; the patient willl not feel the pain of the needle (Ch. 16)

topically administration of drugs to the skin's surface, usually in ointment, lotion, gel, or cream form; in dentistry, topical drugs are sometimes used as anesthesia prior to surgery (Ch. 12)

topographic technique technique used to expose occlusal radiographs (Ch. 17)

tort a wrongful act that results in injury to one person by another (Ch. 31)

transcraniam temporo mandibular joint radiograph radiograph taken with the patient holding a cassette against the side of the head (see pg. 365) (Ch. 17)

transient ischemic attacks a temporary interruption in the supply of blood to the brain; symptoms include weakness, dizziness, and loss of balance (Ch. 13)

transillumination test reflection of fiberoptic light through the crown of a tooth to indicate vertical fractures (Ch. 18)

transverse ridge the union of two triangular ridges produces a single ridge of elevation across the occlusal surface of a posterior tooth (Ch. 6)

treatment room area of the dental office where the actual patient examination is performed (Ch. 14)

Trendelenburg position positioning the patient so the head is low and the legs are slightly elevated (Ch. 13)

triangular ridge a ridge or elevation that descends from the cusp and widens as it runs down to the middle area of the occlusal surface (Ch. 6)

trifurcated when there are three roots coming from the main trunk of the tooth (Ch.6)

triturate to mechanically combine dental materials (Ch. 14)

tubehead where the X-ray tube and step-up and step-down transformers are located (Ch. 17)

ulcer an open sore, usually inflamed and painful, that forms on tissue (Ch. 20)

ultrasonic instruments instruments used to remove hard deposits, stains, and debris through use of high-power vibrations during scaling, curettage, and root planing procedures (Ch. 23)

ultrasonic scaler through a vibrating action, this device removes hard deposits, such as calculus, from teeth (Ch. 14)

unconscious a person who is unable to respond to any sensory stimulation (Ch. 13)

undercuts recessed areas that are wider on the bottom than on the top (Ch. 27)

undernourished lacking the proper nutrients (Ch. 2)

universal distress signal clutching of the throat with the hands (the signal that lets others know you are choking) (Ch. 13)

universal precautions guidelines established by the Centers for Disease Control (CDC) that help protect health care workers and patients from the transmission of infectious diseases (Ch. 9)

Universal/National System for numbering adopted in 1968 by the ADA, this numbering system identifies the teeth. Permanent teeth are numbered (maxillary right to left; mandibular left to right) 1 to 32; primary teeth are labeled A to T (Ch. 7)

urticaria eruption of wheals (welts) on the skin; also known as hives (Ch. 13)

usual, reasonable, and customary fees the amount charged (fee) typically levied by the doctor/dentist for specific procedures; usual is the fee typically charged, reasonable is the midrange of fees charged for the specific procedure, and customary is the average charge physicians levy for the same procedure (Ch. 29)

uvula small soft structure that hangs from the soft palate above the rest of the tongue (Ch. 4)

varnish thin layer of material that is placed to seal the walls and floor of a cavity preparation (Ch. 26)

vasoconstrictors drugs added to anesthetic solutions that constrict blood vessels around the injection site, reducing the blood flow in the area (Ch. 16)

veneers used to cover badly stained teeth and to reshape the anatomy of teeth, veneers are a thin layer of tooth-colored material that covers much of the facial surface (Ch. 24)

ventral cavity the anterior portion of the body (Ch. 3)

vermilion border the line around the lips (Chs. 4 & 11)

vertical angulation the adjustment of angulation from top to bottom; improper vertical angulation shows teeth elongated or foreshortened (Ch. 17)

vertical dimension the space provided by the teeth in normal occlusion, or, with the teeth in occlusion, a measurement of the face at the midline (Ch. 25)

vertical mattress suture used when suturing a flap, goes in and out of the tissue on the same surface; identified by vertical stitch or "bite"; tied with one surgeon's knot on surface where suture procedure began (Ch. 28)

vesicles small, fluid-filled blisters (Ch. 20)

viscosity the ability of liquid to flow (Ch. 26)

vital pulp term used to describe healthy pulp (Ch. 18)

vital signs the basic signs of life; for example, body temperature, pulse, blood pressure, and respiration rate (Ch. 11)

vitamin class of nutrients that do not provide the body with energy but are used to perform other necessary functions (Ch. 2)

walking bleach technique technique utilizing thick paste of hydrogen peroxide, sodium perborate, or a combination of the two, placed in the coronal portion of the nonvital tooth; heat application helps achieve desired results (Ch. 28)

wedge small triangular piece of wood or plastic (Ch. 28)

wettability the ability of a material to flow over a surface (Ch. 26)

Wickham's striae interlacing white lines formed by a grouping of white papules; usually on the buccal mucosa (Ch. 20)

winged clamp clamp with extra projections (wings) that are angled toward the gingiva for better retraction and holding of the dental dam (Ch. 28)

wingless clamp clamp with no projections (wings) and with the letter W in front of the number of the clamp (Ch. 28)

withdrawal the symptoms that occur when a person addicted to a drug stops taking it; nervousness, stomach cramps, diarrhea, shaking, and depression may be symptoms (Ch. 12)

working end part of the instrument that actually performs the specific function (Ch. 15)

xerostomia dryness of the mouth caused by reduction in the amount of saliva (Ch. 2)

x-ray tube part of the dental X-ray unit that houses the coolidge, vacuum tube, filters, collimator, and cone (Ch. 17)

x-rays invisible, odorless electromagnetic radiation (Ch. 17)

yellow stain discoloration of the teeth usually associated with poor oral hygiene and plaque; dull yellow to light brownish in color (Ch. 28)

zinc oxide eugenol type of temporary cementation of crowns, inlays, onlays, and bridges (Ch. 26)

zinc phosphate permanent cement for crowns, inlays, onlays, bridges, and orthodontic bands and brackets (Ch. 26)

zirconium silicate material used for stain removal and polishing on gold restoration, exposed dentin, tooth-colored restoration, and enamel (Ch. 28)

zygomatic bones bones that form the cheeks (Ch. 4)

zygote stage during which cells proliferate (Ch. 5)

REFERENCES

American Dental Assistants Association. (1991). *Introduction to Basic Concepts in Dental Radiography.* Chicago: ADAA.

American Dental Association, Council on Dental Education (1992, revised 1993). *Annual Surveys of Allied Dental Education Programs.* Washington, D.C.: U.S. Department of Health and Human Services, U.S. Department of Labor.

American Dental Association. (1994). *Dental Teamwork,* vol. 7(1). Chicago: The Association.

American Dental Association, Department of Education Surveys. (1993). *Number of Accredited Dental Hygiene Programs* Chicago: The Association.

American Dental Association, Department of Education Surveys. (1993). *Number of CDA Accredited Dental Assisting Programs.* Chicago: The Association.

American Dental Association, Department of Education Surveys. (1992–92). *Allied Dental Education.* Chicago: The Association.

American Dental Association, Department of Legal Affairs. (1992). OSHA: *What You MUST Know.* Chicago: The Association.

American Dental Association. (1994). *OSHA: Refresher Course.* Chicago: The Association.

American Dental Association. (1994). *ADA Principles of Ethics and Code of Professional Conduct.* Chicago: The Association.

American Heart Association. (1992). *Recipes for Low-fat Low-Cholesterol Meals.* Dallas: The Association.

American Heart Association. (1991). *The American Heart Association Diet: An Eating Plan for Healthy Americans.* Dallas: The Association.

Anderson, K.N., Anderson L.E., Ganze W.D. (1993). *Mosby's Medical Nursing, & Allied Health Dictionary,* 4th ed. St. Louis: Mosby.

Anderson, Pauline C., Burkard, Martha R. (1995). *The Dental Assistant,* 6th ed. Albany: Delmar Publishers.

Anderson, P.C., Clifford, S.B. (1981). *Dental Radiology.* Albany, NY: Delmar Publishers.

Appleton & Lange's 1998 Drug Guide (1998). Connecticut: Appleton and Lange.

Ash, M. (1993). *Occlusion,* 4th ed. Philadelphia: W.B. Saunders.

Ash, M.M. (1993). *Wheeler's Atlas of Tooth Form,* 5th ed. Philadelphia: W.B. Saunders.

Babbush, C.A., Fehrenback, M. (1991). *Illustrated Dental Embryology, Histology, and Anatomy.* Philadelphia: W.B. Saunders.

Bath-Balogh, M., Fehrenbach, M.J. (1997). *Illustrated Dental Embryology, Histology, and Anatomy.* Philadelphia: W.B. Saunders.

Beirle, J.W. (1993). *Dental Operatory Water Lines,* 211(2), 13–15. C.D.A.J.

Bergman, R., Adel, K., Heidger, P. (1996). *Histology.* Philadelphia: W.B. Saunders.

Berkovitz, B.K.B., Holland, G.R., Moxham, B.J. (1992). *A Color Atlas and Text of Oral Anatomy, Histology, and Embryology.* St. Louis: Mosby.

Bhaskar, S.N. (1991) *Orban's Oral Histology and Embryology,* 11th ed. St. Louis: Mosby.

Bloodborne Diseases in the Workplace, Trainers Manual (1992). Spokane, WA.: Scenic Bay Publications.

Bork, K. (1996). *Diseases of the Oral Mucosa and the Lips.* Philadelphia: W.B. Saunders.

Bowen, R.F., Marjenhoff, W.A. (1993). *Adhesion of Composites to Dentin and Enamel, 21(6)* 19–22. C.D.A.J.

Brand, R.W., Isselhard, D.E. (1998). *Anatomy of Orofacial Structures,* 6th ed. St. Louis: Mosby.

Bressman, J.K. (1993). Risk Management for the '90s. 124-63-67. J.A.D.A.

Burnstein, L., Burnstein, R.S. (1985). *Interviewing: A Guide for Health Professionals.* Connecticut: Appleton-Century-Crofts.

Burt, B.A., Eklund, S.A. (1992). *Dentistry, Dental Practice, and the Community,* 4th ed. Philadelphia: W.B. Saunders.

Burton, G., Engelkirk, P. (1996). *Microbiology for the Health Sciences,* 5th ed. Philadelphia: J.B. Lippincott Co.

Carranza, F., Newman, M. *Clinical Periodontology,* 8th ed. Philadelphia: W.B. Saunders.

Carter, L.M., Yaman, P. (1981). *Dental Instruments.* St. Louis: Mosby.

Chapman, S. (1998). *Medical & Dental Associates, P.C. Insurance Forms Preparation,* 3rd ed. Albany: Delmar Publishers.

Chasteen, J.E. (1990). *Essentials of Clinical Dental Assisting,* 4th ed. St. Louis: Mosby.

Chernega, J.B. (1994). *Emergency Guide for Dental Auxiliaries,* 2nd ed. Albany: Delmar Publishers

Christensen, G.J. (1994). *A Buyer's Guide to Dentistry.* St. Louis: Mosby.

Christensen, G.J. (1992). *Complex Fixed and Implant Prosthodontics: Making Nearly Foolproof Impressions, 123,* 69–70. J.A.D.A.

Christensen, G.J. (1993). *Removable Prosthodontic Impressions, 124,* 112–113. J.A.D.A.

Corcoran, J.F. (1992). *Endodontics I,* 3rd ed. Ann Arbor, Mich.: University of Michigan. Dental Publications.

Coleman, G.C. (1993). *Principles of Oral Diagnosis.* St. Louis: Mosby.

Commission on Dental Accreditation, Council on Dental Education of the American Dental Association. (1993). *New Faces for Allied Dental Education.* Chicago: The Association.

Cottone, J.A., Terezhalmy, G.T., Molinari, J.A. (1996). *Practical Infection Control in Dentistry,* 2nd ed. Philadelphia: Lea & Febiger.

Council on Dental Materials, Instruments and Equipment. (1994). *Choosing intracoronal restorative materials, 125,* 102–103. J.A.D.A.

Craig, R.G., O'Brien W.J., Powers, J.M. (1996). *Dental Materials: Properties and Manipulation,* 6th ed. St. Louis: Mosby.

Craig, R.G. (1993). *Restorative Dentistry Materials,* 9th ed. St. Louis: Mosby.

Crispin, G.J. (1993). *Expanding the Application of Facial Ceramic Veneers 21(6),* 43–54. C.D.A.J.

Dale, B.G., Ascheim, K.W. (1993). *Esthetic Dentistry: A Clinical Approach to Techniques and Materials.* Philadelphia: Lea & Febiger.

Darby, M., Walsh, M. (1995). *Dental Hygiene Theory and Practice.* Philadelphia: W.B. Saunders.

Dejong, R.H. (1993). *Local Anesthetics.* St. Louis: Mosby.

De Lyre, W.R., Johnson, O.N. (1995). *Essentials of Dental Radiography for Dental Assistants and Hygienists,* 5th ed. Connecticut: Appleton & Lange.

Dental Dam Procedures, 9th ed. (1992). Akron, OH: Hygienic Corp.

Department of Veterans Affairs, American Dental Association, Department of Health and Human Services, Washington, DC: Learning Resources Services.

Dionne, R.A. (1992). *Preventing and treating postoperative pain, 123,* 27–34. J.A.D.A.

Dofka, C. (1996). *Competency Skills for the Dental Assistant.* Albany, NY: Delmar Publishers.

Dorland's Pocket Medical Dictionary, 27th ed. (1995). Philadelphia: W.B. Saunders.

Drafke, M.W. (1994). *Working in Health Care: What You Need to Know to Succeed.* Philadelphia: F.A. Davis.

Dunlap, C., Barker, B.F. (1991). *Oral Lesions,* 3rd ed. Kansas City, Mo: Colgate-Hoyt.

Egelbery, J., Badersten, A. (1994). *Periodontal Examination.* Sweden: Munksgaard.

Ehrlich, A. (1996). *Medical Terminology for Health Professions,* 3rd ed. Albany, NY: Delmar Publishers.

Ehrlich, A. (1994). *Nutrition and Dental Health,* 2nd ed. Albany, NY: Delmar Publishers.

Ehrlich, A., Torres, H.O., Bird, D. (1996). *Essentials of Dental Assisting,* 2nd ed. Philadelphia: W.B. Saunders.

Eversole, L. (1996). *Oral Medicine: A Pocket Guide.* Philadelphia: W.B. Saunders.

Fanning, M. (1997). *HIV Infection: A Clinical Approach,* 2nd ed. Philadelphia: W.B. Saunders.

Fedi, P.F. Jr., Bernino, A.R. (1995). *The Periodontic Syllabus,* 3rd ed. Baltimore: Williams and Wilkins.

Fehrenbach, M., Herring, S. (1996). *Illustrated Anatomy of the Head and Neck.* Philadelphia: W.B. Saunders.

Ferracane, J.L. (1995). *Materials in Dentistry.* Philadelphia: J.B. Lippincott Co.

Finkbeiner B.L., Finkbeiner, C.A. (1996). *Practice Management for the Dental Team,* 4th ed. St. Louis: Mosby.

Finkbeiner, B.L., Johnson, C.S. (1995). *Comprehensive Dental Assisting.* St. Louis: Mosby.

Finkbeiner B.L., Patt J.C. (1990). *Practice Management for the Dental Team,* 3rd ed. St. Louis: Mosby.

Fordney, M.T. (1997). *Insurance Handbook for the Medical Office.* Philadelphia: W.B. Saunders.

Frommer H.H. (1992). *Radiology for Dental Auxiliaries,* 5th ed. St. Louis: Mosby.

Genco, R.J., Goldman, H.M., Cohen, D.W. (1990). *Contemporary Periodontics.* St. Louis: Mosby.

Gershoff, S. (1990). *The Tufts University Guide to Total Nutrition.* New York: Harper & Row.

Glenner, R.A. (1984). *The Dental Office Pictorial History.* Montana: Pictorial Histories Publishing Company.

Gluck, G., Morganstein, W. (1998). *Jong's Community Dental Health,* 4th ed. St. Louis: Mosby.

Gooch, B.F., Cardo, D.M. (1995). *Percutaneous exposures to HIV infected blood 126,* 1237–1242. J.A.D.A.

Goran, K. (1992). *Pedodontics: A Clinical Approach,* 2nd ed. St. Louis: Mosby

Graber, T.M., Vanarsdall R.L. (1994). *Othodontics: Current Principles and Techniques,* 2nd ed. St. Louis: Mosby.

Grembowski, D. (1992). *How fluoridation affects adult dental caries, 123,* 49–54. J.A.D.A.

Guerini, V. (1909). *A History of Dentistry from the Most Ancient Times Until the End of the 18th Century.* Philadelphia: Lea & Febiger.

Hamilton, E.M.N., Whitney, E.N., Sizer, F.S. (1991). *Nutrition: Concepts and Controversies.* St. Paul: West Publishing.

Haring, J.I., Lind, L.J. (1993). *Radiographic Interpretation for the Dental Hygienist.* Philadelphia: W.B. Saunders.

Harris, N., Christen, A. (1995). *Primary Preventive Dentistry,* 4th ed. Stamford: Appleton & Lange.

Haveles, E.B. (1997). *Pharmacology for Dental Hygiene Practice.* Albany, NY: Delmar.

Hazard Communication Program. (1992). Michigan: Health Career Learning Systems, Inc.

Helgeson, B. (1974). *American Dental Assistants Commemorate 50th Anniversary, 89,* 539–544. J.A.D.A.

Herman, W. (1996). *Angina: An update for dentistry, 127,* 98–102. J.A.D.A.

History of the American Dental Assistants Association. (1970). Chicago: American Dental Assistants Association.

Hoag, P.M., Pawlak, E.A. (1990). *Essentials of Clinical Periodontology,* 6th ed. St. Louis: Mosby.

Hodges, K. (1997). *Concepts in Nonsurgical Periodontal Therapy.* Albany: Delmar Publishers.

Houston, W.J.B., Stephens, C.D. (1992). *A Textbook of Orthodontics.* Santa Rosa: Redwood Press.

Hughes, T. (1992). *Electronic claims filing shows dramatic growth, 82(2),* 80–83. Dental Economics.

Ibsen, O.A., Phelan, J. (1996). *Oral Pathology for the Dental Hygienist,* 2nd ed. Philadelphia: W.B. Saunders.

Incorporating New Technologies in Periodontal Diagnosis into Training Programs and Patient Care. (1992). *A Critical Assessment and a Plan for the Future. New England Journal of Medicine 63, (4)* 383–393.

Infection Control in Modern Dental Practice. (1992). Rochester, NY: Eastman Kodak Co.

Ingersoll, B.D. (1986). *Patient Management Skills for Dental Assistants and Hygienists.* Connecticut: Appleton-Century-Crofts.

Intraoral Radiography with Rinn SCP/BAI Instruments. (1993). Elgin, IL: Rinn Corp.

Jablonski, S. (1982). *Illustrated Dictionary of Dentistry.* Philadelphia: W.B. Saunders.

Jacob, J.A. *New technology can remineralize teeth, 23(18)* 27. A.D.A. News

Jocobsen, P., Carpenter, W., Cunny, E. (1992). *Bloodborne exposure incidents: Complying with OSHA regulations, 20,* 8. C.D.A.J.

Karst, N.S., Smith, S.K. (1998). *Dental Anatomy, a Self Instructional program.* Connecticut: Appleton & Lange.

Kasle, M.J. (1989). *An Atlas of Dental Radiographic Anatomy,* 3rd ed. Philadelphia: W.B. Saunders.

Kodak Recommended Dental Films & Intensifying Screens. (1993). Rochester: Eastman Kodak Co.

Kratochbil, F.J. (1988). *Partial Removable Prosthodontics.* Philadelphia: W.B. Saunders.

Kumar, V., Cotran, R.S., Robbins, S.F. (1992). *Basic Pathology,* 5th ed. Philadelphia: W.B. Saunders.

Langlais, R., Miller, C.S. (1992). *Color Atlas of Common Oral Diseases.* Philadelphia: Lea & Febiger.

Langlais, R., Kasle, M. (1992). *Exercises in Oral Radiographic Interpretation,* 3rd ed. Philadelphia: W.B. Saunders.

Leimone, C.A., Earl, E.M. (1988). *Dental Assisting Basic and Dental Sciences.* St. Louis: Mosby.

Lindh,W.Q., Pooler, M.S., Tampero, C.D., & Cerrato, J.U. (1998). *Comprehensive Medical Assisting.* Albany NY: Delmar Publishing.

Little, J., Falace, D., Miller, C., Rhodus, N. (1997). *Dental Management of the Medically Compromised Patient,* 5th ed. St. Louis: Mosby.

Mahan, L.K., Escott-Stump, S. (1996). *Krause's Food, Nutrition, and Diet Therapy,* 9th ed. Philadelphia: W.B. Saunders.

Malamed, S.F. (1997). *Handbook of Local Anesthesia,* 4th ed. St. Louis: Mosby.

Malamed, S.F. (1993). *Managing Medical Emergencies, 124,* 40–52. J.A.D.A.

Malamed, S.F. (1993). *Medical Emergencies in the Dental Office.* St. Louis: Mosby.

Malamed, S.F. (1993). *Pain and anxiety control in dentistry, 21, 10,* 35–41. C.D.A.J.

Malamed, S.F., Sheppard G.A. (1993). *Handbook of Medical Emergencies in the Dental Office,* 4th ed. St. Louis: Mosby.

Manson-Hing, L.R. (1991). *Fundamentals of Dental Radiography.* Philadelphia: Lea & Febiger.

Matteson, S.R., Whaley C., Secrist, V.C. (1988). *Dental Radiology,* 4th ed. Chapel Hill: University of North Carolina Press.

Mauriello, S., Overman, V., Platin, E. (1995). *Radiographic Imaging for the Dental Team.* Philadelphia: J.B. Lippincott Co.

McMinn, R., Hutching, R., Logan, B. (1995). *Color Atlas of Head and Neck Anatomy,* 2nd ed. St. Louis: Mosby-Wolfe.

Meltzer, M., Palau, S.M. (1996). *Acquiring Critical Thinking Skills.* Philadelphia: W.B. Saunders.

Memmler, R.L., Cohen, B.J., Wood, D.L. (1996). *The Human Body in Health and Disease,* 8th ed. Philadelphia: Lippincott-Raven.

Memmler, R.L., Cohen, B.J., Wood, D.L. (1996). *Structure and Function of the Human Body,* 6th ed. Philadelphia: Lippincott-Raven.

Melfi, R.C. (1994). *PERMAR'S Oral Embryology and Microscopic Anatomy.* Pennsylvania: Lea & Febiger.

Miles, D.A., Van Dis, M.L ., Jensen, C.W., Ferretti, A. (1994). *Radiographic Imaging for Dental Auxiliaries,* 2nd ed. Philadelphia: W.B. Saunders.

Miles, D.A., Van Dis, M.L., Jensen, C.W., Feretti, A. (1999). *Radiographic Imaging for Dental Auxiliaries,* 3rd ed. Philadelphia: W. F. Saunders.

Miles D., Van Dis, M., Kaugars, G., Lovas, J. (1991). *Oral and Maxillofacial Radiology: Radiologic/Pathologic Correlations,* Philadelphia: W.B. Saunders.

Miles D.A., Van Dis, M.V., Razmus, T.F. (1992). *Basic Principles of Oral and Maxillofacial Radiology.* Philadelphia: W.B. Saunders.

Miller, B., Keanne, B. (1997). *Encyclopedia and Dictionary of Medicine, Nursing and Allied Health.* Philadelphia: W.B. Saunders.

Mosby's Medical, Nursing, and Allied Health Dictionary, 4th ed. (1994). St. Louis: Mosby.

Miller, C.H., (1993). *Infection Control and Management of Hazardous Material for the Dental Team.* St. Louis: Mosby.

Miller, C.H., Palenik, C. (1994). *Infection Control and Management of Hazardous Materials for the Dental Team.* St. Louis: C.V. Mosby Co.

Movvett, D., Moffett, S., Schauf, D. (1993). *Human Physiology, Foundations and Frontiers,* 2nd ed. St. Louis: Mosby.

Moyers, R.E. (1988). *Handbook of Orthodontics.* Chicago: Year Book Medical Publishers, Inc.

Muma, R.D., Lyons, B.A., Borucki, M.J., Pollard, R.B. (1997). *HIV Manual for Health Care Professional,* 2nd ed. Connecticut: Appleton & Lange.

Neville, B.W., Damm, D.D., White, D.K., Waldron, C.A. (1991). *Color Atlas of Clinical Oral Pathology.* Philadelphia: Lea & Febiger.

Newman, M.G., Nisengard, R. (1988). *Oral Microbiology and Immunology.* Philadelphia: W.B. Saunders.

Nield-Gehrig, J.S., Houseman, G.A. (1996). *Fundamentals of Periodontal Instrumentation,* 3rd ed. Baltimore: Williams & Wilkins.

Nisengard, R., Newman, M. (1994). *Oral Microbiology and Immunology,* 2nd ed. Philadelphia: W.D. Sanders.

Nizel, A.E., Papas, E.S. (1989). *Nutrition in Clinical Dentistry,* 3rd ed. Philadelphia: W.B. Saunders.

Olson, S. (1995). *Dental Radiography Laboratory Manual.* Philadelphia: W.B. Saunders.

Pedersen, G.W. (1988). *Oral Surgery,* Philadelphia: W.B. Saunders.

Periodontal Disease. (1990). *New England Journal of Medicine, 332(6),* 373.

Perry, D., Breemsterboer, P., Carranza, F.A. (1990). *Techniques and Theory of Periodontal Instrumentation.* Philadelphia: W.B. Saunders.

Phillips, R.W., Moore, B.D. (1994). *Elements of Dental Materials for Dental Hygienists and Dental Assistants,* 5th ed. Philadelphia: W.B. Saunders.

Pindborg, J.J. (1993). *Atlas of Diseases of the Oral Mucosa,* 5th ed. Philadelphia: W.B. Saunders.

Poyton, H.G., Pharoah, M.J. (1989). *Oral Radiology.* Toronto, B.C.: Decker Inc.

Profitt W.R. (1993). *Contemporary Orthodontics,* 2nd ed. St. Louis: Mosby.

Reality Information Source for Esthetic Dentistry. (1996). Houston: Reality Publishing Co.

Regezi, J., Sciubba, J.J. (1993). *Oral Pathology: Clinical-Pathologic Correlation's,* 2nd ed. Philadelphia: W.B. Saunders.

Reis, D., (1992). *Dental professionals and the disabled: a new partnership. 26(9),* 14–122. Dental Products Report.

Requa-Clark, B.S., Holroyd, S.V. (1995). *Applied Pharmacology for the Dental Hygienist.* St. Louis: Mosby.

Ring, M.E. (1985). *Dentistry: An Illustrated History.* St. Louis: Mosby-Year Book.

Robinson, H.B.G., Miller, A.S. (1990). *Color atlas of Oral Pathology.* Philadelphia: Lippincott.

Rosenthiel, S.T., Land, M.F., Fujimoto, J. (1994). *Contemporary Fixed Prosthodontics,* 2nd ed. St. Louis: Mosby.

Sarnat, B.G., Laskin, D.M. (1992). *The Tempororomandibular Joint: A Biological Basis for Clinical Practice,* 4th ed. Philadelphia: W.B. Saunders.

Schluger, S., Yuodel, R., Page, R., Johnson, R.H. (1990). *Periodontal Diseases,* 2nd ed. Philadelphia: Lea & Febiger.

Schoen, D., Dean, M. (1996). *Contemporary Periodontal Instrumentation.* Philadelphia: W.B. Sanders.

Schuster, G.M., Wetterhus, G.J., Dryden, P. (1999). *Handbook of Clinical Dental Assisting.* Philadelphia: W.B. Saunders.

Schwartz, M., Lamster, I., Fine, J. (1995). *Clinical Guide to Periodontics.* Philadelphia: W.B. Saunders.

Shaw, L. (1993). *Self-assessment picture tests in dentistry: Pedodontics.* St. Louis: Mosby.

Short, M.J. (1994). *Head and Neck Dental Anatomy,* 2nd ed. Albany: Delmar.

Smith, D.M., Reynard, A.M. (1992). *Textbook of Pharmacology.* Philadelphia: W.B. Saunders.

Smith, R.G. (1993). *Dental Surgery Assistants' Handbook,* 2nd ed. Hong Kong: Mosby.

Snyder, H. (1994). *The rise in latex allergy: Implications for the dentist, 125* 1089–1097. J.A.D.A.

Soloman, E.P. (1992). *Introduction to Human Anatomy and Physiology.* Philadelphia: W.B. Saunders.

Stedman's Concise Medical Dictionary for the Health Professions, 3rd ed. (1997) Baltimore: Williams and Wilkins.

Sturdevant, C.K., Heymann H., Robertson T.M., Sturdevant J.R. (1994). *The Art and Science of Operative Dentistry.* St. Louis: Mosby.

Successful Intraoral Radiography. (1993). Rochester: Eastman Kodak Co.

Taber's cyclopedic medical dictionary. (1993). 17th Edition. Philadelphia: F.A. Davis Company.

Tamparo, Carol D., Lewis, Marsha A. (1995). *Diseases of the Human Body,* 2nd ed. Philadelphia: F.A. Davis.

TenCate, A.R. (1985). *Oral Histology: Development, Structure and Function,* 2nd ed. St. Louis: C.V. Mosby Co.

Thibodeau, G.A., Patton, K.T. (1993). *Anatomy and Physiology,* 2nd ed. St. Louis: Mosby.

Thibodeau, G.A., Patton, K.T. (1992). *The Human Body in Health and Disease.* St. Louis: Mosby.

Tobazin, R.G. , Goldberg, M.H. (1987). *Oral and Maxillofacial Infections,* 2nd ed. Philadelphia: W.B. Saunders.

Torres, H.O., Ehrlich, A. Bird, D., Dietz, E. (1995). *Modern Dental Assisting,* 5th ed. Philadelphia: W.B. Saunders.

U.S. Department of Health and Human Services, Centers for Disease Control and Prevention (1993). Recommended Infection Control Practices for Dentistry.

Waite, I., Strahan, J.D. (1990). *Color Atlas of Periodontology,* 2nd ed. St. Louis: Mosby.

Walton, R.E., Torabinejad, M. (1989). *Principles and Practice of Endodontics.* Philadelphia: W.B. Saunders.

Warden-Tamparo, C., Lewis, M.A. (1989). *Diseases of the Human Body.* Philadelphia, F.A. Davis.

Watson, C.M. Whitehouse, R.L.S. (1993). *Possibility of cross-contamination between dental patients by means of the saliva ejector.* 124-7-80. J.A.D.A.

Weisman, G. (1995). *Scope of applications for lasers in dentistry expanding, 7,* 26–29. Dental Products Report.

White, S.N. (1993). *Adhesive restorative dentistry: Introduction. Many new adhesive materials can offer improved clinical results. 21(6),* 17–18. C.D.A.J.

Williams, S.R. (1994). *Nutrition and Diet Therapy,* 6th ed. St. Louis: Mosby.

Woelfel, J.B. (1990). *Dental Anatomy: Its Relevance to Dentistry,* 4th ed. Connecticut: Lea & Faber.

Wood, J.T. (1996). *Everyday Encounters: An Introduction to Interpersonal Communication.* Belmont: Wadsworth.

Woodall, I.R. (1993). *Comprehensive Dental Hygiene Care,* 4th ed. St. Louis: C.V. Mosby, Co.

Your Teeth Can Be Saved by Endodontic Treatment. (1992). Chicago: American Dental Association, Division of Communications.

Yu, X.Y., Joynt, R.B. (1993). *Adhesion to dentin, 21(6),* 23–28, C.D.A.J.

Zernik, J.H. , Minken, C. (1992). *Genetic control of bone remodeling, 20(12),* 14–19, C.D.A.J.

Zwemer, T.J. (1993). *Boucher's Clinical Dental Terminology,* 4th ed. St. Louis: Mosby.

INDEX

t indicates table
f indicates figure

License Agreement for Delmar
a division of Thomson Learning

Educational Software/Data

You the customer, and Delmar incur certain benefits, rights, and obligations to each other when you open this package and use the software/data it contains. BE SURE YOU READ THE LICENSE AGREEMENT CAREFULLY, SINCE BY USING THE SOFTWARE/DATA YOU INDICATE YOU HAVE READ, UNDERSTOOD, AND ACCEPTED THE TERMS OF THIS AGREEMENT.

Your rights:

1. You enjoy a non-exclusive license to use the software/data on a single microcomputer in consideration for payment of the required license fee, (which may be included in the purchase price of an accompanying print component), or receipt of this software/data, and your acceptance of the terms and conditions of this agreement.

2. You acknowledge that you do not own the aforesaid software/data. You also acknowledge that the software/data is furnished "as is," and contains copyrighted and/or proprietary and confidential information of Delmar or its licensors.

There are limitations on your rights:

1. You may not copy or print the software/data for any reason whatsoever, except to install it on a hard drive on a single microcomputer and to make one archival copy, unless copying or printing is expressly permitted in writing or statements recorded on the diskette(s).

2. You may not revise, translate, convert, disassemble or otherwise reverse engineer the software/data except that you may add to or rearrange any data recorded on the media as part of the normal use of the software/data.

3. You may not sell, license, lease, rent, loan, or otherwise distribute or network the software/data except that you may give the software/data to a student or and instructor for use at school or, temporarily at home.

Should you fail to abide by the Copyright Law of the United States as it applies to this software/data your license to use it will become invalid. You agree to erase or otherwise destroy the software/data immediately after receiving note of Delmar's termination of this agreement for violation of its provisions.

Delmar gives you a LIMITED WARRANTY covering the enclosed software/data. The LIMITED WARRANTY can be found in this product and/or the instructor's manual that accompanies it.

This license is the entire agreement between you and Delmar interpreted and enforced under New York law.

This warranty does not extend to the software or information recorded on the media. The software and information are provided "AS IS." Any statements made about the utility of the software or information are not to be considered as express or implied warranties. Delmar will not be liable for incidental or consequential damages of any kind incurred by you, the consumer, or any other user.

Some states do not allow the exclusion or limitation of incidental or consequential damages, or limitations on the duration of implied warranties, so the above limitation or exclusion may not apply to you. This warranty gives you specific legal rights, and you may also have other rights which vary from state to state. Address all correspondence to:

Delmar / Thomson Learning
3 Columbia Circle
P. O. Box 15015
Albany, NY 12212-5015
Attention: Technology Department